S0-BPO-179

Psychiatry III

STANDARD NOMENCLATURE
OF
DISEASES AND OPERATIONS

FIFTH EDITION

EDWARD T. THOMPSON, M.D., F.A.C.H.A., EDITOR

and

ADALINE C. HAYDEN, C.R.L., ASSOCIATE EDITOR

Published

for

THE AMERICAN MEDICAL ASSOCIATION

The Blakiston Division

McGRAW-HILL BOOK COMPANY, INC.

New York   Toronto   London

STANDARD NOMENCLATURE OF DISEASES
AND OPERATIONS

COPYRIGHT © 1961
BY THE
AMERICAN MEDICAL ASSOCIATION
535 NORTH DEARBORN STREET
CHICAGO 10, ILLINOIS

STANDARD CLASSIFIED NOMENCLATURE OF DISEASE

PRELIMINARY PRINTING APRIL 1932
FIRST EDITION JANUARY 1933
SECOND EDITION JANUARY 1935

STANDARD NOMENCLATURE OF DISEASE
AND
STANDARD NOMENCLATURE OF OPERATIONS

THIRD EDITION JUNE 1942

STANDARD NOMENCLATURE OF DISEASES
AND OPERATIONS

FOURTH EDITION JANUARY 1952

CONTENTS

STANDARD NOMENCLATURE OF DISEASES AND OPERATIONS

STANDARD NOMENCLATURE OF DISEASES
AND OPERATIONS

PREFACE

The purpose of the system of classifying disease employed in this book is to present a logical clinical nomenclature. Work on this Nomenclature was initiated by invitation of the New York Academy of Medicine, March 22, 1928; and at that time the National Conference on Nomenclature of Disease was formed with a membership representing most of the leading medical and public health organizations in the country. Dr. George Baehr served as chairman of the steering committee of this conference, prepared the plan for a dual topographical, etiological classification in accordance with the library coding system, did much of the work in preparing the schema, enlisted the cooperation of national societies, and stimulated development of proper financing for the Nomenclature. The Commonwealth Fund was responsible for a large share of the financial support for this undertaking. A number of individuals, special funds, insurance companies, and medical organizations also contributed to the support of the work. The major credit for completing the book is due to Dr. H. B. Logie, the executive secretary of the National Conference.

The basic plan was adopted officially at the second National Conference on November 24, 1930. The first printing appeared in 1932, the first edition in 1933, and the second edition in 1935. Obviously a nomenclature of this kind must be kept constantly abreast of the progress of medicine, and the responsibility for its periodic revision was therefore taken over by the American Medical Association in 1937. In connection with the third edition, planned after this change in control, a fourth National Conference on Medical Nomenclature was held under the auspices of the American Medical Association in Chicago on March 1, 1940 with Dr. Haven Emerson of New York serving as chairman. About sixty delegates from interested organizations and institutions attended that conference. Abstracts of the conference were published in the *Journal of the American Medical Association.*

The third edition, edited by Dr. Edwin P. Jordan, was published in June, 1942. The fifth National Conference on medical nomenclature was held under the auspices of the American Medical Association in Chicago on June 23, 1948. At this time publication of a new edition was considered and decided upon. Subsequently, on October 1, 1948 the Board of Trustees of the American Medical Association appointed for the fourth edition a new editorial advisory board consisting of Dr. George Baehr, Chairman, New York; Dr. Selwyn D. Collins, Washington; Dr. James R. Miller, Hartford, Conn.; Dr. Halbert L. Dunn, Washington; Dr. Edward T. Thompson, Washington; Dr. Edwin L. Crosby, Baltimore; Dr. Morris Fishbein, Chicago; Dr. R. J. Plunkett, Chicago; and Mrs. Adaline C. Hayden, C.R.L., Chicago.

The editorial advisory board met on December 4, 1948 at the American Medical Association, Chicago. General plans for a new revision were discussed, and individual committees were appointed to consider revision of each section of the Nomenclature. Dr. R. J. Plunkett was designated as editor and Mrs. Adaline C. Hayden, C.R.L., was designated as associate editor for the fourth edition. The fourth edition was published in 1952. Immediately following the publication of the fourth edition, the Editorial Advisory Board was reconstituted under the chairmanship of Dr. George Baehr with the following membership: Dr. Austin Smith, Chicago; Dr. Selwyn D. Collins (deceased), Washington; Dr. Edward T. Thompson, Washington; Dr. Edwin L. Crosby, Chicago; Dr. Richard J. Plunkett, Chicago; and Mrs. Adaline C. Hayden, C.R.L., Chicago. In 1957 Drs. Edwin Jordan and Kenneth Babcock were appointed as additional members of the Editorial Advisory Board.

In December, 1955 Dr. Richard Plunkett resigned as editor of the Nomenclature to assume the position of Associate Director of Administration, Joint Commission of Mental Illness and Health. In February, 1956 the Board of Trustees appointed Dr. Edward T. Thompson, Coordinator of Professional Services, Division of Hospital Facilities, Public Health Service, Washington, editor of the Standard Nomenclature of Diseases and Operations. Dr. Thompson had served as a member of the Editorial Advisory Board since 1948.

The committees appointed for the fifth edition are as follows:

ANATOMY
BARRY J. ANSON, PH.D., *Consultant,* CHICAGO

ANESTHESIOLOGY
HUBERTA M. LIVINGSTONE, M.D., *Chairman,* CHICAGO
EMERY A. ROVENSTINE, M.D., NEW YORK CITY
KENNETH MCCARTHY, M.D., TOLEDO, OHIO
HUGH E. STEPHENSON JR., M.D., COLUMBIA, MO.
RALPH TOVELL, M.D., HARTFORD, CONN.
VINCENT COLLINS, M.D., NEW YORK CITY
O. SIDNEY ORTH, M.D., MADISON, WIS.

BACTERIOLOGY
WILLIAM BURROWS, PH.D., *Chairman,* CHICAGO
NORMAN F. CONANT, M.D., DURHAM, N.C.
GILBERT DALLDORF, M.D., ALBANY, N.Y.
C. E. LANKFORD, PH.D., AUSTIN, TEX.
JAMES P. LEAKE, M.D., WASHINGTON
NORMAN TOPPING, M.D., PHILADELPHIA

BODY AS A WHOLE
PAUL S. RHOADS, M.D., *Chairman,* CHICAGO
GEORGE E. BURCH, M.D., NEW ORLEANS
PAUL STARR, M.D., LOS ANGELES

DENTISTRY
HAROLD HAYES, D.D.S., *Chairman,* CHICAGO
GEORGE B. DENTON, PH.D., CHICAGO
JOHN E. FAUBER, D.D.S., WASHINGTON
HARRY LYONS, D.D.S., RICHMOND, VA.
FLOYD D. OSTRANDER, D.D.S., ANN ARBOR, MICH.
CHARLES M. BELTING, D.D.S., CHICAGO

DIGESTIVE
BURRILL B. CROHN, M.D., *Chairman,* NEW YORK CITY
HENRY L. BOCKUS, M.D., PHILADELPHIA
H. M. POLLARD, M.D., ANN ARBOR, MICH.
HARVEY B. STONE, M.D., BALTIMORE, MD.

DISEASES DUE TO INTOXICATION
ROBERT A. KEHOE, M.D., CINCINNATI, OHIO

EAR, NOSE, AND THROAT
M. M. HIPSKIND, M.D., *Chairman,* CHICAGO
WILLIAM M. S. IRONSIDE, M.D., CHICAGO
JOHN E. MAGIELSKI, M.D., ANN ARBOR, MICH.
CARL H. MCCASKEY, M.D., INDIANAPOLIS
HAROLD F. SCHUKNECHT, M.D., CHICAGO

ENDOCRINE

ARTHUR GROLLMAN, M.D., *Chairman,* DALLAS, TEX.
LOUIS J. SOFFER, M.D., NEW YORK CITY
LAWSON WILKINS, M.D., BALTIMORE, MD.

EYE

JOHN H. DUNNINGTON, M.D., *Chairman,* NEW YORK CITY
JOHN M. MCLEAN, M.D., NEW YORK CITY
FRANK W. NEWELL, M.D., CHICAGO

FEMALE GENITAL

J. P. GREENHILL, M.D., *Chairman,* CHICAGO
LEROY CALKINS, M.D., KANSAS CITY
M. EDWARD DAVIS, M.D., CHICAGO
LOUIS M. HELLMAN, M.D., BROOKLYN, N.Y.
WILLIAM F. MENGERT, M.D., CHICAGO

HEART

HAROLD E. B. PARDEE, M.D., *Chairman,* NEW YORK CITY
MARCUS M. RAVITCH, M.D., BALTIMORE, MD.
CHARLES C. WOLFERTH, M.D., PHILADELPHIA

HEMIC AND LYMPHATIC

LOUIS R. LIMARZI, M.D., *Chairman,* CHICAGO
FRANK J. HECK, M.D., ROCHESTER, MINN.
MAXWELL M. WINTROBE, M.D., SALT LAKE CITY, UTAH

MUSCULOSKELETAL

H. EARLE CONWELL, M.D., *Chairman,* BIRMINGHAM, ALA.
RICHARD H. FREYBERG, M.D., NEW YORK CITY
GEORGE J. GARCEAU, M.D., INDIANAPOLIS

NEUROLOGY

H. HOUSTON MERRITT, M.D., *Chairman,* NEW YORK CITY
FRANCIS M. FORSTER, M.D., WASHINGTON
GEORGE N. RAINES, M.D. (*Deceased*), WASHINGTON

ONCOLOGY

E. CUYLER HAMMOND, PH.D., *Chairman,* NEW YORK CITY
OSCAR AUERBACH, M.D., EAST ORANGE, N.J.
IRA T. NATHANSON, M.D., BOSTON
SHIELDS WARREN, M.D., BOSTON

PARASITOLOGY

W. H. TALIAFERRO, PH.D., *Chairman,* CHICAGO
JUSTIN M. ANDREWS, M.D., WASHINGTON
FREDERICK B. BANG, M.D., BALTIMORE, MD.
HAROLD W. BROWN, M.D., NEW YORK CITY
ERNEST CARROLL FAUST, M.D., NEW ORLEANS
GILBERT F. OTTO, SC.D., CHICAGO

PATHOLOGY

PAUL R. CANNON, M.D., *Chairman,* CHICAGO
JAMES E. ASH, M.D., BETHESDA, MD.
ALFRED S. CONSTON, M.D., SOMERVILLE, N.J.

PSYCHOBIOLOGIC UNIT—PSYCHIATRY

GEORGE N. RAINES, M.D., *Chairman (Deceased),* WASHINGTON
FRANCIS M. FORSTER, M.D., WASHINGTON

M. M. FROHLICH, M.D., ANN ARBOR, MICH.
LAWRENCE C. KOLB, M.D., ROCHESTER, MINN.
H. HOUSTON MERRITT, M.D., NEW YORK CITY
HARVEY J. TOMPKINS, M.D., WASHINGTON

RADIATION

GILBERT H. FLETCHER, M.D., *Chairman,* HOUSTON, TEX.
FRANZ BUSCHKE, M.D., SEATTLE, WASH.
ISADORE LAMPE, M.D., ANN ARBOR, MICH.
NORMAN S. MOORE, M.D., ITHACA, N.Y.

RESPIRATORY

JOHN D. STEELE, M.D., *Chairman,* SAN FERNANDO, CALIF.
H. CORWIN HINSHAW, M.D., SAN FRANCISCO, CALIF.
GORDON M. MEADE, M.D., Saranac Lake, N.Y.

SKIN

HERBERT RATTNER, M.D., *Chairman,* CHICAGO
HERMAN BEARMAN, M.D., PHILADELPHIA
HAMILTON MONTGOMERY, M.D., ROCHESTER, MINN.

TOXICOLOGY

IRVIN KERLAN, M.D., *Chairman,* WASHINGTON
J. A. CALHOUN, M.D., PHILADELPHIA
ROBERT E. GOSSELIN, M.D., HANOVER, N.H.
CAREY P. McCORD, M.D., ANN ARBOR, MICH.
EDWARD PRESS, M.D., EVANSTON, ILL.

UROLOGY

MONTAGUE L. BOYD, M.D., *Chairman,* ATLANTA, GA.
CLYDE L. DEMING, M.D., NEW HAVEN, CONN.
V. J. O'CONOR, M.D., CHICAGO

SURGERY

HILGER PERRY JENKINS, M.D., *Chairman,* CHICAGO
BURRILL B. CROHN, M.D., NEW YORK CITY
MONTAGUE L. BOYD, M.D., ATLANTA, GA.
H. HOUSTON MERRITT, M.D., NEW YORK CITY
JOHN D. STEELE, M.D., MILWAUKEE, WIS.
HAROLD E. B. PARDEE, M.D., NEW YORK CITY
J. P. GREENHILL, M.D., CHICAGO
M. EDWARD DAVIS, M.D., CHICAGO
HAROLD HAYES, D.D.S., CHICAGO
M. M. HIPSKIND, M.D., CHICAGO
ARTHUR GROLLMAN, M.D., DALLAS, TEX.
JOHN H. DUNNINGTON, M.D., NEW YORK CITY
LOUIS R. LIMARZI, M.D., CHICAGO
H. EARLE CONWELL, M.D., BIRMINGHAM, ALA.
HERBERT RATTNER, M.D., CHICAGO

The chairman of each Standard Nomenclature committee was empowered to appoint such additional consultants as were needed for the work of his committee and to collaborate fully with standing committees on nomenclature of other national medical and scientific associations.

Several changes have been made in the general arrangement of this edition to increase the usefulness of the book and to bring about a closer integration of the material presented.

A growing body of scientific knowledge of recent years has required many changes in the scientific material presented. In this revision changes include complete revision of the Neurology, Ophthalmology, and Obstetric and Newborn sections.

The topography and surgery sections have been considerably expanded.

Revision of the other sections of the book has been kept as much as possible to a minimum. Nevertheless, approximately 6,000 changes represented as additions, deletions, or corrections have been required in this edition to compensate for needed consistency changes, advances in knowledge, and new scientific concepts since publication of the fourth edition.

Dr. George Baehr, chairman, and the members of the Editorial Advisory Board express sincere appreciation to the chairmen, committee members, and consultants who have so freely contributed much of their time and effort toward this revision.

EDWARD T. THOMPSON, M.D., *Editor*
ADALINE C. HAYDEN, C.R.L., *Associate Editor*

INTRODUCTION

The Standard Nomenclature attempts to include every disease which is clinically recognizable and to avoid repetition and overlapping. English terms in good usage are employed whenever possible in preference to Latin or Greek terms, although numerous exceptions occur, especially under diseases of the skin and of the eye. This Nomenclature clarifies the distinction between a disease and its manifestations (Supplementary Terms). It has been designed primarily for use by clinicians, as the clinical diagnosis is a most important source of information on prevalence and distribution of disease.

The method of classification is based on two elements: the portion of the body concerned (topographic) and the cause of the disorder (etiologic). These two elements are designated by code numbers separated from each other by a hyphen. The first three digits describe the topographic site; the last three, following the hyphen, describe the etiologic agent. Combined they form a complete diagnostic code number.

TOPOGRAPHIC CLASSIFICATION

The main topographic systems are:

0– Body as a whole (including the psyche and the body generally) not a particular system exclusively
1– Integumentary system (including subcutaneous areolar tissue, mucous membranes of orifices and the breast)
2– Musculoskeletal system
3– Respiratory system
4– Cardiovascular system
5– Hemic and lymphatic systems
6– Digestive system
7– Urogenital system
8– Endocrine system
9– Nervous system
x– Organs of special sense

These major groups are further divided in order to specify a definite organ or part of an organ. Thus, for example, the digestive system is designated by 6. The fourth organ listed in the system being stomach, the digits for the stomach are 64. The pylorus which according to arrangement is the fifth structure under stomach therefore receives the code number 645–. Thus if a lesion involves the whole alimentary tract, it will receive the topographic classification 600–; if the disease involves all of the stomach, it will receive the number 640–; and if it can be positively identified as involving the pylorus, it receives the number 645–.

ETIOLOGIC CLASSIFICATION

A similar system of numbering the causes of disease constitutes the second element of the classification. Thirteen major etiologic categories are included:

–0 Diseases due to prenatal influence
–1 Diseases due to a lower plant or animal parasite
–2 Diseases due to a higher plant or animal parasite
–3 Diseases due to intoxication
–4 Diseases due to trauma or physical agent
–50 Diseases secondary to circulatory disturbance
–55 Diseases secondary to disturbance of innervation or of psychic control

-6   Diseases due to or consisting of static mechanical abnormality (obstruction, calculus, displacement, or gross change in form) due to unknown cause
-7   Diseases due to disorder of metabolism, growth or nutrition
-8   New growths
-9   Diseases due to unknown or uncertain cause with the structural reaction (degenerative, infiltrative, inflammatory, proliferative, sclerotic, or reparative) manifest; hereditary and familial diseases of this nature
-x   Diseases due to unknown or uncertain cause with the functional reaction alone manifest; hereditary and familial diseases of this nature
-y   Diseases of undetermined cause

As in the topographic classification, these major groups are further subdivided to specify particular etiologic agents. For example, a causative agent identified as poison, but with its exact nature undetermined or unspecified, receives the number -300. If identified as a metallic poison, but with the exact metal undetermined, it will receive the number -310. If the metal can be identified as a heavy metal, for example, it will receive the number -311, and if identifiable as mercury, it receives the number -3111, thus indicating the specific etiologic agent. In certain of the etiologic groups it is necessary to insert an added decimal digit to indicate the anatomic or functional disturbance produced by the etiologic agent. If one wishes to indicate that mercury has produced degeneration, the code number assigned would be -3111.9. The digit following the decimal point indicates the resultant degeneration. Similarly, ankylosis of knee due to infection would receive the number 248-100.4; the digit following the decimal represents the ankylosis. The 248- is the topographic number for knee, while -100 indicates infection, generally. More specifically, if the ankylosis was due to tuberculosis, the code would be 248-123.4.

Secondary Diagnoses—The determination of which of two or more diagnoses is primary and which is secondary is influenced by the interpretation of the individual coders. No universal rule can be stated since a diagnosis which is primary in one situation may be secondary in another. This fact invalidates the statistics of primary and secondary diagnoses. Recognition of these facts has influenced many institutions to stop the cross-indexing of primary and secondary diagnoses and to record all conditions, whether primary, secondary, or associated on the appropriate disease-classification card without reference to their relationship.

If an institution wishes to attempt a distinction between primary and secondary diagnoses, this may be done as follows: The secondary diagnoses may be entered with a different color ink or may be placed, if desired, on different color cards.

Symptoms, Manifestations, or *Supplementary Terms*—For the indication of symptoms this edition includes, under the section on Supplementary Terms, code numbers for the coding of symptoms or other manifestations of disease for each of which special cards may be employed if desired. The Supplementary Terms have been grouped in sections that follow the pattern of the sections in the body of the book, i.e., Body as a Whole, Regional and General Diseases, Skin, etc. The terms are listed under the system classification in which they most commonly occur as symptoms or manifestations; however, any of the terms listed in the entire Supplementary Classification may be used if desired as supplements to any of the diagnoses listed in the Nomenclature of Diseases section of the book. This list is probably not complete. Needed additions may be arranged by communication to the editors.

Incomplete Diagnoses—The Use of y—If information for an accurate diagnosis is insufficient, that fact may be indicated at the point in the diagnostic code where the information is lacking. Thus it is possible to code "undiagnosed disease of the heart." This would receive the topographic designation for heart, generally, 410-, and the etiologic code of –y00, signifying an undetermined cause. A lesion known merely to involve an unidentified portion of the digestive tract would receive the topographic code number 6y0-. Similarly, the lesion in an unidentified portion of the stomach but not involving all the stomach would be designated 64y. Therefore y00–y00 would indicate complete ignorance of the nature of a disease both as to location and cause. For similar "nondiagnostic terms for hospital record," see page 481.

Suspected Diagnoses—There is one other purpose for employing y and that is to designate diagnoses which the physician wishes to show are merely suspected. The name and digits of the diagnosis are to be entered as usual, and y is added at the end of the code.

Punch Cards—The system of coding of the Standard Nomenclature is readily adaptable to the use of punch cards.

Eponyms—Eponyms have been avoided in the body of the book as much as possible particularly when an adequate descriptive topographic-etiologic title is available. The common eponymic diseases that appeared in a table in the third edition have been combined with the Disease Index in this edition. The eponyms will now be found in the Disease Index listed in their proper alphabetic sequence with a direct reference to their proper descriptive title as it appears in the Nomenclature.

Index—The index is designed to help the users of this Nomenclature to identify the proper diagnosis. It includes a great many commonly used terms which do not represent acceptable diagnoses. The index is to be used to identify and determine the proper diagnostic title and may not be used as a substitute classification or as an alphabetic nomenclature. The use of the Nomenclature will be simplified if clinicians adapt their thinking to the topographic-etiologic relationship on which the classification is based. An effort has been made whenever possible, to refer the user directly to the page containing the specific diagnosis. Diagnostic cards should be filed in hospital files by strict numeric sequence according to the topographic code number and not by organ arrangement or alphabetical arrangement as the diagnoses occur in the body of the book.

Diseases Occurring in Pregnant State—Any of the diseases of the female genital organs which occur in the pregnant state may be indicated by changing the code approximately, e.g., change 782, Nonpregnant uterus, to 7x2, Pregnant uterus. Vaginitis, acute in pregnant state, would be coded 7x1–100 *Specify organism when known* and not 781–100.

Inactive Tuberculosis—Inactive tuberculosis may be indicated by the addition of the digit 7 to the etiologic code –123.

General—For diagnoses which are not found listed or for which specific provision for coding has not been made, e.g., as in the Regional Classification, it is requested that the user communicate with the editors. Please do not try to improvise new code numbers or titles.

Abridged Statistical Classification for Clinical Indexing Based on Standard Nomenclature of Diseases and Operations—Abridged Statistical Classification Codes have been placed in italics to the right of the diagnosis in the body of the book and in the Appendix as a cross-reference to the Standard code numbers. For use of these numbers, see instructions at the beginning of the Appendix.

EDWARD T. THOMPSON, M.D., *Editor*
ADALINE C. HAYDEN, C.R.L., *Associate Editor*

INSTRUCTIONS TO MEDICAL RECORD LIBRARIANS FOR INSTALLATION OF STANDARD NOMENCLATURE OF DISEASES AND OPERATIONS

The installation of Standard Nomenclature of Diseases and Operations need not be a task beyond the capabilities of the average medical record librarian.

Of prime importance is an understanding of the nomenclature, its principles, its arrangement, and its contents.

A definite installation date must be set. In the interest of harmony of administration it is considered advisable that the date of the installation be determined by the administrator, the medical staff, and the medical record librarian.

The next decision to be made is the determination of the extensiveness of the coding. This should be a joint decision of the administration and the clinic staff.

The success of an installation must be measured by the ease with which clinicians and others may gain access to cases in order to compile an accurate group of cases for study, review, and research.

The classification may be as elaborate or as simple as desired. Consideration must be given the size of the institution, i.e., the number of clinical records to be classified annually and how the records are to be used.

The majority of institutions will find the three digit code both for topographic and etiology satisfactory. This type of installation should meet the needs of all institutions except those using the records for extensive research and group study. These institutions often require a more detailed classification which may be obtained by expending the topographic and etiologic codes to the fourth and fifth position.

Grouping, which is a collection of codes having some mutual relation or dependence, is recommended but extreme care must be exercised in the use of group codes. If you are not conversant with the codes that can be grouped, write the Standard Nomenclature office for the recommended list. No open end, master, or division codes are to be used in your card captions.

Next, a determination must be made of the information, both type and quantity, to be recorded in the indexes. It is advisable to prepare cards only as diagnoses are received by the medical record department. With either visible or vertical equipment, cards must be filed in strict numerical sequence according to topography and not according to book arrangement.

VISIBLE CARD FILING METHOD

Visible card filing cabinet units consist of a number of trays containing individual holders from which cards are suspended. The cards lie flat in the trays, overlapping one another so that the bottom of each is exposed. The exposed portion of each card must bear the classification number and diagnosis. As a tray is pulled forward from the cabinet, the titles of all the cards are plainly visible. With cards arranged in numerical sequence according to code numbers one can instantly locate any particular card. One may then refer, or post, to that card by "lifting" the card above without removing it from its holder.

Cards should be neatly typed, particular care being given to alignment of typing on all cards. This not only improves the appearance of the file but permits faster finding, posting, and reference. Figure 1 illustrates visible record forms correctly and incorrectly typed.

The card filing cabinet should be divided into eleven sections, representing the eleven major topographic classifications. The cards in each section (0 to X) should be arranged in proper numerical sequence.

	Incorrectly typed	
000–x90	Mental deficiency	
014–190	Septicemia, puerperal	
x05–388	Eclampsia	
085–322	Sulfuric acid burn of hand	

	Correctly typed	
000–x90	Mental deficiency	
014–190	Septicemia, puerperal	
015–388	Eclampsia	
085–322	Sulfuric acid burn of hand	

Fig. 1

VERTICAL CARD FILING METHOD

The vertical card filing method requires the conventional card index cabinet drawers. Standard cabinets provided for the purpose may be obtained.

To facilitate the filing and finding of individual diagnostic cards, a suitable set of Standard Nomenclature of Disease index guides should be provided. These guides are available in sizes 8 by 5, 6 by 4, and 5 by 3 inches. A set consists of major subdivision guides for topographic classifications, supplemented with subdivision guides for etiologic classifications. It is suggested that in the beginning only the topographic guides be placed in the cabinet drawer.

As individual cards are made out for each different diagnosis these cards should be filed behind the proper topographic classification index guides. As the accumulation of cards in a particular topographic classification increases, it should be subdivided by inserting suitable etiologic classification index guides. For example, if behind the 330– topographic index guide there are five, six, or more cards accumulated for the –400 etiologic classification (e.g., –401, –441, –496, etc.), a –400 etiologic index guide should be inserted for ease in finding.

Cards for the vertical filing method should have code numbers and diagnoses typed at the extreme top edge of the card, the typing beginning about five spaces from the left edge of the card. Care should be taken to maintain the alignment on all cards.

The cards should be filed strictly by code number, regardless of where the diagnosis is found in the book. For example, diseases of the abdomen, 040–; of the peritoneum, 060–; and of the omentum, 067–, are found in the body of the book under 6– Digestive System; but when the cards are filed, they should be filed in the 0– section.

Recording of Secondary Diagnoses—There are no preferred methods of differentiating between primary and secondary diagnoses. When this differentiation is attempted, however, the use of different color cards is recommended.

Another suggested method is to use only one card but to enter the secondary diagnosis in ink of a different color. The recording of primary and secondary diagnoses is not generally advocated.

Recording of Supplementary Terms—Supplementary Terms may be recorded in one of two ways. A column may be provided for this purpose on the diagnostic card, or each separate supplementary term may have a separate card. When separate cards are used, they should be filed strictly by code number; and a column should be provided on each card for the code number of the primary diagnosis.

Questions—Specific questions should be addressed to Standard Nomenclature of Diseases and Operations, American Medical Association, 535 North Dearborn Street, Chicago 10, Illinois.

SCHEMA OF CLASSIFICATION
TOPOGRAPHIC CLASSIFICATION

TOPOGRAPHIC CLASSIFICATION

SYSTEMS

0 Body as a whole; [including the psyche (mind) and the body generally] not a particular system exclusively

1 Integumentary system (including subcutaneous areolar tissue, mucous membranes of orifices, and the breast)

2 Musculoskeletal system

3 Respiratory system

4 Cardiovascular system

5 Hemic and lymphatic systems

6 Digestive system

7 Urogenital system

8 Endocrine system

9 Nervous system

x Organs of special sense

TOPOGRAPHIC CLASSIFICATION

SYSTEM 0

0 *Body as a whole; [including the psyche (mind) and the body generally]
not a particular system exclusively*

00 PSYCHOBIOLOGIC UNIT

    000 Psychobiologic unit, generally
    001 Integumentary psychobiologic section
    002 Musculoskeletal psychobiologic section
    003 Respiratory psychobiologic section
    004 Cardiovascular psychobiologic section
    005 Hemic and lymphatic psychobiologic section
    006 Digestive psychobiologic section
    007 Urogenital psychobiologic section
    008 Endocrine psychobiologic section
    009 Nervous psychobiologic section
    00x Organs of special sense psychobiologic section
        00x1 Eye psychobiologic section
        00x2 Ear psychobiologic section

01 BODY AS A WHOLE

    010 Diseases affecting the body, generally
    011 Diseases primarily affecting the body, generally
    012 Diseases secondarily affecting the body, generally
    013 ⎤
    014 ⎬ Diseases of two or more systems, variants of 010
    015 ⎦
    016 Mesenchyme tissue
    017 Body fluid
    018 Carrier state
    019 Inoculation state
    01x Collagen

Regions

02 HEAD AND FACE

    020 Head and face, generally
    021 Head, generally
    022 Forehead and frontal region
    023 Parietal region
    024 Occipital region
    025 Temporal region
    026 Scalp
        0261 Subgalea
    027 Face, generally
    028 Cheek
    029 Chin
    02x Head and neck

03 NECK, THORAX, THORACIC WALL, AND MEDIASTINUM

    030 Neck, generally
    031 Superficial structures of neck
    032 Deep structures of neck
    033 Thorax, generally
    034 Thoracic wall, generally
    035 Infraclavicular region
    036 Sternal region
    037 Mammary region
    038 Inframammary region
    039 Mediastinum, generally

04 ABDOMEN, ABDOMINAL WALL, AND PELVIS

    040 Abdomen, generally
    041 Pelvis, generally
    042 Abdominal wall, generally
        0421 Linea semilunaris
    043 Hypochondrium
        0431 Epigastric region
    044 Umbilicus
        0441 Umbilical region
        0442 Lumbar region
    045 Inguinal region (Iliac)
    046 Loin
    047 Pelvic floor
    048 Inguinal ring
    049 Parietal peritoneum
    04x Suprapubic region

05 OTHER AREAS OF TRUNK

    050 Trunk, generally
    051 Back, generally
    052 Shoulder
    053 Scapular region
    054 Interscapular region
    055 Posterior thoracic and abdominal walls
    056 Lumbosacral region
        0561 Lumbovertebral area
    057 Buttock and hip
    058 Sacrococcygeal region
        0581 Sacral area
        0582 Coccygeal area

06 PERITONEUM AND SEROUS SACS

    060 Peritoneum and peritoneal cavity (greater peritoneal sac), generally
        0601 Inguinal region
        0602 Femoral region
        0603 Foramen of Winslow
    061 Omental bursa (lesser peritoneal sac)
    062 Duodenojejunal recess (fossa of Treitz)
    063 Subdiaphragmatic region

064 Subhepatic region
065 Retroperitoneal tissue
    0651 Retrocecal tissue
066 Pelvic peritoneum
    0661 Pelvic peritoneum during pregnancy
    0662 Pelvic peritoneum during puerperium
067 Omentum
    0671 Greater omentum
    0672 Lesser omentum
068 Serous sacs, generally
069 Abdominal contents
06x Other peritoneal regions, local

07 SUPERFICIAL FOSSAE

071 Axilla
072 Groin
073 Popliteal space
074 Perineum
075 Antecubital fossa
076 Supraclavicular fossa

08 UPPER EXTREMITY

080 Upper extremity, generally
081 Arm
082 Elbow
083 Forearm
084 Wrist
085 Hand, generally
086 Fingers, generally
    0861 Thumb
    0862 Index finger
    0863 Middle finger
    0864 Ring finger
    0865 Little finger
089 Palm
08x Intrinsic vessels

09 LOWER EXTREMITY

090 Lower extremity, generally
091 Thigh
092 Knee region
093 Leg
094 Ankle region
095 Heel
096 Foot, generally
    0961 Plantar region; sole
097 Toes, generally
    0971 Great toe
    0972 Second toe
    0973 Third toe
    0974 Fourth toe
    0975 Fifth toe

099   Fingers and toes, generally
09x   Intrinsic vessels

SYSTEM 1

1 *Integumentary system (including subcutaneous areolar tissue, mucous membranes of orifices, and the breast)*

10 COMBINED SITES

100   Skin and mucous membranes, generally
101   Skin and muscle
102   Skin and lymphatic system
103   Skin and subcutaneous tissue
104   Skin and appendages

11 SKIN PROPER

110   Skin, generally
111   Epidermis and papillary body
112   Epidermis
113   Papillary body
114   Cutis
115   Stratum corneum
116   Elastic tissue
117   Deeper cutis and subcutaneous tissue
119   Lymphatics of skin
11x   Blood vessels of skin

12 SUPERFICIAL MUCOUS MEMBRANES

120   Mucous membranes, generally
122   Mucous membrane of mouth
123   Mucous membrane of lip
      1231   Mucous membrane of upper lip
      1233   Mucous membrane of lower lip
      1234   Mucocutaneous junction, upper lip
      1235   Mucocutaneous junction, lower lip
      1236   Philtrum
      1237   Prolabium
124   Mucous membrane of tongue
125   Mucous membrane of nose
      1251   Mucocutaneous junction of nasal vestibule
127   Mucous membrane of anus
128   Mucous membrane of external urinary meatus
      1281   Mucocutaneous junction of penis
129   Mucous membrane of female genital organs
      1291   Mucocutaneous junction of vulva

13 and 14 REGIONS OF SKIN

130   Skin of unspecified region
131   Skin of face and scalp
      1311   Skin of head and neck
132   Skin of eyelid
133   Skin of nose

134 Skin of lip
135 Skin of ear
136 **Skin of neck**
    1361 Skin of neck and shoulder
137 Skin of breast
138 Skin of neck and trunk
    1381 Skin of trunk
139 Skin of arm and elbow
13x Skin of forearm and wrist
    13x1 Skin of arms and hands
141 Skin of hand and fingers
    1411 Skin of thumb
    1412 Skin of index finger
    1413 Skin of middle finger
    1414 Skin of ring finger
    1415 Skin of little finger
    1416 Skin of dorsum of hand
    1417 Skin of palm of hand
142 Skin of perineum
143 Perianal skin; skin of buttock
144 Skin of vulva
    1441 Skin of perineum and lower extremities
145 Skin of penis
146 Skin of inguinal region
147 Skin of leg
148 Skin of foot and toes (*Subdivide if desired by adding an extra digit as under 141*)
149 Skin of hand and foot

15 GLANDS OF SKIN AND SUPERFICIAL MUCOUS MEMBRANES

150 Glands, generally
151 Sebaceous glands
152 Sudoriferous glands
153 Sudoriferous ducts
155 Mucous glands
156 Mucous glands of lip
157 Sebaceous glands of head and face
158 Sebaceous glands of neck
159 Sebaceous glands of trunk

16 HAIR

160 Hair, generally
161 Hair follicles
162 Hair or hair follicles of scalp
163 Eyebrows and their follicles
164 **Cilia** (*including glands of hair follicle*)
165 Hair or hair follicles of face, nose and ear
166 Hair or hair follicles of neck
167 Hair or hair follicles of axilla
168 Hair or hair follicles of trunk
169 Hair or hair follicles of extremities
16x Pubic or perineal hair or hair follicles

17 NAILS
    170 Nails, generally
    171 Nails of fingers (*Subdivide if desired by adding an extra digit as under 141*)
    172 Nails of toes (*Subdivide if desired by adding an extra digit as under 141*)
    173 Nail beds, generally
    174 Nail beds of fingers (*Subdivide if desired by adding an extra digit as under 141*)
    175 Nail beds of toes (*Subdivide if desired by adding an extra digit as under 141*)
    176 Nail folds, generally
    177 Nail folds of fingers (*Subdivide if desired by adding an extra digit as under 141*)
    178 Nail folds of toes (*Subdivide if desired by adding an extra digit as under 141*)

18 SUBCUTANEOUS AREOLAR TISSUE
    180 Subcutaneous areolar tissue, generally
    181 Subcutaneous areolar tissue of face and head
    182 Subcutaneous areolar tissue of neck
    183 Subcutaneous areolar tissue of back
    184 Subcutaneous areolar tissue of trunk
    185 Subcutaneous areolar tissue of arm and elbow
    186 Subcutaneous areolar tissue of forearm
    187 Subcutaneous areolar tissue of hand and fingers (*Subdivide if desired by adding an extra digit as under 141*)
        1878 Lateral palmar space
        1879 Medial palmar space
    188 Subcutaneous areolar tissue of thigh and knee
    189 Subcutaneous areolar tissue of leg and ankle
    18x Subcutaneous areolar tissue of foot and toes (*Subdivide if desired by adding an extra digit as under 141*)

19 BREAST
    190 Breast, generally
    191 Parenchymatous tissue
    192 Interstitial tissue
    193 Ducts
    194 Nipple
    195 Nipple in lactating breast
    196 Premammary (subcutaneous) tissue
    197 Retromammary tissue
    198 Lactating breast
    199 Male breast
    19x Blood vessels of breast

SYSTEM 2

2 *Musculoskeletal system (bones, joints, bursas, cartilages, ligaments, muscles, tendons and fasciae)*

20 BONES, GENERALLY, AND SPECIAL STRUCTURES
    200 Bones, generally

201 Diaphysis
202 Epiphysis
203 Metaphysis
204 Periosteum
205 Cortex
206 Endosteum
207 Synovial membrane of joint
208 Tendon
209 Tendon sheath
20x Sesamoid bones

21 BONES OF CRANIUM,[1] FACE AND NECK (EXCLUSIVE OF VERTEBRAE)

210 Bones of cranium and face, generally
  2101 Skull and spinal column
  2102 Vault of skull
  2103 Base of skull
211 Frontal bones, generally [2]
212 Parietal bone
213 Temporal bone, generally [3]
  2131 Squamous portion
  2132 Tympanic portion
  2133 Styloid process
  2134 Mastoid portion
  2135 Petrous portion
  2136 Subperiosteal portion
214 Occipital bone
215 Sphenoid bone, generally [2]
216 Nasal bones
  2161 Nasal bone
  2162 Ethmoid bone
  2163 Vomer
217 Zygomatic bone
  2171 Zygomatic arch
218 Superior maxilla, generally [2]
  2181 Frontal process
  2182 Palatine process
  2183 Body
  2184 Alveolar process
219 Mandible
  2191 Body
  2192 Ramus
  2193 Condyloid process
  2194 Coronoid process
  2195 Alveolar margin
21x Hyoid bone

22 BONES OF SPINE AND TRUNK

220 Vertebrae, generally
  2201 Body
  2202 Spinous process
  2203 Lamina

[1] Excluding auditory ossicles (Section X).
[2] Accessory sinuses classified in Respiratory System (3).
[3] Mastoid antrum classified in System X.

2204 Transverse process
2205 Vertebral arch
2206 Facets, inferior and superior
2207 Lamina, spinous processes, and pedicles
2208 Lamina and spinous processes
2209 Pedicles
221 Cervical vertebrae. *Indicate part*
2210 Atlas
221x Axis
221x0 Odontoid process
222 Thoracic vertebrae. *Indicate part*
223 Lumbar vertebrae. *Indicate part*
224 Sacrum
225 Coccyx
226 Scapula
2261 Body
2262 Neck
2263 Acromion process
2264 Spine
2265 Coracoid process
2266 Glenoid fossa
227 Clavicle
2271 Outer third
2272 Middle third
2273 Inner third
228 Sternum
2281 Manubrium
2282 Body
2283 Ensiform process
229 Ribs
2291 Costal cartilage
22x Pelvis
22x1 Ilium
22x2 Ischium
22x3 Pubic bone
22x5 Acetabulum

23 BONES OF EXTREMITIES

230 Humerus
2301 Upper extremity
23012 Epiphysis
23013 Anatomic neck
23014 Greater tuberosity
23015 Surgical neck
23016 Lesser tuberosity
2302 Shaft
23021 Upper third
23022 Middle third
23023 Lower third
2303 Lower extremity
23032 Epiphysis
23033 Supracondylar section
23034 Internal condyle
23035 External condyle

```
        23036 Internal and external condyles
        23037 Internal epicondyle
        23038 External epicondyle
        23039 Articular process
231 Radius
    2311 Upper extremity
        23112 Epiphysis
        23113 Head
        23114 Neck
    2312 Shaft
        23121 Upper third
        23122 Middle third
        23123 Lower third
    2313 Lower extremity
        23132 Epiphysis
        23133 Styloid process
232 Ulna
    2321 Upper extremity
        23211 Olecranon process
        23212 Coronoid process
    2322 Shaft
        23221 Upper third
        23222 Middle third
        23223 Lower third
    2323 Lower extremity
        23232 Epiphysis
        23233 Styloid process
        23234 Head
233 Carpal bones
    2331 Navicular
    2332 Pisiform
    2333 Lunate
    2334 Capitate
    2335 Greater multangular
    2336 Triangular
    2337 Lesser multangular
    2338 Hamate
234 Metacarpal bones and phalanges
    2341 First metacarpal
    2342 Second metacarpal
    2343 Third metacarpal
    2344 Fourth metacarpal
    2345 Fifth metacarpal
    2346 Phalanges of thumb
    2347 Phalanges of index finger
    2348 Phalanges of middle finger
    2349 Phalanges of ring finger
    234x Phalanges of little finger
235 Femur
    2351 Upper extremity
        23512 Epiphysis
        23513 Head
        23514 Neck
        23515 Base of neck
```

```
              23516 Lesser trochanter
              23517 Greater trochanter
              23518 Intertrochanteric section
              23519 Subtrochanteric section
        2352  Shaft
              23521 Upper third
              23522 Middle third
              23523 Lower third
        2353  Lower extremity
              23532 Epiphysis
              23533 Lateral condyle
              23534 Medial condyle
              23535 Lateral and medial condyle
              23536 Supracondylar section
236   Patella
        2361  Retropatellar fat pad
237   Tibia
        2371  Upper extremity
              23712 Epiphysis
              23713 Medial condyle
              23714 Lateral condyle
              23715 Medial and lateral condyles
              23716 Intercondyloid eminence
              23717 Tuberosity
        2372  Shaft
              23721 Upper third
              23722 Middle third
              23723 Lower third
        2373  Lower extremity
              23732 Epiphysis
              23733 Anterior lip
              23734 Posterior lip
              23735 Medial malleolus
              23736 Lateral lip
238   Fibula
        2381  Upper extremity
        2382  Shaft
              23821 Upper third
              23822 Middle third
              23823 Lower third
        2383  Lower extremity
              23832 Epiphysis
              23833 Lateral malleolus
239   Tarsal bones
        2391  Calcaneus (os calcis)
        2392  Astragalus (Talus)
        2393  Cuboid
        2394  Navicular
        2395  Cuneiform, external
        2396  Cuneiform, middle
        2397  Cuneiform, internal
23x   Metatarsal bones and phalanges
        23x1  First metatarsal
        23x2  Second metatarsal
```

23x3 Third metatarsal
23x4 Fourth metatarsal
23x5 Fifth metatarsal
23x6 Phalanges of great toe
23x7 Phalanges of second toe
23x8 Phalanges of third toe
23x9 Phalanges of fourth toe
23xx Phalanges of fifth toe

24 JOINTS

240 Joints, generally
    2401 Temporomandibular joint (jaw)
    2402 Sutura sagittalis
    2403 Sutura lambdoidea
    2404 Sutura parietomastoidea
    2405 Sutura occipitomastoidea
    2406 Sutura coronalis
    2407 Sutura sphenoparietalis
    2408 Sutura squamosa
    2409 Sutura sphenosquamosa
    240x Sutura cranial, generally
241 Vertebral joints
    2411 Cervical vertebral joints
    2412 Thoracic vertebral joints
    2413 Lumbar vertebral joints
    2414 Lumbosacral joints
    2415 Sacrococcygeal joint and joints of coccyx
242 Shoulder joint
    2421 Humerus (shoulder joint)
    2422 Acromioclavicular joint
243 Elbow joint
    2431 Humeroradial joint
    2432 Humeroulnar joint
    2433 Proximal radioulnar joint
244 Joints of the wrist
    2441 Distal radioulnar joint
    2442 Radiocarpal joint
    2443 Midcarpal joint
    2444 Carpometacarpal joints
245 Joints of hands and fingers
    2451 Metacarpophalangeal joint of thumb
    2452 Metacarpophalangeal joint of index finger
    2453 Metacarpophalangeal joint of middle finger
    2454 Metacarpophalangeal joint of ring finger
    2455 Metacarpophalangeal joint of little finger
    2456 Interphalangeal joints
246 Joints of trunk
    2461 Sternoclavicular joint
    2462 Sternum, body with manubrium
    2463 Sternum, body with ensiform process
    2464 Costovertebral joint
    2465 Chondrocostal joint
    2466 Chondrosternal joint
    2467 Chondrochondral joint

2468   Sacroiliac joint
2469   Symphysis pubis
247 Hip joint
248 Knee joint
2481   Superior tibiofibular joint
249 Ankle joint
2491   Distal tibiofibular joint
24911 Tibial astragaloid joint
2492   Tarsal joints
24921 Calcaneoastragaloid joint
24922 Calcaneoastragalocuneiform joint
24923 Astragalonavicular joint
2493   Midtarsal joints
24931 Calcaneocuboid joint
24932 Cuneocuboid joint
24933 Intercuneiform joint
24934 Navicularcuneiform joint
2494   Tarsometatarsal joints
2495   Tibioastragaloid joint
2496   Calcaneoastragaloid joint
24x Joints of foot and toes
24x1   Metatarsophalangeal joint of great toe
24x2   Metatarsophalangeal joint of second toe
24x3   Metatarsophalangeal joint of third toe
24x4   Metatarsophalangeal joint of fourth toe
24x5   Metatarsophalangeal joint of fifth toe
24x6   Interphalangeal joints
24x61 Interphalangeal joints of great toe
24x62 Interphalangeal joints of second toe
24x63 Interphalangeal joints of third toe
24x64 Interphalangeal joints of fourth toe
24x65 Interphalangeal joints of fifth toe

25 CARTILAGES [1] AND BURSAS

250 Cartilages, generally
2501   Meniscus of temporomandibular joint
2502   Meniscus of wrist joint
251 Intervertebral cartilages
2511   Nucleus pulposus
252 Xiphoid cartilage
253 Cartilages of knee joint
2531   Medial meniscus
2532   Lateral meniscus
254 Bursas, generally and unspecified
255 Subdeltoid bursa
256 Subcutaneous acromial bursa
2561   Subscapular bursa
257 Olecranon bursa
258 Gluteal bursa
259 Bursas about knee
25x Bursas of ankle and foot

1 Excluding cartilages of eyelids, nose, ear, larynx, and trachea.

26 LIGAMENTS
   260 Ligaments, generally
      2601 Ligaments of neck
   261 Ligaments attached to vertebrae
      2611 Ligaments of lumbosacral joint
      2612 Ligaments of sacrococcygeal joint
   262 Ligaments of shoulder joint
      2621 Ligaments of acromioclavicular joint
   263 Ligaments of elbow joint
      2631 Ligaments of superior radioulnar joint
   264 Ligaments of wrist joint
      2641 Ligaments of inferior radioulnar joint
      2642 Ligaments of radiocarpal joint
      2643 Ligaments of midcarpal joint
      2644 Ligaments of carpometacarpal joints
   265 Ligaments of joints of hand and fingers
      2651 Ligaments of metacarpophalangeal joints
      2652 Ligaments of interphalangeal joints
   266 Ligaments of joints of trunk
      2661 Ligaments of sternoclavicular joint
      2662 Ligaments of sacroiliac joint
   267 Ligaments of hip joint
   268 Ligaments of knee joint
      2681 Ligaments of medial collateral joint
      2682 Ligaments of lateral collateral joint
      2683 Ligaments of anterior crucial joint
      2684 Ligaments of posterior crucial joint
      2685 Ligaments of superior tibiofibular joint
   269 Ligaments of ankle joint
      2691 Ligaments of distal tibiofibular joint
      2692 Ligaments of calcaneoastragaloid joint
      2693 Ligaments of midtarsal joint
      2694 Ligaments of tarsometatarsal joints
      2695 Ligaments of ankle joint, medial
      2696 Ligaments of ankle joint, lateral
   26x Ligaments of joints of foot and toes
      26x1 Ligaments of metatarsophalangeal joints
      26x2 Ligaments of interphalangeal joints

27 STRIATED MUSCLES
   270 Muscles, generally
   271 Muscles of face and head, including eye muscles
      2711 Occipito-frontalis
      2712 Auricularis posterior
      2713 Auricularis superior
      2714 Auricularis anterior
      2715 Orbicularis oculi
      2716 Levator palpebrae superioris
      2717 Rectus superior oculi
      2718 Rectus inferior oculi
      2719 Rectus lateralis oculi
      27110 Rectus medialis oculi

27111 Obliquus superior oculi
27112 Obliquus inferior oculi
27113 Procerus
27114 Nasalis, pars transversa
27115 Nasalis, pars alaris
27116 Depressor septi nasi
27117 Orbicularis oris
27118 Quadratus labii superioris
27119 Quadratus labii superioris, caput zygomaticum
27120 Caninus
27121 Zygomaticus
27122 Risorius
27123 Triangularis
27124 Quadratus labii inferioris
27125 Mentalis
27126 Buccinator
27127 Platysma
27128 Masseter
27129 Temporalis
27130 Pterygoideus externus
27131 Pterygoideus internus
272 Muscles of neck
  2721 Sternocleidomastoideus
  2722 Omohyoideus
  2723 Sternohyoideus
  2724 Sternothyroideus
  2725 Thyrohyoideus
  2726 Digastricus
  2727 Stylohyoideus
  2728 Mylohyoideus
  2729 Geniohyoideus
27210 Genioglossus
27211 Hyoglossus
27212 Intrinsic tongue muscles
27213 Styloglossus
27214 Constrictor pharyngis superior
27215 Constrictor pharyngis medius
27216 Constrictor pharyngis inferior
27217 Stylopharyngeus
27218 Pharyngopalatinus
27219 Musculus uvulae
27220 Levator veli palatini
27221 Tensor veli palatini
27222 Glossopalatinus
27223 Scalenus anterior
27224 Scalenus medius
27225 Scalenus posterior
27226 Longus capitis
27227 Rectus capitis anterior
27228 Longus colli
27229 Rectus capitis lateralis
273 Muscles of trunk (back, thorax, abdomen)
  2731 Splenius
  2732 Sacrospinalis

2733 Iliocostalis
2734 Longissimus
2735 Spinalis dorsi
2736 Semispinalis
2737 Multifidus
2738 Rotatores
2739 Interspinales
27310 Obliquus capitis inferior
27311 Obliquus capitis superior
27312 Rectus capitis posterior major
27313 Rectus capitis posterior minor
27314 Intercostales externi
27315 Intercostales interni
27316 Transversus thoracis
27317 Levatores costarum
27318 Serrati posteriores
27319 Obliquus externus abdominis
27320 Obliquus internus abdominis
27321 Cremaster
27322 Transversus abdominis
27323 Pyramidalis
27324 Quadratus lumborum
27325 Rectus abdominis
      Trapezius ⎫ *See under* Muscles of shoulder
      Latissimus dorsi ⎭
274 Muscles of perineum and pelvis
  2741 Sphincter ani externus
  2742 Transverse perinei superficialis
  2743 Bulbocavernosus
  2744 Ischiocavernosus
  2745 Sphincter urethrae membranaceae
  2746 Transversus perinei profundus
  2747 Levator ani
      27471 Iliococcygeus
      27472 Pubococcygeus
      27473 Puborectalis
  2748 Coccygeus ⎫
      Obturator internus ⎬ *See under* Muscles of hip and knee
      Piriformis ⎮
      Iliacus ⎭
275 Diaphragma
276 Muscles of shoulder and arm
  2761 Trapezius
  2762 Latissimus dorsi
  2763 Levator scapulae
  2764 Rhomboideus major
  2765 Rhomboideus minor
  2766 Serratus anterior
  2767 Pectoralis major
  2768 Pectoralis minor
  2769 Deltoideus
  27610 Supraspinatus
  27611 Infraspinatus
  27612 Teres major

27613 Teres minor
27614 Subscapularis
27615 Biceps brachii
27616 Triceps brachii
27617 Brachialis
27618 Anconeus
27619 Coracobrachialis
27620 Subclavius

277 Muscles of forearm and hand
2771 Pronator teres
2772 Flexor carpi radialis
2773 Palmaris longus
2774 Flexor carpi ulnaris
2775 Flexor digitorum sublimis
2776 Flexor digitorum profundus
2777 Flexor pollicis longus
2778 Pronator quadratus
2779 Brachioradialis
27710 Extensor carpi radialis longus
27711 Extensor carpi radialis brevis
27712 Extensor digitorum communis
27713 Extensor digiti quinti proprius
27714 Extensor carpi ulnaris
27715 Supinator
27716 Abductor pollicis longus
27717 Extensor pollicis longus
27718 Extensor pollicis brevis
27719 Extensor indicis proprius
27720 Palmaris brevis
27721 Abductor pollicis brevis
27722 Opponens pollicis
27723 Flexor pollicis brevis
27724 Adductor pollicis
27725 Abductor digiti quinti manus
27726 Opponens digiti quinti manus
27727 Flexor digiti quinti brevis manus
27728 Lumbricales manus
27729 Interossei volares
27730 Interossei dorsales manus

278 Muscles of hip and knee
2781 Psoas major
2782 Iliacus
2783 Obturator externus
2784 Obturator internus
2785 Gluteus maximus
2786 Gluteus medius
2787 Gluteus minimus
2788 Piriformis
2789 Gemellus superior
27810 Gemellus inferior
27811 Quadratus femoris
27812 Pectineus
27813 Tensor fasciae latae
27814 Sartorius

```
      27815 Adductor brevis
      27816 Adductor longus
      27817 Adductor magnus
      27818 Gracilis
      27819 Quadriceps femoris
      27820 Rectus femoris
      27821 Vastus lateralis
      27822 Vastus medialis
      27823 Vastus intermedius
      27824 Biceps femoris
      27825 Semimembranosus
      27826 Semitendinosus
279   Muscles of leg and foot
      2791  Popliteus
      2792  Gastrocnemius
      2793  Soleus
      2794  Plantaris
      2795  Tibialis anterior
      2796  Extensor hallucis longus
      2797  Extensor digitorum longus pedis
      2798  Peroneus tertius
      2799  Peroneus longus
      27910 Peroneus brevis
      27911 Tibialis posterior
      27912 Flexor digitorum longus
      27913 Flexor hallucis longus
      27914 Abductor hallucis
      27915 Flexor digitorum brevis
      27916 Abductor digiti quinti pedis
      27917 Quadratus plantae
      27918 Lumbricales pedis
      27919 Flexor hallucis brevis
      27920 Adductor hallucis
      27921 Flexor digiti quinti brevis pedis
      27922 Interossei plantares
      27923 Interossei dorsales pedis
```

28 TENDONS

.9 Added to tendon code indicates tendon sheath alone

To indicate the tendon of any particular muscle, choose the specific code from section 27 and change the second digit from 7 to 8, e.g., 27722 Opponens pollicis would become 28722 Tendon of Opponens pollicis.

28x TENDONS AND TENDON SHEATHS

```
      28x1 Tendons and tendon sheaths generally and unspecified
      28x2 Tendo-calcaneous (Tendo Achillis)
      28x3 Conjoined tendon of internal oblique and transversalis muscle
      28x4 Tendons and tendon sheaths about shoulder
      28x5 Tendons and tendon sheaths about elbow
      28x6 Tendons and tendon sheaths about wrist
      28x7 Tendons and tendon sheaths of hand and fingers
      28x8 Tendons and tendon sheaths about knee
      28x9 Tendons and tendon sheaths about ankle
      28xx Tendons and tendon sheaths of foot and toes
```

29 FASCIA

    290 Fascia, generally and unspecified
    291 Fascia of face and head
    292 Fascia of neck
    293 Fascia of trunk
    294 Fascia of arm
    295 Fascia of forearm
    296 Fascia of hands and fingers
        2961 Dorsal subaponeurotic space
        2962 Hypothenar space
        2963 Thenar space
        2964 Middle palmar space
        2966 Distal anterior closed space of finger
    297 Fascia of thigh
    298 Fascia of leg
    299 Fascia of foot and toes

2x MUSCULOSKELETAL STRUCTURES IN COMBINATION

    2x1 Radius and ulna
        2x11 Shafts
            2x111 Upper thirds
            2x112 Middle thirds
            2x113 Lower thirds
        2x12 Lower extremities
            2x122 Epiphyses
    2x2 Tibia and fibula
        2x21 Shafts
            2x211 Upper thirds
            2x212 Middle thirds
            2x213 Lower thirds
        2x22 Lower extremities
            2x222 Epiphyses
            2x223 Supramalleolar sections
            2x224 Bimalleolar sections
            2x225 Trimalleolar sections
    2x3 Muscle and bone
    2x4 Joints in combination
        2x41 Ankle and tarsal joints
        2x42 Calcaneoastragaloid, astragalonavicular, and
            calcaneocuboid joints
        2x43 Tibioastragaloid and calcaneoastragaloid joints
    2x5 Bones in combination (excluding 2x1 and 2x2)
        2x51 Humerus and radius
        2x52 Humerus and ulna
        2x53 Metacarpals combined
    2x6 Tendons and bone
        2x61 Iliacus and psoas major
        2x62 Tibialis anterior and peroneal muscles
        2x63 Flexors of elbow
        2x64 Biceps femoris, semimembranosus and semitendinosus
            (Hamstring muscles)
        2x65 Peroneus longus and brevis

2x7   Muscles in combination
    2x71   Gluteus minimus and gluteus medius
    2x72   Gastrocnemius and soleus
    2x73   Adductor muscles
2x8   Tendons in combination
    2x81   Gastrocnemius and biceps femoris
    2x82   Gastrocnemius and soleus tendon
    2x83   Extensor pollicis longus and extensor digitorum communis
    2x84   Tibialis anterior and peroneus longus and brevis
    2x85   Peroneus longus, medius and brevis
    2x86   Quadriceps femoris and biceps femoris
    2x87   Pectoralis major and biceps brachii
    2x88   Flexor digitorum, profundus, supraspinatus and
          infraspinatus
2x9   Lymphatic structures of bone

For particular designations, a digit with a decimal point is used to indicate structures accessory to bones, joints, and muscles or components of them:
.1 Diaphysis
.2 Epiphysis
.3 Epiphyseal plate (metaphysis)
.4 Periosteum, perimysium, paratenon, capsule of joint
.5 Cortex
.6 Endosteum
.7 Synovial membrane of joint
.8 Epiphysial cartilage
.0 Sesamoid bone
.x Marrow

SYSTEM 3

3 Respiratory system

30   RESPIRATORY SYSTEM
    300   Respiratory system, generally
        3001   Upper respiratory tract
    301   Nose, combined
        3011   Nose and pharynx
    302   Accessory sinuses, combined
        3021   Accessory sinuses and mouth
        3022   Accessory sinuses and pharynx
    303   Larynx, combined
        3031   Larynx and trachea
    304   Trachea, combined
        3041   Trachea and esophagus
        3042   Trachea and bronchi
        3043   Trachea and skin
    305   Bronchi, combined
        3051   Bronchi and pleura
        3052   Bronchi and abdominal viscera
        3053   Bronchi and skin of thorax
        3054   Bronchi and esophagus
        3055   Bronchi and pulmonary vesicles
        3056   Bronchi and liver
    306   Lungs, combined
        3061   Lung and peritoneum
        3062   Lung and liver
        3063   Lung and tracheobronchial lymph nodes

307   Pleura, combined
     3071   Pleura and pericardium
     3072   Pleura and peritoneum
     3073   Pleura and liver
     3074   Pleura and thoracic wall
     3075   Pleural cavity
        30751   Pneumothorax
        30752   Hydropneumothorax
        30753   Pyopneumothorax
        30754   Hemopneumothorax
     3076   Pleura and esophagus

31   NOSE

310   Nose,[1] generally
311   Vestibule
312   Naris
313   Septum
314   Cartilages
     3141   Alar
     3142   Upper lateral
     3143   Septal
315   Turbinates, generally
316   Middle turbinate
317   Inferior turbinate
318   Nasopharynx
     3181   Pharyngeal bursa
31x   Intrinsic vessels

32   ACCESSORY SINUSES

320   Accessory sinuses, generally
321   Maxillary sinus
322   Frontal sinus
323   Ethmoid sinus
324   Sphenoid sinus

33   LARYNX

330   Larynx, generally
     3301   Subglottic larynx
331   Epiglottis; glossoepiglottic folds and valleculae; petiolus
332   Arytenoid cartilages; aryepiglottic folds
333   Thyroid cartilage
334   Cricoid cartilage
335   Perichondrium
336   Vocal cords
     3361   Ventricular fold
337   Laryngeal ventricle
338   Articulations
     3381   Cricoarytenoid articulation
     3382   Cricothyroid articulation
339   Intrinsic muscles
33x   Intrinsic vessels

[1] Excluding skin and mucous membrane proper (System 1).

34 TRACHEA

- 340 Trachea, generally
- 341 Cartilages
- 342 Mucosa
- 343 Bifurcation
- 34x Intrinsic vessels

35 BRONCHI AND BRONCHIOLES

- 350 Bronchi and bronchioles, generally
- 351 Bronchi
- 352 Cartilages
- 353 Bronchioles
  - 3531 Bronchioles of upper lobe, right lung
  - 3532 Bronchioles of middle lobe, right lung
  - 3533 Bronchioles of lower lobe, right lung
  - 3534 Bronchioles of upper lobe, left lung
  - 3535 Bronchioles of lower lobe, left lung
- 354 Mucosa
- 35x Intrinsic vessels

36 LUNG

- 360 361 Lung, generally
- 362 Alveoli, primarily
- 363 Upper lobe of right lung
  - 3631 Apical segment
  - 3632 Anterior segment
  - 3633 Posterior segment
- 364 Middle lobe of right lung
  - 3641 Medial segment
  - 3642 Lateral segment
- 365 Lower lobe of right lung
  - 3651 Superior segment
  - 3652 Anterior basal segment
  - 3653 Posterior basal segment
  - 3654 Lateral basal segment
  - 3655 Medial basal segment
- 366 Upper lobe of left lung
  - 3661 Lingula
  - 3662 Anterior segment, upper division
  - 3663 Apical posterior segment, upper division
  - 3664 Superior segment, lower division
  - 3665 Inferior segment, lower division
- 367 Lower lobe of left lung
  - 3671 Superior segment
  - 3672 Anterior medial basal segment
  - 3673 Posterior basal segment
  - 3674 Lateral basal segment
- 368 Interstitial tissue
- 369 Lymphatic structures
- 36x Intrinsic vessels

37 PLEURA

    370 Pleura, generally
    371 Parietal pleura
    372 Visceral pleura
    373 Interlobar pleura
    374 Diaphragmatic pleura
    375 Other pleural zones
    376 Subpleural tissues

SYSTEM 4

4 *Cardiovascular system*

40 CARDIOVASCULAR SYSTEM

    400 Cardiovascular system, generally
    401 Vascular system, generally
    402 Arteries and veins combined
        4020 Hepatic artery and portal vein
        4021 Arteries and veins of head
        4022 Large vessels of neck
        4023 Subclavian artery and vein
            40231 Pulmonary vein and subclavian artery
            40232 Splenic artery and vein
            40233 Coronary sinus and systemic arterial circulation
            40234 Visceral pericardium and mitral valve
            40235 Systemic circulation and myocardium
            40236 Visceral pericardium and cardiac septums
        4024 Axillary artery and vein
        4025 Brachial artery and vein
        4026 Radial and ulnar vessels
        4027 Iliac vessels
        4028 Femoral vessels
        4029 Popliteal vessels
        402x Other vessels of leg
    403 Aorta, combined
        4031 Aorta and pulmonary vessels
        4032 Aorta and great vein
        4033 Aorta and trachea
        4034 Aorta and esophagus
        4035 Aorta and subclavian artery
        4036 Aorta and bronchus
        4037 Aorta and intestinal tract
        4038 Aorta and iliac artery
    404 Pericardium and mediastinum
    405 Pulmonary arteries, combined
        4051 Pulmonary artery and aorta
        4052 Pulmonary artery and subclavian artery
        4053 Pulmonary artery and innominate artery
        4054 Pulmonary artery and right ventricle
    406 Veins, combined
        4061 Vena cava and portal vein
        4062 Vena cava and superior mesenteric vein

4063 Splenic vein and renal vein
4064 Pulmonary vein and azygos vein
4065 Pulmonary vein and left auricle
4066 Pulmonary vein and right auricle
4067 Inferior vena cava and left auricle
4068 Superior vena cava and left auricle
4069 Superior vena cava and pulmonary artery
406x Superior vena cava and right auricle
407 Endothelium of cardiovascular system
408 Carotid sinus
409 Omentum and myocardium
40x Ductus arteriosus

41 HEART

410 Heart, generally
    4101 Left side
    4102 Right side
411 Cardiac septums, generally
412 Interatrial septum
413 Interventricular septum
414 Chambers, generally
415 Right atrium
    4151 Auricular appendage, right
    4152 Eustachian valve
416 Right ventricle
417 Left atrium
    4171 Auricular appendage, left
418 Left ventricle
419 Veins of heart
    4191 Great cardiac vein
    4192 Middle cardiac vein
    4193 Small cardiac vein
    4194 Coronary sinus
    4195 Valve of coronary sinus
41x Coronary arteries
    41x1 Right
    41x2 Left

42 PERICARDIUM

420 Pericardium, generally
421 Visceral pericardium
422 Parietal pericardium
423 Pericardial cavity

43 MYOCARDIUM

430 Myocardium, generally
431 Atria, generally
432 Right atrium
433 Left atrium
434 Ventricles, generally
435 Right ventricle
436 Left ventricle

437   Papillary muscles
438   Interstitial tissue, predominantly

44   Conduction system

440   Conduction system, generally
441   Sinoatrial node
442   Atrionodal junction (atrial node)
443   Atrioventricular node
444   Atrioventricular bundle, generally
    4441   Bundle branches, generally
    4442   Right bundle branch
    4443   Left bundle branch
447   Purkinje fibers
448   Transitional fibers

45   Endocardium, valves, and chordae tendineae

450   Endocardium, generally
451   Valves, generally
452   Tricuspid valve
453   Pulmonary valve
454   Mitral valve
455   Aortic valve
456   Mural endocardium
457   Chordae tendineae

46 and 47   Arteries [1]

460   Arteries, generally
    4601   Adventitial coat of artery
    4602   Middle coat of artery
    4603   Intimal coat of artery
461   Aorta, generally
    4611   Ascending aorta
    4612   Right aortic sinus
    4613   Right aortic arch
    4614   Transverse aortic arch
    4615   Descending thoracic aorta
    4616   Abdominal aorta
462   Branches of thoracic aorta
    4621   Innominate artery
    4622   Common carotid, left
    4623   Subclavian artery, left
    4624   Intercostal arteries
    4625   Internal mammary artery
463   Subclavian artery, right
464   Common carotid artery, right
466   Hepatic artery
467   Splenic artery
468   Renal artery

[1] For particular designations a digit with a decimal point is used to indicate accessory or component structures of arteries and veins:
    .1 Adventitial coat
    .2 Middle muscular coat
    .3 Intimal coat
Intrinsic vessels are included in the component structures of the organ concerned.

 4681 Left renal artery
 4682 Right renal artery
469 Mesenteric arteries
46x Iliac arteries
 46x1 Left iliac artery
 46x2 Right iliac artery
471 Pulmonary arteries, generally
 4711 Pulmonary artery
 4712 Infundibulum of pulmonary artery
 4713 Left pulmonary artery
 4714 Right pulmonary artery
472 Other arteries of trunk (except intrinsic arteries of organs)
473 Internal carotid artery and its branches
 4731 Left internal carotid artery
 4732 Right internal carotid artery
474 External carotid artery and its branches
 4741 Left temporal artery
 4742 Right temporal artery
 4743 Left external carotid artery
 4744 Right external carotid artery
475 Other arteries of neck
476 Arteries of face and scalp
477 Arteries of brain
 4771 Circle of Willis
 4772 Anterior cerebral artery
 4773 Anterior communicating artery
 4774 Middle cerebral artery (Sylvian)
 4775 Posterior communicating artery
 4776 Posterior cerebral artery
 4777 Lenticulostriate artery
 4778 Lenticulo-optic artery
 4779 Anterior choroid artery
 47710 Internal carotid artery (intracranial portion)
 47711 Vertebral artery (intracranial portion)
 47712 Basilar artery
 47713 Pontine artery
 47714 Superior cerebellar artery
 47715 Anterior inferior cerebellar artery
 47716 Posterior inferior cerebellar artery
478 Axillary artery
 4781 Brachial artery
 4782 Radial and ulnar arteries and branches
479 Femoral artery
 4791 Profunda femoris artery
 4792 Popliteal artery
 4793 Posterior tibial artery
 4794 Anterior tibial artery
47x Peripheral arterioles, generally

48 VEINS [1]

480 Veins, generally
 4801 Valves of veins

[1] Intrinsic vessels are included in the component structures of the organ concerned.

481 Veins of thorax
    4811 Superior vena cava
    4812 Subclavian vein
    4813 Azygos vein
482 Portal vein
483 Splenic veins
484 Renal veins
485 Mesenteric veins and other abdominal veins
    4851 Inferior vena cava
    4852 Iliac veins
486 Pulmonary veins
487 Jugular veins
    4871 Sinus of external jugular vein
488 Brachial vein
    4881 Antecubital vein
489 Femoral vein
    4891 Popliteal vein
    4893 Long saphenous vein
    4894 Short saphenous vein
    4895 Communicating veins of legs
48x Superficial veins and venules, generally

49 CAPILLARIES

490 Capillaries, generally

SYSTEM 5

5 *Hemic and lymphatic systems*

50 BLOOD AND BLOOD-FORMING ORGANS

500 Blood and blood-forming organs, generally
501 Erythrocytic tissue (Erythropoietic)
502 Granulocytic tissue (Myeloid)
    5021 Neutrophilic granulocytic tissue
    5022 Eosinophilic granulocytic tissue
    5023 Basophilic granulocytic tissue
503 Lymphocytic tissue (Lymphoid)
504 Plasmocytic tissue
505 Histiocytic tissue (Reticuloendothelial tissue)
506 Monocytic tissue (Parent tissue of monocytes)
507 Thrombocytic tissue (Megakaryocytic tissue)

51 PLASMA CONSTITUENTS

510 Plasma or serum, generally
511 Electrolytes
512 Proteins
    5121 Albumin
    5122 Globulins
513 Plasma components affecting coagulation, generally

```
    5131  Fibrinogen
    5132  Prothrombin
    5133  Thrombin
    5134  Antihemophilic globulin
    5135  Accelerator factors
    5136  Anticoagulants
514 Hemoglobin pigments
    5141  Hemoglobin
    5142  Methemoglobin
    5143  Sulfhemoglobin
    5144  Carbon monoxide hemoglobin
    5145  Myoglobin
515 Porphyrins
```

52 Spleen (fixed cells)

```
520 Spleen (fixed cells), generally
521 Perilienal tissue
```

53 Marrow

```
530 Marrow (fixed cells), generally
```

54 Lymphatic channels and lymph

```
540 Lymphatic channels and lymph, generally and unspecified
541 Thoracic duct
542 Right lymphatic trunk
543 Other lymphatic channels of thorax
544 Other lymphatic channels of abdomen
545 Lymphatic channels of genital organs
546 Lymphatic channels of lower extremity
547 Lymphatic channels of upper extremity
548 Lymphatic channels of neck
549 Lymphatic channels of face, scalp, and cranium
```

55 Lymph nodes (fixed cells)

```
550 Lymph nodes, generally and unspecified
551 Lymph nodes of head and face
    5510  Occipital lymph nodes
    5511  Mastoid lymph nodes
    5512  Parotid lymph nodes, superficial
    5513  Parotid lymph nodes, deep
    5514  Preauricular lymph nodes
    5515  Mandibular lymph nodes
    5516  Infraorbital lymph nodes
    5517  Buccal lymph nodes
    5518  Lingual lymph nodes
    5519  Submental lymph nodes
    551x  Submandibular lymph nodes
552 Infraclavicular lymph nodes
553 Cervical lymph nodes
    5530  Superior deep cervical lymph nodes
```

    5531 Inferior deep cervical lymph nodes (supraclavicular)
    5532 Jugulodigastric lymph nodes
    5534 Jugulo-omohyoid lymph nodes
    5535 Jugular lymph nodes
    5536 Retropharyngeal lymph nodes
    5537 Anterior cervical lymph nodes
    5538 Infrahyoid lymph nodes
    5539 Prelaryngeal lymph nodes
    553x Pretracheal lymph nodes
554 Mediastinal lymph nodes
    5540 Intercostal lymph nodes
    5541 Posterior mediastinal lymph nodes
    5542 Diaphragmatic lymph nodes
    5543 Internal mammary lymph nodes
    5544 Retrosternal lymph nodes
555 Tracheobronchial lymph nodes
    5550 Hilus lymph nodes
    5551 Pulmonary lymph nodes
    5552 Bronchopulmonary lymph nodes
    5553 Superior tracheobronchial lymph nodes
    5554 Inferior tracheobronchial lymph nodes
    5555 Paratracheal lymph nodes
    5556 Innominate lymph nodes
556 Mesenteric lymph nodes
    5560 Celiac lymph nodes
    5561 Right suprapancreatic lymph nodes
       55610 Biliary lymph nodes (hepatic)
       55611 Cystic lymph nodes
       55612 Suprapyloric lymph nodes
    5562 Middle suprapancreatic lymph nodes
       55620 Subpyloric lymph nodes
       55621 Right gastroepiploic lymph nodes
       55622 Left gastric lymph nodes
       55623 Paracardial lymph nodes
    5563 Left suprapancreatic lymph nodes
       55630 Splenic lymph nodes
       55631 Left gastroepiploic lymph nodes
    5564 Superior mesenteric lymph nodes
       55640 Superior mesenteric root lymph nodes
       55641 Ileocolic lymph nodes
       55642 Right colic lymph nodes
       55643 Middle colic lymph nodes
       55644 Main mesenteric lymph nodes
       55645 Cecal lymph nodes
       55646 Appendicular lymph nodes
    5565 Inferior mesenteric lymph nodes
       55650 Epicolic lymph nodes
       55651 Paracolic lymph nodes
       55652 Intermediate mesenteric lymph nodes
       55653 Main colic lymph nodes
557 Lymph nodes of upper extremity
    5570 Brachial lymph nodes
    5571 Axillary lymph nodes

5572 Central axillary lymph nodes
5573 Lateral axillary lymph nodes
5574 Anterior axillary (pectoral) lymph nodes
5575 Posterior axillary (subscapular) lymph nodes
5576 Supratrochlear lymph nodes
5577 Deltopectoral lymph nodes
5578 Interpectoral lymph nodes
5579 Cubital, deep lymph nodes
558 Lymph nodes of lower extremity
5580 Inguinal lymph nodes
5581 Superficial inguinal lymph nodes
5582 Popliteal lymph nodes
5584 Common iliac lymph nodes
5585 External iliac lymph nodes
    55850 Epigastric lymph nodes
    55851 Circumflex lymph nodes
5586 Internal iliac lymph nodes
    55860 Gluteal lymph nodes
    55861 Pudendal lymph nodes
    55862 Obturator lymph nodes
5587 Anterior tibial lymph nodes
5588 Cloquet's (Rosenmuller) lymph nodes
5589 Presymphysial lymph nodes
559 Retroperitoneal lymph nodes
5590 Aortic lymph nodes
    55901 Right lateral aortic lymph nodes
    55902 Left lateral aortic lymph nodes
    55903 Preaortic lymph nodes
    55904 Retroaortic lymph nodes
5591 Lateral lumbar lymph nodes
5592 Sacral lymph nodes
5593 Lateral sacral lymph nodes
5594 Mid-rectal lymph nodes
5596 Vesical lymph nodes
5597 Parauterine lymph nodes

SYSTEM 6

6 *Digestive system*

60 DIGESTIVE SYSTEM, GENERALLY AND UNSPECIFIED

600 Alimentary tract, generally
6001 Esophagus and stomach
6002 Esophagus and duodenum
6003 Esophagus and jejunum
6004 Esophagus and abdominal or thoracic wall
6005 Esophagus and ileum
6006 Esophagus and colon
601 Stomach, combined
6011 Stomach and abdominal wall
6012 Stomach and duodenum
6013 Stomach and jejunum
6014 Stomach and colon

      6015 Stomach, jejunum, and colon
      6016 Stomach and ileum
  602 Small intestine, combined
      6021 Duodenum and jejunum
      6022 Duodenum and ileum
      6023 Jejunum and ileum
      6024 Small intestine and mesenteric lymph nodes
      6025 Duodenum and abdominal wall
      6026 Jejunum and abdominal wall
      6027 Ileum and abdominal wall
  603 Large intestine, combined
      6031 Cecum and colon
      6032 Cecum and sigmoid colon
      6033 Cecum and rectum
      6034 Colon and sigmoid colon
      6035 Colon and rectum
      6036 Sigmoid colon and rectum
      6037 Cecum and abdominal wall
      6038 Colon and abdominal wall
      6039 Sigmoid colon and abdominal wall
      603x Rectum and abdominal wall
  604 Small and large intestines combined
      6041 Jejunum and cecum
      6042 Jejunum and colon
      6043 Jejunum and sigmoid colon
      6044 Jejunum and rectum
      6045 Ileum and cecum
      6046 Ileum and colon
      6047 Ileum and sigmoid colon
      6048 Ileum and rectum
      6049 Intestine and abdominal wall
  605 Gallbladder, combined
      6051 Gallbladder and stomach
      6052 Gallbladder and intestine, generally
      6053 Gallbladder and duodenum
      6054 Gallbladder and jejunum
      6055 Gallbladder and colon
  606 Pancreas, combined
      6061 Pancreas and stomach
      6062 Pancreas and duodenum
      6063 Pancreas and jejunum
  609 Bile ducts and alimentary tract
      6091 Bile ducts and stomach
      6092 Bile ducts and duodenum
      6093 Bile ducts and jejunum
      6094 Intrahepatic ducts and intestines
      6095 Liver and abdominal wall
  60x Intrinsic vessels

61 MOUTH [1]

  610 Mouth, generally
      6101 Mouth and pharynx

[1] Excluding mucous membrane (System 1).

6102 Floor of mouth
6103 Vestibule of mouth
611 Lips [1]
6111 Frenulum labii
6112 Upper lip
6113 Lower lip
612 Tongue [1,2]
6121 Frenulum linguae
6122 Body anterior two-thirds
6123 Base posterior one-third
6124 Median rhomboid, area and foramen cecum
613 Teeth
6131 Cementum
6132 Pulp canal
6133 Enamel
6134 Dentin
6135 Dental arches
61351 Maxillary arch, complete
61352 Maxillary arch, partial
61353 Mandibular arch, complete
61354 Mandibular arch, partial
6136 Root
6137 Crown
614 Supporting structures, tooth (periodontium)
6141 Gums
6142 Gingiva
6143 Alveolar bone
61431 Upper alveolus
61432 Lower alveolus
6144 Periodontal membrane
6145 Alveolar arches
616 Palate [1]
6161 Premaxilla
6162 Hard palate
6163 Soft palate
617 Uvula [1]
618 Cheek
61x Intrinsic vessels

62 SALIVARY GLANDS

620 Salivary glands and ducts, generally
6201 Sublingual and submaxillary ducts
621 Parotid gland and duct
6211 Stensen's duct
622 Sublingual gland and duct
623 Submaxillary gland and duct
6231 Wharton's duct
624 Salivary ducts

63 PHARYNX AND ESOPHAGUS

630 Pharynx and esophagus, generally

[1] Excluding mucous membrane (System 1).
[2] Including muscles.

631 Oral pharynx
    6311 Branchial vestiges
632 Pharyngeal lymphadenoid tissue
633 Adenoids
634 Tonsil
635 Lingual tonsil
636 Peritonsillar tissue (including pillars of fauces)
637 Esophagus
    6371 Cervical portion of esophagus
    6372 Thoracic portion of esophagus
    6373 Abdominal portion of esophagus
    6374 Esophagocardiac junction
    6375 Ampulla phrenic
    6376 Inferior esophageal sphincter
638 Mucosa of esophagus
639 Retropharyngeal lymphadenoid tissue
63x Intrinsic vessels

64 STOMACH

640 Stomach, generally
641 Cardiac region
    6411 Cardiac orifice
642 Fundus; acid secreting structures
643 Greater curvature
644 Lesser curvature
645 Pyloric region
    6451 Pyloric antrum
646 Gastric glands
647 Mucosa, generally
648 Muscular coat, generally
649 Perigastric tissue
64x Intrinsic vessels

65 SMALL INTESTINE AND MESENTERY

650 Small intestine, generally
651 Duodenum
    6511 Sphincter of Oddi
    6512 Papilla of Vater
653 Jejunum
654 Ileum
655 Ileocecal valve
656 Mucosa, generally; lymphatic structures
657 Serosa, generally
658 Meckel's diverticulum
659 Mesentery
    6591 Mesentery of duodenum
    6592 Mesocolon
    6593 Mesosigmoid
65x Intrinsic vessels

66 LARGE INTESTINE; APPENDIX

    660 Colon, generally
        6601 Serosa of colon
        6602 Subserosa of colon
    661 Appendix
        6611 Lymphatic tissue of appendix
        6612 Nerves of appendix
        6613 Periappendicular tissue
    662 Cecum
    663 Ascending colon
    664 Hepatic flexure of colon, transverse colon, and splenic flexure of colon
        6641 Hepatic flexure
        6642 Transverse colon
        6643 Splenic flexure
    665 Descending colon (splenic flexure to crest of ilium)
    666 Sigmoid colon (crest of ilium to third sacral vertebra)
        6661 Serosa of sigmoid colon
        6662 Rectosigmoid
        6663 Sigmoid flexure
        6664 Iliac segment
        6665 Pelvic segment
    667 Appendices epiploicae
    668 Rectum
        6681 Rectosigmoid junction at third sacral vertebra
    669 Perirectal tissue
        6691 Pelvirectal tissue
        6692 Submucous tissue
        6693 Retrorectal tissue
    66x Intrinsic vessels

67 ANUS

    670 Anus, generally
    671 Internal sphincter
    672 External sphincter
        6721 Superficial portion
        6722 Deep portion
        6723 Subcutaneous portion
    673 Anal canal
        6731 Anoderm
        6732 Anorectal line
        6733 Anal verge
    675 Crypts of Morgagni
    676 Anal papillae
    677 Perianal cellular tissue
        6771 Ischiorectal tissue
        6772 Subcutaneous tissue
        6773 Posterior anal triangle tissue
    67x Intrinsic vessels

68 LIVER AND BILIARY TRACT

    680 Liver, generally
    681 Perihepatic tissue
    682 Bile passages, generally
    683 Intrahepatic ducts and canaliculi
    684 Hepatic ducts
    685 Common bile duct
    686 Cystic duct
    687 Gallbladder
        6871 Pericholecystic tissue
    688 Ampulla of Vater
    689 Intrahepatic vessels, generally
    68x Hepatic veins

69 PANCREAS

    690 Pancreas, generally [1]
    691 Acinar tissue
    692 Pancreatic ducts
    69x Intrinsic vessels

SYSTEM 7

7 Urogenital system

70 UROGENITAL SYSTEM, GENERALLY

    700 Urinary system and genital system combined
    701 Urinary system combined
        7011 Ureter and bladder
        7013 Bladder and urethra
    702 Ureter and genital or vascular systems combined
        7021 Ureter and vulva
        7022 Ureter and vagina
        7023 Ureter and common iliac artery
    703 Bladder and genital system
        7031 Bladder and vagina (vesicovaginal)
        7032 Bladder and uterus
        7033 Bladder and seminal vesicles
    704 Urethra and genital system
        7041 Urethra and vulva
        7042 Urethra and vagina (urethrovaginal)
        7043 Urethra and scrotum
        7044 Urethra and perineum
    705 Genital system, generally
        7051 Vagina and cervix
        7052 Vagina and vulva
        7053 Vagina and abdominal wall
    706 Urogenital system and intestinal tract
        7061 Vagina, bladder and intestine
        7062 Uterus, vagina, bladder and intestine
        7063 Kidney and intestine
    707 Ureter and intestine

[1] Insular tissue classified under Endocrine System (8).

7071 Ureter and duodenum
7072 Ureter and cecum
7073 Ureter and colon
7074 Ureter and sigmoid colon
7075 Ureter and rectum
7076 Ureter and ileum
708 Bladder and intestine
7081 Bladder and ileum
7082 Bladder and cecum
7083 Bladder and colon
7084 Bladder and sigmoid colon
7085 Bladder and rectum
709 Urethra and rectum
70x Genital system and intestinal tract
70x1 Rectum and vulva
70x2 Rectum and vagina
70x21 Vaginorectal septum
70x3 Rectum and uterus
70x4 Rectum and labia
70x5 Rectum and perineum
70x6 Ileum and vagina
70x7 Uterus and abdominal wall

71 KIDNEY

710 Kidney, generally
711 Parenchyma, generally
712 Glomeruli, primarily or predominantly
713 Tubules, primarily or predominantly
714 Interstitial tissue, primarily or predominantly
715 Capsule
716 Perirenal tissue
717 Papillae
718 Hilus
719 Kidney and renal pelvis
71x Intrinsic vessels

72 RENAL PELVIS AND URETER

720 Renal pelvis and ureter, generally
721 Renal calices
722 Renal pelvis
723 Ureter, generally
724 Ureteropelvic junction
725 Periureteral tissue
726 Ureterovesical junction; distal portion of ureter
727 Ureterovesical orifice

73 BLADDER

730 Bladder, generally
7301 Urachus
7302 Bladder and abdominal wall
7303 Bladder and perineum

731 Trigone
    7311 Interureteral ridge
732 Neck of bladder
733 Urethral orifice and internal sphincter
734 Fundus
735 Body
736 Mucosa
737 Submucosa
738 Muscularis
739 Perivesical tissue
73x Intrinsic vessels

74 URETHRA

740 Urethra, generally
    7401 Submucosa
    7402 Utriculus masculinus
    7403 Paraurethral ducts
741 Prostatic portion
742 Membranous portion
743 Bulbous portion
744 Penile portion
745 Verumontanum
746 Meatus
    7461 Skene's gland
747 Bulbourethral (Cowper's) glands
    7471 Urethral (Littré's) glands
748 Periurethral tissue
749 Intrinsic muscle; external sphincter
74x Intrinsic vessels

75 EXTERNAL MALE ORGANS

750 External male organs, generally
751 Penis, generally
752 Glans penis
753 Prepuce
754 Corpora cavernosa (including fascia and septums)
    7541 Corpus spongiosum
755 Testis [1]
    7551 Appendix of testis
756 Epididymis
    7561 Appendix of epididymis
757 Tunica vaginalis
758 Scrotum
759 Spermatozoa
75x Intrinsic vessels

76 INTERNAL MALE ORGANS

760 Internal male organs, generally
761 Vas deferens
762 Spermatic cord
763 Seminal vesicles
    7631 Perivesicular tissue

[1] Excluding endocrine diseases (System 8).

764 Prostate
765 Ejaculatory ducts
766 Periprostatic tissue
767 Intrinsic vessels of prostate
76x Other intrinsic vessels

77 EXTERNAL FEMALE ORGANS

770 External female organs, generally
772 Labia majora
773 Labia minora
774 Vulva
    7741 Vulva and deep structures
775 Clitoris
776 Hymen
777 Bartholin's glands
778 Intrinsic muscles
779 Canal of Nuck
77x Intrinsic vessels

78 INTERNAL FEMALE ORGANS

780 Internal female organs, generally
    7801 Uterus and tubes combined
    7802 Vestigial remnant mesonephritic duct
    7803 Ovaries and tubes
    7804 Tubes and abdominal wall
781 Vagina
    7811 Vagina and perineum
    7812 Anterior vaginal wall
    7813 Posterior vaginal wall
782 Uterus, generally, corpus
    7820 Fundus uteri
783 Cervix uteri
    7831 Glands of cervix uteri
784 Parametrium
785 Endometrium
786 Myometrium
787 Uterine tube (oviduct)
    7871 Serous coat of uterine tube (oviduct)
788 Ovary
    7881 Graafian follicle
    7882 Corpus luteum
    7883 Epoophoron
    7884 Paroophoron
    7885 Interstitial tissue
    7886 Serous coat
    7887 Testicular tissue (hermaphroditic)
    7888 Corpus albicans
789 Supporting and associated structures
    7891 Round ligament
    7892 Broad ligament
    7893 Sacrouterine ligament
78x Intrinsic vessels

79 FETAL STRUCTURES
    790 Fetus, generally
        7901 Scalp
        7902 Head
        7903 Neck
        7904 Thorax
        7905 Shoulder
        7906 Arm
        7907 Abdomen
        7908 Back
        7909 Buttocks
        790x Leg
        790x1 Foot
    792 Ovum
    793 Site of implantation of ovum
    794 Placenta
        7941 Placenta and membranes
        7942 Placental fragment
    795 Amnion; membranes, generally
    796 Chorion
    797 Chorionic villi
    798 Syncytium
    799 Umbilical cord
        7991 Omphalomesenteric duct (Vitelline duct)
    79x Placental vessels

7x FEMALE GENITAL ORGANS DURING PREGNANCY, PARTURITION, AND PUERPERIUM
    7x0 Pregnant organs, generally and unspecified
    7x1 Vagina
    7x2 Uterus
    7x3 Cervix uteri
    7x4 Vulva
        7x41 Fourchette
    7x5 Endometrium
        7x51 Decidua
        7x52 Decidual fragment
    7x6 Placental site
    7x7 Uterine tube
    7x8 Ovary
    7x9 Supporting ligaments and cellular tissue
    7xx Pelvic floor

SYSTEM 8

8 *Endocrine system*

80 ENDOCRINE SYSTEM
    800 Endocrine glands, generally

81 THYROID GLAND
    810 Thyroid gland, generally
    811 Right lobe

812   Left lobe
813   Isthmus
814   Aberrant thyroid; lingual thyroid
    8141   Substernal thyroid
815   Thyroglossal duct
81x   Intrinsic vessels

82   PARATHYROID GLANDS

820   Parathyroid gland, generally

83   THYMUS GLAND

830   Thymus gland, generally

84   PITUITARY GLAND

840   Pituitary gland, generally
841   Anterior lobe
842   Posterior lobe
843   Pars intermedia
844   Pituitary stalk
845   Craniobuccal (Rathke's) pouch

85   PINEAL GLAND

850   Pineal gland, generally

86   ADRENAL GLANDS

860   Adrenal glands, generally
861   Cortex
862   Medulla
86x   Intrinsic vessels

87   PANCREAS [1]

870   Insular tissue, generally

88   GONADS

880   Gonads, generally
See also page 38

89   CAROTID GLAND

890   Carotid gland, generally

SYSTEM 9

9 *Nervous system*

90   NERVOUS SYSTEM, GENERALLY

900   Nervous system, generally
901   Brain and meninges, generally
9011 Meninges, brain and spinal cord
902   Gray matter, generally or predominantly

[1] Pancreas (generally) classified in Digestive System (6).

903   White matter, generally or predominantly
904   Upper and lower motor neurons
     9041   Pyramidal system
     9042   Striatorubrospinal system
     9043   Cerebellorubrospinal system
     9044   Vestibulospinal system
     9045   Other extrapyramidal systems
     9046   Pyramidopallidonigral system
905   Ascending pathways
906   Brain and spinal cord
     9061   Brain, spinal cord and nerve roots
     9062   Brain, optic pathway and spinal cord
     9063   Brain, spinal cord, and peripheral nerves
907   Spinal cord and nerve roots or peripheral nerves
     Subdivide as under 97021 to 97062 (page 47)
908   Cortex and basal ganglia
909   Spinal cord and meninges
     Subdivide as under 97021 to 97062 (page 47)
90x   Intrinsic vessels

91   COVERINGS

     Meninges, cerebrospinal
910   Meninges, cerebral, combined regions, generally
     91001   Frontoparietal
     91002   Frontotemporal
     91003   Parietotemporal
     91004   Parietooccipital
     91005   Occipitotemporal
     9101   Frontal
     9102   Parietal
     9103   Temporal
     9104   Occipital
     9105   Falx cerebri
     9106   Falx cerebri, frontoparietal
     9107   Falx cerebri, occipital
     9108   Tentorium, upper surface
     9109   Tentorium, lower surface
     91010   Orbital
     91011   Cerebellar
     91012   Diaphragma sellae
     91013   Falx cerebelli
     91014   Of olfactory groove
     91015   Of optic groove (optic nerve and chiasm)
     91016   Of sphenoid ridge
     91017   Of sphenoid wing
     91018   Suprasellar
     91019   Parasagittal
     9101x   Tuberculum sellae
91020   Meninges, spinal, generally
     Meninges, spinal, locally
     91021   Cervical, generally
     91022   Cervical, upper
     91023   Cervical, middle

      91024 Cervical, lower
      91025 Of cervicothoracic junction
      91030 Thoracic, generally
      91031 Thoracic, upper
      91032 Thoracic, middle
      91033 Thoracic, lower
      91034 Of thoracolumbar junction
      91040 Lumbosacral, generally
      91041 Lumbar, upper
      91042 Lumbar, lower
      91043 Of lumbosacral junction
      91061 Sacral, upper
      91062 Sacral, lower
      91063 Of cauda equina
      91064 Of filum terminale

911 Pachymeninges, cerebral; locally. *Subdivide as under 91001 to 91019*

      Pachymeninges, spinal; locally. *Subdivide as under 91021 to 91064*

912 Leptomeninges, cerebral; locally. *Subdivide as under 91001 to 91019*

      Leptomeninges, spinal; locally. *Subdivide as under 91021 to 91064*

913 Subdural space, cerebral; locally. *Subdivide as under 91001 to 91019 where applicable*

914 Arachnoid, cerebral; locally. *Subdivide as under 91001 to 91019*

      Arachnoid spinal; locally. *Subdivide as under 91021 to 91064*

914x Pacchionian granulations

915 Epidural space, cerebral; locally. *Subdivide as under 91001 to 91019 where applicable*

916 Epidural space, spinal; locally. *Subdivide as under 91021 to 91064*

917 Subarachnoid space and cisternae, generally; pacchionian bodies
      9171 Subarachnoid space, cranial
      91711 Cisterna basalis
      91712 Cisterna medullocerebellaris (magna)
      91713 Cisterna ambiens
      9172 Subarachnoid space, spinal, generally

918 Cerebrospinal fluid

91x Intrinsic vessels
      91x1 Middle meningeal artery
      91x2 Superior longitudinal sinus
      91x3 Lateral sinus
      91x4 Sigmoid sinus
      91x5 Cavernous sinus
      91x6 Straight sinus
      91x7 Other sinuses
      91x8 Venous plexus

92 VENTRICLES AND CENTRAL CANAL

  920 Ventricles, generally
  921 Lateral ventricles, both
  922 Lateral ventricle, right or left

923   Third ventricle
    9231   Mesencephalic aqueduct (Sylvius)
924   Fourth ventricle
925   Lateral medullary recess
926   Cavum septi pellucidi
927   Ependyma, generally
    9271   Of right or left lateral ventricle
    9272   Of third ventricle
    9273   Of mesencephalic aqueduct (Sylvius)
    9274   Of fourth ventricle
928   Foramens, generally
    9281   Interventricular foramen (Monro) right or left
    9282   Lateral apertures of fourth ventricle (Luschka)
          (Retzius and Key)
    9283   Median aperture of fourth ventricle (Magendie)
929   Central canal, generally
    Central canal, locally. *Subdivide as under 91021 to 91063*
    Meninges, spinal (*page 42*)
92x   Choroid plexus, lateral ventricle, right or left, generally
    92x1   Of body, right or left
    92x2   Of temporal horn, right or left
    92x3   Of third ventricle
    92x4   Of fourth ventricle

93, 94, and 95 BRAIN

930   Brain, generally
931   Gray matter, generally or predominantly
932   Cortex, generally
    Cortex, locally. *Subdivide as follows*:
933   Frontal lobe, generally
    9331   Right or left pole
    9332   Intermediate precentral (premotor) area, right or left
    9333   Posteroinferior (Broca's), convolution, right or left
    9334   Precentral convolution, right or left
    9335   Orbital convolutions
934   Parietal lobe, generally
    9341   Postcentral convolution
    9342   Superior lobule
    9343   Inferior lobule (angular, supramarginal, and postparietal
          convolutions)
935   Temporal lobe, generally
    9351   Dorsal surface
    9352   Lateral surface
    9353   Ventral surface
936   Occipital lobe, generally
    9361   Mesial surface, cuneus
    9362   Mesial surface, calcarine cortex (area striata)
    9363   Lateral surface
    9364   Ventral surface
937   Rhinencephalic lobe, generally
    9371   Cingular gyrus
    9372   Hippocampal gyrus
    9373   Uncus

938 Subcortex
    9381 Frontal area
    9382 Parietal area
    9383 Temporal area
    9384 Occipital area
    9385 Combined areas
939 Lobes in various combinations
    9391 Interfrontal
    9392 Interparietal
    9393 Interoccipital
    9394 Frontoparietal
    9395 Parietooccipital
    9396 Occipitotemporal
    9397 Frontoparietotemporal
    9398 Temporoparietooccipital
    9399 Frontotemporal
    939x Temporoparietal
93x Insula
940 Structures in various fossae, generally
    9401 In anterior fossa
    9402 In middle fossa
    9403 In posterior fossa
942 White matter, generally or predominantly
943 Corpus callosum
    9431 Rostrum
    9432 Genu
    9433 Truncus (corpus)
    9434 Splenium
944 Corticopontocerebellar tracts
    9441 Corticostriatal system
    9442 Corticocerebral striatal system
945 Internal capsule
946 Basal ganglia, generally
    9461 Caudate nucleus
    9462 Lenticular nucleus
    9463 Putamen
    9464 Globus pallidus
    9465 Substantia nigra
    9466 Red nucleus
    9467 Corpus subthalamicum
    9468 Others
947 Optic thalamus
948 Striatal system
949 Pallidal system
950 Striatopallidal system
951 Hypencephalon, generally
    9511 Supraopticohypophyseal connections
952 Brain stem, generally
953 Brain stem, upper part
954 Brain stem, lower part
    9541 Cerebellopontine angle
955 Midbrain (mesencephalon)
956 Pons (metencephalon)

957 Medulla oblongata (myelencephalon)
 9571 Medulla oblongata and spinal cord
958 Cerebellum, generally
 9581 Lateral hemisphere, superior
 9582 Lateral hemisphere, inferior
 9583 Superior vermis
 9584 Inferior vermis
 9585 Intrinsic nuclei
 9586 Cortex
 9587 Superior peduncle
 9588 Middle peduncle
 9589 Inferior peduncle
959 Cerebellum and brain stem
 9591 Olivopontocerebellar system
 Intrinsic arteries. See 477, page 27
95x Intrinsic vessels, generally

96 CRANIAL NERVES [1]

961 Olfactory pathway
 9611 Fila olfactoria
 9612 Olfactory bulb
 9613 Olfactory tract
962 Optic pathway
 9621 Papillomacular bundle
 9622 Peripheral fibers
 9623 Retrobulbar portion
 9624 Intracranial portion of nerve
 9625 Canalicular portion of nerve
 9626 Optic chiasm
 9627 Optic tract
963 Oculomotor nerves
 9631 Third nerve (oculomotor)
 9632 Fourth nerve (trochlear)
 9633 Sixth nerve (abducens)
964 Fifth nerve (trigeminal)
 9641 First division (ophthalmic)
 9642 Second division (maxillary)
 9643 Third division (mandibular)
 9644 Combinations of divisions
 9645 Gasserian ganglion
 9646 Motor trigeminal root
 9647 Sensory trigeminal root
965 Seventh nerve (facial)
 9651 Geniculate ganglion
966 Eighth nerve (auditory; cochlear; vestibular)
 9661 Cochlear division
 9662 Vestibular division
 End organs. See Organs of special sense, page 49
967 Ninth nerve (glossopharyngeal)
 9671 Ganglia
968 Tenth nerve (vagus)
 9681 Ganglia

[1] Autonomic fibers classified in section 99 System (9).

9682 Superior laryngeal nerve
969 Eleventh nerve (spinal accessory)
96x Twelfth nerve (hypoglossal)

97 SPINAL CORD

970 Spinal cord, generally
Spinal cord, locally. *Subdivide as follows*
97021 Cervical, upper
97022 Cervical, middle
97023 Cervical, lower
97024 Cervicothoracic
97031 Thoracic, upper
97032 Thoracic, middle
97033 Thoracic, lower
97034 Thoracolumbar
97041 Lumbar, upper
97043 Lumbar, lower
97044 Lumbosacral
97061 Sacral, upper
97062 Sacral, lower (conus terminalis)
97063 Filum terminale
971 Gray columns, generally
Gray columns, locally 21-62. *Subdivide as under 970*
972 Ventral horn cells, generally
Ventral horn cells, locally 21-62. *Subdivide as under 970*
973 Gray and white columns combined
974 Lateral gray columns
975 Dorsal white columns
976 Lateral white columns
977 Dorsal and lateral white columns combined
978 Combined ventral and dorsal roots. *Subdivide 21-62 as under 970*
9781 Ventral roots. *Subdivide 21-62 as under 970*
9782 Dorsal roots. *Subdivide 21-62 as under 970*
9783 Dorsal root ganglions. *Subdivide 21-62 as under 970*
9784 Combined roots and ganglia. *Subdivide 21-62 as under 970*
97844 Cauda equina (lumbosacral roots)
979 Spinal cord and nerve roots
97x Intrinsic vessels, at different levels. *Subdivide 21-62 as under 970*
97x1 Anterior spinal artery. *Indicate region*
97x2 Posterior spinal artery. *Indicate region*
97x3 Lateral spinal arteries. *Indicate region*
97x4 Spinal veins. *Indicate region*

98 PERIPHERAL NERVES AND PLEXUSES

980 Peripheral nerves, generally (cranial and spinal)
981 Spinal nerves, generally
982 Cervical plexus, generally
9821 Great occipital nerve
9822 Ansa cervicalis
9823 Great auricular nerve
9824 Phrenic nerve

983 Brachial plexus, generally
     9831 Lateral cord
     9832 Posterior cord
     98321 Subscapular nerve
     98322 Thoracodorsal nerve
     9833 Medial cord
     9834 Musculocutaneous nerve
     9835 Median nerve
     98351 Volar interosseous nerve
     98352 Median digital nerves
     9836 Ulnar nerve
     98362 Ulnar digital nerves
     9837 Radial nerve
     98371 Radial nerve, deep ramus
     98372 Radial nerve, superficial ramus
     9838 Suprascapular nerve
     9839 Dorsal scapular nerve
     98310 Long thoracic nerve
     98311 Lateral and medial anterior thoracic nerves
     98312 Medial cutaneous nerve of arm or forearm
     98313 Axillary nerve
984 Nerves of cervical and brachial plexus (various combinations).
986 Thoracic nerves
     9861 Intercostobrachial nerve
     9862 Intercostal nerves, second to eleventh.
     9863 Twelfth thoracic nerve
987 Lumbosacral plexus, generally
     98701 Iliohypogastric nerve
     98702 Ilioinguinal nerve
     9871 Genitofemoral nerve
     9872 Obturator nerve
     9873 Femoral nerve
     98731 Intermediate cutaneous nerve
     98732 Medial cutaneous nerve
     98733 Saphenous nerve
     9874 Lateral cutaneous nerve
988 Sciatic nerve
     9881 Common peroneal nerve
     98811 Deep peroneal nerve
     98812 Superficial peroneal nerve
     9884 Tibial nerve
     98841 Medial plantar nerve
     98842 Lateral plantar nerve
     9886 Medial cutaneous nerve of leg
989 Pudendal plexus, generally
     9891 Posterior cutaneous nerve of thigh
     9892 Pudendal nerve
         98921 Muscular
         98922 Sensory

99 Vegetative nervous system: sympathetic and parasympathetic (autonomic), including mixed ganglia

    990 Vegetative nervous system, generally
    991 Sympathetic nervous system, generally
    992 Parasympathetic (autonomic) nervous system, generally
    993 Suprasegmental neuron of either system
    994 **Preganglionic segmental neuron.** *Subdivide as under 970 (page 47)*
    995 Ganglionated chain (sympathetic system)
        9951 Superior cervical ganglion
        9952 Middle cervical ganglion
        9953 Inferior cervical ganglion (stellate ganglion)
        9954 Thoracic ganglia
        9955 Lumbar ganglia
        9956 Sacral ganglia
    996 Postganglionic segmental neurons
        9961 Great splanchnic nerve
    997 Mixed plexuses, generally
        9971 Cardiac plexuses
        9972 Solar plexus
        9973 Semilunar ganglions
        9974 Celiac plexus
        9975 Aortic plexus
        9976 Mesenteric plexus
        9977 Hypogastric plexus
        9978 Pelvic plexuses
        9979 Carotid body
        997x Renal plexus
    998 Parasympathetic fibers of cranial nerves
    999 Parasympathetic fibers of pelvic nerves
    99x Mixed ganglia associated with cranial nerves
        99x1 Ciliary ganglion, associated with the third nerve and the ophthalmic division of the fifth nerve
        99x2 Sphenopalatine (Meckel's) ganglion, associated with the maxillary division of the fifth nerve and the seventh nerve
        99x3 Otic ganglion, associated with the mandibular division of the fifth and the seventh and ninth nerves
        99x4 Submaxillary ganglion, associated with the fifth and seventh nerves

SYSTEM X

x *Organs of special sense*

    x00 Olfactory sense
    x01 Gustatory sense

x1, x2, x3, and x4 Structures concerned in vision

    x10 Structures concerned in vision, generally and unspecified
    x11 Eyeball, generally
        x111 Fascia bulbi (Tenon's capsule)
    x12 Cornea
        x121 Superficial layers
        x122 Stroma

  x123 Deep layers
  x124 Descemet's membrane
  x125 Endothelium
  x126 Limbus
  x127 Cornea and conjunctiva
  x128 Bowman's membrane
  x129 Epithelium
 x13 Sclera
 x14 Uveal tract
 x15 Iris
  x151 Iris and cornea
  x152 Iris and capsule of lens
 x16 Ciliary body
 x17 Choroid
 x18 Aqueous
 x19 Anterior chamber
 x1x Intrinsic veins of retina
  x1x1 Central retinal vein
  x1x2 Superior nasal retinal vein
  x1x3 Inferior nasal retinal vein
  x1x4 Superior temporal retinal vein
  x1x5 Inferior temporal retinal vein
 x20 Crystalline lens
  x201 Polar
   x2011 Anterior polar
   x2012 Posterior polar
  x202 Subcapsular
   x2021 Anterior subcapsular
   x2022 Posterior subcapsular
  x203 Cortical
   x2031 Anterior cortical
   x2032 Posterior cortical
  x204 Nuclear
   x2041 Perinuclear
  x205 Equatorial
 x21 Capsule of lens
 x22 Vitreous
 x23 Retina
 x24 Choroid and retina
 x25 Central area of retina
 x26 Peripheral part of retina
 x27 Inner layer
 x28 Outer layer
 x29 Optic papilla
 x2x Vessels of retina
  x2x1 Central retinal vessels
  x2x2 Superior nasal retinal vessels
  x2x3 Inferior nasal retinal vessels
  x2x4 Superior temporal retinal vessels
  x2x5 Inferior temporal retinal vessels
 x30 General neuromuscular mechanism for binocular vision
 x31 Mechanism for conjugate lateral movement
 x32 Mechanism for convergence

x33   Mechanism for divergence
x34   Mechanism for conjugate movement upward
x35   Mechanism for conjugate movement downward
x36   Mechanism for disjunctive vertical movement
x37   Mechanism for cyclovergence
x38   Mechanism for pupil
x39   Mechanism for accommodation
x3x   Intrinsic arteries of eye retina
     x3x1   Central retinal artery
     x3x2   Superior nasal retinal artery
     x3x3   Inferior nasal retinal artery
     x3x4   Superior temporal retinal artery
     x3x5   Inferior temporal retinal artery
x40   Extrinsic muscles of eye, generally
x41   Intrinsic veins of eye
x42   Intrinsic arteries of eye
x43   Intrinsic vessels of eye
x44   Extrinsic veins of orbit
x45   Extrinsic arteries of orbit
x46   Extrinsic vessels of orbit
x48   Intrinsic muscles, iris and ciliary body
x4x   Hyaloid artery

x5 and x6   STRUCTURES AUXILIARY TO THE EYE

x50   Orbit
x51   Orbital tissues and contents, generally
x52   Eyelids [1]; palpebral fissure
     x521   Medial palpebral ligament
     x522   Lateral palpebral ligament
x53   Upper lid
x54   Lower lid
x55   Tarsus
x56   Conjunctiva
     x56x   Vessels of conjunctiva
x57   Tarsal conjunctiva
x58   Bulbar conjunctiva
x59   Caruncle
x60   Generally and unspecified glands of lid
x61   Meibomian glands
x62   Lacrimal gland and ducts
x63   Lacrimal passages
x64   Lacrimal punctum
x65   Lacrimal canaliculus
x66   Lacrimal sac
x67   Lacrimonasal duct
x68   Canthi
     x681   Inner canthus
     x682   Outer canthus
x6x   Vessels of eyelids

[1] The code number of skin of eyelids is 132.

x7 and x8   ACOUSTIC SENSE

    x70   Acoustic sense, generally
    x71   Ear, generally
    x72   Auricle
    x74   Cartilage of auricle
    x75   External acoustic meatus (canal)
    x76   Osseous meatus
    x77   Tympanic membrane
    x78   Lobule
    x79   Cartilagenous meatus
    x80   Middle ear, generally
    x81   Auditory ossicles
    x82   Muscles of tympanum
    x83   Auditory tube (Eustachian tube)
    x84   Mastoid antrum and mastoid air cells
    x85   Internal ear
    x86   Osseous labyrinth
    x87   Cochlea
    x88   Organ of Corti
    x89   Perilabyrinthine tissues
    x8x   Petrous portion

x9   VESTIBULAR EQUILIBRATORY SENSE

    x90   Vestibular equilibratory sense, generally
    x91   Vestibule
    x93   Semicircular canals
    x94   Utricle and saccule

ETIOLOGIC CLASSIFICATION

ETIOLOGIC CLASSIFICATION

CATEGORIES

0   Diseases due to genetic and prenatal influence

1   Diseases or infections due to a lower plant or animal parasite

2   Diseases or infections due to a higher plant or animal parasite

3   Diseases due to intoxication

4   Diseases due to trauma or physical agent

50   Diseases secondary to circulatory disturbance

55   Diseases secondary to disturbance of innervation or of psychic control

6   Diseases due to or consisting of static mechanical abnormality (such as obstruction, calculus, displacement, or gross change in form) due to unknown cause

7   Diseases due to disorder of metabolism, growth, or nutrition

8   New growths

9   Diseases due to unknown or uncertain cause with the structural reaction (degenerative, infiltrative, inflammatory, proliferative, sclerotic, or reparative) manifest; hereditary and familial diseases of this nature

x   Diseases due to unknown or uncertain cause with the functional reaction alone manifest; hereditary and familial diseases of this nature

y   Diseases of undetermined cause

ETIOLOGIC CLASSIFICATION

CATEGORY 0

0 *Diseases due to genetic and prenatal influence*

00 DISEASES DUE TO ABNORMALITY OF BONE DEVELOPMENT

    000 Generally and unspecified
    001 Retardation of endochondral bone growth
    002 Cartilaginous inclusions
    003 Osteocartilaginous exostosis
    004 Generalized increased density
    005 Disseminated spotted increased density
    006 Diminished strength
  · 007 Replacement by fibrous tissue
    008 Multiple eccentric centers of ossification

01 and 02 ABNORMALITIES IN STRUCTURE OR ANATOMIC RELATIONSHIP

    010 Generally or unspecified
    011 Entire absence; aplasia; agenesis
    012 Partial absence
    013 Hypertrophy; enlargement; elongation
    014 Hyperplasia
    015 Dilatation
    016 Hypoplasia; atrophy; shortening
    017 Contracture; stricture
    018 Atresia; occlusion
    019 Persistence of fetal form
    01x Anomaly of structure due to persistence or distortion of fetal characteristics
    021 Displacement
    022 Distortion
    023 Inclusion; ectopic rest
    024 Fusion
    025 Adhesion
    026 Dislocation, ectopia
    027 Hernia, protrusion
    028 Persistence of fetal position
    029 Fistula
    02x Transposition

03 SUPERNUMERARY PART; DUPLICATION; DIVISION; BIFURCATION; DIVER-TICULATION

    031 Supernumerary parts
    032 Duplication
    033 Triplication
    034 Division; abnormal degree of division
    035 Bifurcation

036   Diverticulation
037   Nonfusion
038   Fissure
039   Anomalous bands and folds
03x   Failure of segmentation

04 ABNORMALITIES OF FUNCTION

040   Generally or unspecified
041   Absence of function
042   Decrease of function
043   Increase of function
044   Other disturbance of function
045   Inherent defective tendency
046   Persistence of fetal characteristics
047   Anomaly of function due to persistence or distortion of fetal
      characteristics
048   Abnormal function due to asphyxiation at birth

05 DISEASES DUE TO INFECTION, INTOXICATION, OR TRAUMA BEFORE OR
   DURING BIRTH; ABNORMALITIES OF PREGNANCY AND LABOR

050   Injury during birth
      Abnormalities of pregnancy and labor are listed on page 377
052   Due to maternal infection [1]
053   Due to maternal intoxication [1]
054   Injury prior to birth
057   Due to maternal metabolic disturbances [1]
059   Due to genetic disturbances prior to birth

06 DISEASES DUE TO OR CONSISTING OF OBSTRUCTION OR PRESSURE

061   Foreign body; stone
062   Valve formation
063   Dilatation
064   Cyst
065   Torsion
066   Strangulation
067   Incarceration
068   Pressure

07 DISEASES DUE TO METABOLIC, NUTRITIONAL, OR TROPHIC DISTURBANCE
   BEFORE BIRTH

070   Generally or unspecified
071   Disorder of general metabolism
072   Disorder of calcium metabolism
073   Deprivation of vitamins
074   Disorder of pigment
075   Overdevelopment
076   Underdevelopment
077   Other abnormal development; dysplasia
079   Reduction of pigment

[1] Record secondary diagnosis.

09 DISEASES DUE TO NONINFECTIVE INFLAMMATORY OR DEGENERATIVE PROCESS BEFORE BIRTH

090 Generally or unspecified
091 Process predominantly inflammatory
092 Process predominantly degenerative
093 Simple hyperplasia
094 Hyperplasia and degeneration
095 Effusion
096 Infiltration
097 Proliferation

00 DISEASES DUE TO ABNORMALITY OF BONE DEVELOPMENT

000 Generally and unspecified
001 Retardation of endochondral bone growth
002 Cartilaginous inclusions
003 Osteocartilaginous exostosis
004 Generalized increased density
005 Disseminated spotted increased density
006 Diminished strength
007 Replacement by fibrous tissue
008 Multiple eccentric centers of ossification

0x DEFECTS OF CARDIAC SEPTUMS. (*See under* Diseases of cardiovascular system). *Also used for classification of* Color blindness (*page 446*)

CATEGORY 1

1 *Diseases or infections due to a lower plant (bacteria, rickettsiae, or viruses) or animal parasite (bacteria, rickettsiae, and viruses)*

PREFERRED NAME	COMMON NAME
100 General or unspecified (acute infection, purulent infection)	
101 Diplococcus pneumoniae	Pneumococcus
102 Streptococcus (including anaerobic streptococci and enterococcus)	
1026 Alpha hemolytic (green or viridans type)	
10261 Streptococcus fecalis	
10262 Streptococcus salivarius	
10263 Streptococcus mitis	
1027 Beta hemolytic	
10271 Streptococcus pyogenes (group A)	

PREFERRED NAME	COMMON NAME

          10272 Streptococcus
                 equisimilis
                 (human group
                 C)
   1028 Nonhemolytic
103 Neisseria gonorrheae   Gonococcus
104 Neisseria meningitidis   Neisseria intracellularis
                                     (Meningococcus)
105 Staphylococcus pyogenes   Staphylococcus
     1051 Staphylococcus
           aureus, hemolytic
           type
     1052 Staphylococcus
           aureus, nonhemolytic
           type
106 Pasteurella pestis   Bacillus pestis
                                     (plague bacillus)
107 Pasteurella tularensis   Bacillus tularense
108 Hemophilus pertussis   Bacillus pertussis
109 Pasteurella pseudotubercu-
     losis
10x Hemophilus ducreyi   Ducrey's bacillus
110 Hemophilus influenzae   Influenza bacillus
                                     (Pfeiffer's bacillus)
     1101 Hemophilus aegypti   Koch-Weeks bacillus
111 Moraxella lacunata   Morax-Axenfeld bacillus
112 Coliform bacteria
     1121 Escherichia coli   Bacterium coli
           11211 Nonhemolytic
                  112111 Serotype 055
                  112112 Serotype 0111
                  112113 Other serotypes
           11212 Hemolytic
     1122 Atypical coliform bacteria
           11221 Intermediate forms
           11222 Paracolon bacilli
                  112221 Arizona group
                  112222 Bethesda-Ballerup group
                  112223 Providence group
     1123 Aerobacter-Klebsiella
113 Salmonella—Animal origin
     1131 Salmonella enteritidis
     1132 Salmonella typhi-   Bacillus aertryke
           murium
     1133 Salmonella choler-   Bacillus suipestifer
           aesuis
114 Salmonella—Human origin
     1141 Salmonella paratyphi   Paratyphoid A
           A
     1142 Salmonella paratyphi   Paratyphoid B
           B   Salmonella Schottmuelleri

PREFERRED NAME	COMMON NAME
1143 Salmonella paratyphi C	Paratyphoid SC Salmonella hirschfeldii
115 Salmonella typhi (typhosa)	Eberthella typhi Bacillus typhosus (typhoid bacillus)
116 Shigella	
1161 Shigella dysenteriae	Shiga's bacillus
1162 Shigella paradysenteriae	Flexner-Strong bacilli
1163 Shigella sonnei	
1165 Shigella ambigua	Shigella schmitzii Schmitz's bacillus
117 Brucella	
1171 Brucella melitensis	
1172 Brucella abortus	
1173 Brucella suis	
118 Bacillus anthracis	Anthrax bacillus
119 Clostridium tetani	Bacillus tetani Tetanus bacillus
11x Clostridium novyi	Bacillus oedematiens
120 Clostridium botulinum	Bacillus botulinus
121 Clostridium septicum	Vibrion septique
122 Clostridium perfringens	Bacillus welchii Clostridium welchii
123 Mycobacterium tuberculosis	Bacillus tuberculosis tubercle bacillus
124 Mycobacterium leprae	Bacillus leprae Leprosy bacillus Hansen's bacillus
125 Corynebacterium diphtheriae	Bacillus diphtheriae Diphtheria bacillus
126 Actinobacillus mallei	Bacillus mallei Glanders bacillus Malleomyces mallei
127 Pseudomonas pseudomallei	Bacillus whitmori Whitmore's bacillus Malleomyces pseudomallei
128 Pseudomonas aeruginosa	Bacillus pyocyaneus
129 Vibrio cholerae	Vibrio comma
130 Generally or unspecified (alternative with 100 or 190); organisms of doubtful or rare pathogenicity; newly discovered organisms.	
131 Klebsiella pneumoniae	Friedländer's bacillus
132 Proteus vulgaris	Bacillus proteus
134 Streptobacillus moniliformis	Haverhillia multiformis
135 Bacteroides	
136 Bartonella bacilliformis	
137 Donovania granulomatis (inguinal granuloma)	

14 DISEASES OR INFECTIONS DUE TO A SPIROCHETE (INCLUDING
    SPIRILLA)

PREFERRED NAME	COMMON NAME
140 Generally or unspecified	
141 Borrelia	
1411 Borrelia recurrentis	
1412 Borrelia duttonii	
1413 Borrelia vincentii	Spirochaeta vincenti
1414 Borrelia parkeri	
142 Leptospira	
1421 Leptospira icterohem- orrhagiae	
1422 Leptospira hebdomadis	
1423 Leptospira canicola	
1424 Leptospira pomona	
146 Treponema pertenue	Spirochaeta pallida
147 Treponema pallidum	Spirochaeta pallida
149 Treponema carateum	Treponema pintae

15 DISEASES OR INFECTONS DUE TO PROTOZOON

150 Generally or unspecified
151 Amoeba
   1510 Endamoeba (Entamoeba) histolytica
   1511 Endolimax nana
   1512 Iodamoeba williamsi (I. bütschlii)
   1513 Dientamoeba fragilis
   1514 Endamoeba (Entamoeba) coli
   1515 Endamoeba (Entamoeba) gingivalis
152 Leishmania
   1521 Leishmania donovani
   1522 Leishmania brasiliensis
   1523 Leishmania tropica
153 Trypanosoma
   1531 Trypanosoma gambiense
   1532 Trypanosoma cruzi
   1533 Trypanosoma rhodesiense
154 Trichomonas
   1541 Trichomonas hominis
   1542 Trichomonas tenax (T. buccalis)
   1543 Trichomonas vaginalis
155 Giardia lamblia
156 Chilomastix mesnili
157 Haemosporidia
   1571 Plasmodium vivax
   1572 Plasmodium malariae
   1573 Plasmodium falciparum
   1574 Plasmodium ovale
   1577 Toxoplasma gondii
158 Isospora hominis
159 Balantidium coli

16, 17, 18, and 19 DISEASES OR INFECTIONS DUE TO A SPECIFIC VIRUS, A RICKETTSIA, OR AN UNKNOWN OR UNCLASSIFIED OR-GANISM

PREFERRED NAME	COMMON NAME

160 Generally or unspecified
162 Dengue
163 Encephalomyocarditis virus
164 Epidemic hiccup virus
165 Rubella (German measles) virus
166 Herpes virus
168 Influenza virus, unspecified
    1681 Influenza virus, type A
    1682 Influenza virus, type A (A prime, A1)
    1683 Influenza virus, type A (A double prime, A2, Asian)
    1684 Influenza virus, type B
    1685 Pneumonitis virus, unspecified
    1686 Newcastle disease virus (NDV, avian pneumoencephalitis)
169 Rubeola (measles) virus
16x Miliary fever virus
170 Mumps virus
171 Poliovirus (poliomyelitis virus)
    1711 Poliovirus type 1
    1712 Poliovirus type 2
    1713 Poliovirus type 3
172 Sandfly (pappataci) fever virus
173 Psittacosis-lymphogranuloma venereum virus, unspecified
    1731 Psittacosis ornithosis virus (parrot fever, ornithosis)
    1732 Lymphogranuloma venereum virus (esthiomene)
174 Rabies virus
175 Equine encephalomyelitis, virus unspecified
    1751 Western
    1752 Eastern
    1753 St. Louis
    1754 Venezuelan
    1755 Japanese B
    1756 Murray valley (Australian X)
    1757 West Nile
    1758 Rift valley fever (enzootic hepatitis) virus
176 Pox virus, unspecified
    1761 Variola (smallpox) virus
    1762 Vaccinia (cowpox) virus
    1763 Varicella (chickenpox) virus
    1764 Zoster virus
177 Lymphocytic choriomeningitis virus
178 Yellow fever virus
179 Verruca virus
17x Coxsackie virus, unspecified
    17x1 Coxsackie virus, type A
    17x2 Herpangina
    17x3 Coxsackie virus, type B
    17x4 Epidemic pleurodynia virus   Bornholm disease (epidemic myalgia)

PREFERRED NAME	COMMON NAME

17x5 Aseptic meningitis virus

180 Rickettsiosis, unspecified

181 Spotted fever rickettsia

    1811 Rickettsia rickettsiae (Dermocentroxenus rickettsiae) — Spotted fever (Sao Paulo typhus) (Tobia fever)

    1812 Rickettsia conori — Boutonneuse fever (Mediterranean tick fever) (tick typhus)

    1813 Rickettsia australis — North Queensland tick typhus

    1814 Rickettsia akari — Rickettsialpox

183 Tsutsugamushi (scrub typhus) rickettsia

    1831 Rickettsia tsutsugamushi (Rickettsia orientalis); (Rickettsia nipponica); (Rickettsia akamushi) — Tsutsugamushi disease (Japanese river fever); (Kedani fever); (scrub typhus); (rural typhus)

    1832 Coxiella burneti (Rickettsia burneti, Rickettsia diaporica) — Q fever

    1833 Rickettsia quintana (Rickettsia pediculi, Rickettsia wolhynica) — Trench fever (Wolhynian fever)

184 Typhus fever rickettsia

    1841 Rickettsia prowazeki — Epidemic typhus (classic typhus) (louse-borne typhus)

    1842 Rickettsia typhi — Endemic typhus (murine typhus) (flea-borne typhus)

185 Molluscus contagiosum virus

186 Colorado tick fever virus

187 Salivary gland disease virus — Cytomegalic inclusion disease

188 ECHO (enteric cytopathogenic human orphan) virus, unspecified

    1881 ECHO virus, type A

    1882 ECHO virus, type B

189 Hepatitis virus, unspecified

    1891 Hepatitis virus A — Infectious hepatitis

    1892 Hepatitis virus B — Serum hepatitis

18x Adenovirus, unspecified

    18x1 Pharyngoconjunctival fever virus

    18x2 Epidemic kerato-conjunctivitis virus

190 Unknown or unclassified organism, generally (nonsuppurative infection unspecified)

PREFERRED NAME

192 Exanthema subitum (roseola infantum) virus
193 Epidemic hemorrhagic fever virus
194 Trachoma
195 Diffuse endothelioangiitis
196 Chorea
197 Inclusion conjunctivitis virus

1x STRUCTURAL AND FUNCTIONAL CHANGES DUE TO INFECTION; TOXIC EFFECTS OF REMOTE INFECTION

1x0 (100.0) Generally and unspecified; localized inflammatory lesion; chronic inflammation; inflammation due to remote infection
1x1 (100.1) Loss of substance; gangrene
1x2 (100.2) Abscess
1x3 (100.3) Fistula; sinus; perforation
1x4 (100.4) Adhesion; contracture; distortion; constriction; compression; obstruction; ankylosis; embolism
1x5 (100.5) Rupture; fracture; dislocation
1x6 (100.6) Proliferation; fibrosis; hypertrophy; dilatation
1x7 (100.7) Circulatory disturbance (hemorrhage)
1x8 (100.8) Effusion; cyst formation
1x9 (100.9) Degeneration; atrophy; calcification; ulceration
1xx (100.x) Impairment; disturbance or loss of function

Note: The code in parentheses is simply an amplification of the code which precedes it. In both cases the final digit is sometimes used arbitrarily.

CATEGORY 2

2 Diseases or infections due to fungus or animal parasite

20, 21, 22, and 23 DUE TO A FUNGUS PARASITE

200 Generally and unspecified
201 Nocardia
  2011 Nocardia minutissima
  2012 Nocardia asteroides
  2013 Nocardia tenuis
  2014 Nocardia brasiliensis
  2015 Streptomyces (Nocardia) madurae
  2016 Streptomyces (Nocardia) pelletieri
  2017 Streptomyces (Nocardia) somaliensis
202 Actinomyces
  2022 Actinomyces bovis
  2023 Actinomyces israeli
204 Trichosporon
  2041 Trichosporon beigelii
205 Madurella
206 Monosporium apiospermum (Allescheria boydii)
208 Malassezia furfur

209 Candida
  2091 Candida albicans
  2092 Candida parapsilosis
  2093 Candida guilliermondi
210 Cladosporium (Hormodendrum)
  2101 Cladosporium carionii
  2102 Cladosporium trichoides
211 Trichophyton
  2111 Trichophyton mentagrophytes
  2112 Trichophyton concentricum
  2113 Trichophyton violaceum
  2114 Trichophyton schoenleinii
  2115 Trichophyton rubrum
  2116 Trichophyton tonsurans
212 Phialophora
  2121 Phialophora verrucosa
  2122 Phialophora pedrosoii (Hormendendrum pedrosoii)
  2123 Phialophora compactum (Hormendendrum compactum)
213 Microsporum
  2131 Microsporum audouini
  2132 Microsporum canis (lanosum)
  2133 Microsporum gypseum
214 Geotrichum
215 Epidermophyton
  2151 Epidermophyton floccosum
216 Sporotrichum
  2162 Sporotrichum schenckii
217 Blastomyces
  2171 Blastomyces dermatitidis
  2172 Paracoccidioides brasiliensis (Blastomyces brasiliensis)
218 Cryptococcus
  2181 Cryptococcus neoformans (Torula histolytica)
219 Coccidioides
  2191 Coccidioides immitis
220 Histoplasma
  2201 Histoplasma capsulatum
  2202 Histoplasma capsulatum dubosoii
  2203 Histoplasma farciminosum
226 Aspergillus
  2261 Aspergillus fumigatus
227 Penicillium
231 Rhinosporidium
  2311 Phinosporidium seeberi
232 Mucor
235 Rhizopus

23 and 25 DUE TO A NEMATODE (ROUNDWORM)

240 Generally and unspecified
241 Ascaris lumbricoides (large intestinal roundworm)
242 Enterobius (Oxyuris) bermicularis (pinworm, seatworm)
243 Ancylostomatidae (hookworm)
  2431 Ancylostoma duodenale
  2432 Necator americanus

2433 Ancylostoma ceylanicum
2434 Ancylostoma brasiliense
244 Nematode larvae
245 Toxocara
    2451 Toxocara canis (dog ascaris)
    2452 Toxocara felis (cat ascaris)
246 Stronglidae of mammals
    2461 Ternidens diminutus
    2462 Oesophagostomum apiostomum
    2463 Oesophagostomum stephanostomum
    2464 Strongyloides stercoralis (threadworm)
    2465 Strongyloides fulleborni
248 Trichostrongylus orientalis
254 Trichuroidea
    2541 Trichuris trichiura (whipworm)
    2542 Trichinella spiralis (trichina worm)
    2543 Capillaris hepatica
257 Filaria
    2571 Wuchereria bancrofti (Bancroft's filaria)
    2572 Acanthocheilonema perstans
    2573 Loa loa (eye worm)
    2574 Onchocerca volvulus (convoluted filaria)
    2575 Mansonella ozzardi
    2576 Wuchereria malayi (Malayan filaria)
    2577 Acanthocheilonema streptocerca
258 Dracunculus medinensis (Guinea worm)

26 DUE TO A CESTODE (TAPEWORM)

260 Generally and unspecified
261 Taenia (large tapeworm)
    2611 Taenia solium (pork tapeworm)
    2612 Taenia saginata (beef tapeworm)
262 Hymenolepis (small tapeworm)
    2621 Hymenolepis nana (dwarf tapeworm)
    2622 Hymenolepis diminuta (rat tapeworm)
263 Dipylidium caninum (dog tapeworm)
264 Diphyllobothrium (dibothriocephalus) latum (fish tapeworm)
265 Sparganum mansoni (encystic-stage fish tapeworm)
266 Cysticercus cellulosae (encystic-stage pork tapeworm)
267 Echinococcus
    2671 Echinococcus granulosus (unilocular hydatid)
    2672 Echinococcus multilocularis (alveolar hydatid)

27 DUE TO A TREMATODE (FLUKE)

270 Generally and unspecified
271 Fasciola (liver fluke)
    2711 Fasciola hepatica (sheep liver fluke)
    2712 Fasciola gigantica (giant liver fluke)
272 Fasciolopsis buski (large intestinal fluke)
273 Clonorchis sinensis (Chinese liver fluke)
274 Opisthorchis
    2741 Opisthorchis felineus (cat liver fluke)
    2742 Opisthorchis viverrini

275   Heterophyidae (small intestinal flukes)
    2751   Heterophyes heterophyes
    2752   Metagonimus yokogawai
277   Paragonimus westermani (lung fluke)
278   Schistosoma (blood fluke)
    2781   Schistosoma haematobium
    2783   Schistosoma mansoni
    2784   Schistosoma yokogawai
279   Echinostomatidae (echinostome flukes)
27x   Trematode larvae
    27x1   Trichobilharzia

28   DUE TO ARACHNIDS (MITES, TICKS, MYRIAPODS, ETC.)

280   Generally and unspecified
281   Chilopoda (centipedes)
282   Diplopoda (millipedes)
283   Acari (mites)
    2831   Sarcoptes scabiei (scabic mite)
    2832   Demodex folliculorum (follicular mite)
    2833   Thrombiculid mite (chigger)
    2834   Liponyssus bacoti
    2835   Dermanyssus gallinae
    2836   Allodermanyssus sanguineus
    2837   Pediculoides ventricosus
284   Ixodoidea (ticks)
285   Linguatulidae (pentastomes, porocephalus, tongue worms)
    2851   Armillifer moniliformis
    2852   Linguatula serrata
286   Scorpiones (scorpions)

4 *Venom poisoning due to any member of this group is to be classified under poisoning by venom*

287   Araneae (spiders)
    2871   Latrodectus mactans (black widow spider)
    2872   Loxosceles (brown spider)
    2873   Other

29   DUE TO AN HEXAPOD (INSECT)

291   Pediculus
    2911   Pediculus humanus capitis (head louse)
    2912   Pediculus humanus corporis (body louse)
292   Phthirius pubis (pubic louse)
294   Pulicidae (fleas)
    2941   Pulex irritans (human flea)
    2942   Nosopsyllus fasciatus (rat flea)
    2943   Xenopsyllus cheopsis (rat flea)
    2944   Ctenocephalides canis (dog flea)
    2945   Tunga penetrans
295   Diptera (generally and unspecified)
    2952   Dipterous larvae
    2953   Dermatobia hominis
296   Culicidae (mosquitoes)

297   Hymennoptera (bees, wasps, ants)
298   Cimex (bedbug)
299   Lepidoptera (caterpillars)

CATEGORY 3

This category includes exogenous chemical substances and mixtures which cause intoxication. Inorganic substances are listed in Sections 31 and 32. When two or more constituents of an inorganic substance may cause intoxication, as in lead arsenate, the poisoning should be coded under the constituent which has caused the observed reactions. Organometallic compounds in which the intoxications are obviously caused by the metallic constituents are classified under the respective metals.

Simple organic compounds with many uses are grouped according to their dominant molecular structural features in Section 33. The following sections contain more complex organic substances subdivided into various use categories. Thus, Sections 34 and 35 include complex organic substances used as drugs. The classification of drugs is similar to that in "New and Nonofficial Drugs," a compilation published for the American Medical Association.

3 *Diseases due to chemicals*

    300   Due to undetermined or unspecified substance

31   DUE TO INORGANIC SUBSTANCES (e.g., no carbon-to-hydrogen, carbon-to-carbon, or carbon-to-halogen covalent bonds)

    310   Generally, not listed or unspecified
    311   Corrosive mineral acids
        3110   Unspecified or unlisted. See also 3144, 314x, 3167, 3174, 3175
        3111   Hydrobromic acid
        3112   Hydrochloric acid (muriatic)
        3113   Hydrofluoric acid
        3114   Nitric acid
        3115   Phosphoric acid (orthophosphoric acid)
        3116   Sulfuric acid (oil of vitriol)
    312   Caustic alkalis—oxides, hydroxides, carbonates, bicarbonates, and basic carbonates. Also of lithium, rubidium, cesium, and strontium
        3122   Of sodium
        3123   Of potassium
        3126   Of calcium
        3128   Of barium
    313   Neutral compounds [1] (chlorides, sulfates, nitrates, phosphates) —exclusive of 3224
        3132   Of sodium
        3133   Of potassium
        3137   Of calcium
        3139   Of barium
    314   Strong oxidizing compounds [1]
        3141   Oxygen
        3142   Ozone

[1] If symptoms are caused chiefly by one radical of a compound, classify poisoning according to that radical.

    3143   Hydrogen peroxide
    3144   Hypochlorous acid and hypochlorites
    3145   Permanganates
    3146   Chromates and dichromates
    3147   Chlorates and perchlorates
    3148   Bromates and perbromates
    3149   Iodates and periodates
    314x   Other peroxides, oxy- and peroxy-salts and their acids—not elsewhere classified

315   Inorganic compounds [1] of carbon—exclusive of 311 and 312
    3151   Carbon monoxide
    3152   Carbon dioxide and carbonic acid
    3153   Hydrogen cyanide (hydrocyanic acid)
    3154   Other inorganic cyanides
    3155   Cyanate and thiocyanate salts
    3156   Cyanamide and its salts
    3157   Carbon disulfide

316   Inorganic compounds [1] of nitrogen—exclusive of 311, 312, 313, and 315; including hydroxylamine, azide salts, nitrogen halides, and nitrosyl halides.
    3162   Ammonia and annomia water (ammonium hydroxide)
    3163   Hydrazine
    3166   Nitrous oxide
    3167   Other oxides of nitrogen—e.g., nitric oxide, nitrogen dioxide, and their acids—exclusive of 3114
    3168   Nitrite and nitrate salts

317   Inorganic compounds [1] of sulfur—exclusive of 311, 313, and 315; including sulfur, sulfite and bisulfite salts, sulfate and thiosulfate salts, sulfur halides, inorganic thiophosphates
    3172   Hydrogen sulfide
    3173   Other inorganic sulfides and polysulfides
    3174   Sulfur dioxide and sulfurous acid
    3175   Other oxides of sulfur and their acids

318   Inorganic compounds [1] of boron, silicon, and phosphorus [2]—exclusive of 311 and 313. Also other compounds of boron (perborates, boron hydrides, etc.) and of phosphorus (oxides and acids of phosphorus exclusive of 3115, and metaphosphites, phosphorus halides, etc.)
    3181   Boric acid and borates
    3184   Silicon compounds
    3185   Phosphorus
    3188   Phosphine and phosphides

319   Inorganic halogen compounds [1]—exclusive of 311, 313, 314, 315, 316, 317, and 318.
    3191   Fluorine and hydrogen fluoride (as a gas)
    3192   Chlorine and hydrogen chloride (as a gas)
    3193   Bromine and hydrogen bromide (as a gas)
    3194   Iodine and hydrogen iodine (as a gas or in solution)
    3195   Fluoride salts

---

[1] If symptoms are caused chiefly by one radical of a compound, classify poisoning according to that radical.

[2] For simple organic compounds containing these elements, see 339; also 3691.

3196   Bromide salts
3197   Iodide salts

32 DUE TO METALS, METALLOIDS, AND THEIR COMPOUNDS, inorganic and organic—exclusive of 312, 313, 314

   321 Arsenic, selenium, tellurium, and their compounds
       3211 Arsenic trioxide, arsenites, and other inorganic trivalent arsenic compounds
       3212 Arsenates and other inorganic pentavalent arsenic compounds
       3213 Arsine and other organic compounds with trivalent arsenic
          32131 Arsine
          32134 Chlorovinyldichloroarsine (lewisite)
          32136 Diphenylaminochloroarsine (adamsite)
       3214 Organic compounds with pentavalent arsenic; e.g., sodium cacodylate, sodium arsanilate, carbasone, carbasone oxide, and thiocarbasone
          32143 Tryparasamide
       3215 Selenium and its compounds
       3216 Tellurium and its compounds
 322, 323, 324, 325, and 326   Nonradioactive metals and their compounds
       3221 Aluminum and its compounds
       3222 Antimony and its compounds
       3223 Barium and its compounds—exclusive of 3128 and 3139
       3224 Beryllium and its compounds
       3225 Bismuth and its compounds
       3227 Cadmium and its compounds
       3231 Copper and its compounds
       3232 Chromium and its compounds—exclusive of 3146
       3237 Iron (ferrous and ferric) and its compounds
       3238 Lead and its compounds
          Inorganic lead compounds, e.g.
          32382 Lead oxides
          Organic lead compounds, e.g.
          32384 Tetraethyl lead
          32385 Lead acetate
       3243 Mercury and its compounds
          32431 Inorganic mercuric salts
          32432 Inorganic mercurous salts
          32433 Alkyl mercury salts
          32434 Phenyl mercury salts and esters
          32435 Organic mercurial diuretics
          32436 Organic mercurial antiseptics
          32437 Organic mercury compounds—not elsewhere classified
       3245 Nickel and its compounds
       3249 Potassium and its compounds—exclusive of 3123 and 3133
       3250 Rare earths and their compounds
       3253 Silver and its compounds
       3257 Thallium and its compounds
       3258 Tin and its compounds
       3260 Uranium (nonenriched) and its compounds
       3263 Zinc and its compounds

33   SIMPLE ORGANIC SUBSTANCES, OTHER THAN THOSE SPECIFIED IN CATE-
GORIES 34 to 39

     330   Generally, not listed, or unspecified
     331   Hydrocarbons and halogenated hydrocarbons
         3311   Aliphatic saturated hydrocarbons
             33111   Methane
             33112   Ethane
             33113   Propane; butane; or higher alkanes
             33114   Cyclopropane
             33115   Petroleum ether (naptha, petroleum benzin, lighter fluid)
             33116   Gasoline
             33117   Kerosene (mineral spirits)
             33118   Mineral oil
             33119   Paraffins
             3311x   Cyclobutane or higher cyclic alkanes
         3312   Aliphatic, unsaturated hydrocarbons such as propylene; butene; higher alkanes, butadiene or other polyenes
             33121   Ethylene
             33122   Acetylene
         3313   Aromatic hydrocarbons including styrene and biphenyl
             33131   Benzene (benzol)
             33132   Toluene (toluol)
             33133   Xylene; ethylbenzene; or other alkyl benzenes
         3314   Polycyclic aromatic hydrocarbons such as tetralin; decalin and anthracene, phenanthrene, benzpyrene and methylcholanthrene
             33141   Naphthalene
         3315   Halogenated aliphatic hydrocarbons
             33151   Methyl chloride (chloromethane); methyl bromide; methyl iodide
             33152   Chloroform
             33153   Bromoform; iodoform
             33154   Carbon tetrachloride
             33155   Ethyl chloride; ethyl bromide; ethyl iodide
             33156   Ethylene dichloride; ethylene dibromide
             33157   Methyl chloroform; trichloroethane; tetrachloroethane
             33158   Trichloroethylene; tetrachloroethylene; butylidene chloride
             ^3159   Fluorinated aliphatic hydrocarbons; freons; halothane
         3316   Halogenated aromatic hydrocarbons
             33161   Chlorobenzene
             33162   Dichlorobenzene, ortho and para
     332   Simple alcohols, glycols, phenols, ethers, and oxides
         3321   Alcohols
             33211   Methyl alcohol (methanol, wood alcohol)
             33212   Ethyl alcohol (ethanol, grain alcohol)
             33213   Isopropyl alcohol; propyl alcohol
             33214   Amyl alcohol: isoamyl alcohol; amylene hydrate; fusel oil

33215 Benzyl alcohol
3322 Phenols such as thymol, naphthols, resorcinol, hydroquinone, pyrogallol (pyrogallic acid) and asphalt, coal and oil tar
33221 Phenol (carbolic acid)
33222 Cresol (cresylic acid, tricresol)
3323 Ethers and oxides
33231 Ethyl ether (diethyl ether)
33232 Vinyl ether
33233 Ethylene oxide
3324 Glycols, glycol ethers, glycol esters, glycol ether-esters
33241 Ethylene glycol
33242 Diethylene glycol; triethylene glycol
33243 Propylene glycol
33244 Polyethylene glycols (carbowaxes)
33247 Diethylene glycol monoethyl ether
333 Simple aldehyde, ketones, and quinones
3331 Formaldehyde (formalin; paraformaldehyde; trioxymethylene)
3332 Acetaldehyde; paraldehyde; metaldehyde
3333 Acrolein (acrylic aldehyde)
3338 Acetone
334 Simple carboxylic acids, their salts, anhydrides, and acid chlorides
3341 Carboxylic acids and their salts [1]
33411 Formic acid; formate salts
33416 Oxalic acid; oxalate salts
33417 Chloroacetic acids (monochloroacetic acid; dichloroacetic acid; trichloroacetic acid)
33418 Fluoroacetic acid; fluoracetate salts
3342 Acetic anhydride
3343 Acetyl chloride
3344 Benzoyl chloride
335 Simple esters and lactones
3351 Methyl formate
3353 Isoamyl acetate (banana oil)
3355 Benzyl benzoate
3357 Coumarin
336 Simple amines and amides
3361 Amines, e.g., ethylamine and other aliphated amines, ethylenediamine, methylaniline, other aromatic amines
33613 Aniline
33615 Ethylenediamine tetra-acetate
3362 Amides, e.g., formamide, dimethylformamide, urea, and urethane
337 Other simple nitrogenous organic substances
3371 Nitro compounds
33711 Nitromethane; tetranitromethane; nitroethane; nitropropane
33712 Nitrobenzene
33713 Dinitrobenzene
33714 Trinitrotoluene (TNT)

[1] If symptoms are caused chiefly by one radical of a compound (salt), classify poisoning according to that radical.

33715 Dinitrochlorobenzene
33716 Nitrophenol; dinitrophenol
33717 Trinitrophenol (picric acid)
33718 Trinitroaniline
33719 Tetryl (trinitrophenyl methyl nitramine)
3372 Nitroso compounds
3373 Hydrazine derivatives (for hydrazine, see 3163)
3374 Nitrogen heterocycles, e.g., pyridine, collidine, quinoline, and 8-hydroxyquinoline (oxyquinoline)
3375 Simple nitriles
33751 Acrylonitrile
338 Simple organic substances containing sulfur
3381 Mercaptans
3382 Sulfides
33821 Disulfiram
3383 Sulfones
33831 Sulfonmethane; sulfonethymethane
3384 Sulfonic acids and their chlorides
3385 Sulfur heterocycles
33851 Thiophene
33852 Phenothiazine
3386 Thiourea and its derivatives
339 Simple organic substances containing phosphorus, silicon, or boron
—exclusive of 3615, 3616. See also 318
3391 Silicones

34 ORGANIC SUBSTANCES USED AS DRUGS

340 Generally not listed or unspecified
341 Local anesthetics
3411 Esters of para-aminobenzoic acid
34111 Ethyl aminobenzoate
34112 Procaine
3412 Other local anesthetics
34127 Lidocaine
34128 Pramoxine
34129 Cocaine
342 Antihistamines
3421 Motion sickness drugs
34211 Cyclizine
34212 Dimenhydrinate
34213 Meclizine
3422 Psychotherapeutic antihistamines
34221 Hydroxyzine
3423 to 3424 Histamine-antagonizing drugs
34235 Chlorpheniramine
34236 Diphenhydramine
34246 Tripelennamine
343 to 344 Anti-infectives
3431 Antibacterial drugs
34311 Para-amino salicylic acid; aminosalicylate salts
34312 Isoniazid (isonicotinyl hydrazine)
34313 Iproniazid

        34314 Chlorquinaldol
        34315 Methenamine (hexamethylenetetramine)
3432 Sulfonamides
        34321 Sulfonilamide
        34322 Sulfadiazine
        34323 Sulfamerazine
        34324 Sulfamethazine
        34325 Sulfisomidine
        34326 Sulfacetamide
        34327 Sulfathiazole
        34328 Paranitrosulfathiazole
        34329 Phthalylsulfathiazole
        34330 Succinylsulfathiazole
        34331 Sulfamethizole
        34332 Salicylazosulfapyridine
        34333 Sulfisoxazole
        34334 Acetyl sulfisoxazole
        34335 Sulfamethoxypyridazine
3434 Sulfones
        34341 Glucosulfone
        34342 Sulfoxone
        34343 Thiazolsulfone
3435 to 3436   Antibiotics
        34351 Bacitracin
        34352 Carbomycin
        34353 Chloramphenicol
        34354 Cycloserine
        34355 Erythromycin
        34356 Furmagillin
        34357 Neomycin
        34358 Novobiocin
        34359 Nystatin
        34360 Penicillin
        34361 Polymyxin
        34362 Streptomycin; dihydrostreptomycin
        34363 Chlortetracycline
        34364 Oxytetracycline
        34365 Tetracycline
        34366 Tyrothricin
        34367 Viomycin
        34368 Oleandomycin
        34369 Ristocetin
3437 Antifungal drugs. See also Fungicides (366)
        34371 Coparaffinate
        34372 Diamthazole
        34373 Hexetidine
        34374 Salicylic acid and salicylate salts
        34375 Salicylanilide
3438 Antimalarial drugs
        34381 Quinidine and its salts
        34382 Quinine and other cinchona alkaloids;
                 ethylhydrocupreine
        34383 Quinacrine

34384 Chloroquine
34385 Chloroguanide
34386 Pyrimethamine
34387 Pamaquine
3439 Antiprozoan drugs
  34391 Stilbamidine; hydroxystilbamidine
  34392 Propamidine, pentamidine
  34393 Suramin
  34394 Diiodohydroxyquin
3440 Antiseptics and disinfectants. See also Organic mercurial antiseptics (32436)
  34401 Hexachlorophene
  34402 Thymol iodide
  34403 Mandelic acid
  34409 Other cationic germicides (with quaternary nitrogen)
3441 Vermifugal Drugs
  34411 Diethylcarbamazine
  34412 Piperazine
  34413 Pyruvinium chloride
  34414 Methylrosaniline chloride (gentian violet, crystal violet, methyl violet)
  34415 Hexylresorcinol
  34416 Chenopodium oil
  34417 Aspidium
  34418 Pelletierine
  3441x Santonin
345 Antineoplastic drugs
  3451 Aminopterin
  3452 Busulfan
  3453 Mechlorethamine
  3454 Mercaptopurine
346 Autonomic drugs
  3461 Sympathomimetic (adrenergic) drugs
    34611 Epinephrine
    34612 Levarterenol
    34613 Amphetamine
    34616 Ephedrine, racephedrine
    34617 Isoproterenol
    34620 Methamphetamine
    34622 Phenylephrine
  3463 Sympatholytic (adrenergic-blocking) drugs
    34631 Dibenzylchlorethylamine
    34632 Phenoxybenzamine
    34637 Ergonovine; ergotamine, and other ergot alkaloids
  3464 Parasympathomimetic (cholinergic) drugs
    34647 Neostigmine
    34648 Physostigmine
    34649 Pilocarpine
  3465 Parasympatholytic (cholinergic-blocking) drugs
    34651 Atropine (hyoscyamine), scopolamine (hyoscine), and other belladonna alkaloids
    34652 Homatropine

        34657 Methantheline
        34663 Ethopropazine
        34675 Benactyzine
   3468 Ganglionic blocking agents. See also 3473
        34681 Tetraethylammonium chloride

347 Cardiovascular drugs
   3471 Digitalis and related drugs
        34710 Digitalis whole leaf
        34711 Digitoxin
        34712 Digoxin
        34715 Ouabain (G-strophanthin)
   3472 Heart muscle depressants—For quinidine, see 34381
        34721 Procainamide
   3473 Hypotensive drugs
        34731 Amyl nitrite
        34732 Glyceryl trinitrate; mannitol hexanitrate; erythrityl tetranitrate; pentaerythritol tetranitrate; aminotrate
              Sodium nitrite, see 3168
              Thiocyanates, see 3155
        34733 Protoveratrine; cryptenamine; and other *Veratrum viride* alkaloids
        34734 Hydrazaline
   3474 Sclerosing drugs
        34741 Sodium morrhuate
        34742 Sodium recinoleate

348 Central nervous system depressants
   For anesthetics, general, see cyclopropane (33114); chloroform (33152); ethyl ether (33231); vinyl ether (33232); ethylene oxide (33233); nitrous oxide (3166); trichloroethylene (33158); halothane (33159)
   3481 Analgesics
        34811 Acetylsalicylic acid (aspirin)—for sodium salicylate, see 34374
        34812 Salicylamide
        34813 Methyl salicylate (wintergreen oil)
        34814 Acetanilid
        34815 Acetophenetidin (phenacetin)
        34817 Aminopyrine
        34818 Antipyrine
        34819 Aconitine
   3482 Narcotic antagonists
        34821 Nalorphine
        34822 Levallorphan
   3483 Opium, its alkaloids, and their derivatives
        34831 Morphine; opium; paregoric
        34832 Codeine; ethylmorphine
        34833 Heroin (diacetylmorphine)
        34834 Dihydromorphinone
        34835 Dihydrocodeine
        34837 Papaverine
   3484 Synthetic opiumlike drugs
        34841 Dextrometorphan

        34842 Levorphanol
        34843 Meperidine
   3485 Hypnotics and sedatives—for paraldehyde, see 3332
        34850 Chloral hydrate
        34851 Barbital, phenobarbital, or barbituric acid derivatives
        3485x Tribromethanol
   3486 Anticonvulsants
        34861 Diphenylhydantoin
        34862 Paramethadione
   3487 Antitussives
        34871 Carbetapentane
   3488 Central sympathetic suppressants (tranquilizers)
        34881 Chlorpromazine
        34885 Prochlorperazine
        34886 Other phenothiazine tranquilizers
        34887 Reserpine; rescinnamine; or other *Rauwolfia* alkaloids
   3489 Skeletal muscle relaxants
        34891 Zoxazolamine
        34892 Meprobamate
        34899 Tubocurarine and other curare bases (chondodendron)
 349 Central nervous system stimulants
          Camphor. See Essential oils (373)
          Amphetamine. See Sympathomimetic drugs (34613)
          Iproniazid. See Anti-infectives (34313)
        34911 Methylphenidate
        34912 Nikethamide
        34913 Picrotixin
        34915 Aminophyllin
        34916 Caffeine, theobromine, theophylline, and other xanthine derivatives (including dyphylline)
        34917 Pentylenetetrazol
        34918 Nux vomica, brucine, and related alkaloids—exclusive of strychnine (36731)

 35 DIAGNOSTIC AIDS

      3501 Histamine
      3502 Evans blue
      3503 Betazole hydrochloride
      3504 Mannitol
      3505 Sodium para-aminohippurate
      3506 Iodine compounds for roentgenography
         35061 Chloriodized oil
         35068 Iodopyracet
      3507 Enzymes
         35071 Hyaluronidase
         35072 Trypsin
         35073 Streptodornase
         35074 Streptokinase

351 Gastrointestinal drugs
Antacids. See 31 and 32
   3511 Hydrocholeretics
      35111 Bile and bile salts
      35112 Dehydrocholic acid; desoxycholic acid and other
            cholic acid derivatives
   3512 Fecal moistening agents
      35122 Methyl cellulose; carboxymethylcellulose
      35124 Psyllium
   3513 Laxatives and cathartics
      35131 Cascara
      35132 Phenolphthalein
      35133 Castor oil
      35134 Podophyllum; podophyllin
      35135 Croton oil
      35136 Senna
      35137 Aloin and aloes
      35138 Rhubarb
      35139 Colocynth
   3514 Emetics. For nicotine and its salts, see 36171
      35141 Apomorphine
      35142 Ipecac; emetine; other ipecac alkaloids
      35143 Lobelia and its alkaloids
352 Hematological drugs
   3521 Anticoagulants
      35213 Bishydroxycoumarin
          For warfarin sodium, see rodenticides (36711)
   3522 Hemostatics
      35224 Thrombin
   3523 Blood and blood derivatives
   3524 Plasma substitutes
      35241 Dextran
354 Renal-acting and edema-reducing agents
   3541 Carbonic anhydrase inhibitors
      35411 Acetazolamide
      35412 Ethoxyzolamide
      35413 Chlorothiazide; hydrochlorothiazide. For Organic
            mercurial diuretics, see 32435
   3542 Drugs affecting renal tubular resorption and secretion
      35423 Probenecid
355 Therapeutic Nutrients and Substitutes
   3551 Carbohydrate substitutes
      35511 Cyclamate
      35512 Saccharine
   3552 Protein hydrolysates and amino acids
   3553 Fats and antagonists
356 Vitamins
   3562 Vitamin A
   3565 Vitamin D
   3566 Vitamin K and its analogues

36 ECONOMIC POISONS [1] AND CHEMICAL WARFARE AGENTS

    360   Unlisted,[1] unclassifiable, or unspecified economic poison

    361 to 362   Insecticides and poisons against other invertebrate pests (miticides, hematocides, etc.). See also 363, 364, and 365.

        3611 to 3612   Halogenated hydrocarbon insecticides

            36111 Aldrin

            36112 Benzene hexachloride

            36113 Chlordane

            36114 Dichlorodiphenyl trichloroethane (DDT)

            36116 Heptachlor

            36121 Lindane

            36123 Toxaphene

        3613   Halogenated hydrocarbon insecticides containing organic oxygen

            36134 Dieldrin

            36135 Methoxychlor

        3614   Halogenated hydrocarbon insecticides (miticides) containing organic sulfur (with or without oxygen)

            36141 Aramite

            36145 Ovex (Ovotran)

        3615 to 3616   Organic phosphorus insecticides

            36158 Malathion

            36162 Para-oxon

            36163 Parathion

        3617   Insecticides from botanical sources (and related synthetic substances)

            36171 Nicotine and its salts

            36173 Pyrethrum

            36174 Rotenone

        3619   Miscellaneous insecticides

            Organic thiocyanates. See also: fumigants (363), repellents (364), petroleum oils (3311), dinitrophenol derivatives (3655)

    363   Fumigants for space, soil, and grain

        3631   Nitriles exclusive of acrylonitrile (33751) and hydrogen cyanide (3153)

        3632   Chlorinated aliphatic compounds. See also carbon tetrachloride (33154), methyl bromide (33151), ethylene dichloride and dibromide (33156), trichloroethylene (33158)

            36321 Dichloroethyl ether

            36324 Tetrachloro and hexachloro-ethane

        3633   Chlorinated aromatic compounds exclusive of ortho- and para-dichlorobenzene (33162)

        3634   Organic oxides exclusive of ethylene oxide (33233)

        3635   Naphthalene and derivatives used as fumigants

        3636   Sulfur-containing fumigants except carbon disulfide (3157)

        3637   Miscellaneous fumigants

            36371 Nitroparaffins

            36372 Allyl alcohol

---

[1] For germicides, sanitizers, disinfectants, antiseptics, and other chemicals that attack microorganisms, see 343 and 344.

364 Repellents
  3641 Simple esters and diesters except benzyl benzoate (3355)
    36416 Dimethyl phthalate
  3642 Amides
    36421 Diethyl toluamide
  3643 Glycols and glycol ethers
    36433 Ethyl hexanediol
  3644 Miscellaneous repellents
    36441 Butopyronoxyl
365 Herbicides (weed killers, defoliants, desiccants, soil sterilants) and plant growth regulators
  3651 Chlorophenol and chlorophenoxy derivatives
    36517 Pentachlorophenol
  3652 Chloralkyl compounds
    36521 Trichloroacetic acid and sodium salts (TCA)
  3653 Derivatives of urea
    36531 Monuron
    36532 Diuron
    36533 Fenuron
  3654 Carbamates and other amides—exclusive of 3653
    36541 Isopropyl-N-phenyl carbamate (IPC)
    36545 Ammonium sulfamate
  3655 Dinitro alkyl phenols except 33716 dinitrophenol
    36551 Dinitro-o-cresol (DNC)
  3656 Inorganic and metallo-organic compounds
    For specific classification, see 31 and 32
  3657 Miscellaneous except allyl alcohol (36372), acrolein (3333), potassium cyanate (3175)
    36571 Aminotriazole
    36572 Triazines
366 Fungicides [1, 2]
  3661 General
    For specific classification, see 31 and 32
  3662 Dithiocarbamates and related fungicides
    36621 Nabam
    36622 Ferbam
    36623 Maneb
    36626 Thiram
  3663 Quinones
    36631 Dichlone
    36632 Chloranil
  3664 Derivatives of phenol—exclusive of 3663, pentachlorophenol (36517), hexachlorophene (34401), salicylic acid (34374)
    36643 Dichlorophene
    36645 o-Phenylphenol
    36646 Tri- and tetrachlorophenol
  3665 Heterocyclic nitrogen compounds
    36652 Captan
    36653 Cycloheximide
    36656 Glyodin

[1] For volatile fungicides, see Fumigants (363).
[2] See also Antifungal drugs (3427).

3666 Nitrogenous organic fungicides—exclusive of 3662 and
3665 and except dinitrophenol (3655), quaternary am-
monium surfactants and germicides (see 3440), tetra- and
pentachloronitrobenzene (36331), salicylamide (34375)
3667 Miscellaneous organic fungicides
    36671 Biphenyl
    36672 Carboxylic acids and salts
    36673 Dehydroacetic acid (DHA)
367 Rodenticides [1] and other vertebrate poisons
3671 Inhibitors of prothrombin formation except bishydroxy-
coumarin (35213)
    36711 Warfarin
    36712 Pivalyl indandione
3672 Inorganic poisons
    For specific classification, see 31 and 32
3673 Poisons of botanical origin except rotenone (36174)
    36731 Strychnine and its salts
    36732 Red squill
    36733 Ricin
3674 Miscellaneous
    36741 A-Naphthylthiourea
    36742 Sodium fluoracetate
    36743 Castrix
369 Chemical warfare agents
3691 Nerve gases
3692 Vesicants
    36921 Mustard (B,B'-dichloroethyl sulfide)
    36922 Nitrogen mustards
    36923 Phosgene oxime
    36924 Others—exclusive of lewisite (chlorovinyl-dichloro-
           arsine) (32134) and phenyldichloroarsine (32135)
3693 Lung irritants
    36931 Phosgene (carbonylchloride)
    36932 Chloropicrin (nitrochloroform)
    36933 Cyanogen and cyanogen chloride
    36934 Others—exclusive of chlorine (3192), nitrous fumes
           (3167), sulfur dioxide (3173)
3694 Systemic poisons—exclusive of hydrogen cyanide (3153),
cyanogen chloride (36933), and carbon monoxide (3151)
3695 Sternutators (nose gases)—exclusive of diphenylamino-
chloroarsine (adamsite) (32136), diphenylchloroarsine
(32137), and diphenylcyanoarsine (32137)
3696 Lacrimators (tear gases)
    36961 Chloroacetophenone
    36962 Brombenzyl cyanide
    36963 Others—exclusive of chloropicrin (36932) and
           cyanogen chloride (36933)
3697 Screening smokes—if not classifiable elsewhere

[1] For volatile rodenticides, see Fumigants (363).

37 SURFACE ACTIVE AGENTS—SOAP, DETERGENTS, WETTING AGENTS, AND EMULSIFIERS [1]

370 Generally and unspecified
371 Soaps
    3711 Soluble soaps (household soaps)
    3715 Insoluble soaps (industrial soaps)
372 Detergents, wetting agents, and emulsifiers
    3721 Anionic agents
    3722 Cationic agents
    3723 Organic nonionic agents
    3724 Inorganic agents
373 Natural essential oils
    3731 Of plant origin
    3732 Of animal origin
374 Synthetic essential oils

38 DUE TO ANIMAL, PLANT, OR FOOD POISON

380 Generally, not listed or unspecified
381 Poisoning by venom
    3813 By jelly fish (coelenterata)
    3814 By snake
    3815 By scorpion
    3816 By spider (araneae)
    3817 By wasp, bee, hornet, or ant
    3818 By centipede (myriapoda)
        38181 Scolopendra heros
        38182 Scolopendra morsitans
        38183 Scolopendra gigantea
    3819 By tick (exodidae)
382 Hormones, synthetic substitutes, and antagonists
    3825 Adrenal cortex hormones
        38251 Adrenal cortex extract
        38252 Desoxycorticosterone acetate
        38253 Cortisone; Hydrocortisone
        38256 Prednisolone
        38257 Prednisone
    3826 Female sex hormones
        38261 Progesterone
        38264 Estradiol
        38266 Estrone
        38268 Diethylstilbestrol or related synthetic estrogen
    3827 Insulin and synthetic substitutes
        38271 Insulin
        38272 Tolbutamide
        38273 Chlorpropamide
    3824 Pituitary hormones
        38241 Corticotropin
        38242 Vasopressin
    3828 Hormones, gonadal
        38281 Gonadotropin

[1] If the radical of a compound is known as the toxic agent, classify according to that radical.

    3829 Testicular hormones and synthetic substitutes
          38292 Methyltestosterone
          38294 Testosterone and its derivatives
    3821 Thyroid, synthetic substitutes, and antagonists
          38211 Thyroid
          38212 Sodium levothroxyine
          38214 Thiouracil
  383 Poisoning by food, type undetermined
  384 Poisoning by naturally toxic food (mushrooms or toadstools and plants)
    3842 Fava bean
    3843 Castor bean
    3844 Tobacco (leaf)
    3845 Filex mas
  388 Toxin due to pregnancy
  389 Toxin of azotemia
  38x Reaction following blood transfusion

39 DUE TO ANAPHYLAXIS OR ALLERGY

  390 Generally or unspecified
  391 Due to ingestion of foreign protein
  392 Due to inhalation of foreign protein
  393 Due to injection of foreign protein
    3931 Serum
    3932 Vaccine
  394 Due to fungus
  395 Due to idiosyncrasy to food
  396 Due to heat
  397 Due to cold
  398 Due to ultraviolet radiation
  399 Due to Rh sensitization
    3991 Hemolytic disease of (fetus and) newborn
    3992 Transfusion hemolysis
  39x Due to transfusion of blood, unspecified

3x STRUCTURAL OR FUNCTIONAL CHANGE DUE TO INTOXICATION

  3x0 (300.0) Generally or unspecified; inflammation
  3x1 (300.1) Loss of substance; gangrene
  3x2 (300.2) Abscess
  3x3 (300.3) Fistula; sinus; perforation
  3x4 (300.4) Adhesion; contracture; distortion; constriction; compression; obstruction; ankylosis
  3x5 (300.5) Rupture
  3x6 (300.6) Proliferation; hypertrophy; dilatation; fibrosis
  3x7 (300.7) Circulatory disturbance (hemorrhage)
  3x8 (300.8) Effusion
  3x9 (300.9) Degeneration; ulceration; hypoplasia
  3xx (300.x) Impairment; disturbance or loss of function

Note: The code in parentheses is simply an amplification of the code which precedes it. In both cases the final digit is sometimes used arbitrarily.

CATEGORY 4

4 *Diseases due to trauma or physical agent*

40 and 41   DUE TO SUDDEN TRAUMA

400   Generally or unspecified
401   Abrasion
402   Contusion
403   Compression; depression
404   Crushing
405   Amputation; severance
    4051   Incomplete amputation
406   Dislocation; extrusion (of viscus)
407   Open dislocation
    Fracture-dislocation. Diagnose both fracture and dislocation
408   Incomplete dislocation (subluxation); diastasis
409   Avulsion
    4091   Stretching or traction
40x   Habitual dislocation
410   Wound, general
    4101   Perforating wound
411   Incised wound; stab wound
    4111   Penetrating wound
412   Lacerated wound
    4121   Wound caused directly by explosive
413   Bite
    4131   Human bite
    4132   Animal bite
    4133   Spider bite
414   Gunshot wound (missile)
    4141   Penetrating wound
    4142   Perforating wound
415   Operative wound: instrumentation wound
416   Closed fracture [1]: rupture
    4161   Incomplete
    4162   Transverse
    4163   Oblique
    4164   Spiral
    4165   Comminuted
    4167   Chip
417   Injury during birth [1]
418   Open fracture [2]
    4182   Transverse
    4183   Oblique
    4184   Spiral
    4185   Comminuted
419   Intrauterine injury

[1] Restricted to bones only.
[2] Add to the code number the digit 4 for impacted fracture; the decimal digit 9 for depressed fracture.

42 REMOTE [1] EFFECTS OF TRAUMA

  420 Generally or unspecified
  421 Asphyxiation
  422 Strangulation
  423 Drowning
  424 Hernia
  425 Embolism, postoperative
  426 Fat embolism
  427 Air embolism; accumulation of air (in cavity or tissue)
  428 Concussion; dilatation
  429 Foreign body embolism

43 DISEASES DUE TO CONSTANT OR INTERMITTENT TRAUMA [2]

  430 Generally or unspecified
  431 From posture or pressure
  432 From occupation
  433 From clothing
  434 From abnormal position of anatomic structures
  435 From distortion of adjacent structures
  436 From fractured bone
  437 From opposed surfaces; from abscess or granuloma
  438 From foreign body
    4380 Aluminum (bauxite)
    4381 Asbestos
    4382 Coal dust
    4383 Cotton dust
    4384 Diatomaceous earth
    4385 Fine stone dust
    4386 Silica dust
    4387 Sugar cane dust
    4388 Tobacco dust
    4389 Welding fumes (iron dust)
  439 From contiguous neoplasm
  43x From overstrain; from contiguous hematoma

44 DISEASES DUE TO HEAT, INCLUDING FRICTION, AND COLD

  440 Generally or unspecified
  441 Burn from heat directly
  442 Burn from friction
  443 Dissolution: incineration
  444 Scald
  445 Effects of radiant heat; heatstroke (prostration)
  446 Chillblain
  447 Exhaustion from cold
  448 Freezing; frostbite
  449 Indirect effect of heat
  44x Indirect effect of cold

45 DISEASES DUE TO LIGHT

  450 Generally or unspecified
  451 Immediate effects of ultraviolet ray

[1] Anatomically.
[2] Excluding trauma from accretion or stone. (Category 6).

452 Late effects of ultraviolet ray
453 Sunstroke

46 DISEASES DUE TO ELECTRICITY

460 Generally or unspecified
461 Burn
462 Electric shock
463 Lightning stroke
464 Incineration
465 Remote effect
466 Late effect
467 Effect of ultraviolet rays from electric light

47 DISEASES DUE TO X-RAYS, RADIUM, OR OTHER RADIOACTIVE SUBSTANCE

470 Generally or unspecified
 4701 Remote effect of radioactive substance unspecified
 4702 Late effect of radioactive substance unspecified
471 Roentgen ray (x-ray)
 4711 Remote effect of roentgen ray (x-ray)
 4712 Late effect of roentgen ray (x-ray)
472 Radium or radium compound
 4721 Remote effect of radium
 4722 Late effect of radium
473 Plutonium or plutonium compound
 4731 Remote effect of plutonium
 4732 Late effect of plutonium
474 Thorium or thorium compound
 4741 Remote effect of thorium
 4742 Late effect of thorium
475 Uranium or uranium compound
 4751 Remote effect of uranium
 4752 Late effect of uranium

48 DISEASES DUE TO ABNORMAL PRESSURE

480 Atmospheric pressure, generally
481 Effect of high altitude
482 Blast injury (air and submersion)
485 Loss of cerebrospinal fluid

49 DISEASES DUE TO ANOTHER PHYSICAL AGENT

490 Generally or unspecified
491 Injury by powdered glass
492 Suffocation by gas or vapor (nonpoisonous)
493 Suffocation by smoke
494 Other injury produced by gas, vapor or smoke (nonpoisonous)
495 Irritation by filth
496 Presence of foreign body; aspiration of foreign body
 4961 Aspiration of oil
 4962 Tattoo (ink, gunpowder, etc.)
497 Presence of coal dust
 4971 Presence of asbestos dust
498 Presence of stone dust

499   Immersion
49x   Submersion

4x   STRUCTURAL AND FUNCTIONAL CHANGE DUE TO TRAUMA

4x0   (400.0)   Generally unspecified; inflammation
4x1   (400.1)   Loss of substance; gangrene; necrosis
4x2   (400.2)   Abscess; infection
4x3   (400.3)   Fistula; sinus; perforation
4x4   (400.4)   Adhesion; contracture; distortion; constriction; compression; obstruction; ankylosis; embolism
4x5   (400.5)   Rupture; fragmentation
4x6   (400.6)   Proliferation; exostosis; accumulation; hypertrophy; dilatation; fibrosis
4x7   (400.7)   Circulatory disturbance (hemorrhage, hematoma); failure of healing
4x8   (400.8)   Effusion; accumulation of secretion; cyst formation
4x9   (400.9)   Herniation; degeneration; atrophy; ulceration
4xx   (400.x)   Impairment, disturbance or loss of function

Note: The code in parentheses is simply an amplification of the code which precedes it. In both cases the final digit is sometimes used arbitrarily.

CATEGORY 50

50-54 *Diseases secondary to circulatory disturbance*

50   DISEASES DUE TO CHANGE IN PLASMA OR LYMPH

500   Due to disturbance of blood supply
501   Due to obstruction of lymph circulation
502   Due to extravasation of lymph
505   Due to chemical change in plasma

51   DISEASES DUE TO DIMINISHED BLOOD SUPPLY

510   Generally or unspecified
511   Due to thrombosis of nutritional artery
512   Due to embolism of the nutritional artery
513   Due to spasm of the nutritional artery
514   Due to section, ligation, compression, or constriction of the nutritional artery
515   Due to arteritis or endarteritis
516   Due to sclerosis of the nutritional artery
517   Due to sclerosis of the intrinsic arterioles
518   Due to reflex or other disturbance of vasomotor control
519   Due to disorder of heart beat
51x   Due to arteritis or phlebitis

52   DISEASES DUE TO INCREASED BLOOD SUPPLY OR BLOOD CONTENT

520   Generally or unspecified
521   Due to dilatation of arteriolar-capillary bed
522   Due to venous obstruction or stasis
523   Due to increased capillary bed

53 DISEASES DUE TO ABNORMAL PRESSURE OF THE BLOOD

530 Generally or unspecified
531 Due to aneurysm
532 Due to extravasated blood
533 Due to increased pressure
534 Due to decreased pressure
535 Due to increased pressure in lesser circulation
536 Due to increased pressure in portal circulation; congestive splenomegaly

54 DISEASES DUE TO CYTOLOGIC CHANGE IN THE BLOOD

540 Generally or unspecified
541 Due to increase in number of erythrocytes
542 Due to decrease in number of erythrocytes
543 Due to increase in number of granulocytic cells
544 Due to decrease in number of granulocytic cells
545 Due to increase in number of lymphocytes
546 Due to decrease in number of lymphocytes
547 Due to increase in number of thrombocytes (platelets)
548 Due to decrease in number of thrombocytes (platelets)
549 Due to disturbance of clotting mechanism

5x STRUCTURAL AND FUNCTIONAL CHANGES DUE TO DISTURBANCE OF CIRCULATION, INNERVATION, OR PSYCHIC CONTROL

5x0 (500.0) Generally or unspecified; inflammation
5x1 (500.1) Gangrene; necrosis; myelopthisis
5x2 (500.2) Passive congestion; abscess
5x3 (500.3) Fistula; sinus
5x4 (500.4) Adhesion; embolism; obstruction; distortion of cell structure
5x5 (500.5) Rupture; dislocation; disintegration; hemolysis
5x6 (500.6) Hypertrophy; hyperplasia; dilatation; fibrosis
5x7 (500.7) Infarction; hemorrhage (internal or external) blood loss; thrombosis
5x8 (500.8) Effusion; edema; accumulation of secretion; cyst formation
5x9 (500.9) Atrophy; hypoplasia; degeneration; ulceration
5xx (500.x) Disturbance of function; impairment

Note: The code in parentheses is simply an amplification of the code which precedes it. In both cases the final digit is sometimes used arbitrarily.

CATEGORY 55

55-59 *Diseases secondary to disturbance of innervation or of psychic control*

55 DISEASES DUE TO DISTURBANCE OF PSYCHIC CONTROL

550 Generally or unspecified
551 With sensory manifestations
552 With anesthesia
553 With hyperesthesia
554 With paresthesia

555 With motor manifestations
556 With motor excitation
557 With sympathetic manifestations
558 With sympathetic preponderance
559 With parasympathetic preponderance
55x Due to nervous shock

56 DISEASES DUE TO DISTURBANCE OF EFFERENT INNERVATION
560 With flaccid paralysis or paresis; with incoordination
561 With spastic paralysis or paresis, spasm or contracture
562 With undue fatigability
563 Due to bacterial toxin
    5631 Diphtheria toxin
    5632 Tetanus toxin
    5633 Botulinum
564 Due to ancient poliomyelitis or encephalitis
565 Due to trophic disturbance
566 Due to trophic disturbance caused by syphilis
567 Due to central lesion
568 With paralysis due to exogenous intoxication
569 With paralysis due to pressure on or lesion of nerve

57 DISEASES DUE TO DISTURBANCE OF SENSORY INNERVATION
570 Generally or unspecified
571 With diminution or loss of sensation
572 With exaltation of sensation or pain
573 With other abnormality of sensation
576 Due to disturbance of vestibular sense

58 DISEASES DUE TO DISTURBANCE OF SYMPATHETIC OR PARASYMPATHETIC INNERVATION
580 Generally or unspecified
581 With diminution or loss of sympathetic control
582 With excitation of sympathetic control
583 With diminution or loss of parasympathetic control
584 With excitation of parasympathetic control
585 With fluctuation of parasympathetic control
586 With sympathetic preponderance
587 With parasympathetic preponderance
588 Due to central lesion
589 Due to trauma of nervous system

59 DISEASES DUE TO REFLEX DISTURBANCE
590 Generally or unspecified
591 From trauma
592 From trauma to sympathetic nervous system
593 With sensory manifestations
594 With motor manifestations compensated
595 With excitation of motor manifestations compensated
596 With depression of motor manifestations compensated
597 With motor excitation uncompensated
598 With periodic motor manifestations
599 With dilatation

CATEGORY 6

6 *Diseases due to or consisting of static mechanical abnormality (e.g., obstruction, calculus, displacement, or gross change in form) due to unknown cause*

61 MECHANICAL OBSTRUCTION OR ABNORMALITY
  - 610 Generally or unspecified; remote obstruction
  - 611 Foreign body
  - 612 Hair ball
  - 613 Extravasated urine
  - 614 Products of conception (retained)
  - 615 Calculus; concretion; calcareous fragment
  - 616 Impaction of contents
  - 617 Indigestible food
  - 618 Embolus
  - 619 Thrombus
  - 61x Extravasated blood

62 OTHER MECHANICAL ABNORMALITY
  - 621 Fat embolism
  - 622 Air embolism

63 DISPLACEMENT AND DISTORTION (OF UNKNOWN OR UNCERTAIN CAUSE)
  - 630 Generally or unspecified
  - 631 Displacement caudally; prolapse; ptosis
  - 632 Displacement cephalically
  - 633 Displacement to right
  - 634 Displacement to left
  - 635 Displacement ventrally
  - 636 Displacement dorsally
  - 637 Torsion; rotation
  - 638 Distortion; inversion
  - 639 Extrusion; hernia

64 GROSS DEFORMITY (OF UNKNOWN OR UNCERTAIN CAUSE)
  - 640 Deformity
  - 641 Dilatation
  - 642 Diverticulation
  - 643 Angulation
  - 644 Valvulation
  - 645 Partial protrusion
  - 646 Constriction
  - 647 Atresia; conglutination
  - 648 Collapse; shrinking
  - 649 Elongation
  - 64x Perforation

65 ABNORMAL DIMENSION
  - 650 Abnormal relative dimension
  - 651 Relative shortening
  - 652 Relative lengthening
  - 653 Abnormal curvature

654 Aspherical curvature
655 Shortening with aspherical curvature
656 Lengthening with aspherical curvature
657 Irregular curvature
658 Normal dimensions

66, 67, 68, and 69 RESERVED FOR PRESENTATION OF FETUS (*see page 382*)

6x STRUCTURAL AND FUNCTIONAL CHANGES DUE TO STATIC MECHANICAL ABNORMALITY

6x0 (600.0) Generally or unspecified; inflammation
6x1 (600.1) Loss of substance; gangrene
6x2 (600.2) Infection; abscess
6x3 (600.3) Perforation; fistula; sinus
6x4 (600.4) Constriction; adhesion
6x5 (600.5) Rupture
6x6 (600.6) Distention; dilatation; fibrosis
6x7 (600.7) Hemorrhage
6x8 (600.8) Accumulation of secretion; cyst formation
6x9 (600.9) Transplantation of tissue from other region or organ; atrophy; ulceration
6xx (600.x) Disturbance of function

Note: The code in parentheses is simply an amplification of the code which precedes it. In both cases the final digit is sometimes used arbitrarily.

CATEGORY 7

7 *Diseases due to disorder of metabolism, growth, or nutrition*

70 DISTURBANCE OF GENERAL NUTRITION

701 Deprivation of food
    7011 Deprivation of protein
702 Lack of intrinsic factor; pernicious anemia
703 Deprivation of anti-pernicious-anemia factors
704 Deprivation of oxygen, generally (anoxemia)
705 Deprivation of oxygen by asphyxiation
706 Deprivation of oxygen by strangulation
707 Deprivation of oxygen by drowning
708 Deprivation of water
709 Unsuitable food
70x Excess of food
70x2 Excess of water

71 DISTURBANCE OF GENERAL METABOLISM OR ABSORPTION OF FOOD

711 Disturbance of assimilation of food
712 Overexertion; exhaustion
713 Disuse
714 Disturbance of absorption of carbohydrate
715 Disturbance of absorption of protein
716 Disturbance of absorption of fat
717 Disturbance of absorption of calcium
718 Disturbance of absorption of vitamin

72 DISTURBANCE OF ACID-BASE EQUILIBRIUM

  720 Generally or unspecified
  721 Acidosis
  722 Alkalosis

73 DISTURBANCE OF METABOLISM OF SPECIFIC ELECTROLYTES

  730 Generally or unspecified
  731 General disturbance of calcium metabolism
  734 General disturbance of phosphate metabolism
  735 General disturbance of chloride metabolism
  736 General disturbance of iron metabolism
  737 General disturbance of sodium metabolism
  738 General disturbance of potassium metabolism
  739 Deficiency of iodine

74 DISTURBANCE OF NITROGEN METABOLISM

  740 Generally or unspecified
  741 Associated with purine bodies
  742 Associated with homogentisic acid
  743 Associated with cystine
  744 Associated with disturbance of pigment metabolism, generally
  745 Associated with melanin metabolism
  746 Associated with dioxyphenylalanine (propigment)
  747 Associated with lack of pigment oxidase
  748 Associated with hemoglobin metabolism
  749 Associated with formation of porphyrins

75 DISTURBANCE OF CARBOHYDRATE, FAT, OR WATER METABOLISM

  750 General disturbance of carbohydrate (dextrose) metabolism
  751 Tissue excess of carbohydrate (localized)
  752 Disturbance of metabolism of other carbohydrates
  753 Disturbance of metabolism of fats
  754 Tissue excess of fat (localized)
  755 Disturbance of metabolism of lipoids
  756 Disturbance of metabolism of lipoids with deposition of kerasin
  757 Disturbance of metabolism of cholesterol
  758 Disturbance of metabolism of phosphatides
  759 Disturbance of metabolism of water
  75x Disturbance of metabolism of carotene

76 DEPRIVATION OF A VITAMIN

  760 Generally or in combination
  761 Vitamin A
  7611 Carotene
  7621 Vitamin B_1 (thiamine)
  7622 Riboflavin (vitamin B_2 or G)
  7623 Nicotinic acid
  7624 Vitamin B_6 (pyridoxine)
  7625 Other factors of B complex, B_{12}
  763 Ascorbic acid (vitamin C)
  764 Vitamin D

765   Vitamin E
766   Vitamin K
767   Deprivation of enzyme
       7671   Diaphorase
768   Presence of abnormal enzyme
769   Other vitamins

77 and 78   DISTURBANCE OF SPECIFIC ENDOCRINE ORGANS OR HORMONES

770   Generally or unspecified
771   Thyroid gland, increased or perverted function
772   Thyroid gland, decreased function
773   Parathyroid glands, increased function
774   Parathyroid glands, decreased function
775   Thymus gland
776   Pituitary gland, anterior lobe, increased or perverted function
777   Pituitary gland, anterior lobe, decreased function
778   Pituitary gland, posterior lobe, increased or perverted function
779   Pituitary gland, posterior lobe, decreased function
77x   Pituitary gland, perverted function
780   Pineal gland, perverted function
781   Adrenal cortex, increased function
782   Adrenal cortex, decreased function
783   Adrenal medulla, increased function
7831 Adrenal medulla, decreased function
784   Insular tissue, increased function
785   Insular tissue, decreased function
       7851   Parenchyma of pancreas, decreased function (lipocaic deficiency)
786   Gonads, increased function
       7861   Increase in estrogen
       7862   Increase in progesterone
787   Gonads, decreased function
       7871   Decrease in estrogen
       7872   Decrease in progesterone
788   Excessive administration of hormone
789   Hormones of placenta, perverted function; pregnancy
78x   Chromaffin system, increased function
78x1 Chromaffin system, decreased function

79   OTHER DISTURBANCE OF GROWTH OR DEVELOPMENT; INVOLUTION OR ABNORMALITY OF INVOLUTION

790   Arrest or retardation of growth
791   Arrest or retardation of development
792   Abnormal increase in growth
793   Abnormal increase in development
794   Other abnormalities of development
795   Failure of normal involution
796   Abnormal involution
797   Senile change, generally
       7971   Presenile change
798   Senile atrophy
799   Senile hyperplasia
79x   Senile dysfunction

7x STRUCTURAL OF FUNCTIONAL CHANGES SECONDARY TO DISTURBANCE OF METABOLISM, GROWTH, OR NUTRITION

7x0	(700.0)	Localized inflammatory lesion
7x1	(700.1)	Structural change due to depression of function
7x2	(700.2)	Structural change due to increase of function
7x4	(700.4)	Adhesion; distortion; obstruction; ankylosis; deformity
7x5	(700.5)	Rupture; fracture
7x6	(700.6)	Hyperplasia; hypertrophy; dilatation; fibrosis
7x7	(700.7)	Circulatory disturbance
7x8	(700.8)	Accumulation of secretion
7x9	(700.9)	Degeneration
7xx	(700.x)	Impairment, disturbance or loss of function

Note: The code in parentheses is simply an amplification of the code which precedes it. In both cases the final digit is sometimes used arbitrarily.

CATEGORY 8

8 *New growths*

80 and 81 TUMORS OF EPITHELIUM

Tumors of Glandular Epithelium
Ductal tumors
   8001 Paget's disease except bone

Tumors of Mucinous Secreting Epithelium
   8011 Pseudomucinous cystic tumor
   8012 Mucinous carcinoma
   8013 Krukenberg tumor

Papillary tumors
   8021 Serous papillary cystic tumor
   8023 Papillary or polypoid tumor, not otherwise specified

Neoplastic cysts
   8031 Intracystic papillary carcinoma (breast)
   8032 Multiple benign cystic epithelioma
   8033 Cystadenoma

Functionally active tumors
   8041 Virilizing tumor
   8042 Arrhenoblastoma
   8043 Interstitial cell tumor
   8044 Functioning islet cell tumor
   8045 Eosinophilic tumor
   8046 Functionally hyperactive parathyroid tumor
   8047 Functionally hyperactive thyroid tumor
   8051 Feminizing tumor
   8052 Thecoma (theca cell tumor)
   8053 Granulosa cell tumor

8054   Adrenal cortical rest tumor (testis)
8055   Basophilic tumor

Other specific glandular tumors
8061   Sweat gland tumor
8062   Medullary carcinoma with lymphoid stroma
8063   Hepatoma
8064   Gynandroblastoma
8065   Hürthle cell tumor
8066   Giant cell carcinoma
8067   Chromophobe tumor
8068   Sertoli cell tumor
8072   Bronchiolar carcinoma
8073   Cholangioma
8074   Nonfunctioning islet cell tumor
8075   Sebaceous tumor
8076G   Scirrhous carcinoma
8077   Rete cell tumor
8078G   Small cell carcinoma (thyroid)
8079G   Carcinoma with osseous metaplasia (breast)

Unspecified tumors of glandular epithelium origin
8091   Adenocarcinoma
8091A   Adenoma
8092   Endometrial carcinoma
8093   Pseudomyxoma peritonei
8096   Follicular carcinoma (thyroid)

Tumors of nonglandular epithelium
811   Transitional cell carcinoma
812   Basal cell carcinoma
813   Baso-squamous carcinoma
814A   Squamous cell papilloma
814   Epidermoid carcinoma

Tumors of melanoblast
8170   Pigmented nevus (mole)
8171   Nonpigmented nevus
8173   Melanoma
8174   Melanoblastoma
8175   Amelanotic melanoma

Unspecified tumors of epithelial origin
8191   Carcinoma, not otherwise specified
8192   Epithelioma, not otherwise specified

82 and 83   TUMORS OF HEMATOPOIETIC TISSUE

Leukemias
820   Lymphocytic leukemia
821   Monocytic leukemia
822   Granulocytic leukemia
        8221 Neutrophilic leukemia

	8222 Eosinophilic leukemia
	8223 Basophilic leukemia
826	Compound leukemia
827	Leukemia and lymphoma
	8271 Polycythemia vera
	8272 Erythroblastoma
	8273 Leukosarcoma
828	Other specific leukemias
	8281 Megakaryocytic leukemia
	8282 Plasmacytic leukemia
	8283 Stem cell leukemia
829	Leukemia, type not specified

Lymphomas and myelomas

830	Lymphosarcoma
831	Reticulum cell sarcoma
832	Hodgkin's disease
833	Plasma cell myeloma
834	Giant follicular lymphoma
836	Compound lymphomas
838A	Benign lymphoid polyp
839	Lymphoma

84 TUMORS OF NERVE TISSUE AND ASSOCIATED STRUCTURES

Tumors of ganglia

840A	Ganglioneuroma
840H	Malignant ganglioneuroma

Tumors of sympathicoblast

841F	Sympathicoblastoma
841G	Sympathicogonioma

Tumors of neuro-epithelium

842F	Neuro-epithelioma
842G	Medulloblastoma

Tumors of paraganglion

8431	Pheochromocytoma
8432	Paraganglioma

Tumors of argentaffin tissue

844	Argentaffinoma

Tumors of peripheral nerve sheaths

8451	Neurofibroma
8452	Schwannoma
8453	Neurofibromatosis
	8453B Plexiform neuroma

Tumors of meninges

846	Meningioma

Tumors of glial tissue
8471   Ganglioglioma
8472   Oligodendroma
8473   Astrocytoma
8474   Glioblastoma multiforme
8475   Glioma, not otherwise specified

Other specified tumors of nerve tissue
848   Ependymoma

Unspecified tumors of nerve tissue
849   Neuroma, not otherwise specified

85 TUMORS OF VASCULAR TISSUE

Tumors of blood vessels
850A   Hemangioma (angioma)
850B   Hemangioendothelioma
850G   Hemangiosarcoma
851   Hemangiomatosis
852   Multiple hemorrhagic hemangioma of **Kaposi**

Tumors of specialized vascular structures
8531   Hemangiopericytoma
8532   Glomangioma

Tumors of lymph vessels
854A   Lymphangioma
854B   Lymphendothelioma (lymphangio-endothelioma)
854G   Lymphangiosarcoma

86 TUMORS OF MUSCLE TISSUE

Tumors of smooth muscle
866A   Leiomyoma (fibro-myoma)
866F   Leiomyosarcoma

Tumors of striated muscle
867A   Rhabdomyoma
867F   Rhabdomyosarcoma

Other specified tumors of muscle origin
868A   Granular cell myoblastoma

Unspecified tumors of muscle
8690A   Myoma
8690F   Myosarcoma

87 TUMORS OF CONNECTIVE TISSUE

Tumors of fibrous tissue
870A   Fibroma
         8701A   Keloid
870F   Fibrosarcoma
870G   Fibroblastoma

Tumors of mucinous connective tissue
871B   Myxoma
871G   Myxosarcoma

Tumors of lipoid tissue
872A   Lipoma
872B   Fetal fat cell lipoma
872F   Liposarcoma

Tumors of cartilage
873A   Chondroblastoma
873B   Chondroma
873F   Chondrosarcoma

Giant cell tumors
874   Giant cell tumor of bone
8741   Giant cell tumor except bone (epulis)

Ewing's sarcoma
875G   Ewing's sarcoma

Tumors of osseous tissue
876A   Osteoma
876B   Osteochondromatosis
876F   Osteosarcoma (osteogenic sarcoma)
876G   Osteoblastoma

Tumors of serous and synovial surfaces
8771A   Synovialoma
8771B   Synovioma
8771F   Synovial sarcoma
8772A   Mesothelioma
8772G   Mesothelial sarcoma

Specific nonepithelial tumors
8782A   "Ganglion" of tendon sheath

Unspecified tumors of nonepithelial tissue
879   Sarcoma, not otherwise specified

88   TUMORS OF EMBRYONAL AND MIXED TISSUES

Tumors of trophoblast
880B   Hydatiform mole
880E   Chorioadenoma
880F   Choriocarcinoma

Tumors of embryonal gonadal tissue
881   Disgerminoma (seminoma)

Tumors of teratoid structures
882   Teratoma

Tumors of epithelial and mesodermal tissues
8831A   Adenofibroma
8831F   Carcinosarcoma
8832   Cystosarcoma phyllodes

8833   Hepatoblastoma
8834   Nephroblastoma
8835   Embryonal carcinoma of testis
8836   Brenner tumor

Tumors of epithelial and lymphoid tissues
8841   Thymoma
8842   Adenolymphoma

Tumors of mixed tissue, salivary gland type
8851A   Myoepithelial tumor
8852   Mixed tumor, salivary gland type

Tumors of dental structures
886A   Odontogenic tumor, benign
886E   Ameloblastoma
886F   Adamantinocarcinoma

Tumors of mesenchyme
887   Mesenchymoma
8871   Mesenchymal mixed tumor

Other specific tumors of embryonal and mixed tissues
8881A   Adenomyosis (adenomyoma)
8881F   Adenomyosarcoma
8882   Hamartoma
8883   Branchioma
8884   Mesonephroma
8886   Chordoma
8887   Craniopharyngioma

Unspecified tumors of embryonal and mixed tissues
8891F   Embryonal sarcoma
8892   Dysontogenetic tumor
8893   Malignant embryonic rest
8894   Embryoma, not otherwise specified
8895   Mixed tumor, not otherwise specified

89   TUMORS NOT ELSEWHERE CLASSIFIED
8981   Carotid body tumor
8982   Pinealoma

8▲▲   STRUCTURAL AND FUNCTIONAL CHANGES DUE TO NEOPLASM
8▲▲.0   Neoplasm with metastasis
8▲▲.1   Neoplasm with loss of substance
8▲▲.2   Neoplasm with abscess
8▲▲.3   Neoplasm with fistula or sinus
8▲▲.4   Neoplasm with constriction or obstruction
8▲▲.5   Neoplasm with rupture or fracture
8▲▲.6   Neoplasm with inflammatory reaction or colloid formation
8▲▲.7   Neoplasm with circulatory disturbance or hemorrhage
8▲▲.8   Neoplasm with effusion, accumulation of secretion or cyst formation
8▲▲.9   Neoplasm with ulceration

MALIGNANCY CODE (BEHAVIOR)

A   Benign—no premalignant significance
B   Benign neoplasm—having premalignant significance
C   Diagnosis not completed—suspected malignancy
D   Neoplasm, malignancy not determined
E   Malignant neoplasm, noninfiltrating (including carcinoma in situ)
F   Malignant neoplasm, differentiated
G   Malignant neoplasm, undifferentiated (anaplastic)
H   Malignant neoplasm, differentiation not determined
I   Malignant neoplasm metastatic site

LEUKEMIA MALIGNANCY CODE (BEHAVIOR)
Used with 820 to 829

E   Aleukemic
F   Chronic
G   Acute
H   Not determined whether acute or chronic

LYMPHOMA MALIGNANCY CODE (BEHAVIOR)
Used with 830 to 839

A   Specified as benign
F   Single
G   Multiple
H   Multiplicity not determined

CATEGORY 9

9   *Diseases due to unknown or uncertain cause with the structural reaction (degenerative, infiltrative, inflammatory, proliferative, sclerotic or reparative) manifest; hereditary and familial diseases of this nature.*

90   GENERALLY OR UNSPECIFIED

91   DISEASES IN WHICH THE REACTION IS PRINCIPALLY DEGENERATIVE
    910   Generally or unspecified
    911   Degeneration of a primary or principal structure predominating
    912   Degeneration of a supporting structure predominating
    913   Simple ulceration
    914   With vesicle formation
    915   Necrosis
    917   Fatty degeneration

92   DISEASES IN WHICH THE REACTION IS PRINCIPALLY INFILTRATIVE OR PERMEATIVE
    920   Generally or unspecified
    921   Infiltration with fat or fatty substance
    922   Amyloid infiltration
    923   Infiltration with a calcium salt
    924   Infiltration with an iron compound
    925   Cellular infiltration (not inflammatory or neoplastic)

926   Production of connective tissue (noninflammatory)
928   Hyaline degeneration
929   Mucinous (mucoid) degeneration; colloid degeneration
92x   Mucinoid or myxomatous degeneration

93 DISEASES IN WHICH THE REACTION IS PRINCIPALLY ACUTELY INFLAM-
    MATORY
    930   Generally or unspecified
    931   Affecting a primary or parenchymatous structure predominantly
    932   Affecting a supporting structure predominantly
    933   With effusion or vesicle formation

94 DISEASES IN WHICH THE REACTION IS PRINCIPALLY PROLIFERATIVE,
    REPARATIVE, OR SCLEROTIC (CHRONIC INFLAMMATION)
    940   Generally or unspecified
    941   Affecting a specialized structure predominantly
    942   Affecting a supporting structure predominantly
    943   Simple proliferation predominantly
    944   Simple polyp formation (nonneoplastic)
    945   Granuloma (noninfectional)
    946   With effusion or vesicle formation
    947   With softening
    948   With scale formation

95 DISEASES IN WHICH A COMBINED REACTION PREDOMINATES
    950   Generally or unspecified
    951   Gross necrosis with inflammatory reaction
    952   Degeneration and proliferation
    953   Degeneration and gliosis
    954   Hyperplasia and infiltration
    955   Degeneration, fibrosis and/or gliosis
    956   Proliferation and degeneration
    957   Chronic inflammation followed by degeneration
    958   Metaplasia and proliferation
    959   Transposition or implantation and proliferation

96
97 } DISEASES OF SKIN OF UNKNOWN CAUSE, NOT CLASSIFIABLE IN GENERAL
98   TERMS

99 HEREDITARY AND FAMILIAL DISEASES OF THIS NATURE
    991   Hereditary disease
    992   Hereditary degenerative disease
    993   Hereditary proliferative disease
    995   Familial disease
    996   Familial degenerative disease
    997   Familial proliferative or sclerotic disease

9x STRUCTURAL AND FUNCTIONAL CHANGES RESULTING FROM UNKNOWN
    CAUSE
    9x0   (900.0)   Generally or unspecified; inflammation
    9x1   (900.1)   Loss of substance
    9x3   (900.3)   Fistula; sinus; perforation

9x4 (900.4) Adhesion; distortion; constriction; obstruction; ankylosis

9x5 (900.5) Rupture

9x6 (900.6) Hypertrophy; dilatation; aneurysm; fibrosis; hyperplasia

9x7 (900.7) Circulatory disturbance; thrombosis; infarction; hemorrhage

9x8 (900.8) Exudation; effusion; cyst formation

9x9 (900.9) Atrophy; hypoplasia; degeneration

9xx (900.x) Disturbance of function

Note: The code in parentheses is simply an amplification of the code which precedes it. In both cases the final digit is sometimes used arbitrarily.

CATEGORY X

x *Diseases due to unknown or uncertain cause with the functional reaction alone manifest; hereditary and familial diseases of this nature*

It is impossible to define functional manifestations of different organs in specific terms. The arrangement of this category is therefore arbitrary.

x00
x10
x20
x30
x40
x50 Disturbances of function
x60
x70
x80
x90

CATEGORY Y

y *Diseases of undetermined cause*

The subdivisions and the two additional digits in the code are used largely arbitrarily. In general, —Y00 signifies a disease of undetermined cause and —10 an inflammation of undetermined nature. The significance of the code letter Y and its uses in filing records are explained in the Introduction.

NOMENCLATURE OF DISEASES

0– DISEASES OF THE PSYCHO-BIOLOGIC UNIT

INTRODUCTION

The basic division of the section of the nomenclature is into those mental disorders associated with organic brain disease and those occurring without such association with a primary disturbance of brain function. Other categorizations are secondary to the basic divisions.

This nomenclature permits the modification of any of the primary psychiatric diagnoses by qualifying phrases which are intended to describe any major alterations of the clinical picture of a diagnosed condition whenever further mental symptoms are superimposed on those of the basic disorders.

Qualifying Phrases

.x0   Unqualified
.x1   With psychotic manifestation
.x2   With neurotic manifestation
.x3   With behavioral manifestation
.x4   With mental deficiency
.x5   With mental deficiency and psychotic manifestation
.x6   With mental deficiency and neurotic manifestation
.x7   With mental deficiency and behavioral manifestation
.x8   With psychophysiologic manifestation
.x9   With mental deficiency and psychophysiologic manifestation

> The above qualifying phrases may be added to any diagnosis in the Psychobiologic Unit when needed but should be appended to any diagnosis in the Acute or Chronic Brain Disorder groups to define further or describe the clinical picture. They will not be used where redundant. In general, the phrase will be redundant when it repeats the major heading of any group of diagnosis, for example:

.x1   is redundant when used with a diagnosis listed under Psychotic Disorders
.x2   is redundant when used with Psychoneurotic Disorders
.x3   is redundant when used with Personality Disorders

> The degree may be indicated by an additional digit as, for example, "with psychotic manifestations":

.x11   mild
.x12   moderate
.x13   severe

DISORDERS CAUSED BY OR ASSOCIATED WITH IMPAIRMENT OF BRAIN TISSUE FUNCTION

Acute Brain Disorders

—I DISORDERS DUE TO OR ASSOCIATED WITH INFECTION

0000–100	Acute brain syndrome associated with intra-cranial infection. *Specify infection*	*0001*
000–100	Acute brain syndrome associated with systemic infection. *Specify infection*	*0001*

—3 DISORDERS DUE TO OR ASSOCIATED WITH INTOXICATION

000–3▲▲	Acute brain syndrome, drug or poison intoxication. *Specify drug or poison*	*0001*
000–33212	Acute brain syndrome, alcohol intoxication	*0001*
000–332121	Acute hallucinosis	*0001*
000–332122	Delirium tremens	*0001*

—4 DISORDERS DUE TO OR ASSOCIATED WITH TRAUMA

000–4▲▲	Acute brain syndrome associated with trauma. *Specify trauma*	*0001*

—50 DISORDERS DUE TO OR ASSOCIATED WITH CIRCULATORY DISTURBANCE

000–5▲▲	Acute brain syndrome associated with circulatory disturbance. (*Indicate cardiovascular disease as additional diagnosis*)	*0001*

—55 DISORDERS DUE TO OR ASSOCIATED WITH DISTURBANCE OF INNERVATION OR OF PSYCHIC CONTROL

000–550	Acute brain syndrome associated with convulsive disorder. (*Indicate manifestation by Supplementary Term*)	*0001*

—7 DISORDERS DUE TO OR ASSOCIATED WITH DISTURBANCE OF METABOLISM, GROWTH OR NUTRITION

000–7▲▲	Acute brain syndrome with metabolic disturbance. *Specify disturbance*	*0001*

—8 DISORDERS DUE TO OR ASSOCIATED WITH NEW GROWTH

000–8▲▲	Acute brain syndrome associated with intra-cranial neoplasm. *Specify neoplasm*	*0001*

000–900   Acute brain syndrome with disease of un-
               known or uncertain cause. (*Indicate*
               disease as additional diagnosis)   *0001*

000–xx0   Acute brain syndrome of unknown cause   *0001*

Chronic Brain Disorders [1]

009–0▲▲   Chronic brain syndrome associated with
               congenital cranial anomaly. *Specify*
               anomaly   *0009*
009–016   Chronic brain syndrome associated with
               congenital spastic paraplegia   *0009*
009–071   Chronic brain syndrome associated with
               mongolism   *0009*
009–052   Chronic brain syndrome due to prenatal
               maternal infectious diseases   *0009*

009–147   Chronic brain syndrome associated with
               central   nervous   system   syphilis.
               Specify type as   *0009*
0091–147   Meningoencephalitic   *0009*
0092–147   Meningovascular   *0009*
0095–147   Other central nervous system syphilis   *0009*
009–1▲▲   Chronic brain syndrome associated with
               intracranial infection. *Specify infec-*
               tion [2]   *0009*

009–300   Chronic brain syndrome associated with
               intoxication.   *0009*
009–3▲▲   Chronic brain syndrome, drug or poison
               intoxication. *Specify drug or poison*   *0009*
009–33212   Chronic brain syndrome, alcohol intoxi-
               cation. *Specify reaction* .x1, .x2,
               .x3 *when known*   *0009*

---

[1] The qualifying phrase "Mental Deficiency" .x4 (mild .x41, moderate .x42, or severe .x43) should be added at the end of the diagnosis in disorders of this group which present mental deficiency as the major symptom of the disorder. Include intelligence quotient (I. Q.) in the diagnosis.

[2] When infection is more important than the reaction or mental deficiency, specify the infection. If both infection and reaction or mental deficiency are important, two diagnoses are required.

—4 DISORDERS ASSOCIATED WITH TRAUMA

009–050	Chronic brain syndrome associated with birth trauma	*0009*
009–400	Chronic brain syndrome associated with brain trauma	*0009*
009–4▲▲	Chronic brain syndrome, brain trauma, gross force. *Specify.* (*Other than operative*)	*0009*
009–415	Chronic brain syndrome following brain operation	*0009*
009–462	Chronic brain syndrome following electrical brain trauma	*0009*
009–470	Chronic brain syndrome following irradiational brain trauma	*0009*

—50 DISORDERS ASSOCIATED WITH CIRCULATORY DISTURBANCES

009–516	Chronic brain syndrome associated with cerebral arteriosclerosis	*0009*
009–5▲▲	Chronic brain syndrome associated with circulatory disturbance other than cerebral arteriosclerosis. *Specify disturbance*	*0009*

—55 DISORDERS ASSOCIATED WITH DISTURBANCE OF INNERVATION OR OF PSYCHIC CONTROL

009–550	Chronic brain syndrome associated with convulsive disorder	*0009*

—7 DISORDERS ASSOCIATED WITH DISTURBANCE OF METABOLISM, GROWTH, OR NUTRITION

009–79x	Chronic brain syndrome associated with senile brain disease	*0009*
009–700	Chronic brain syndrome associated with other disturbance of metabolism, growth or nutrition (Includes presenile sclerosis, glandular, pellagra, familial amaurosis)	*0009*
009–746.x4	Chronic brain syndrome due to phenylketonuria with mental deficiency	*0009*

—8 DISORDERS ASSOCIATED WITH NEW GROWTH

009–8▲▲	Chronic brain syndrome associated with intracranial neoplasm. *Specify neoplasm*	*0009*

—9 DISORDERS ASSOCIATED WITH UNKNOWN OR UNCERTAIN CAUSE

009–900   Chronic brain syndrome associated with diseases of unknown or uncertain cause (Includes multiple sclerosis, Huntington's chorea, cortical cerebral atrophy localized and other diseases of a familial or hereditary nature). *Indicate disease by additional diagnosis*   *0009*

—X DISORDERS DUE TO UNKNOWN OR UNCERTAIN CAUSE WITH THE FUNCTIONAL REACTION ALONE MANIFEST

009–xx0   Chronic brain syndrome of unknown cause   *0009*

MENTAL DEFICIENCY [1]

000–x90	Mental deficiency (familial or hereditary)	*0002*
000–x91	Mild	*0002*
000–x92	Moderate	*0002*
000–x93	Severe	*0002*
000–x95	Mental deficiency, idiopathic	*0002*
000–x96	Mild	*0002*
000–x97	Moderate	*0002*
000–x98	Severe	*0002*

Psychotic Disorders

—X PSYCHOTIC DISORDERS WITHOUT CLEARLY DEFINED STRUCTURAL CHANGE

000–x10	Affective psychotic reactions	*0051*
000–x11	Manic depressive reaction, manic type	*0051*
000–x12	Manic depressive reaction, depressive type	*0051*
000–x13	Manic depressive reaction, other	*0051*
000–x14	Psychotic depressive reaction	*0051*
000–x15	Involutional psychotic reaction	*0051*
000–x20	Schizophrenic reactions (not otherwise specified)	*0052*
000–x21	Schizophrenic reaction, simple type	*0052*
000–x22	Schizophrenic reaction, hebephrenic type	*0052*
000–x23	Schizophrenic reaction, catatonic type	*0052*
000–x24	Schizophrenic reaction, paranoid type	*0052*
000–x25	Schizophrenic reaction, acute undifferentiated type	*0052*
000–x26	Schizophrenic reaction, chronic, undifferentiated type	*0052*
000–x27	Schizophrenic reaction, schizo-affective type	*0052*
000–x28	Schizophrenic reaction, childhood type	*0052*
000–x29	Schizophrenic reaction, residual type	*0052*
000–x2x	Schizophrenic reaction, other	*0052*
000–x30	Paranoid reactions	*0053*
000–x39	Psychotic reaction, other than above	*0050*
000–x3x	Psychotic reaction, unclassified	*0050*

[1] Include intelligence quotient (I. Q.) in the diagnosis.

Psychophysiologic Disorders

—55 DISORDERS DUE TO DISTURBANCE OF INNERVATION OR OF PSYCHIC CONTROL

000–580	Psychophysiologic reaction, generally or unclassified. (*Indicate manifestation by Supplementary Term or by additional diagnosis.*)	*0006*
001–580	Psychophysiologic skin reaction. (*Indicate manifestation by Supplementary Term*)	*0006*
002–580	Psychophysiologic musculoskeletal reaction. (*Indicate manifestation by Supplementary Term*)	*0006*
003–580	Psychophysiologic respiratory reaction. (*Indicate manifestation by Supplementary Term*)	*0006*
004–580	Psychophysiologic cardiovascular reaction. (*Indicate manifestation by Supplementary Term*)	*0006*
005–580	Psychophysiologic hemic and lymphatic reaction. (*Indicate manifestation by Supplementary Term*)	*0006*
006–580	Psychophysiologic gastrointestinal reaction. (*Indicate manifestation by Supplementary Term*)	*0006*
007–580	Psychophysiologic genito-urinary reaction. (*Indicate manifestation by Supplementary Term*)	*0006*
008–580	Psychophysiologic endocrine reaction. (*Indicate manifestation by Supplementary Term*)	*0006*
009–580	Psychophysiologic nervous system reaction. (*Indicate manifestation by Supplementary Term*)	*0006*
00x–580	Psychophysiologic reaction of organs of special sense. (*Indicate manifestation by Supplementary Term*)	*0006*

Psychoneurotic Disorders

—X DISORDERS OF PSYCHOGENIC ORIGIN OR WITHOUT CLEARLY DEFINED TANGIBLE CAUSE OR STRUCTURAL CHANGE

000–x00	Psychoneurotic reactions	*0007*
000–x01	Anxiety reaction	*0007*
000–x02	Dissociative reaction	*0007*

000–x03	Conversion reaction	0007
000–x04	Phobic reaction	0007
000–x05	Obsessive compulsive reaction	0007
000–x06	Depressive reaction	0007
000–x09	Psychoneurotic reaction, other	0007

Personality Disorders

—X PERSONALITY DISORDERS WITHOUT CLEARLY DEFINED TANGIBLE CAUSE OR STRUCTURAL CHANGE

000–x40	Personality pattern disturbance (not further specified)	0008
000–x41	Inadequate personality	0008
000–x42	Schizoid personality	0008
000–x43	Cyclothymic personality	0008
000–x44	Paranoid personality	0008
000–x45	Immature personality	0008
000–x46	Emotionally unstable personality	0008
000–x465	Passive-aggressive type	0008
000–x466	Passive-dependent type	0008
000–x467	Aggressive type	0008
000–x47	Compulsive personality	0008
000–x48	Hysterical personality	0008
000–x59	Personality pattern disturbance, other	0008
000–x60	Sociopathic personality (not further specified)	0008
000–x61	Antisocial personality (unspecified)	0008
000–x615	Violent type	0008
000–x616	Stealing type	0008
000–x617	Cheating type	0008
000–x619	Other specified types	0008
000–x62	Dyssocial personality	0008
000–x63	Sexual deviation (unspecified)	0008
000–x635	Homosexual type	0008
000–x636	Voyeur-exhibitionist type	0008
000–x639	Other types	0008
000–x64	Addiction	0030
000–x641	Alcohol addiction chronic	0031
000–x642	Drug addiction	0032
000–x643	Alcohol and drug addiction, combined types	0033
000–x70	Special symptom disturbance (not further specified)	0008
000–x71	Hearing disturbance	0008
000–x72	Speech disturbance	0008
000–x73	Enuresis, persistent	0008
000–x74	Somnambulism	0008
000–x79	Other special symptom disturbance	0008

Transient Stress Disorders without Clearly Defined Structural Change in the Brain

000–x80	Transient stress reactions (not further specified)	*0008*
000–x81	Gross stress reaction	*0008*
000–x82	Adult situational reaction	*0008*
000–x83	Adjustment reaction of infancy (first year of life, or through weaning)	*0008*
000–x84	Adjustment reaction of childhood	*0008*
000–x85	Adjustment reaction of adolescence	*0008*
000–x86	Adjustment reaction of late life	*0008*
000–x87	Transient stress reaction, other	*0008*

01– DISEASES OF THE BODY
AS A WHOLE

010– BODY GENERALLY

—0 DISEASES DUE TO GENETIC AND PRENATAL INFLUENCES

013–010	Arachnodactyly	*0101*
010–032	Composite monster	*0101*
010–076	Congenital dwarfism	*0101*
010–013	Congenital hemihypertrophy	*0101*
010–025	Double monster	*0101*
010–012	Dysostosis cleidocranialis	*0101*
090–012	Hemimelus anomaly	*0101*
015–077	Laurence-Moon-Biedl syndrome	*0101*
010–070	Lipochondrodystrophy	*0101*
010–071	Mongolism	*0101*
011–076	Prematurity. To be used only in the case of infants admitted after birth. *See premature birth, page 380*	*0101*
014–02x	Situs transversus	*0101*
014–02x1	Situs inversus	*0101*

—I DISEASES DUE TO INFECTION WITH LOWER ORGANISM

010–100.2	Abscess multiple. *Specify important organs affected, by additional diagnosis*	*0110*
010–151	Amebiasis. *Specify organ affected when possible, by additional diagnosis*	*0110*
014–100.9	Amyloid degeneration, due to infection. *Specify organism (page 57) when known*	*0110*
014–123.9	Amyloid degeneration, due to tuberculosis	*0110*
012–118	Anthrax infection, generalized	*0110*
012–100	Bacteremia. *Specify organism (page 57) when known*	*0110*
010–136	Bartonellosis (oroya fever, verruga peruana)	*0110*
010–120	Botulism	*0110*
010–117▲	Brucellosis (undulant fever). *Specify type (page 57) when known*	*0117*
018–1▲▲	Carrier state. *Specify organism (page 57)*	*0110*
010–1763	Chickenpox	*0110*
010–129	Cholera	*0110*
012–158	Coccidiosis, generalized	*0110*

114

010–186	Colorado tick fever	*0110*
012–187	Cytomegalic inclusion disease, generalized	*0110*
010–162	Dengue	*0110*
016–195	Endothelioangiitis, diffuse	*0110*
010–134	Epidemic arthritic erythema (Haverhill fever)	*0110*
010–190	Epidemic diarrhea of the newborn, organism unknown	*0110*
010–160	Epidemic vomiting of childhood	*0110*
010–1605	Erythema infectiosum (fifth disease)	*0110*
010–192	Exanthema subitum	*0110*
010–113	Food poisoning due to Salmonella	*0110*
010–126	Glanders	*0110*
010–193	Hemoglobinuric fever (nonmalarial)	*0110*
013–166	Herpes simplex, systemic	*0110*
010–168	Influenza	*0118*
019–100	Inoculation, *Specify. Code is taken from Category I so that organism directly or remotely responsible may be indicated*	*0111*
0191–100	Triple	*0111*
0192–100	Before traveling	*0111*
0193–100	During pregnancy	*0111*
0194–100	Mass	*0111*
019–125	Antidiphtheria	*0111*
019–171	Poliomyelitis	*0111*
019–119	Antitetanus	*0111*
019–169	Measles	*0111*
019–108	Pertussis	*0111*
010–142	Jaundice, spirochetal	*0110*
010–152	Kala-azar	*0110*
010–166.0	Kaposi's varicelliform eruption	*0110*
010–124	Leprosy	*0110*
010–1302	Lymphocytosis, infectious	*0110*
010–157▲	Malaria. *Specify type (page 57)*	*0110*
010–169	Measles	*0116*
010–127	Melioidosis	*0110*
012–104	Meningococcemia	*0110*
010–16x	Miliary fever	*0110*
010–1301	Mononucleosis, infectious	*0113*
010–170	Mumps (epidemic parotitis)	*0110*
013–160	Myalgic encephalomyelitis benign	*0110*
010–172	Pappataci fever	*0110*
010–114▲	Paratyphoid (*specify*)	*0110*
010–109	Pasteurella pseudotuberculosis infection	*0110*
010–108	Pertussis (whooping cough) systemic	*0110*
010–106	Plague	*0110*

010–1686	Pneumoencephalitis, avian	*0110*
010–197	Pretibial fever	*0110*
010–1603	Pseudorabies	*0110*
010–173	Psittacosis (ornithosis)	*0110*
010–1832	Q fever	*0110*
010–174	Rabies	*0110*
010–1341	Rat bite fever	*0110*
013–100.0	Reiter's disease (urethritis, conjunctivitis, arthritis)	*0110*
010–1411	Relapsing fever, louse-borne	*0110*
010–1412	Relapsing fever, tick-borne	*0110*
010–1814	Rickettsialpox	*0110*
010–1811	Rocky Mountain spotted fever	*0110*
010–165	Rubella	*0110*
010–1x0	Sarcoidosis, generalized. *See also Regional Diseases, page 122 and under Diseases of the Skin, page 131*	*0110*
010–102	Scarlet fever; scarlatina	*0112*
013–190	Septicemia. *Specify organism (page 57) when known*	*0119*
014–190	Septicemia, puerperal	*5750*
010–1761	Smallpox	*0110*
012–147	Syphilis, generalized	*0114*
014–147	Syphilis, tertiary multiple	*0114*
010–119	Tetanus	*0110*
010–1577	Toxoplasma infection, generalized	*0110*
010–1833	Trench fever	*0110*
010–146	Treponematosis; yaws (Frambesia tropica)	*0110*
010–153	Trypanosomiasis	*0110*
010–1531	Trypanosomiasis, African	*0110*
010–1532	Trypanosomiasis, American	*0110*
010–183	Tsutsugamushi fever	*0110*
012–123	Tuberculosis, miliary, acute	*0110*
010–107	Tularemia	*0110*
010–115	Typhoid	*0110*
018–115	Typhoid carrier state	*0110*
010–184	Typhus	*0110*
010–1762	Vaccinia	*0110*
010–19y	Virus infection of undetermined type	*0110*
010–178	Yellow fever	*0110*

—2 DISEASES DUE TO HIGHER PLANT OR ANIMAL PARASITE

012–219	Coccidioidomycosis, generalized	*0120*
010–220	Histoplasmosis, generalized	*0121*
012–2▲▲	Mycosis, generalized. *Specify parasite (page 63) when known, as*	*0120*
012–201	Nocardiosis, generalized	*0120*

—3 DISEASES DUE TO INTOXICATION

014–393▲	Anaphylactic reaction, generalized. *Specify*	*0130*
010–390	Anaphylactic shock	*0130*
010–3843	Favism	*0131*
010–395	Food allergy	*0130*
011–300	Infusion reaction	*0130*
010–3990	Isoimmunization due to ABO factor incompatibility	*0130*
010–399	Isoimmunization due to Rh factor incompatibility	*0130*
010–3141	Oxygen toxicity	*0131*
010–3▲▲.x	Physiological (functional) reaction following poisoning by . . . . *Specify poison*	*0131*
010–382	Poisoning by glandular extract. *Specify extract (page 67)*	*0131*
010–38271	Insulin shock	*0131*
010–38211	Thyroxin shock	*0131*
010–3▲▲	Poisoning, general. *Specify poison (page 67)*	*0131*
010–33▲	Anesthetic gas. *Specify anesthetic (page 67) if possible*	*0131*
010–33613	Aniline	*0131*
010–34814	Acetanilid	*0131*
010–321	Arsenic (acute)	*0131*
011–321	Arsenic (chronic)	*0131*
010–34851	Barbital	*0137*
010–3196	Bromine (acute bromism)	*0131*
011–3196	Bromine (chronic bromism)	*0131*
010–3151	Carbon monoxide	*0135*
010–33152	Chloroform (acute). *For delayed chloroform poisoning see under liver (page 287)*	*0131*
010–34129	Cocaine	*0131*
010–315▲	Cyanide	*0131*
010–33231	Ether	*0131*
010–33212	Ethyl alcohol (acute)	*0131*
011–33212	Ethyl alcohol (chronic)	*0131*
010–33156	Ethylene	*0131*
010–33111	Illuminating gas	*0131*
010–3238	Lead	*0131*
010–3243	Mercury	*0131*
010–33211	Methyl alcohol	*0131*
010–3483	Opium (including morphine, codeine and heroin)	*0131*
010–33221	Phenol (carbolic acid)	*0131*

010–34648	Physostigmine	*0131*
010–34651	Scopolamine	*0131*
010–3253	Silver	*0131*
010–36731	Strychnine	*0131*
010–3432	Sulfanilamide	*0131*
010–3257	Thallium	*0131*
010–3485x	Tribromethanol (avertin) with amylene hydrate	*0131*
010–369	War gases	*0131*
010–391	Protein sickness	*0130*
010–38x	Reaction following transfusion of blooɑ	*0131*
010–3▲▲.0	Sensitivity to poison. *Specify poison* (*page 67*)	*0130*
014–390	Serum reaction, accelerated	*0130*
010–3931	Serum sickness	*0130*
010–388	Toxemia of pregnancy	*5630*
015–388	Eclampsia	*5630*
013–388	Pernicious vomiting (hyperemesis gravidarum)	*5630*
014–388	Preeclampsia	*5630*
010–3932	Vaccination reaction, general	*0130*
010–381▲	Venom poisoning. *Specify venom* (*page 67*)	*0139*

—4 DISEASES DUE TO TRAUMA OR PHYSICAL AGENT

014–421	Asphyxiation due to trauma	*0149*
010–482	Blast injury (air blast or submersion blast)	*0141*
010–414	Bullet wounds, multiple	*0140*
010–480	Caisson disease	*0140*
010–402	Contusion, multiple	*0140*
010–404	Crushing, general	*0141*
010–423	Drowning due to trauma	*0142*
010–460	Electric shock	*0146*
010–462	Electrocution	*0146*
010–447	Exhaustion from cold	*0144*
010–448	Freezing, general	*0144*
010–445	Heat prostration	*0145*
010–481	Hypobaropathy	*0140*
010–499	Immersion. *See also cramps* (*page 168*)	*0142*
010–443	Incineration	*0140*
010–464	Incineration by electricity	*0146*
010–400	Injuries. *Specify* (*page 83*)	*0140*
010–463	Lightning stroke	*0146*
010–47▲1	Poisoning by radioactive substance, generalized. *Specify radioactive substance*	*0147*

010–47▲	Radioactive substances, general effects.	
	Specify radioactive substance, e.g.,	*0147*
010–471	Roentgen rays (x-rays), general effects	*0147*
010–4xx	Shock due to trauma or following operation	*0140*
010–411	Stab wounds, multiple	*0140*
010–422	Strangulation	*0149*
010–49x	Submersion	*0142*
010–433	Suffocation from clothing	*0149*
010–492	Suffocation by nonpoisonous gases or vapors	*0149*
010–493	Suffocation by smoke	*0149*
010–453	Sunstroke	*0145*

—55 DISEASES DUE TO DISTURBANCE OF INNERVATION OR OF PSYCHIC CONTROL

| 010–576 | Motion sickness; air, car, sea | *0155* |

—6 DISEASES DUE TO OR CONSISTING OF STATIC MECHANICAL ABNORMALITY

| 010–640 | Abnormal posture | *0160* |

—7 DISEASES DUE TO OR ASSOCIATED WITH DISORDER OF METABOLISM, GROWTH, OR NUTRITION

Record primary diagnosis when possible

DISORDERS OF GENERAL NUTRITION AND METABOLISM

010–707	Anoxia due to drowning	*0170*
010–705	Asphyxiation due to cause other than trauma	*0170*
010–7011	Deprivation of protein (Kwashiorkor) (familial)	*0170*
010–708	Deprivation of water	*0170*
017–735	Edema due to excessive administration of sodium chloride	*0170*
010–712	Exhaustion	*0170*
011–709	Feeding, improper, of child under 2 years	*0171*
012–709	Feeding, improper, of person over 2 years	*0171*
010–718	Hypervitaminosis	*0170*
013–711	Malnutrition in child under 2 years	*0171*
014–711	Malnutrition in person over 2 years	*0171*
010–711	Marasmus	*0170*
010–70x	Obesity due to excess of food	*0175*
010–70y	Obesity of undetermined cause	*0175*
010–701	Starvation; inanition	*0171*
010–701.8	Inanition with edema	*0171*

010–717.x	Tetany due to deficient absorption of calcium	*0170*

DISORDERS OF ACID-BASE EQUILIBRIUM

010–721	Acidosis due to cause other than diabetes	*0170*
010–722	Alkalosis	*0170*
010–722.x	Tetany due to alkalosis	*0170*

DISORDERS OF METABOLISM OF ELECTROLYTES

012–731	Calcinosis	*0170*
010–731	Tetany of nephritis	*0170*
010–73▲	Tetany of newborn. *Specify*	*0170*
010–736	Transfusion siderosis	*0170*

DISORDERS OF NITROGEN METABOLISM

010–743	Cystinosis	*0170*
010–741	Gout	*0170*
010–742	Ochronosis	*0170*
010–740	Oxalosis (inborn error of oxalate metabolism)	*0170*
010–746	Phenylketonuria	*0170*
010–749	Porphyria, acquired, due to unknown cause. *See also under blood, page 237*	*0170*

DISORDERS OF CARBOHYDRATE, FAT, AND WATER METABOLISM

010–754	Adiposis dolorosa	*0170*
010–75x	Carotenemia	*0170*
013–755	Eosinophilic granuloma of skin and bone	*0170*
010–7551	Familial hyperlipemia	*0170*
013–752	Galactosemia, idiopathic	*0170*
010–751	Glycogenosis; Von Gierke's disease	*0170*
010–755	Histiocytosis X	*0170*
010–757	Hands-Schuller-Christian disease	*0170*
010–759	Letterer-Siwe's disease	*0170*
010–753	Obesity, constitutional	*0175*
010–752	Pentosuria. *See page 307 for other urinary abnormalities*	*0170*
010–70x2	Water intoxication	*0170*

DISEASES DUE TO DEPRIVATION OF VITAMINS

010–7621	Beriberi	*0176*
010–761	Deficiency of vitamin A	*0176*
010–766	Deficiency of vitamin K	*0176*
010–760	Hypovitaminosis, multiple or undefined	*0176*
010–7623	Pellagra	*0176*

010–7622	Riboflavin deficiency (cheilosis)	*0176*
010–764	Rickets	*0176*
010–764.x	Tetany associated with rickets	*0176*
010–763	Scurvy; Avitaminosis due to deprivation of vitamin C.	*0176*
010–76▲	Vitamin deficiency. *Specify. See page 67*	*0176*

DISORDERS OF DEVELOPMENT

| 014–797 | Progeria | *0170* |
| 010–797 | Senility | *0170* |

—8 NEW GROWTHS

| 012–8▲▲▲ | Carcinomatosis. *Specify neoplasm and behavior (page 93 only codes 80 and 81)* | *0180* |
| 012–8▲▲▲ | Generalized neoplastic disease. *Specify neoplasm and behavior (page 93 except codes 80 and 81)* | *0180* |

—9 DISEASES DUE TO UNKNOWN OR UNCERTAIN CAUSE WITH THE STRUCTURAL REACTION MANIFEST

011–940	Acrodermatitis entropathia	*0190*
014–922	Amyloidosis, generalized, due to unknown cause	*0192*
013–955	Lupus erythematosus disseminatus	*0195*
013–997	Pachydermoperiostosis	*0190*
013–930	Periodic disease, familial	*0190*
010–932	Rheumatic fever	*0193*
010–971	Sclerosis, systemic, progressive (scleroderma)	*0190*

—X DISEASES DUE TO UNKNOWN OR UNCERTAIN CAUSE WITH THE FUNCTIONAL REACTION ALONE MANIFEST

| 010–x30 | Lymphatism | *0190* |

—Y DISEASES DUE TO CAUSES NOT DETERMINABLE IN THE PARTICULAR CASE

Y signifies an incomplete diagnosis. It is to be replaced whenever possible by a code digit signifying the specific diagnosis

01x–y00	Collagen disease	*0910*
y00–y10	Fever of undetermined origin	*0910*
y00–y00	Undiagnosed disease (diagnosis deferred). *Change as many of first three digits as possible to indicate site.*	*0910*

REGIONAL AND GENERAL DISEASES

(DISEASES NOT ASSOCIATED WITH A SINGLE ANATOMIC SYSTEM)

Indicate region or organ by inserting first three digits. See Topographic Classification, *pages 3 to 52. See also under organ affected.*

—0 DISEASES DUE TO GENETIC AND PRENATAL INFLUENCES

▲▲▲–011	Absence, congenital, of . . .	*0▲01*
▲▲▲–025 ,	Adhesions, congenital, of . . .	*0▲01*
▲▲▲–0▲▲	Anomaly, congenital. *Specify site and anomaly*	*0▲01*
▲▲▲–0y0	Anomaly, congenital, undiagnosed, of . . .	*0▲01*
▲▲▲–050	Birth injury of . . .	*0▲01*
▲▲▲–050.0	Birth injury, infected, of . . .	*0▲01*
▲▲▲–050.7	Hematoma due to birth injury	*0▲01*
039–064	Bronchogenic cyst of mediastinum	*0301*
▲▲▲–039	Constriction of . . . by anomalous bands	*0▲01*
021–01x	Craniosynostosis, congenital	*0201*
0211–01x	Acrocephalia (closure of coronal suture)	*0201*
0212–01x	Oxycephalia (closure of coronal and lamboid sutures)	*0201*
0213–01x	Scaphocephalia (closure of sagittal suture)	*0201*
096–034	Division abnormal of foot; lobster claw foot	*0901*
085–034	Division abnormal of hand; lobster claw hand	*0801*
▲▲▲–013	Elephantiasis, congenital, of . . .	*0▲01*
083–013	Arm and hand	*0801*
027–019	Facial clefts, congenital	*0201*
027–076	Facial dystrophy, congenital	*0201*
027–022	Scaphoid face (dishface; bird face)	*0201*
0▲▲–03x	Failure of segmentation of parts	*0▲01*
086–03x	Fingers (syndactyly)	*0801*
097–03x	Toes	*0901*
099–03x	Fingers and toes	*0901*
0▲▲–075	Hypertrophy, congenital	*0▲01*
096–075	Foot	*0901*
097–075	Toes	*0901*
▲▲▲–014	Hyperplasia, congenital. *Specify region or organ*	*0▲01*
090–016	Leg, shortening of, congenital	*0901*
0582–029	Pilonidal sinus (or cyst)	*0501*
0▲▲–076	Rudimentary part; hypoplasia of part, congenital	*0▲01*
080–076	Arm	*0801*

0▲▲–031	Supernumerary parts	*0▲01*
086–031	Fingers	*0801*
0861–031	Thumb	*0801*
097–031	Toes	*0801*
097–022	Toes, overlapping, congenital	*0901*
0975–022	Overlapping fifth toe, congenital (with clubfoot)	*0901*

—I DISEASES DUE TO INFECTION WITH LOWER ORGANISM

▲▲▲–100.2	Abscess, of . . . . *Specify organism (page 57) when known*	*0▲12*
	Palmar abscess. *See under abscess of fascia, page 173*	
0261–100.2	Subgaleal abscess	*0212*
▲▲▲–100.3	Fistula of . . . due to infection. *Specify organism (page 57) when known*	*0▲10*
▲▲▲–100.1	Gangrene of . . . due to infection. *Specify organism (page 57) when known*	*0▲11*
▲▲▲–103	Gonococcus infection . . . . *Specify site*	*0▲10*
▲▲▲–100.6	Granuloma of . . . due to infection. *Specify organism (page 57) when known*	*0▲10*
044–100.6	Granuloma, umbilical	*0410*
▲▲▲–147.6	Gumma of . . .	*0▲10*
0▲▲–100	Infection of . . . ; cellulitis. *Specify organism (page 57) when known*	*0▲10*
0▲▲–125	Diphtheritic infection of wound	*0▲10*
0▲▲–11x	Malignant edema	*0▲10*
0▲▲–122	Bacillus welchi or gas bacillus infection of wound	*0▲10*
039–190	Mediastinitis, nonsuppurative	*0310*
039–100	Mediastinitis, suppurative, general or localized. *Specify organism (page 57) when known*	*0310*
039–123	Mediastinum, tuberculosis of	*0310*
▲▲▲–1x0	Sarcoidosis of . . .	*0▲10*
▲▲▲–100.4	Scar of . . . due to infection. *Specify organism (page 57) when known. See also scar of skin due to infection, page 133*	*0▲10*
▲▲▲–147.4	Stricture of . . . due to syphilis. *Specify site*	*0▲10*
▲▲▲–147	Syphilis of . . . . *Specify site*	*0▲10*
▲▲▲–1471	Syphilis, congenital of . . . . *Specify site*	*0▲10*
▲▲▲–147.3	Syphilitic perforation of . . . . *Specify site*	*0▲10*
▲▲▲–154	Trichomonas infection of . . . . *Specify site*	*0▲10*

▲▲▲–1236	Tuberculoma of . . .	0▲10
▲▲▲–123	Tuberculosis of . . . . *Specify site*	0▲10
▲▲▲–1237	Tuberculosis, inactive. *Specify site*	0▲10
0▲▲–100.9	Ulcer of . . . due to infection. *Specify organism (page 57) when known*	0▲10
0▲▲–1762	Vaccinia, localized	0▲10

—2 DISEASES DUE TO HIGHER PLANT OR ANIMAL PARASITE

▲▲▲–202	Actinomycosis of . . . . *Specify region or organ*	0▲20
▲▲▲–243	Ancylostomiasis of . . . . *Specify site*	0▲20
▲▲▲–241	Ascariasis of . . . . *Specify site*	0▲20
▲▲▲–226	Aspergillosis of . . . . *Specify region or organ*	0▲20
▲▲▲–2171	Blastomycosis (N.A.) of . . . . *Specify region or organ*	0▲20
▲▲▲–2172	Blastomycosis (S.A.) of . . . . *Specify region or organ*	0▲20
▲▲▲–219	Coccicioidomycosis of . . . . *Specify region or organ*	0▲20
▲▲▲–218	Cryptococcosis of . . . . *Specify region or organ*	0▲20
▲▲▲–258	Dracunculosis of . . . . *Specify site*	0▲20
▲▲▲–257	Filariasis of . . . . *Specify site*	0▲20
▲▲▲–214	Geotrichosis of . . . . *Specify region or organ*	0▲20
▲▲▲–2161	Hemisporosis of . . . . *Specify region or organ*	0▲20
▲▲▲–220	Histoplasmosis of . . . . *Specify region or organ*	0▲20
▲▲▲–20▲	Maduromycosis (mycetoma) of . . . . *Specify region or organ and parasite*	0▲20
093–205	Mycetoma of leg	0920
096–205	Madura foot	0920
▲▲▲–209	Moniliasis of . . . . *Specify region or organ*	0▲20
▲▲▲–232	Mucormycosis of . . . . *Specify region or organ*	0▲20
▲▲▲–2▲▲	Mycotic or parasitic infection of . . . . *Specify region or organ and parasite*	0▲20
▲▲▲–24▲	Nematode disease of . . . . *Specify site and nematode (page 63)*	0▲20
▲▲▲–201	Nocardiosis of . . . . *Specify region or organ*	0▲20
▲▲▲–231	Rhinosporidiosis of . . . . *Specify region or organ*	0▲20
▲▲▲–278	Schistosomiasis. *Specify organ or tissue affected*	0▲20

▲▲▲–216	Sporotrichosis of . . . . *Specify region or organ*	0▲20
▲▲▲–26▲	Tapeworm infection of . . . . *Specify tapeworm and site*	0▲20
▲▲▲–266	Cysticerosis of . . . . *Specify region or organ*	0▲20
▲▲▲–267	Echinococcosis of . . . . *Specify region or organ*	0▲20
▲▲▲–265	Sparganosis of . . . . *Specify region or organ*	0▲20
▲▲▲–270	Trematodiasis (distomiasis). *Specify fluke and organ or tissue affected (page 63)*	0▲20
▲▲▲–2542	Trichinosis of . . . . *Specify site*	0▲20
▲▲▲–240	Visceral larva migrans of . . . . *Specify parasite if known (page 63) and organ affected*	0▲20

—3 DISEASES DUE TO INTOXICATION

0▲▲–393	Anaphylactic reaction, local	0▲30
0▲▲–382	Autodigestion of . . .	0▲30
▲▲▲–32▲	Chemical burn. *Specify poison (page 67)*	0▲30
096–3126	Lime (quicklime) burn of foot	0930
085–3116	Sulfuric acid burn of hand	0830
▲▲▲–300.4	Cicatrix of . . . due to chemical burn. *Specify poison (page 67) when known. See also Cicatrix of skin due to chemical burn, page* ▲▲	0▲30
▲▲▲–3▲▲.1	Gangrene of . . . due to poison. *Specify poison (page 67) when known*	0▲30
▲▲▲–312▲.1	Due to chemical burn	0▲30
▲▲▲–33221.1	Due to phenol (carbolic acid)	0▲30
▲▲▲–34637.1	Due to ergot	0▲30
▲▲▲–3▲▲	Poisoning of . . . . *Specify site and poison*	0▲30
▲▲▲–300.3	Sinus of . . . due to chemical burn. *Specify poison (page 67)*	0▲30

—4 DISEASES DUE TO TRAUMA OR PHYSICAL AGENT

▲▲▲–415.2	Abscess of operative wound	0▲40
▲▲▲–400.2	Abscess of . . . due to trauma	0▲40
▲▲▲–415.x	Absence of . . . following operation	0▲40
▲▲▲–400.x	Absence of . . . due to trauma	0▲40
0▲▲–405	Amputation of . . . due to accident	0▲40
0▲▲0–4xx	Amputation stump, abnormal, as:	0▲40
0860–4xx	Abnormal amputation stump of finger	0▲40

0▲▲–413▲	Bite. *Specify type (page 83)*	0▲40
▲▲▲–461	Burn of . . . electric	0▲44
0▲▲–4413	Burn of skin, third degree. *Specify region*	0▲40
0▲▲–446	Chilblain (pernio)	0▲40
034–415.4	Collapse of thorax following operation	0340
020–405	Decapitation	0240
▲▲▲–400.4	Deformity of . . . due to trauma	0▲40
▲▲▲–415.4	Deformity of . . . following operation	0▲40
▲▲▲–441.4	Deformity of . . . due to burn (from heat). *If deformity affects skin and subcutaneous tissue only, diagnose Cicatrix of skin due to burn (page 136)*	0▲40
039–435.4	Depression of mediastinum	0340
0▲▲–400.8	Edema of . . . due to trauma	0▲40
0▲▲–427	Emphysema of . . . . *See also* Subcutaneous emphysema, *page 137*	0▲40
039–427	Emphysema of mediastinum	0340
069–4x9	Evisceration	0640
▲▲▲–47▲.3	Fistula of . . . due to radioactive substance. *Specify (page 83)*	0▲40
▲▲▲–415.3	Fistula of . . . following operation	0▲40
034–415.3	Fistula of chest wall following operation	0340
▲▲▲–400.3	Fistula of . . . due to trauma	0▲40
▲▲▲–496	Foreign body of . . . due to trauma	0▲40
▲▲▲–438.6	Foreign body granuloma of . . .	0▲40
0▲▲–448	Frostbite	0▲40
▲▲▲–400.1	Gangrene of . . . due to trauma	0▲40
0▲▲–448.1	Gangrene of . . . due to cold	0▲40
0▲▲–461.1	Gangrene of . . . due to electric burn	0▲44
0▲▲–441.1	Gangrene of . . . due to heat	0▲40
▲▲▲–402.7	Hematoma of . . . due to trauma	0▲43
▲▲▲–4x7	Hematoma of . . . following operation	0▲43
▲▲▲–400.7	Hemorrhage[1] of . . . due to trauma	0▲43
▲▲▲–415.7	Hemorrhage[1] of . . . following operation	0▲43
0▲▲–415.9	Hernia of incision following operation	0▲45
	Hernia of incision, strangulated. *See under organ affected, strangulation of, due to hernia*	
0▲▲–44x	Immersion syndrome. *Specify region*	0▲40
▲▲▲–4▲▲	Injury of . . . . *Specify injury (page 83)*	0▲40
▲▲▲–47▲2	Late effect of radioactive substance. *Specify site and radioactive substance (page 83)*	0▲40

[1] For hemorrhage from a large vessel, see pages 216 to 226.

▲▲▲–4712	Late effect of roentgen ray (x-ray). *Specify site*	0▲40
▲▲▲–4722	Late effect of radium. *Specify site*	0▲40
▲▲▲–47▲.1	Necrosis of . . . due to radioactive substance. *Specify site and radioactive substance (page 83)*	0▲40
097–433	Overlapping of toes due to footwear	0▲40
▲▲▲–400.6	Ossification of . . . due to trauma	0▲40
▲▲▲–47▲	Radioactive injury. *Specify site and radioactive substance (page 83)*	0▲40
▲▲▲–471	Roentgen ray injury. (*X-ray.*) *Specify site*	0▲40
▲▲▲–472	Radium injury. *Specify site*	0▲40
▲▲▲–47▲.0	Radiation burn. *Specify site and radioactive substance (page 83)*	0▲40
▲▲▲–47▲1	Remote effect of radioactive substance (poisoning). *Specify site and radioactive substance*	0▲40
▲▲▲–4711	Remote effect of roentgen ray (x-ray). *Specify site*	0▲40
▲▲▲–4721	Remote effect of radium. *Specify site*	0▲40
▲▲▲–444	Scald of . . . *if superficial, diagnose Burn of skin (page 136)*	0▲40
▲▲▲–400.4	Scar of . . . due to trauma. *See also scar of skin due to trauma, page 137*	0▲40
▲▲▲–415.4	Scar of . . . following operation	0▲40
0▲▲–43x	Strain of . . .	0▲40
▲▲▲–415.9	Status following operation. *Specify organ*	0▲40
0▲▲–410	Wound of . . .	0▲41
034–410	Wound of chest wall	0341
042–410	Wound of abdominal wall	0441
0▲▲–410.0	Wound of . . . [1] infected	0▲41
0▲▲–415.5	Wound of . . . operative, disruption of	0▲41
0▲▲–4111	Wound of . . . penetrating	0▲41
033–4111	Wound of thorax, penetrating	0341
040–4111	Wound of abdomen, penetrating	0441
0▲▲–415	Wound of . . . postoperative	0▲41
0▲▲–415.0	Wound of . . . postoperative, infected [1]	0▲41

–50 DISEASES DUE TO CIRCULATORY DISTURBANCE
Record primary diagnosis when possible

099–518	Acrocyanosis	0950
▲▲▲–520.2	Congestion of . . . due to disturbance of circulation	0▲50

---

[1] When infection is more important than the wound, especially when the causative organism is determined, classify as infection. If both injury and infection are important, two diagnoses are required.

▲▲▲–522	Edema localized of . . . due to venous obstruction	0▲50
▲▲▲–501	Elephantiasis of . . . due to lymph-angiectasis	0▲50
▲▲▲–522.6	Elephantiasis of . . . due to venous thrombosis	0▲50
▲▲▲–502	Extravasion of lymph . . . . *Specify site*	0▲50
▲▲▲–500.1	Gangrene of . . . due to disturbance of circulation	0▲50
▲▲▲–515.1	Due to angiitis	0▲50
▲▲▲–516.1	Due to arteriosclerosis	0▲50
▲▲▲–512.1	Due to embolism	0▲50
▲▲▲–513.1	Due to Raynaud's disease	0▲50
▲▲▲–514.1	Due to section or constriction of artery	0▲50
▲▲▲–51x.1	Due to thromboangiitis obliterans	0▲50
▲▲▲–511.1	Due to thrombosis	0▲50
▲▲▲–549.7	Hematoma of . . . due to hemophilia	0▲50
▲▲▲–520.6	Hypertrophy of . . . due to increased blood supply	0▲50
▲▲▲–510	Infarction of . . . . *Specify site*	0▲50
090–522.8	Phlegmasia alba dolens; milk leg	0950
0▲▲–516.9	Ulcer of . . . due to arteriosclerosis	0▲50

—55 DISEASES DUE TO DISTURBANCE OF INNERVATION OR OF PSYCHIC CONTROL

Record primary diagnosis when possible

08x–572	Causalgia of arm	0855
09x–572	Causalgia of leg	0955
0▲▲–565.9	Ulcer of . . . due to trophic disturbance	0▲55

—6 DISEASES DUE TO OR CONSISTING OF STATIC MECHANICAL ABNORMALITY

▲▲▲–639	Herniation of . . . . *Specify site*	0▲63
069–631	Splanchnoptosis	0660
▲▲▲–641	Varix of . . . . *Specify vein or intrinsic vessels*	0▲60

—7 DISEASES DUE TO DISORDER OF METABOLISM, GROWTH, OR NUTRITION

086–704	Clubbed fingers	0870
0▲▲–785.1	Diabetic gangrene of . . .	0▲70
0▲▲–785.9	Diabetic ulcer of . . .	0▲70
▲▲▲–754	Fatty infiltration	0▲70
▲▲▲–748	Hemochromatosis	0▲70
0▲▲–753	Obesity of . . .	0▲70
069–776	Splanchnomegaly	0670
▲▲▲–755	Xanthomatosis (histiocytosis X) of . . .	0▲70

—8 NEW GROWTHS

040–8▲▲▲I	Generalized abdominal carcinomatosis. *Specify neoplasm when possible*	*0480*
▲▲▲–8532	Glomangioma. *Specify site and behavior*	*0▲80*
▲▲▲–850B	Hemangioendothelioma	*0▲80*
▲▲▲–850A	Hemangioma. *Specify site*	*0▲80*
▲▲▲–851	Hemangiomatosis	*0▲80*
▲▲▲–8531	Hemangiopericytoma. *Specify site and behavior (page 99)*	*0▲80*
▲▲▲–832	Hodgkin's [1] disease. *Specify site and behavior*	*0▲80*
▲▲▲–854A	Lymphangioma. *Specify site*	*0▲80*
▲▲▲–852	Multiple hemorrhagic hemangioma of Kaposi. *Specify site and behavior*	*0▲80*
▲▲▲–8▲▲▲I	Neoplasm metastatic. *Specify site and neoplasm (page 99)*	*0▲80*
▲▲▲–882	Teratoma of . . . . *Specify site and behavior*	*0▲80*
039–882	Mediastinal teratoma. *Specify behavior*	*0380*
058–882	Sacrococcygeal teratoma. *Specify behavior*	*0580*
▲▲▲–8▲▲▲	Unlisted tumor of region or organ. *Specify site and behavior*	*0▲80*

—9 DISEASES DUE TO UNKNOWN OR UNCERTAIN CAUSE WITH THE STRUCTURAL REACTION MANIFEST

097–9x1	Ainhum (dactylolysis spontanea)	*0990*
▲▲▲–922	Amyloidosis of . . . due to unknown cause	*0▲90*
▲▲▲–923	Calcification of . . . due to unknown cause	*0▲90*
▲▲▲–921	Cholesterosis of . . .	*0▲90*
▲▲▲–910	Chondromalacia due to unknown cause. *Specify cartilage*	*0▲90*
▲▲▲–959	Endometriosis of . . . due to unknown cause	*0▲90*
▲▲▲–943	Keratosis due to unknown cause	*0▲90*
▲▲▲–941	Leukoplakia of . . . due to unknown cause	*0▲90*
▲▲▲–92x	Mucinoid degeneration; myxomatous degeneration	*0▲90*
▲▲▲–929	Mucinous degeneration; colloid degeneration	*0▲90*
▲▲▲–944	Polyp formation, simple. *Specify site*	*0▲90*
▲▲▲–913	Ulcer of, simple. *Specify site*	*0▲90*

1 Use lymphoma behavior code (page 99).

—Y DISEASES DUE TO CAUSE NOT DETERMINABLE IN THE PARTICULAR CASE

Y signifies an incomplete diagnosis. It is to be replaced whenever possible by a code digit signifying the specific diagnosis

▲▲▲–yx8   Cyst of . . . due to undetermined cause   *00*▲▲

1– DISEASES OF THE SKIN, SUBCUTANEOUS AREOLAR TISSUE, AND SUPERFICIAL MUCOUS MEMBRANES

110– Skin
130–⎫
13x–⎭ Regions of skin
160– Hair
170– Nails
180– Subcutaneous areolar tissue

For detailed list of structures of skin, see page 6

—0 DISEASES DUE TO GENETIC AND PRENATAL INFLUENCES

112–079	Albinismus	*1101*
160–011	Alopecia congenital	*1600*
170–011	Anonychia	*1700*
13▲–012	Defect, ectodermal, congenital. *Specify* site	*1301*
114–077	Dermatomegaly (cutis laxa)	*1101*
114–092	Edema neonatorum	*1101*
13▲–023.8	Epidermoid cyst (epidermal)	*1301*
116–076	Epidermolysis bullous	*1101*
110–077	Epidermodysplasia verruciformis	*1101*
111–014	Erythroderma ichthyotic congenital	*1101*
131–014	Gyrate scalp	*1301*
160–075	Hypertrichosis, congenital	*1600*
170–092	Hypoplasia, unguinal, congenital (atrophia unguium)	*1700*
112–014	Ichthyosis	*1101*
110–097	Keratosis congenital	*1101*
149–097	Keratosis palmar and plantar	*1301*
149–093	Keratosis punctate	*1301*
112–074	Lentigo	*1101*
160–077	Monilethrix	*1600*
170–021	Nails, displacement of, congenital	*1700*
170–022	Nails, malformation of, congenital	*1700*
170–014	Pachyonychia congenital	*1700*
114–074	Pigmented spots (mongolian)	*1101*
170–031	Polyunguia	*1700*
111–070	Sclerema neonatal	*1101*
12▲▲–023	Sebaceous glands of mucocutaneous junction, aberrant. *Specify* (*page 6*)	*1200*
110–1471	Syphilis of skin, congenital	*1101*
161–034	Trichostasis spinulosa	*1600*

131

110–045	Urticaria pigmentosa (mastocytosis)	*1101*
141–03x	Webbed fingers	*1301*
148–03x	Webbed toes	*1301*
110–044	Xeroderma pigmented	*1101*
150–042	Xerosis of skin (asteatosis)	*1500*

—I DISEASES DUE TO INFECTION WITH LOWER ORGANISM

18▲–100.2	Abscess of subcutaneous areolar tissue of . . . . *Specify site and organism (page 57) when known*	*1813*
161–1x3	Acne conglobate	*1610*
141–100	Acrodermatitis persistent	*1310*
162–190	Alopecia postfebrile	*1610*
162–115.9	Due to typhoid fever	*1610*
162–147.9	Due to syphilis	*1610*
162–168.9	Due to influenza	*1610*
13▲–151	Amebiasis of skin. *Specify region*	*1310*
110–118	Anthrax	*1110*
116–147.9	Atrophy of skin, macular due to syphilis	*1110*
111–1005	Bacterid. *Specify organism (page 57) when known*	*1110*
18▲–100.3	Carbuncle. *Specify site and organism (page 57) when known*	*1812*
18▲–100	Cellulitis. *Specify site and organism (page 57) when known*	*1811*
13▲–10x	Chancroid (ulcus molle cutis). *Specify site. See also under other organs affected*	*1310*
110–105	Dermatitis infectious eczematoid	*1110*
110–130	Dermatitis vegetative	*1110*
111–190	Dermatitis seborrheic	*1110*
13▲–125	Diphtheria of skin. *Specify region*	*1310*
110–105.1	Ecthyma	*1110*
13▲–102	Erysipelas. *Specify region*	*1313*
13▲–130	Erysipeloid. *Specify region*	*1313*
11x–190	Erythema multiform	*1110*
114–1x0	Erythema nodose	*1110*
161–1x6	Folliculitis decalvans (alopecia cicatricial, pseudopelade)	*1610*
161–190	Folliculitis keloidal	*1610*
161–100.2	Folliculitis, pyodermal	*1610*
16▲–100.0	Furuncle. *Specify site and organism (page 57) when known*	*1611*
161–100.0	Furunculosis	*1611*
13▲–100.1	Gangrene of skin due to infection. *Specify region and organism (page 57) when known*	*1310*

146–137	Granuloma inguinale	*1310*
13▲–100.6	Granuloma telangiectaticum (granuloma pyogenicum). *Specify region and organism (page 57) when known*	*1310*
1▲▲–166	Herpes simple. *Specify region*	*1316*
152–100	Hidradenitis suppurativa. *Specify organism (page 57) when known*	*1500*
111–105	Impetigo. *Specify organism (page 57) if not staphylococcus*	*1111*
111–105.8	Impetigo, bullous	*1111*
13▲–105	Impetigo, localized. *Specify site*	*1111*
110–1021	Impetigo neonatal	*1111*
13▲–152	Leishmaniasis. *Specify type when known*	*1310*
13▲–124	Leprosy of skin. *Specify region*	*1310*
13▲–1x9	Lupus erythematosus of skin, localized. *Specify site*	*1310*
110–1x9	Lupus erythematosus of skin	*1110*
110–1x91	Lupus erythematosus discoid	*1110*
	Lupus erythematosus, systemic. *See page 121*	
	Lymphopathia, venereal. *See under Lymph nodes and other organs involved.*	
111–185	Molluscum	*1110*
18▲–190	Nodular nonsuppurative panniculitis. *Specify site*	*1810*
130–147.6	Nodules, juxta-articular due to syphilis	*0114*
173–100	Onychia	*1700*
176–100	Paronychia	*1700*
110–190	Pemphigus	*1110*
162–130	Perifolliculitis dissecting of scalp (dissecting cellulitis)	*1610*
122–190	Perleche. *Specify organism (page 57) when known*	*1200*
110–149	Pinta	*1110*
111–130	Pityriasis simple	*1110*
1▲▲–100.1	Pyoderma gangrenous. *Specify region*	*1111*
114–130	Rhinoscleroma	*1110*
117–1x0	Sarcoidosis of skin	*1110*
13▲–100.4	Scar of skin due to infection. *Specify site*	*1310*
161–105	Sycosis pyogenic	*1610*
110–147	Syphilis of skin, primary or secondary	*0114*
110–147.6	Syphilis of skin, tertiary, gumma	*0114*
166–133	Trichomycosis axillarix (lepothrix)	*1610*
102–123	Tuberculosis lichenoides (lichen scrofulosus)	*1110*
114–123	Tuberculosis verrucous of skin	*1110*

110–123	Tuberculosis of skin	*1110*
110–1230	Tuberculosis luposa (lupus vulgaris)	*1110*
110–1231	Tuberculosis due to inoculation	*1110*
110–1232	Tuberculosis orificialis	*1110*
110–1233	Tuberculosis miliaris disseminated	*1110*
110–1234	Tuberculosis miliaris disseminated of face	*1110*
110–1235	Tuberculid (rosacea-like)	*1110*
110–1236	Tuberculosis colliquative (scrofuloderma)	*1110*
110–1238	Tuberculosis indurative (erythema induratum)	*1110*
110–1239	Tuberculosis papulonecrotic	*1110*
13▲–179	Wart (verruca). *Specify region*	*1310*
13▲–1791	Verruca plana. *Specify region*	*1310*
13▲–1792	Verruca acuminata. *Specify region*	*1310*
	Verruga peruana (oroya fever, bartonellosis). (*See page 114*)	
1▲▲–1764	Zoster. *Specify skin region or mucous membrane*	*1310*

—2 DISEASES DUE TO HIGHER PLANT AND ANIMAL PARASITE

110–283	Acarodermatitis (grain itch)	*1120*
162–213.9	Alopecia due to favus	*1620*
13▲–210	Chromomycosis of skin. *Specify region*	*1320*
110–218	Cryptococcosis of skin	*1120*
13▲–266	Cysticercosis of skin. *Specify region* ·	*1320*
13▲–299	Dermatitis, caterpillar	*1320*
13▲–2833	Dermatitis, chigger	*1320*
16▲–2832	Dermatitis, demodex	*1620*
13▲–2▲▲	Dermatomycosis. *Specify fungus*	*1320*
112–211	Dermatophytosis. *Change 3d digit to indicate organism when known*	*1120*
112–2011	Erythrasma	*1120*
162–213	Favus capitis	*1620*
13▲–213	Favus corporis. *Specify region*	*1320*
110–240	Ground itch	*1120*
110–29▲	Infestation with bedbug, flea, chigger or other parasite. *Specify (page 63)*	*1120*
131–211	Kerion	*1320*
110–244	Larva migrans. *Specify nematode if known*	*1120*
110–292.0	Maculae ceruleae	*1120*
141–209	Moniliasis (erosio interdigitalis blastomycetica)	*1320*
13▲–209	Moniliasis of skin. *Specify region*	*1320*
114–211	Nodular granulomatous perifolliculitis	*1120*

170–2▲▲	Onychomycosis. *Specify parasite (page 63)*	*1720*
13▲–2172	Paracoccidioidomycosis (Blastomycosis S.A.). *Specify region*	*1320*
110–2911	Pediculosis capitis	*1120*
110–2912	Pediculosis corporis	*1120*
164–292	Pediculosis palpebrarum	*1620*
110–292	Pediculosis pubis	*1120*
160–204	Piedra	*1620*
110–2831	Scabies	*1120*
110–216	Sporotrichosis of skin	*1120*
165–211	Tinea of beard	*1620*
162–211	Tinea capitis. *Specify parasite if not Trichophyton (page 63)*	*1620*
130–211	Tinea corporis. *Specify parasite if not Trichophyton (page 63)*	*1320*
146–215	Tinea of groin. *Specify parasite if not Epidermophyton (page 63)*	*1320*
13▲–211	Tinea imbricated. *Specify region*	*1320*
112–208	Tinea versicolor	*1120*

—3 DISEASES DUE TO INTOXICATION

162–388	Alopecia due to pregnancy	*1600*
113–3253	Argyria	*1130*
110–321.6	Arsenical keratosis	*1130*
13▲–300.4	Cicatrix of skin due to chemical burn. *Specify region and poison (page 67) when known*	*1330*
13▲–320	Dermatitis escharotic. *Specify region and poison (page 67)*	*1330*
113–3▲▲	Dermatitis medicamentosa. *Specify drug (page 67)*	*1132*
110–3▲▲	Dermatitis photomelanotic (Berlock dermatitis). *Specify agent*	*1132*
110–300	Dermatitis venenata. *Specify irritant or allergen (page 67) when known*	*1131*
111–394	Dermatophytid	*1130*
111–390	Eczema. *Specify allergen (page 67) when known*	*1130*
116–300.8	Epidermolysis bullous, acquired (porphyria cutanea tarda). *Specify poison*	*1130*
143–3001	Erythema gluteal	*1330*
11x–3x7	Erythema multiform, toxic	*1130*
113–3x1	Erythema scarlatiniform	*1130*
113–3x0	Erythema toxic	*1130*
149–300	Keratosis palmar and plantar, acquired. *Specify poison when known*	*1330*

110–396	Physical allergy	*1130*
18▲–3▲▲	Subcutaneous inflammation due to extra-vasated drug. *Specify site and drug (page 67)*	*1800*
18▲–3▲▲.9	Subcutaneous atrophy due to extravasated drug. *Specify site and drug (page 67), e.g.,*	*1800*
185–3827.9	Of arm due to injection of insulin	*1800*
11x–390	Urticaria	*1133*
11x–3901	Urticaria papular	*1133*

—4 DISEASES DUE TO TRAUMA OR PHYSICAL AGENT

13▲–401	Abrasion. *Specify region*	*1342*
18▲–400.2	Abscess due to stitch. *Specify region*	*1800*
162–409	Avulsion of hair of scalp	*1600*
13▲–4x8	Blister due to trauma. *Specify region*	*1340*
13▲–4411	Burn of skin, first degree. *Specify region*	*1343*
13▲–4412	Burn of skin, second degree. *Specify region*	*1344*
112–430	Callositas (callus)	*1140*
13▲–441.4	Cicatrix of skin due to burn (from heat). *Specify region*	*1340*
13▲–433	Clavus. *Specify region*	*1340*
13▲–430	Decubitus ulcer. *Specify region*	*1341*
110–470	Dermatitis actinica due to roentgen rays (x-rays) or radioactive substance	*1140*
110–451	Dermatitis actinica due to ultraviolet radiation	*1140*
110–400	Dermatitis factitial	*1140*
13▲–450	Elastosis solar (actinic)	*1340*
11x–445	Erythema caloricum (from heat)	*1140*
180–4x9	Fat necrosis, neonatal (adiponecrosis neonatorum)	*1800*
13▲–49▲▲	Foreign body in skin. *Specify region and foreign body*	*1340*
13▲–4962	Tattoo. *Specify region*	*1340*
112–451	Freckles (ephelides)	*1140*
13▲–448	Frostbite (congelatic). *Specify region*	*1340*
13▲–400.1	Gangrene of skin due to trauma or physical agent. *Specify region and agent when known*	*1340*
13▲–441.1	Due to heat	*1340*
13▲–448.1	Due to cold	*1340*
18▲–4x7	Hematoma, subcutaneous. *Specify region*	*1800*
18▲–4x8	Implantation cyst due to trauma. *Specify region*	*1800*
111–437	Intertrigo	*1140*

11x–440	Marble skin (cutis marmorata)	*1140*
153–445	Miliaria (prickly heat)	*1500*
153–4451	Rubra	*1500*
153–4452	Crystallina	*1500*
170–4▲▲	Nail, injury of. *Specify injury (page 83)*	*1740*
110–446	Pernio	*1140*
110–452	Sailor's skin	*1140*
13▲–400.4	Scar of skin due to trauma. *Specify region. For deeper scar, see Regions, page 127*	*1340*
18▲427	Subcutaneous emphysema due to trauma. *Specify region*	*1800*
181–427	Of face	*1800*
182–427	Of thoracocervical region	*1800*
184–427	Of trunk	*1800*
184–415.6	Subcutaneous emphysema of trunk following operation	*1800*
173–4x7	Subungual hemorrhage due to trauma	*1740*
13▲–4x9	Ulcer due to trauma. *Specify region*	*1340*
176–433	Unguis incarnatus (ingrown nail)	*1743*
13▲–410	Wound of skin. *Specify region*	*1340*

—50 DISEASES DUE TO CIRCULATORY DISTURBANCE OR BLOOD DYSCRASIA

Record primary diagnosis when possible

099–518	Acrocyanosis	*0950*
110–521.6	Angiokeratoma	*1150*
110–5x0	Dermatitis hypostatica	*1150*
110–515	Dermatosis, progressive pigmentary; purpuric lichenoid dermatitis; purpura annularis telangiectodes	*1150*
110–518	Dermographia	*1150*
170–518	Eggshell nails	*1700*
114–501	Elephantiasis nostras	*1150*
147–5xx	Erythrocyanosis crurum	*1350*
13▲–501	Induration due to phlebitis. *Specify region, e.g.,*	*1350*
147–501	Of leg	*1350*
147–5x2	Livedo reticularis	*1350*
133–521.6	Rhinophyma	*1350*
131–521.0	Rosacea with acne	*1350*
173–549	Subungual hemorrhage in blood dyscrasia	*1700*
13▲–544.9	Ulcer of skin in granulocytopenia. *Specify region*	*1350*
13▲–522.9	Ulcus hypostatic. *State site, e.g.,*	*1352*
147–522.9	Of skin of leg	*1352*

—55 DISEASES DUE TO DISTURBANCE OF INNERVATION OR OF PSYCHIC CONTROL
Record primary diagnosis when possible

149–573	Acroparesthesia	*1355*
160–580	Alopecia areata	*1600*
162–580	Alopecia capitis total	*1600*
160–5801	Alopecia disseminated	*1600*
160–5802	Alopecia universal	*1600*
11x–580	Angioneurotic edema; giant urticaria	*1155*
152–565	Anhidrosis	*1500*
110–565	Atrophoderma neuritic (glossy skin)	*1155*
110–572	Dermatalgia	*1155*
170–565	Dystrophy of nails	*1700*
152–580	Hyperhidrosis	*1500*
110–573	Pruritus	*1155*
13▲–565.9	Ulcer, neurogenic. *Specify region, e.g.,*	*1355*
148–565.9	Of foot	*1355*
148–5651.9	Due to leprosy. *Record primary diagnosis*	*1355*
148–567.9	Due to lesion of central nervous system. *Record primary diagnosis*	*1355*
148–566.9	Due to syphilis of nervous system. *Record primary diagnosis*	*1355*

—6 DISEASES DUE TO OR CONSISTING OF STATIC MECHANICAL ABNORMALITY

18▲–639	Herniation of fascial fat. *Specify tissue site*	*1800*
112–6x8	Milium	*1160*

—7 DISEASES DUE TO DISORDERS OF METABOLISM, GROWTH, OR NUTRITION

151–7x0	Acne	*1500*
110–776	Acromegaly of skin	*1170*
170–796	Atrophia of nails	*1700*
110–798	Atrophy of skin, involutional	*1170*
152–7xx1	Bromhidrosis	*1500*
160–747	Canities	*1600*
110–718	Carotenosis of skin	*1170*
112–770	Chloasma (melasma)	*1170*
152–7xx	Chromhidrosis	*1500*
161–7x8	Comedo	*1600*
133–7x0	Granulosis rubra nasi	*1370*
	Granuloma, eosinophilic. *See histiocytosis (page 120)*	
110–749	Hydroa vacciniform	*1170*
160–792	Hypertrichosis, acquired	*1600*

112–799	Keratosis seborrheic	*1170*
111–799	Keratosis senile	*1170*
112–745	Leukoderma	*1170*
180–770	Lipodystrophy, progressive	*1800*
13▲–754	Lipid proteinosis (hyalinosis cutis). *Specify region*	*1370*
13▲–772	Myxedema of skin	*1370*
170–700	Nails, transverse furrowing of	*1700*
13▲–785	Necrobiosis lipoidic diabetic. *Specify region*	*1370*
110–742	Ochronosis. *File also under Diseases of the Body as a Whole (page 120)*	*1170*
110–770	Poikiloderma	*1170*
160–744	Ringed hair (thrix annulata)	*1600*
160–794	Trichorrhexis nodosa	*1600*
152–740	Urhidrosis	*1500*
112–747	Vitiligo	*1170*
114–785	Xanthoma diabeticorum	*1170*
114–7571	Xanthoma disseminatum	*1170*
114–7572	Xanthoma eruptive	*1170*
114–757	Xanthoma tuberosum multiplex	*1170*

—8 NEW GROWTHS

13▲–8175	Amelanotic melanoma. *Specify region and behavior*	*1382*
13▲–812	Basal cell carcinoma. *Specify region and behavior*	*1382*
13▲–814	Epidermoid carcinoma of skin. *Specify region and behavior*	*1381*
13▲–814E	Epidermoid carcinoma in situ of skin (Bowen's disease). *Specify region*	*1381*
13▲–8192	Epithelioma of skin, not otherwise specified	*1380*
13▲–834	Giant follicular lymphoma of skin. *Specify region and behavior*	*1380*
13▲–8532	Glomangioma of skin. *Specify region and behavior*	*1380*
13▲–868A	Granular cell myoblastoma	*1380*
13▲–8882	Hamartoma. *Specify region and behavior*	*1380*
13▲–850B	Hemangioendothelioma. *Specify region*	*1380*
13▲–850A	Hemangioma of skin. *Specify region*	*1380*
13▲–850G	Hemangiosarcoma of skin. *Specify region*	*1380*
13▲–832	Hodgkin's disease of skin. *Specify region and behavior*	*1380*
13▲–8701A	Keloid. *Specify region*	*1380*
13▲–866A	Leiomyoma. *Specify region and behavior*	*1380*
114–829	Leukemia cutis	*1380*
18▲–872A	Lipoma. *Specify region*	*1880*

13▲–854A	Lymphangioma. *Specify region*	*1380*
13▲–830	Lymphosarcoma of skin. *Specify region and behavior*	*1380*
13▲–8173	Melanoma. *Specify region and behavior*	*1383*
13▲–8895	Mixed tumor of skin. *Specify region and behavior*	*1380*
13▲–8032A	Multiple benign cystic epithelioma. *Specify region*	*1380*
13▲–852	Multiple hemorrhagic hemangioma of Kaposi. *Specify region and behavior*	*1380*
13▲–8851A	Myoepithelial tumor. *Specify region*	*1380*
13▲–8451	Neurofibroma of skin. *Specify region and behavior*	*1384*
110–8453	Neurofibromatosis. *Specify behavior*	*1384*
13▲–8171	Nonpigmented nevus of skin. *Specify region and behavior*	*1380*
13▲–814A	Papilloma of skin. *Specify region*	*1380*
13▲–8170	Pigmented nevus of skin. *Specify region and behavior*	*1385*
13▲–831	Reticulum cell sarcoma	*1380*
13▲–879	Sarcoma of skin. *Specify region and behavior*	*1380*
13▲–8075	Sebaceous carcinoma of skin. *Specify region and behavior*	*1380*
13▲–8061	Sweat gland adenoma (hidradenoma) of skin. *Specify region and behavior*	*1380*
1▲▲–8▲▲▲	Unlisted tumor of skin. *Specify region, neoplasm and behavior*	*1380*

—9 DISEASES DUE TO UNKNOWN OR UNCERTAIN CAUSE WITH THE STRUCTURAL REACTION MANIFEST: HEREDITARY AND FAMILIAL DISEASES OF THIS NATURE

110–960	Acanthosis nigricans (dystrophy papillary pigmented)	*1190*
161–940	Acne varioliformis	*1600*
110–910	Acrodermatitis atrophic chronic	*1190*
162–992	Alopecia hereditary (premature and senile)	*1600*
110–922	Amyloidosis of skin	*1190*
116–973	Atrophoderma macular, striae atrophic	*1190*
123–943	Cheilitis exfoliative	*1200*
155–900	Cheilitis glandular	*1500*
114–929	Colloid degeneration of skin	*1190*
115–943	Cutaneous horn	*1190*
116–9x6	Cutis hyperelastic	*1190*
110–966	Dermatitis exfoliative	*1190*
110–969	Dermatitis exfoliative of newborn	*1190*
110–985	Dermatitis gangrenous of newborn	*1190*
111–985	Dermatitis herpetiform	*1190*

131–943	Dermatosis papulosa nigra	*1390*
110–943	Dyskeratosis, benign (keratosis folliculosis)	*1190*
110–96x	Erythema annulare centrifugum	*1190*
110–974	Erythema elevatum diutinum	*1190*
11x–943	Erythema induratum (nodular vasculitis)	*1190*
11x–971	Erythema multiform exudative	*1190*
111–964	Erythroderma psoriatic	*1190*
1▲▲–9x6	Erythroplasia of Queyrat. *Specify region*	*1190*
131–976	Folliculitis ulerythematosus reticulated	*1390*
152–977	Fox-Fordyce disease	*1500*
13▲–975	Granuloma annular. *Specify region*	*1390*
111–984	Impetigo herpetiform	*1190*
13▲–954	Keratocanthoma. *Specify site*	*1390*
149–988	Keratolysis exfoliativa	*1390*
161–943	Keratosis pilaris	*1600*
170–961	Koilonychia (spoon nails)	*1700*
12▲–943	Kraurosis of. *Specify mucous membrane*	*1200*
170–962	Leukonychia	*1700*
12▲–941	Leukoplakia of . . . . *Specify mucous membrane*	*1200*
113–978	Lichen nitidus	*1190*
110–965	Lichen planus	*1190*
12▲–965	Lichen planus. *Specify mucous membrane*	*1200*
13▲–965.9	Lichen sclerosus et atrophicis. *Specify region*	*1390*
161–952	Lichen spinulosus	*1600*
111–9662	Lichen striata	*1190*
111–966	Neurodermatitis localized (lichen chronicus simplex)	*1190*
111–9661	Neurodermatitis, disseminata, dermatitis atopic	*1190*
130–943	Nodules, juxta-articular, not due to syphilis or yaws	*1390*
170–943	Onychauxis (hypertrophy of nail)	*1700*
170–961	Onychomadesis	***1700***
170–960	Onychorrhexis	*1700*
111–963	Parapsoriasis	*1190*
111–989	Pemphigus benign of Hailey and Hailey	*1190*
111–983	Pemphigus erythematosus	*1190*
111–981	Pemphigus foliaceus	*1190*
111–982	Pemphigus vegetans	*1190*
111–980	Pemphigus; pemphigoid	*1190*
111–987	Pemphigus, South American (fogo seluagem)	*1190*
11x–931	Periarteritis nodosa of skin	*1190*
110–986	Pityriasis lichenoides et varioliformis acuta	*1190*
111–962	Pityriasis rosea	*1190*

110–968	Pityriasis rubra pilaris	*1190*
112–970	Pompholyx	*1190*
112–995	Porokeratosis	*1190*
110–963	Prurigo mitis	*1190*
110–964	Prurigo nodularis	*1190*
116–911	Pseudoxanthoma elastic	*1190*
111–961	Psoriasis	*1196*
111–9611	Generalized	*1196*
111–9612	Exfoliative	*1196*
111–9613	Guttate	*1196*
111–9614	Flexural	*1196*
111–9615	Pustular	*1196*
110–971	Scleroderma, generalized of skin and mucous membranes	*1190*
114–971	Scleroderma, generalized, progressive	*1190*
114–970	Scleroderma, localized (morphea)	*1190*
162–940	Tinea (asbestos-like)	*1600*
110–9x1	Veldt sore (desert sore)	*1190*

—X DISEASES DUE TO UNKNOWN OR UNCERTAIN CAUSE WITH THE FUNCTIONAL REACTION ALONE MANIFEST

104–x90	Dysplasia, ectodermal, anhydrotic type (hereditary)	*1190*
11x–x95	Familial or hereditary edema	*1190*

—Y DISEASES DUE TO CAUSES NOT DETERMINABLE IN THE PARTICULAR CASE

Y signifies an incomplete diagnosis. It is to be replaced whenever possible by a code digit signifying the specific diagnosis

162–y00	Alopecia due to undetermined cause	*0061*
110–y10	Dermatitis due to undetermined cause	*0061*
161–yx2	Folliculitis due to undetermined cause	*0061*
13▲–yx1	Gangrene of skin due to undetermined cause. *Specify region*	*0061*
13▲–yx9	Ulceration of skin due to undetermined cause	*0061*

DISEASES OF THE BREAST

For male breast, change first three digits to 199

190– Breast
191– Parenchymatous tissue
192– Interstitial tissue
193– Duct
194– Nipple
195– Nipple in lactating breast
196– Premammary tissue
197– Retromammary tissue
198– Lactating breast
199– Male breast
19x– Blood vessels of breast

—0 DISEASES DUE TO GENETIC AND PRENATAL INFLUENCES

190–021	Aberrant breast	*1901*
190–012	Absence of one breast	*1901*
190–016	Hypoplasia of areola or entire breast	*1901*
194–023	Inversion of nipple	*1901*
199–075	Overdevelopment of breast in male	*1901*
190–031	Supernumerary breast	*1901*
194–031	Supernumerary nipple	*1901*

—I DISEASES DUE TO INFECTION WITH LOWER ORGANISM

190–100.2	Abscess of breast. *Specify organism (page 57) when known*	*1912*
198–100.2	Puerperal abscess of breast	*5750*
196–100.2	Abscess, premammary. *Specify organism (page 57) when known*	*1912*
197–100.2	Abscess, retromammary. *Specify organism (page 57) when known*	*1912*
193–100.8	Cyst, retention, of breast due to infection	*1910*
198–100.8	Galactocele due to infection	*5750*
190–100.3	Fistula, mammary	*1910*
198–100.3	Puerperal mammary fistula	*5750*
190–190	Mastitis, acute. *Specify organism (page 57) when known*	*1911*
198–100	Puerperal mastitis	*5750*
190–170	Mastitis with mumps	*1911*
190–190.0	Mastitis, chronic	*1911*
	Mastitis, chronic, cystic. *See* Cystic breast due to unknown cause, *following*	
192–190	Mastitis, interstitial	*1911*

190–100	Mastitis, suppurative. *Specify organism (page 57) when known*	*1911*
193–100.4	Occlusion of duct due to infection	*1910*
19x–100.7	Thrombophlebitis of veins of breast	*1910*
194–100	Thelitis. *Specify organism (page 57) when known*	*1910*
195–100	Puerperal thelitis	*5750*

—2 DISEASES DUE TO HIGHER PLANT OR ANIMAL PARASITE

194–209	Thrush of nipple	*1900*

—3 DISEASES DUE TO INTOXICATION

190–32▲	Chemical burn of breast. *Specify poison (page 67)*	*1900*

—4 DISEASES DUE TO TRAUMA OR PHYSICAL AGENT

193–400.8	Cyst of breast due to trauma	*1940*
198–400.8	Galactocele due to trauma	*5750*
190–4x9	Fat necrosis of breast	*1940*
190–4x7	Hematoma of breast due to trauma	*1940*
190–4▲▲	Injury of breast. *Specify (page 83)*	*1940*
194–4x0	Thelitis due to trauma	*1940*

—50 DISEASES DUE TO CIRCULATORY DISTURBANCE

190–510	Infarction of breast	*1900*

—6 DISEASES DUE TO OR CONSISTING OF STATIC MECHANICAL ABNORMALITY

190–6x8	Cystic breast due to unknown cause	*1968*
19x–641	Varicose veins of breast	*1960*

—7 DISEASES DUE TO DISORDER OF METABOLISM, GROWTH, OR NUTRITION

199–788	Gynecomastia due to administration of estrogens	*1970*
199–793	Gynecomastia	*1970*
191–789	Hypertrophy of breast in newborn infant	*1970*
193–796	Involution cyst of breast	*1970*
190–7x0	Mastitis of adolescence	*1970*
190–786	Mastopathy of ovarian origin	*1970*
190–793	Overdevelopment of breast in female	*1970*
190–789	Pregnancy changes, breast	*1970*

—8 NEW GROWTHS

190–8091	Adenocarcinoma of breast. *Specify behavior (page 99)*	*1981*
190–8831A	Adenofibroma of breast	*1982*
190–8832	Cystosarcoma phyllodes of breast. *Specify behavior (page 99)*	*1980*
190–850G	Hemangiosarcoma of breast	*1980*
193–8031F	Intracystic papillary carcinoma of breast	*1981*
190–830	Lymphosarcoma [1] of breast	*1980*
190–8062G	Medullary carcinoma with lymphoid stroma of breast	*1981*
190–879	Sarcoma of breast. *Specify behavior*	*1980*
190–8061	Sweat gland carcinoma of breast. *Specify behavior (page 99)*	*1981*
190–8▲▲▲	Unlisted tumor of breast. *Specify neoplasm and behavior*	*1980*

—9 DISEASES DUE TO UNKNOWN OR UNCERTAIN CAUSE WITH THE STRUCTURAL REACTION MANIFEST

190–940	Adenomatosis of breast	*1990*
193–957	Comedo mastitis	*1990*
192–956	Fibrosis of breast due to unknown cause	*1990*
194–9x5	Fissure of nipple	*1995*
190–993	Hypertrophy of breast, hereditary	*1990*
193–958	Plasma cell mastitis	*1990*

—X DISEASES DUE TO UNKNOWN OR UNCERTAIN CAUSE WITH THE FUNCTIONAL REACTION ALONE MANIFEST

198–x30	Abnormal quality of milk	*1990*
198–x40	Abnormal secretion of milk	*1990*
198–x10	Agalactia	*1990*
198–x20	Galactorrhea	*1990*

—Y DISEASES DUE TO CAUSE NOT DETERMINABLE IN THE PARTICULAR CASE

Y signifies an incomplete diagnosis. It is to be replaced whenever possible by a code digit signifying the specific diagnosis

198–yx8	Galactocele due to undetermined cause	*0061*

[1] Use lymphoma behavior code (page 99).

2– DISEASES OF THE MUSCULO-SKELETAL SYSTEM

DISEASES OF THE BONES

200– Bones
220– Vertebrae

For detailed list of bones, see page 8

—0 DISEASES DUE TO GENETIC AND PRENATAL INFLUENCES

2▲▲–011	Absence, congenital, of . . . . *Specify bone, e.g.*	2101
235–011	Femur	2101
2▲▲–012	Absence, partial, congenital of . . . . *Specify bone, e.g.*	2101
220–012	Vertebra; hemivertebra	2101
220–012.4	Scoliosis due to hemivertebra	2101
2▲▲–031	Accessory: supernumerary. *Specify bone, e.g.*	2101
2394–031	Accessory navicular of tarsus	2101
2331–031	Accessory navicular of carpus	2101
229–031	Supernumerary rib, cervical	2101
220–031	Supernumerary vertebra	2101
200–001	Achondroplasia, complete (dwarfism) or incomplete	2101
237–0221	Anterior bowing of tibia	2101
2101–038	Craniorachischisis	2101
2▲▲–077	Deformity, congenital of . . . . *Specify bone and type, e.g.*	2101
221–077	Cervical portion of spine, multiple congenital deformities of	2101
	Femur	
2351–077	Femur, anteversion of neck of, congenital	2101
2351–0776	Coxa vara, congenital	2101
2351–0777	Coxa valga, congenital	2101
231–077	Radius, idiopathic curvature of	2101
237–022	Torsion of tibia, congenital	2101
229–077	Pigeon breast, congenital	2101
229–0771	Funnel chest, congenital	2101
2▲▲–026	Dislocation; or subluxation, complete or incomplete, congenital, of . . . . (*Bone to be specified only if joint cannot be specified*)	2101
236–026	Patella	2101

146

200–002	Dyschondroplasia (skeletal enchondromatosis)	*2101*
220–077	Dysplasia of vertebrae, multiple	*2101*
2▲▲–007	Dysplasia monostotic, fibrous of . . . . *Specify bone*	*2101*
200–008	Eccentro-osteochondrodysplasia	*2101*
2133–013	Elongation of styloid process of temporal bone	*2101*
200–003	Exostoses, multiple osteocartilaginous (metaphysial aclasis)	*2101*
2▲▲–097	Exostosis, congenital, of . . . . *Specify bone*	*2101*
200–006	Fragilitas ossium	*2101*
2▲▲–037	Fusion defect of . . . . *Specify bone, e.g.*	*2101*
236–037	Patella biparta •	*2101*
23x1.0–037	Sesamoid bone of first metatarsal, fusion defect of	*2101*
2205–037	Vertebral arch, fusion defect of	*2101*
220▲–037	Spina bifida. *Specify site. If clubfoot is associated record as separate diagnosis. See page 156*	*2101*
2203–037	Spondylolisthesis (fusion defect between laminas and pedicles)	*2102*
2203–0371	Spondylolysis (fusion defect between laminas and pedicles without displacement of body)	*2102*
2x51–024	Synostosis of humerus and radius, congenital	*2103*
2▲▲.4–014	Hyperostosis cortical, congenital	*2101*
215–013	Hypertelorism (congenital enlargement of sphenoid bone)	*2101*
2▲▲–016	Hypoplasia, congenital of . . . . *Specify bone, e.g.*	*2101*
23x1–016	Short first metatarsal segment	*2101*
2▲▲–021	Misplacement, congenital of . . . . *Specify bone, e.g.*	*2101*
226–021	Scapula, congenital elevation of	*2101*
200–004	Osteopetrosis (marble bones)	*2101*
200–005	Osteopoikilosis	*2101*
200–007	Polyostotic fibrous dysplasia	*2101*
200–0071	Albright's syndrome	*2101*
2▲▲–076	Rudimentary . . . . *Specify bone, e.g.*	*2101*
236–076	Patella	*2101*
2▲▲–03x	Segmentation, incomplete (synostosis) of . . . . *Specify bone, e.g.*	*2101*
2x51–03x	Humerus and radius	*2101*
223–03x	Lumbosacral vertebra, transitional	*2101*
2x1–03x	Radius and ulna	*2101*

—I DISEASES DUE TO INFECTION WITH LOWER ORGANISM

2▲▲–100.2	Abscess of . . . . *Specify bone and organism (page 57) when known, e.g.*	2110
237–105.2	Abscess of tibia due to staphylococcic infection	2311
2▲▲–130.2	Abscess of . . . chronic (Brodie's abscess)	2110
2▲▲–100.7	Atrophy of . . . due to infection. *Specify bone and organism (page 57) when known, e.g.*	2110
220–100.7	Vertebra	2110
2135–100.9	Caries of petrous bone	2110
2▲▲–100.4	Deformity of . . . due to infection. *Specify bone and organism (page 57) when known, e.g.*	2110
2351–100.4	Coxa vara due to infection	2110
2▲▲▲2–100.4	Epiphysis, slipping of . . . due to infection.[1] *Specify bone and organism (page 57) when known*	2110
235▲2–100.4	Femur	2110
2▲▲–100.6	Exostosis of . . . due to infection. *Specify bone and organism (page 57) when known*	2110
2391–103.6	Calcaneus (os calcis), exostosis of, due to gonococcic infection	2110
2▲▲–100.3	Fistula leading to . . . due to infection. *Specify bone and organism (page 57) when known*	2110
2▲▲–100.5	Fracture of . . . due to infection. *Specify bone and organism (page 57) when known, e.g.*	2110
230–147.5	Humerus, fracture of, due to syphilis	2110
2▲▲–100.x	Growth arrest of . . . due to infection. *Specify bone and organism (page 57) when known, e.g.*	2110
235–102.x	Femur, arrest of growth of, due to streptococcic osteomyelitis	2110
2▲▲–124	Leprosy of . . . . *Specify bone*	2110
2▲▲–190.6	Osteitis, sclerotic nonsuppurative, of . . . . *Specify bone*	2110
2▲▲–100	Osteomyelitis, acute of . . . . *Specify bone and organism (page 57) when known, e.g.*	2311
23514–105	Osteomyelitis of neck of femur, due to staphylococcic infection	2311
237–115	Osteomyelitis of tibia, due to typhoid	2311

[1] If specific topographic code number is not listed, use .2 to indicate epiphysis.

2▲▲–100.0	Osteomyelitis, chronic, of . . . . *Specify bone and organism (page 57) when known*	2311
2▲▲.4–100	Periostitis, acute, of . . . . *Specify bone and organism (page 57) when known,* e.g.	2110
230.4–102	Humerus, acute periostitis of, due to streptococcic infection	2110
2▲▲.4–100.0	Periostitis, chronic, of . . . . *Specify bone and organism (page 57) when known*	2110
2▲▲–100.1	Rarefaction of . . . due to infection. *Specify bone and organism (page 57) when known*	2110
2361–100.6	Retropatellar fat pad, hypertrophy of, due to infection	2110
2▲▲–100.9	Sequestrum formation of . . . due to infection. *Specify bone and organism (page 57) when known*	2311
20x–100	Sesamoiditis	2110
2▲▲.2–147	Syphilitic osteochondritis of . . . . *Specify bone*	2110
220–123	Tuberculosis of vertebra	2212

—2 DISEASES DUE TO HIGHER PLANT OR ANIMAL PARASITE

2▲▲–2▲▲	Mycosis of bone. *Specify bone and fungus*	2120

—3 DISEASES DUE TO INTOXICATION

2▲▲–38253	Changes in bone associated with hypercortisonism induced by medication	2130
2▲▲–3▲▲	Poisoning of . . . by . . . . *Specify bone and poison (page 67),* e.g.	2130
200–3195	Fluorine poisoning of bones	2130
200–3238	Lead osteosclerosis	2130
219–3185	Phosphorus poisoning of mandible	2130
2▲▲–3185.1	Phosphorus necrosis of . . . . *Specify bone*	2130
200–3185.6	Phosphorus osteosclerosis	2130

—4 DISEASES DUE TO TRAUMA OR PHYSICAL AGENT

2▲▲–437	Atrophy of . . . due to pressure. *Specify bone,* e.g.	2140
210–437	Skull	2140
2▲▲▲2–409	Avulsion of epiphysis of[1] . . . . *Specify bone,* e.g.	2140

[1] If specific topographic code number is not listed, use .2 to indicate epiphysis

235.2–409	Femur	2140
2▲▲–480	Caisson disease of . . . . *Specify bone or joint*	2140
2▲▲.4–402.9	Calcification, subperiosteal, of . . . due to trauma. *Specify bone*	2140
2▲▲–416.0	Callus, excessive of . . . following fracture. *Specify bone*	2140
236–4x9	Chondromalacia of patella due to trauma	2140
2▲▲–400.4	Deformity of . . . due to trauma. *Specify deformity and bone, e.g.*	2140
2351–400.4	Coxa vara due to trauma	2140
2351–4001.4	Coxa valga due to trauma	2140
210–431	Deformity of skull due to posture	2140
210–408	Diastasis of cranial bones	2140
2▲▲–406	Dislocation of . . . . *Specify bone. Express in terms of joint when possible*	2140
2▲▲–407	Dislocation open of . . . . *Specify bone. Express in terms of joint when possible*	2140
2▲▲–408	Dislocation incomplete (subluxation) of . . . . *Specify bone. Express in terms of joint when possible*	2140
2▲▲–400.6	Exostosis of . . . due to trauma or pressure. *Specify bone*	2140
2▲▲–496	Foreign body in . . . . *Specify bone*	2140
2▲▲–4167	Fracture, chip of . . . . *Specify bone*	2347
2▲▲–416▲	Fracture, closed of . . . . *Specify bone and type of fracture*	2347
2▲▲–417	Fracture of . . . due to birth injury. *Specify bone*	2347
2▲▲–417.5	Nonunion of fracture of . . . due to birth injury. *Specify bone*	2347
2▲▲–419	Fracture, intrauterine of . . . . *Specify bone*	2347
2▲▲–418▲	Fracture, open of . . . . *Specify bone and type of fracture*	2347
2▲▲–4185	Fracture, open, comminuted of . . . . *Specify bone*	2347
2▲▲–403.5	Fracture, compression, of . . . . *Specify bone*	2347
2▲▲–41▲.9	Fracture, depressed, of . . . . *Specify bone and type of fracture*	2347
2▲▲–41▲.4	Fracture, impacted, of . . . . *Specify bone and type of fracture*	2347
2▲▲–414.5	Fracture, gunshot, of . . . . *Specify bone*	2347
2x12–41▲▲	Fracture, Colles's. *For other fractures of radius and ulna, see page 83*	2341

2x1–41▲▲	Fracture, Monteggia's	*2341*
2x22–41▲▲	Fracture, Pott's. *For other fractures of tibia and fibula see page 83*	*2346*
2x225–41▲▲	Fracture, trimalleolar, of ankle	*2346*
2x▲–41▲.4	Fracture of . . . with cross union following. *Specify bone and type of fracture*	*2347*
2▲▲–41▲.7	Fracture of . . . with delayed union following. *Specify bone and type of fracture*	*2347*
2▲▲–41▲.6	Fracture of . . . with malunion following. *Specify bone and type of fracture*	*2347*
2▲▲–41▲.5	Fracture of . . . without union following. *Specify bone and type of fracture*	*2347*
2▲▲–415.5	Fracture of graft of . . . . *Specify bone*	*2347*
2▲▲–41▲.x	Growth, arrest of, of . . . following fracture. *Specify bone*	*2140*
2▲▲.4–4x7	Hematoma, subperiosteal, of . . . . *Specify bone, e.g.*	*2140*
21▲.4–4x7	Cephalhematoma. *Specify bone*	*2140*
2▲▲–4▲▲	Injury of . . . . *Specify bone and type of injury (page 83)*	*2140*
2▲▲–400.1	Loss of substance of . . . due to trauma. *Specify bone*	*2140*
2▲▲–438.1	Necrosis of . . . due to foreign body. *Specify bone*	*2140*
2▲▲–47▲.1	Necrosis of . . . due to radioactive substance. *Specify bone and radioactive substance*	*2140*
229–4x0	Osteochondritis of rib due to trauma	*2140*
2▲▲–400.0	Osteomyelitis of . . . due to trauma. *Specify bone. If infection is important especially if organism is determined, make a secondary diagnosis*	*2140*
2▲▲–400.9	Osteoporosis of . . . due to trauma. *Specify bone*	*2140*
2▲▲.4–400.0	Periostitis due to trauma. *Specify bone*	*2140*
236–40x	Recurrent dislocation of patella	*2140*
2▲▲–4x5.5	Refracture of . . . following fracture. *Specify bone*	*2347*
2361–4x6	Retropatellar fat pad, hypertrophy of, due to trauma	*2140*
2▲▲▲2–400.4	Slipping of epiphysis of[1] . . . due to trauma. *Specify bone, e.g.*	*2347*
23512–400.4	Slipping of capital epiphysis of femur due to trauma	*2346*

[1] If specific topographic code number is not listed, use .2 to indicate epiphysis.

—50 DISEASES DUE TO CIRCULATORY DISTURBANCE
Record primary diagnosis when possible

2▲▲–510	Atrophy of . . . due directly to interference with blood supply infarction. *Specify bone, e.g.*	2150
2▲▲–516.9	Atrophy of . . . due to arteriosclerosis. *Specify bone*	2150
2▲▲–512	Due to embolism. *Specify bone*	2150
2▲▲–515.9	Atrophy of . . . due to endarteritis. *Specify bone*	2150
2▲▲–511	Due to thrombosis. *Specify bone*	2150
2▲▲–510.1	Necrosis of bone, aseptic, due to deficient blood supply. *Specify bone, e.g.*	2150
2▲▲▲2–510.1	Epiphyseal [1]	2150

—55 DISEASES DUE TO DISTURBANCE OF INNERVATION OR OF PSYCHIC CONTROL
Record primary diagnosis when possible

210–565	Hemiatrophy of face	2155
2▲▲–565	Neurogenic atrophy of . . . due to syringomyelia. *Specify bone*	2155
2▲▲–566	Neurogenic atrophy of . . . due to tabes dorsalis. *Specify bone, e.g.*	2155
220–566	Vertebra	2155
2▲▲–564.9	Postpoliomyelitic atrophy of . . . with shortening. *Specify bone*	2155

—6 DISEASES DUE TO OR CONSISTING OF MECHANICAL ABNORMALITY OF UNKNOWN ORIGIN

229–630	Slipping rib	2160
226–630	Slipping scapula; snapping scapula	2160
237–637	Torsion of tibia due to unknown cause	2160

—7 DISEASES DUE TO DISORDER OF METABOLISM, GROWTH, OR NUTRITION
Record primary diagnosis when possible

DISEASES DUE TO DISTURBANCE OF GENERAL METABOLISM

2▲▲–713	Atrophy of . . . due to disuse. *Specify bone*	2170
2▲▲–711	Osteoporosis of bone due to prolonged malnutrition	2170
200–704	Secondary hypertrophic osteoarthropathy	2170

DISEASES DUE TO DISTURBANCE OF ACID-BASE EQUILIBRIUM

200–720	Renal osteodystrophy	2170

DISEASES DUE TO METABOLISM OF SPECIFIC ELECTROLYTES

200–734	Hypophosphatasia	2170

DISEASES DUE TO DISTURBANCE OF FAT METABOLISM

2▲▲–755.6	Granuloma, eosiniphilic. *Specify bone*	*2170*
2▲▲–755	Xanthomatosis of bone, unclassified. *Specify bone*	*2170*

DISEASES DUE TO DEPRIVATION OF VITAMINS

2▲▲–7641	Changes in . . . associated with rachitis tarda; juvenile osteomalacia. *Specify bone*	*2170*
2▲▲.4–763	Changes in periosteum, due to scurvy. *Specify bone*	*2170*
2▲▲–764.4	Deformity of bone . . . due to rickets. *Specify bone*	*2170*
2x2–764.4	Genu varum (bowlegs) due to rickets	*2170*
2▲▲–7642.5	Fracture of . . . due to osteomalacia	*2170*
2▲▲–764.5	Fracture of . . . due to rickets. *Specify bone*	*2170*
200–7642	Osteomalacia	*2170*
200–7644	Osteomalacia associated with pregnancy or puerperium	*2170*
200–7643	Senile osteomalacia	*2170*

DISEASES DUE TO ENDOCRINE DISTURBANCE

2▲▲–781	Changes in and associated with hyperfunction of adrenal cortex. *Specify bone*	*2170*
2▲▲–776	Changes in . . . associated with pituitary basophilism. *Specify bone*	*2170*
	Osteitis fibrosa cystica, generalized. *See secondary hyperplasia parathyroid (page 391)*	*2170*
2351–773.4	Coxa vara due to osteitis fibrosa cystica	*2170*
2▲▲–773.5	Fracture of . . . due to osteitis fibrosa cystica. *Specify bone*	*2170*
2▲▲–770	Osteoporosis of bone due to endocrine disorders	*2170*
2▲▲–787	Osteoporosis of bone, postmenopausal	*2170*

INVOLUTIONAL DISEASES

22▲–798	Senile atrophy ; senile osteoporosis of . . . . *Specify bone, e.g.*	*2170*
220–798	Vertebra, senile atrophy of	*2170*
220–798.4	Round back due to senile atrophy	*2170*

DEVELOPMENTAL DISEASES

210–794	Craniotabes, due to cause other than rickets	*2170*
219–791	Micrognathism ; microgenia ; opisthognathism	*2170*

216–793.   Overdevelopment of nasal bones   2170
21▲–792   Prognathism. *Specify maxilla or mandible*   2170

—8 NEW GROWTHS

2▲▲–873A   Chondroblastoma of . . . . *Specify bone*   2180
2▲▲–873B   Chondroma of . . . . *Specify bone*   2180
2▲▲–873F   Chondrosarcoma of . . . . *Specify bone*   2180
2▲▲–875G   Ewing's sarcoma of . . . . *Specify bone*   2182
2▲▲.4–870A   Fibroma, periosteal, of . . . . *Specify bone*   2180
2▲▲–870F   Fibrosarcoma of . . . . *Specify bone*   2180
2▲▲–874   Giant cell tumor of . . . . *Specify bone*   2180
2▲▲–874F   Giant cell tumor, malignant, of . . . .
                      Specify bone   2180
2▲▲–850A   Hemangioma of . . . . *Specify bone*   2180
2▲▲–850G   Hemangiosarcoma of . . . . *Specify
                      bone*   2180
2▲▲–8451   Neurofibroma of . . . . *Specify bone and
                      behavior (page 99)*   2180
2▲▲–876A   Osteoma of . . . . *Specify bone*   2187
2▲▲–833   Plasma cell myeloma[1] of . . . . *Specify
                      bone and behavior*   2180
2▲▲–831   Reticulum cell sarcoma of . . . . *Specify
                      bone and behavior (page 99)*   2180
2▲▲–8▲▲▲   Unlisted tumor of . . . . *Specify site,
                      neoplasm and behavior (page 93)*   2180

**—9 DISEASES DUE TO UNKNOWN OR UNCERTAIN CAUSE WITH THE
STRUCTURAL REACTION MANIFEST**

22x5–9x9   Acetabulum, pelvic protrusion of   2190
2▲▲–922   Amyloid infiltration of . . . . *Specify bone*   2190
2▲▲–9▲▲.8   Cyst, localized, of . . . . *Specify bone and
                      predominating process (page 99)*   2190
  2▲▲–9x8.5   Fracture of . . . due to localized cyst.
                      Specify bone   2190
2▲▲–947   Dysplasia, progressive. *Specify site*   2190
2▲▲▲2–942   Epiphysitis of . . . due to unknown
                      cause.[2] *Specify bone*   2190
2▲▲▲2–912   Epiphysiolysis of . . . due to unknown
                      cause.[2] *Specify bone, e.g.*   2190
  23512–912   Of upper end of femur   2190
231–950   Idiopathic curvature of radius progressive   2190
2▲▲–911.5   Fracture of . . . due to osteochondrosis.
                      Specify bone   2191
216–952   Goundou   2190
2▲▲–943   Hyperostosis due to unknown cause   2190

[1] Use lymphoma behavior code (page 99).
[2] If specific typographic code number is not used, use .2 to indicate epiphysis.

DISEASES OF THE JOINTS

240– Joints
241– Joints of spine
206– Capsule of joint
207– Synovial membrane
250– Cartilages
251– Intervertebral cartilages
260– Ligaments

For detailed lists of joints, cartilages and ligaments, see page 13

—0 DISEASES DUE TO GENETIC AND PRENATAL INFLUENCES

26▲–017	Contraction, congenital, of ligaments of . . . . *Specify ligaments, e.g.*	2600
	Toe	
26x–017	Hammer toe, congenital	2600
	Spine	
261–017	Scoliosis, congenital	2600
240–022	Deformity, congenital, of joints, multiple; arthrogryposis	2401
24▲–022	Deformity, congenital, of . . . . *Specify joint, e.g.*	2402
	Hand	
245–022	Club hand, congenital	2402
	Lumbosacral joint	
2414–022	Lumbosacral joint, unstable	2402
2414–0221	Lumbosacral joint, unstable, with posterior displacement of sacrum	2402
2414–0224	Lumbosacral joint, transitional (incomplete sacralization)	2402
2414–025	Sacralization of the fifth lumbar vertebra with sciatica and scoliosis (Bertolotti's syndrome)	2402
	Knee	
248–022	Genu recurvatum, congenital	2402
248–0224	Genu valgum, congenital	2402
248–0223	Genu varum, congenital	2402
	Foot	
2493–022	Talipes, congenital. *Specify type*	2404
2493–0227	Talipes, calcaneovalgus	2404
2493–0226	Talipes calcaneovarus	2404
2493–0221	Talipes calcaneus	2404
2493–0228	Talipes cavus	2404
2493–0225	Talipes equinovalgus	2404

2493–0220	Talipes, equinovarus (clubfoot)	*2404*
2493–0224	Talipes equinus	*2404*
2493–0222	Talipes planovalgus	*2404*
2493–0223	Talipes varus (clubfoot)	*2404*
24x–042	Clubfoot, congenital paralytic (in spina bifida)	*2404*
26x–042	Flatfoot, congenital due to paralysis	*2600*
24x1–0221	Hallux valgus, congenital	*2402*
24x1–022	Hallux varus, congenital	*2402*
2494–0229	Metatarsus adductus, congenital	*2404*
2494–022	Metatarsal varus, congenital	*2402*
24x5–022	Toe, fifth, varus, congenital	*2402*
24▲–042	Deformity, congenital paralytic, of . . . . *Specify joint; if deformity is important, specify as additional diagnosis*	*2402*
24▲–026	Dislocation, congenital, complete or partial, of . . . . *Specify joint*	*2402*
247–026	Hip	*2402*
2493–026	Midtarsal joints	*2402*
253–013	Hypertrophy of meniscus of knee, congenital	*2401*
26▲–013	Relaxation of ligaments of joint, congenital. *Specify ligaments, e.g.*	*2600*
268–013	Knee	*2600*

—I DISEASES DUE TO INFECTION WITH LOWER ORGANISM

24▲–100	Arthritis due to infection. *Specify joint and organism (page 57) when known, e.g.*	*2411*
241–123	Of spine due to tuberculosis	*2411*
248–103	Of knee due to gonococcic infection	*2411*
244–101	Of wrist due to pneumococcic infection	*2411*
25▲–100.2	Cartilage, abscess of . . . . *Specify cartilage and organism (page 57) when known*	*2510*
25▲–100.1	Atrophy of cartilage due to infection. *Specify cartilage and organism (page 57) when known*	*2510*
251–100.9	Cartilage, intervertebral, calcification of, due to infection	*2510*
251–123	Cartilage, intervertebral, tuberculosis of	*2512*
25▲–190	Chondritis of . . . . *Specify cartilage, e.g.*	*2510*
251–190	Intervertebral cartilage	*2510*
26▲–100.4	Contracture of . . . due to infection. *Specify joint and organism (page 57) when known*	*2600*

24▲–100.4   Deformity (of bony parts) of . . . due to
infection. *Specify deformity, joint
and organism (page 57) when known,
e.g.*   *2400*

24x1–100.4   Hallux rigidus due to infection   *2410*

241–123.4   Kyphosis due to tuberculosis   *2412*

24▲–100.5   Dislocation (complete or partial) of . . .
due to infection. *Specify joint*   *2410*

24▲–100.3   Fistula into joint due to infection. *Specify
joint and organism (page 57) when
known*   *2410*

Synovitis. *Diagnose under* Arthritis
preceding

—3 DISEASES DUE TO INTOXICATION

24▲–390   Arthritis due to allergy   *2430*

—4 DISEASES DUE TO TRAUMA OR PHYSICAL AGENT

24▲–4x4   Adhesions of . . . due to trauma. *Specify joint*   *2440*

24▲–400.4   Ankylosis, bony or fibrous of . . . due to
trauma. *Specify joint*   *2440*

24▲–415.4   Ankylosis, bony or fibrous, of . . . following operation. *Specify joint*   *2440*

24▲–400.0   Arthritis of . . . due to direct trauma.
Specify joint and trauma, e.g.   *2440*

248–402.0   Of knee due to contusion   *2440*

243–40x.0   Of elbow due to habitual dislocation   *2440*

243–416.0   Of elbow due to fracture involving joint   *2440*

24x1–4x0.0   Bunion. *Specify site*   *2540*

2681–400.9   Calcification of medial collateral ligament
of knee due to trauma   *2600*

25▲–430   Cartilage, atrophy of, due to trauma.
Specify cartilage   *2540*

25▲–402.9   Cartilage, calcification of, due to trauma.
Specify cartilage   *2540*

25▲–4x9   Chondromalacia of . . . due to trauma.
Specify cartilage   *2540*

26▲–400.4   Contracture (of soft parts) of . . . due to
trauma. *Specify ligaments, e.g.*   *2600*

267–400.4   Hip   *2600*

267–4001.4   Adduction contracture   *2600*

267–4002.4   Flexion contracture   *2600*

24▲–400.9   Deformity (of bony parts) of . . . due to
trauma. *Specify joint and deformity*   *2440*

241–400.9   Kyphosis due to trauma   *2440*

241–4001.9	Scoliosis due to trauma	2440
241–435	Scoliosis due to thoracic disease	2440
	Dislocation of joint. *See under* Injury of joint, *following*	
	Dislocation of cartilage. *See under* Injury of cartilage, *following*	
24▲–496	Foreign body in . . . . *Specify joint*	2440
24▲–4x4.5	Fracture of ankylosed joint. *Specify joint*	2440
	Fracture-dislocation. *Diagnose both fracture and dislocation*	
248–40x	Habitual dislocation of knee	2441
24x1–400.9	Hallux rigidus due to trauma	2440
24x1–433	Hallux valgus due to pressure	2440
24x1–4001.9	Hallux valgus due to acute trauma	2440
24x1–400.6	Hallux varus due to scar tissue	2440
24▲–4x7	Hemarthrosis due to trauma. *Specify joint*	2440
2511–400.9	Herniation of nucleus pulposus due to trauma	2541
24▲–4▲▲	Injury of . . . . *Specify injury and joint, e.g.*	2440
269–412	Ankle, sprain of	2440
243–407	Elbow, open dislocation of	2443
247–406	Hip, dislocation of	2444
242–408	Shoulder, incomplete dislocation of	2442
25▲–4▲▲	Injury of . . . . *Specify injury and cartilage of joint, e.g.*	2540
2531–409	Detachment of medial meniscus of knee	2540
2532–412	Tear of lateral meniscus of knee	2540
24▲–4x9	Instability of . . . due to trauma. *Specify joint*	2440
24▲–415.9	Instability of . . . following operation. *Specify joint*	2440
2414–415.7	Pseudarthrosis of lumbosacral spine following fusion (or arthrodesis)	2440
24▲–415.7	Pseudarthrosis following fusion (or arthrodesis) of . . . . *Specify joint*	2440
	Sprain of joint. *See* Sprain of ligaments of joint, *following*	
26▲–412	Sprain of ligament of . . . . *Code ligament and state joint, e.g.*	2640
2681–412	Knee, medial collateral ligament of	2640
2682–412	Knee, lateral collateral ligament of	2640
2683–412	Knee, anterior crucial ligament of	2640
2684–412	Knee, posterior crucial ligament of	2640
24▲–400.x	Stiffness (slight limitation of motion) of . . . due to trauma. *Specify joint*	2440

24▲–415.x	Stiffness of . . . following operation. *Specify joint*	2440
24x–43x	Strained foot (due to constant or inter- mittent trauma)	2440
	Synovitis due to trauma. *Diagnose* Ar- thritis due to direct trauma (*page 158*)	
2493–408	Subluxation of midtarsal joints, due to trauma	2441
24x–415.9	Talipes equinus following operation	2440
24▲.4–412	Tear of capsule of . . . . *Specify joint,* *e.g.*	2440
242.4–412	Shoulder	2440
	Tear of cartilage. *See under* Injury of cartilage, *preceding*	
24x5–433	Toe, fifth, varus, due to trauma	2440
26x–434	Toe, hammer	2640

—55 DISEASES DUE TO DISTURBANCE OF INNERVATION OR OF PSYCHIC CONTROL

Record primary diagnosis when possible

24▲–564	Contracture of . . . due to flaccid paraly- sis following poliomyelitis. *Specify joint and deformity, e.g.*	2455
	Foot	
24x–564	Talipes due to flaccid paralysis follow- ing poliomyelitis	2455
24x–5641	Talipes calcaneus	2455
24x–5647	Talipes calcaneovalgus	2455
24x–5646	Talipes calcaneovarus	2455
24x–5648	Talipes cavus	2455
24x–5644	Talipes equinus	2455
24x–5645	Talipes equinovalgus	2455
24x–5640	Talipes equinovarus (clubfoot)	2455
24x–5642	Talipes planovalgus	2455
24x–5643	Talipes varus (clubfoot)	2455
247–564	Hip	2455
247–5643	Abduction contracture of hip follow- ing poliomyelitis	2455
247–5644	Adduction contracture of hip follow- ing poliomyelitis	2455
247–5642	Extension contracture following poliomyelitis	2455
247–5646	External rotation contracture of hip following poliomyelitis	2455
247–5641	Flexion contracture following polio- myelitis	2455

247–5645	Internal rotation contracture of hip following poliomyelitis	*2455*
248–564	Knee. *Indicate type and add 7th digit*	*2455*
241–564	Spine	*2455*
241–5642	Kyphosis following poliomyelitis	*2455*
2413–564	Lordosis following poliomyelitis	*2455*
241–5641	Scoliosis following poliomyelitis	*2455*
	Toe	
24x1–564	Hallux valgus following poliomyelitis	*2455*
26x–5641	Hammer toe following poliomyelitis	*2455*
241–569	Contracture of spine due to flaccid paralysis resulting from spina bifida	*2455*
24▴–560	Contracture of . . . due to other type of flaccid paralysis (not following poliomyelitis or not due to spina bifida). *Specify joint and deformity, e.g.*	*2455*
	Foot	
24x–560	Talipes flaccid. *Specify type and code, as under* Contracture of . . . due to flaccid paralysis following poliomyelitis	*2455*
247–560	Hip. *Specify type and code, as under* Contracture of . . . due to flaccid paralysis following poliomyelitis	*2455*
248–560	Knee. *Specify type and code, as under* Contracture of . . . due to flaccid paralysis following poliomyelitis	*2455*
2468–560	Pelvis	*2455*
2468–5601	Pelvic obliquity, not fixed	*2455*
2468–5602	Pelvic obliquity, fixed	*2455*
2468–5603	Tilt of pelvis (in sagittal plane)	*2455*
241–560	Spine	*2455*
	Toe	
24x1–560	Hallux valgus due to other type of paralysis	*2455*
24▴–561	Contracture of . . . due to spastic paralysis. *Specify joint, as:*	*2455*
	Foot	
24x–561	Talipes due to spastic paralysis. *Specify type and add 7th digit as under* Contracture of . . . due to flaccid paralysis following poliomyelitis, *preceding*	*2455*
	Hand	
245–561	Clawhand	*2455*
2468–561	Pelvis. *Specify type and add 7th digit, as under* Contracture of . . . due to flaccid paralysis fol-	

	lowing poliomyelitis, *preceding*	2455
242–561	Shoulder. *Specify type and add 7th digit, as under* Contracture of . . . due to flaccid paralysis following poliomyelitis, *preceding*	2455
241–561	Spine. *Specify type and add 7th digit, as under* Contracture of . . . due to flaccid paralysis following poliomyelitis, *preceding*	2455
244–561	Wrist. *Specify type and add 7th digit, as under* Contracture of . . . due to flaccid paralysis following poliomyelitis, *preceding*	2455
24▲–564.5	Dislocation of . . . due to paralysis following poliomyelitis. *Specify joint*	2455
24▲–560.5	Dislocation of . . . due to other type of flaccid paralysis. *Specify joint*	2455
24▲–561.5	Dislocation of . . . due to spastic paralysis. *Specify joint*	2455
24▲–569.5	Dislocation of . . . due to spina bifida. *Specify joint*	2455
24▲–564.x	Flail joint due to paralysis from poliomyelitis. *Specify joint*	2455
24▲–565	Neurogenic arthropathy (Charcot joint). *Specify joint*	2455
245–565	Clawhand, syringomyelic	2455
248–566	Tabetic arthropathy of knee	2455
24▲–564.9	Relaxation of . . . due to paralysis following poliomyelitis. *Specify joint*	2455
248–564.9	Genu recurvatum	2455
24▲–560.9	Relaxation of . . . due to other type of flaccid paralysis. *Specify joint*	2455
248–560.9	Genu recurvatum	2455

—6 DISEASES DUE TO OR CONSISTING OF MECHANICAL ABNORMALITY OF UNKNOWN ORIGIN

253–600.8	Cyst of meniscus of knee (snapping knee)	2500
2501–630	Displacement of meniscus of jaw (snapping jaw)	2500
24▲.7–600.8	Ganglion of . . . . *Specify joint, e.g.*	2460
248.7–600.8	Ganglion of knee joint	2460
248–639	Hernia of knee joint	2460
24▲–611	Loose bodies in . . . . *Specify joint, e.g.*	2460
248–611	Knee (joint mice)	2460

—7 DISEASES DUE TO DISORDER OF METABOLISM, GROWTH, OR NUTRITION
Record primary diagnosis

24▲–741	Arthritis due to gout. *Specify joint. Record* gout (*page 120*) *as primary diagnosis invariably*	2470
25▲–731	Calcification of . . . (not due to infection or trauma). *Specify cartilage*	2570
24▲–764.4	Deformity of . . . due to rickets. *Specify joint*	2470
248–764.4	Genu valgum due to rickets (knock knee)	2470
24▲–7642	Deformity of . . . due to osteomalacia. *Specify joint*	2470
24▲▲–794	Premature closure of cranial sutures. *Specify suture* (*page 13*)	2470
24▲.7–755	Pigmented villo-nodular synovitis	2470
25▲–797	Senile ossification of . . . . *Specify cartilage*	2570
24▲–755	Xanthoma of . . . . *Specify joint*	2470

—8 NEW GROWTHS

25▲–873B	Chondroma of . . . . *Specify cartilage, e.g.*	2580
251–873B	Chondroma of intervertebral cartilage	2580
25▲–873F	Chondrosarcoma of cartilage. *Specify cartilage*	2580
24▲–871B	Myxoma of . . . . *Specify joint*	2480
24▲–8771	Synovioma of . . . . *Specify joint and behavior*	2480
2▲▲–8▲▲▲	Unlisted tumor of joint. *Specify joint, neoplasm and behavior*	2480

—9 DISEASES DUE TO UNKNOWN OR UNCERTAIN CAUSE WITH THE STRUCTURAL REACTION MANIFEST

240–932	Arthritis due to rheumatic fever. *Record* rheumatic fever *as primary diagnosis invariably*	2490
24▲–952	Arthritis rheumatoid of . . . . *Specify, e.g.*	2490
240–952	Arthritis rheumatoid multiple	2490
241–952	Arthritis rheumatoid of spine	2490
25▲–911	Cartilage, atrophy of, due to unknown cause. *Specify cartilage*	2590
25▲–943	Cartilage, hypertrophy of, due to unknown cause. *Specify cartilage, e.g.*	2590
253–943	Knee	2590
26x–9x6	Clawfoot	2590

240–912	Degenerative joint disease, multiple, due to unknown cause; osteoarthritis	2491
26x–900.4	Flatfoot, fixed type due to unknown cause (contracture of ligaments has occurred)	2600
248–9x6	Genu valgum due to unknown cause	2490
24x1–940	Hallux rigidus due to unknown cause	2490
24x1–9x4	Hallux valgus due to unknown cause	2490
26x–9x4	Hammer toe due to unknown cause	2600
2511–9x9	Herniation of nucleus pulposus due to unknown cause	2590
24▲–9x8	Hydrarthrosis, intermittent, of . . . . *Specify joint*	2490
261–9x6	Hypertrophy of ligamenta flava	2600
24▲–911	Osteochondritis dissecans of . . . . *Specify joint*	2490
24▲–930	Palindromic rheumatism	2490
240–991	Polyarthritis due to sickle cell anemia	2490
241–9x4	Scoliosis due to unknown cause	2490
24x–9x4	Talipes cavus due to unknown cause	2490

—X DISEASES DUE TO UNKNOWN OR UNCERTAIN CAUSE WITH THE FUNCTIONAL REACTION ALONE MANIFEST

24▲–x90.4	Deformity of joint due to hemophilia. *Specify joint. Diagnose disease*	2490
24▲–x90.7	Deformity of joint due to hemorrhage. *Specify joint. Diagnose disease*	2490
26x–x10	Flatfoot due to posture (capable of restitution)	2600
26x–x30	Flatfoot, spastic, due to muscle spasm (not paralytic)	2600
24▲–x40	Periarticular fibrositis. *Specify joint*	2490

—Y DISEASES DUE TO CAUSE NOT DETERMINABLE IN THE PARTICULAR CASE

Y signifies an incomplete diagnosis. It is to be replaced whenever possible by a code digit signifying the specific diagnosis

25▲–yx9	Calcification of . . . due to unknown cause	0062

DISEASES OF BURSAS

254— Bursas generally or unspecified

For detailed list of bursas, see page 14

—I DISEASES DUE TO INFECTION WITH LOWER ORGANISM

25▲–190	Acute bursitis. *Specify bursa and organism (page 57) when known*	2510
25▲–100	Acute suppurative bursitis. *Specify bursa and organism (page 57)*	2510
25▲–190.0	Chronic bursitis. *Specify bursa and organism (page 57)*	2510

—4 DISEASES DUE TO TRAUMA OR PHYSICAL AGENT

25▲–4x0	Acute bursitis of . . . due to trauma. *Specify bursa*	2540
25▲–43x	Adventitious bursa. *Specify bursa*	2540
25▲–4x0.0	Chronic bursitis of . . . due to trauma. *Specify bursa, e.g.*	2540
25▲–4x0.9	Chronic bursitis of . . . with calcification. *Specify bursa*	2540
258–430	Gluteal bursitis	2540
25▲–4▲▲	Injury of . . . . *Specify bursa and injury (page 83)*	2540
257–430	Olecranon bursitis; miner's elbow; tennis elbow	2540
259–430	Prepatellar bursitis	2540

—7 DISEASES DUE TO DISORDER OF METABOLISM, GROWTH, OR NUTRITION
Record primary diagnosis

25▲–741	Bursitis of . . . due to gout. *Specify bursa*	2570

—8 NEW GROWTHS

25▲–873B	Chondroma of . . . . *Specify bursa*	2580
25▲–870A	Fibroma of . . . . *Specify bursa*	2580
25▲–871B	Myxoma of . . . . *Specify bursa*	2580
25▲–879	Sarcoma of . . . . *Specify bursa and behavior*	2580
25▲–8▲▲▲	Unlisted tumor of . . . . *Specify bursa, neoplasm, and behavior*	2580

**—9 DISEASES DUE TO UNKNOWN OR UNCERTAIN CAUSE WITH THE
STRUCTURAL REACTION MANIFEST**

25▲–930   Bursitis of . . . due to unknown cause.
                          Specify bursa   2590
25▲–923   Deposits of calcium in . . . *Specify*
                          bursa   2590

DISEASES OF MUSCLES

270– Striated muscles

For detailed list of muscles, see page 15

—0 DISEASES DUE TO GENETIC AND PRENATAL INFLUENCES

27▲–011	Absence of . . . . *Specify muscle*	2701
27▲–031	Accessory; supernumerary . . . . *Specify muscles*	2701
270–090	Amyoplasia congenita	2701
	Amyotonia congenita. *See page 421*	
27▲–017	Contracture of . . . congenital. *Specify muscle*	2701
278–017	Contracture of hamstring muscles, congenital	2701
27▲–037	Diastasis, congenital, of . . . . *Specify muscle, e.g.*	2701
27325–037	Rectus abdominis	2701
28819–013	Ligamentum patallae, elongation of	2701
270–044	Myotonia congenita	2701
270–0441	Myotonia congenita intermittens	2701
27▲–050	Obstetric paralysis. *Specify muscle. Diagnose injury of nerve. See page 429*	2701
270–043	Paramyotonia congenita	2701
272–017	Torticollis, congenital	2701
2x72–042	Weakness of muscles of calf (gastrocnemius and soleus), congenital	2701

—I DISEASES DUE TO INFECTION WITH LOWER ORGANISM

27▲–100.2	Abscess of . . . . *Specify muscle and organism (page 57) when known*	2710
27▲–100.4	Contracture of . . . due to infection. *Specify muscle*	2710
27▲–100	Myositis, acute, of . . . . *Specify muscle and organism (page 57) when known*	2711
27▲–100.0	Myositis, chronic (chronic myogelosis), of . . . . *Specify muscle*	2711

—4 DISEASES DUE TO TRAUMA OR PHYSICAL AGENT

27▲–402	Contusion of . . . . *Specify muscle*	2740
27▲–400.4	Contracture of . . . due to trauma. *Specify muscle and trauma when known, e.g.*	2740
279–431.4	Short Achilles tendon due to posture	2740

279–400.4	Short Achilles tendon due to unspecified trauma	*2740*
270–499	Cramps, general muscular, due to immersion	*2740*
270–445	Cramps, general muscular due to radiant heat: heat cramps	*2740*
27▲–4▲▲.5	Diastasis of . . . . *Specify muscle and cause, e.g.*	*2740*
27325–43x.5	Of rectus abdominis due to pregnancy	*2740*
27325–415.5	Of rectus abdominis following operation	*2740*
27▲–438	Foreign body reaction of muscle. *Specify muscle*	*2740*
27▲–4x7	Hematoma of . . . . *Specify muscle*	*2740*
27▲–4x9	Hernia of . . . . *Specify muscle*	*2740*
27▲–44x	Myositis (myogelosis) of . . . due to cold. *Specify muscle*	*2740*
27▲–432	Myositis (myogelosis) of . . . due to occupation. *Specify muscle*	*2740*
27x–432	Writer's cramp	*2740*
27▲–4x6	Myositis ossificans of . . . . *Specify muscle, e.g.*	*2740*
276–4x6	Brachialis anticus	*2740*
	Adductors of thigh	
27817–4x6	Rider's bone	*2740*
27819–4x6	Quadriceps femoris	*2740*
27▲–43x	Myositis of . . . due to overstrain. *Specify muscle*	*2740*
27▲–430	Myositis of . . . due to trauma. *Specify muscle. Not to be diagnosed in cases of simple healing injury*	*2740*
27▲–416	Rupture, complete of . . . . *Specify muscle*	*2740*
27▲–412	Rupture, incomplete, of . . . . *Specify muscle*	*2740*
27▲–415.4	Scar of muscle following operation. *Specify muscle*	*2740*
27▲–400.4	Scar of muscle due to trauma. *Specify muscle*	*2740*
272–44x	Torticollis, acute, due to cold	*2740*
272–4x4	Torticollis, chronic, due to trauma	*2740*
27▲–410	Wound of . . . . *Specify muscle*	*2740*
27▲–410.0	Wound, infected,[1] of . . . . *Specify muscle*	*2740*

---

[1] When the infection is more important than the wound, especially when the organism is determined, classify as infection. If both injury and infection are important, two diagnoses are required.

—50 DISEASES DUE TO CIRCULATORY DISTURBANCE
Record primary diagnosis when possible

27▲–514   Contracture of . . . due to ischemia.
              Specify muscle   *2750*

—55 DISEASES DUE TO DISTURBANCE OF INNERVATION OR OF PSYCHIC CONTROL
Record primary diagnosis when possible

2747–551   Irritability of levator ani muscle (coc-
              cygodynia)   *2755*
27▲–590.x   Muscular dystrophy, reflex type   *2755*
270–562   Myasthenia gravis   *2755*
27▲–564   Paralysis, residual of . . . following polio-
              myelitis. *Specify muscle or group of*
              muscles   *2755*
27▲–568   Paralysis, flaccid, of . . . due to poison.
              Specify muscle or group of muscles.
              Specify poison in primary diagnosis   *2755*
27▲–567   Paralysis, flaccid, of . . . due to lesion of
              central nervous system. *Specify*
              muscle or group of muscles. Record
              primary diagnosis when applicable   *2755*
27▲–569   Paralysis, flaccid, of . . . due to nerve le-
              sion. *Specify muscle or group of mus-*
              cles. Record primary diagnosis when
              applicable   *2755*
27▲–561   Paralysis, spastic, of . . . . *Specify mus-*
              cle or group of muscles   *2755*
272–550   Spasmus nutans   *2755*
272–590   Torticollis due to ocular imbalance   *2755*

—7 DISEASES DUE TO DISORDER OF METABOLISM, GROWTH OR NUTRITION
Record primary diagnosis

27▲–713   Atrophy of . . . due to disuse. *Specify*
              muscle   *2770*
270–731   Progressive ossifying myositis   *2770*
270–712   Recurrent rhabdomyolysis, exertional type
              (recurrent myoglobinuria)   *2770*
270–748   Recurrent rhabdomyolysis, nonexertional
              type (idiopathic myoglobinuria)   *2770*

—8 NEW GROWTHS

27▲–870A   Fibroma of . . . (desmoid). *Specify mus-*
              cle   *2780*
27▲–870F   Fibrosarcoma of . . . . *Specify muscle*   *2780*
27▲–850A   Hemangioma of . . . . *Specify muscle*   *2780*

—9 DISEASES DUE TO UNKNOWN OR UNCERTAIN CAUSE WITH THE STRUCTURAL REACTION MANIFEST

—X DISEASES DUE TO UNKNOWN OR UNCERTAIN CAUSE WITH THE FUNCTIONAL REACTION ALONE MANIFEST

DISEASES OF THE DIAPHRAGM

275– Diaphragm

—0 DISEASES DUE TO GENETIC AND PRENATAL INFLUENCES

275–012	Defect of diaphragm, congenital	2701
275–027	Diaphragmatic hernia, congenital	2701
275–021	Elevation of diaphragm, congenital	2701
275–037	Enlargement of normal apertures in diaphragm, congenital	2701
275–037.9	Esophageal hiatus hernia, congenital	2701
275–016	Eventration of diaphragm, congenital	2701

—I DISEASES DUE TO INFECTION WITH LOWER ORGANISM
For subdiaphragmatic peritonitis see page 299.

275–100	Diaphragmitis. *Specify organism (page 57) when known*	2711
275–100.3	Fistula of diaphragm. *Specify organism (page 57) when known*	2710
3052–100.3	Bronchovisceral fistula (abnormal opening in diaphragm between bronchi and abdominal organs). *Specify organism (page 57) when known*	2710
3072–100.3	Pleuroperitoneal fistula. *Specify organism (page 57) when known*	2710
3061–100.3	Pulmonoperitoneal fistula. *Specify organism (page 57) when known*	2710
2750–100	Infection at congenital abnormal apertures in diaphragm. *Specify organism (page 57) when known*	2710

—4 DISEASES DUE TO TRAUMA

275–409	Avulsion of diaphragm, peripheral	2740
275–414	Gunshot wound of diaphragm	2740
275–424	Hernia of diaphragm due to trauma.	2740
275–43x	Inversion of diaphragm (due to abnormal intrathoracic tension)	2740
275–436	Puncture of diaphragm by fractured rib	2740
275–415	Puncture of diaphragm by instrument	2740
275–416	Rupture of diaphragm	2740
275–411	Stab wound of diaphragm	2740

—55 DISEASES DUE TO DISTURBANCE OF INNERVATION OR OF PSYCHIC CONTROL

Record primary diagnosis when possible

275–560	Flaccid paralysis of diaphragm	2755
275–564	Following poliomyelitis	2755
275–569	Due to section of phrenic nerve	2755
275–595	Reflex spasm of diaphragm (hiccup)	2755

—6 DISEASES DUE TO OR CONSISTING OF STATIC MECHANICAL ABNORMALITY OF UNKNOWN ORIGIN

2751–639	Paraesophageal hiatal hernia	2760
275–639	Sliding esophageal hiatal hernia	2760

—8 NEW GROWTHS

See under Muscles, *page 169.   Make necessary change in 3d digit*

DISEASES OF TENDONS, FASCIA, ETC.

280 – Tendons
280.9– Tendon sheaths
290 – Fascia
28x – Tendons and tendon sheaths

> *To indicate the tendon of any particular muscle, choose the specific code from section 27 and change the second digit from 7 to 8; e.g., 27722 Opponens pollicis would become 28722 Tendon of Opponens pollicis. To indicate tendon sheath add .9 to end of tendon code.*

—0 DISEASES DUE TO GENETIC AND PRENATAL INFLUENCES

287–017	Stenosis of tendon sheath of finger, congenital; trigger finger, congenital	*2801*

—I DISEASES DUE TO INFECTION WITH LOWER ORGANISM

29▲–100.2	Abscess of . . . . *Specify fascia or fascial space and organism (page 57) when known*	*2910*
2964–100.2	Palmar abscess	*2910*
28▲.9–100.2	Abscess of . . . . *Specify tendon sheath*	*2810*
29▲–100	Fasciitis of . . . due to infection. *Specify fascia and organism (page 57) when known*	*2910*
2966–100	Infection of distal closed space of finger (felon). *Specify organism (page 57) when known*	*2910*
28▲–100.1	Sloughing of . . . . *Specify tendon and organism (page 57) when known*	*2810*
29▲–100.1	Sloughing of . . . . *Specify fascia and organism (page 57) when known*	*2910*
28▲–100	Tendonitis, acute	*2810*
28▲–100.0	Tendonitis, chronic	*2810*
28▲.9–100	Tenosynovitis, acute, of . . . due to infection. *Specify tendon sheath and organism (page 57) when known*	*2810*
28▲.9–100.4	Tenosynovitis, adhesive, of . . . . *Specify tendon sheath and organism (page 57) when known*	*2810*

—4 DISEASES DUE TO TRAUMA OR PHYSICAL AGENT

29▲–400.4	Contracture of . . . due to trauma.	
	Specify fascia	*2940*
29▲–430	Fasciitis due to trauma. *Specify fascia*	*2940*
296–430	Palmar fasciitis	*2940*
299–430	Plantar fasciitis due to stress	*2940*
28▲–4▲▲	Injury of . . . . *Specify tendon and injury (page 83)*	*2840*
28▲–406	Dislocation of . . . . *Specify tendon*	*2840*
28▲–405	Division (partial or complete) of . . . . *Specify tendon*	*2840*
28▲–416	Rupture of . . . . *Specify tendon*	*2840*
293–424	Pannicular lumbosacroiliac hernia	*2940*
28▲.9–43x	Tenosynovitis of . . . due to trauma. *Specify tendon sheath*	*2840*

—6 DISEASES DUE TO OR CONSISTING OF MECHANICAL ABNORMALITY OF UNKNOWN ORIGIN

297–630	Snapping hip	*2460*
287–646	Trigger finger, acquired	*2860*

—7 DISEASES DUE TO DISORDER OF METABOLISM, GROWTH, OR NUTRITION

28▲–755	Xanthoma of . . . . *Specify tendon*	*2870*

—8 NEW GROWTHS

28▲–873B	Chondroma of . . . . *Specify tendon*	*2880*
28▲–870A	Fibroma of . . . . *Specify tendon*	*2880*
28▲–8741A	Giant cell tumor of . . . benign. *Specify tendon sheath*	*2880*
28▲–850A	Hemangioma of . . . . *Specify tendon*	*2880*
28▲–872A	Lipoma of . . . . *Specify tendon*	*2880*
28▲–8▲▲▲	Unlisted tumor of . . . . *Specify tendon, neoplasm and behavior*	*2880*

—9 DISEASES DUE TO UNKNOWN OR UNCERTAIN CAUSE WITH THE STRUCTURAL REACTION MANIFEST

28▲.9–923	Calcification of . . . . *Specify tendon sheath*	*2890*
29▲–9x4	Contracture	*2990*
296–9x6	Dupuytren's	*2990*
28▲.9–940	Tenosynovitis crepitans of . . . . *Specify tendon sheath*	*2890*
28▲.9–952	Tenosynovitis, villous, of . . . . *Specify tendon sheath*	*2890*

3- DISEASES OF THE RESPIRATORY SYSTEM

30- Respiratory System

DISEASES OF THE NOSE

310– Nose
312– Nostril
313– Septum
315– Turbinates, generally
316– Middle turbinate
317– Inferior turbinate
318– Nasopharynx
31x– Intrinsic vessels
125– Mucous membrane of nose
133– Skin of nose
216– Nasal bones
x100– Olfactory sense

(For detailed list of structures of nose, see page 22)

—0 DISEASES DUE TO GENETIC AND PRENATAL INFLUENCES

310–011	Absence of nose, congenital	3101
31▲–012	Absence of part of nose, congenital. *Specify part*	3101
312–018	Atresia of choana, congenital	3101
310–037	Bifid nose	3101
313–022	Deflection of nasal septum, congenital	3101
310–022	Deformity of nose; notching of tip of nose, congenital	3101
310–010	Flattening of nose, congenital (with harelip)	3101
312–017	Stenosis of nares, congenital	3101

—I DISEASES DUE TO INFECTION WITH LOWER ORGANISM

318–100.2	Abscess, nasopharyngeal. *Specify organism (page 57) when known, e.g.*	3110
3181–100.2	Abscess of pharyngeal bursas. *Specify organism (page 57) when known*	3110
313–100.2	Abscess of septum. *Specify organism (page 57) when known*	3110
312–100.4	Adhesions in nose (anterior or posterior portion) due to infection	3110
x00–100.x	Anosmia due to infection	3110
3181–100.8	Cyst of pharyngeal bursas, due to infection	3110
310–147.4	Deformity of nose and nasal bones due to syphilis	3110
310–100.4	Deformity of nose due to infection	3110
313–100.4	Deflection of septum due to infection	3110
318–125	Diphtheria, nasopharyngeal	3111

125–100.0	Furuncle of vestibule	*3110*
317–190	Gangosa	*3110*
310–126	Glanders of nose	*3110*
310–124	Leprosy of nose	*3110*
318–100	Nasopharyngitis	*3111*
313–100.3	Perforation of septum due to infection	*3110*
313–147.3	Perforation of septum due to syphilis	*3110*
313–123.3	Perforation of septum due to tuberculosis	*3110*
316–1x6	Polyp of middle turbinate, due to infection	*3110*
310–100	Rhinitis, acute. *Specify organism (page 57) when known; diagnose ordinarily as common cold (page 175)*	*3110*
310–16▲	Rhinitis, acute, associated with exanthem. *Specify exanthem (page 57)*	*3110*
310–1x6	Rhinitis, hypertrophic, due to infection	*3110*
133–130	Rhinoscleroma	*3110*
310–123	Tuberculosis of nose	*3110*
310–100.9	Ulcer of nose due to infection. *Specify organism (page 57) when known*	*3110*

—2 DISEASES DUE TO HIGHER PLANT OR ANIMAL PARASITE

3011–200.3	Fistula of nasopharynx due to fungus. *Specify fungus when known (page 63)*	*3120*
310–231	Rhinosporidiosis	*3120*

—3 DISEASES DUE TO INTOXICATION

310–3▲▲	Acute rhinitis due to chemical poison. *Specify poison (page 67), e.g.*	*3130*
310–319	Due to poisonous gases	*3130*
310–391	Allergic rhinitis (hay fever)	*3139*
310–300.6	Chronic hypertrophic rhinitis due to chemical irritant. *Specify irritant when known*	*3130*

—4 DISEASES DUE TO TRAUMA OR PHYSICAL AGENT

312–400.4	Adhesions in nose (anterior or posterior portion), due to trauma	*3140*
312–415.4	Adhesions in nose (anterior or posterior portion), following operation	*3140*
313–400.4	Deflection of septum due to trauma	*3142*
216–400.4	Deformity of nose and nasal bones due to trauma	*3140*
216–408	Dislocation of nose	*3140*
310–400.7	Epistaxis due to trauma	*3141*
310–496	Foreign body in nose	*3143*

310–448	Frostbite of nose	*3140*
310–402.7	Hematoma of nose due to trauma. . . .	
	Specify part of nose, if desired	*3140*
31▲–4▲▲	Injury of nose . . . . *Specify injury*	
	(page 83) and part of nose	*3140*
313–430.3	Perforation of septum due to repeated	
	trauma	*3140*
313–415.3	Perforation of septum following operation	*3140*
310–438	Rhinitis, acute, due to foreign body	*3140*
310–438.0	Rhinitis, chronic, due to foreign body	*3140*
313–4x6	Spur of septum due to trauma	*3140*
318–415.4	Stenosis of nasopharynx following opera-	
	tion	*3140*
310–400.9	Ulcer of nose due to trauma	*3140*

—50 DISEASES DUE TO CIRCULATORY DISTURBANCE
Record primary diagnosis when possible

31x–533.5	Epistaxis due to hypertension	*3150*
310–518	Hydrorrhea due to vasomotor disturbance	*3150*
313–522.9	Varicose ulcer of septum	*3150*

—6 DISEASES DUE TO OR CONSISTING OF STATIC MECHANICAL AB-
NORMALITY

318–600.8	Cyst of nasopharynx	*3160*
313–640	Deflection of septum due to unknown	
	cause	*3164*
316–6x8	Mucocele of middle turbinate	*3160*
312–611	Obstruction of nose due to foreign body	*3160*
310–615	Rhinolith	*3160*
31x–641	Varicose veins of septum	*3160*

—7 DISEASES DUE TO DISORDER OF METABOLISM, GROWTH, OR NUTRITION

216–794	Deformity of nose and nasal bones, de-	
	velopmental	*3170*
310–786	Vicarious menstruation, nasal	*3170*

—8 NEW GROWTHS

310–8091	Adenocarcinoma of nose. *Specify behavior*	*3180*
310–8091A	Adenoma of nose	*3180*
310–814	Epidermoid carcinoma of nose. *Specify*	
	behavior (page 99)	*3180*
310–870	Fibrosarcoma of nose. *Specify behavior*	
	(page 99)	*3180*
310–850A	Hemangioma of nose	*3180*
310–830	Lymphosarcoma of nose	*3180*

310–8451	Neurofibroma of nose. *Specify behavior*	*3180*
310–833	Plasma cell myeloma[1] of nose. *Specify behavior*	*3180*
310–814A	Squamous cell papilloma of nose	*3180*
310–811	Transitional cell carcinoma of nose. *Specify behavior*	*3180*
310–8▲▲▲	Unlisted tumor of nose. *Specify neoplasm and behavior*	*3180*

—9 DISEASES DUE TO UNKNOWN OR UNCERTAIN CAUSE WITH THE STRUCTURAL REACTION MANIFEST

310–957	Atrophic rhinitis	*3190*
313–900.6	Exostosis of nasal septum	*3190*
31▲–940	Hypertrophic rhinitis due to unknown cause. *Specify part of nose*	*3190*
31▲–944	Polyp of nose, simple. *Specify part of nose*	*3194*
310–951	Ulcer of nose due to unknown cause	*3190*

—X DISEASES DUE TO UNKNOWN OR UNCERTAIN CAUSE WITH THE FUNCTIONAL REACTION ALONE MANIFEST

x00–x10	Anosmia due to unknown cause	*3190*
31x–x30	Epistaxis due to unknown cause	*3190*
310–x30	Hydrorrhea due to unknown cause	*3190*

—Y DISEASES DUE TO CAUSE NOT DETERMINABLE IN THE PARTICULAR CASE

Y signifies an incomplete diagnosis. It is to be replaced whenever possible by a code digit signifying the specific diagnosis

| 310–yx7 | Epistaxis due to undetermined cause | *0063* |

---

[1] Use lymphoma behavior code (page 99).

DISEASES OF THE ACCESSORY SINUSES

320–   Accessory sinuses
321–   Maxillary sinus
322–   Frontal sinus
323–   Ethmoid sinus
324–   Sphenoid sinus

—0 DISEASES DUE TO GENETIC AND PRENATAL INFLUENCES

32▲–039	Anomalous sinus. *Specify sinus*	*3201*
32▲–032	Duplication of sinus. *Specify sinus*	*3201*
32▲–014	Hyperplasia of sinus system. *Specify sinus*	*3201*
32▲–012	Partial absence of sinus. *Specify sinus*	*3201*
32▲–019	Persistence of fetal form. *Specify sinus*	*3201*

—I DISEASES DUE TO INFECTION WITH LOWER ORGANISM

302▲–100.3	Fistula of . . . due to infection. *Specify combined parts as*	*3210*
3021–100.3	Bucomaxillary fistula	*3210*
32▲–100.6	Granuloma of sinus due to infection. *Specify sinus*	*3210*
32▲–100.8	Mucocele of sinus. *Specify organism (page 57) when known*	*3210*
32▲–100	Sinusitis, acute. *Specify sinus and organism (page 57) when known*	*3211*
32▲–100.0	Sinusitis, chronic. *Specify sinus and organism (page 57) when known*	*3211*
320–100	Sinusitis, pansinusitis, acute (including subacute). *Specify organism (page 57) when known*	*3211*
320–190	Sinusitis (pansinusitis), nonpurulent, chronic. *Specify sinus and organism (page 57) when known*	*3211*
32▲–130	Sinusitis, purulent, acute. *Specify sinus and organism (page 57) when known*	*3211*
320–100.0	Sinusitis, pansinusitis, purulent, chronic. *Specify sinus when known and organism (page 57) when known*	*3211*
32▲–123	Tuberculosis of sinus. *Specify sinus*	*3211*

—2 DISEASES DUE TO HIGHER PLANT OR ANIMAL PARASITE

32▲–2952	Myiasis of sinus. *Specify sinus*	*3220*

—3 DISEASES DUE TO INTOXICATION

320–3▲▲   Sinusitis (pansinusitis) due to chemical
                 irritant. *Specify irritant (page 67)*
                 when known   *3230*

—4 DISEASES DUE TO TRAUMA OR PHYSICAL AGENT

321–481.0   Barosinusitis   *3248*
3021–415.3   Fistula of maxillary sinus following opera-
                 tion. *Including dental extraction*   *3240*
32▲–400.6   Granuloma of sinus due to trauma.
                 Specify sinus   *3240*
32▲–4▲▲   Injury of sinus. *Specify sinus and injury*
                 (page 83)   *3240*

**—6 DISEASES DUE TO OR CONSISTING OF STATIC MECHANICAL AB-
NORMALITY**

32▲–615   Rhinolith in sinus. *Specify sinus*   *3260*
32▲–600   Vacuum in sinus. *Specify sinus*   *3260*

—8 NEW GROWTHS

*See under Nose, page 178. Make necessary changes in 2d and
3d digits.*

**—9 DISEASES DUE TO UNKNOWN OR UNCERTAIN CAUSE WITH THE
STRUCTURAL REACTION MANIFEST**

32▲–9x8   Cystic degeneration of sinus. *Specify*
                 sinus   *3290*
32▲–944   Polyp formation, simple. *Specify sinus*   *3294*

DISEASES OF THE LARYNX

330– Larynx
331– Epiglottis
336– Vocal cord
338– Articulations
339– Intrinsic muscles
33x– Intrinsic vessels

For detailed list of structures of larynx, see page 22

—0 DISEASES DUE TO GENETIC AND PRENATAL INFLUENCES

33▲–011	Absence of larynx or of a part, congenital. *Specify part*	3301
330–018	Atresia of larynx, congenital	3301
330–017	Constriction of larynx, congenital; congenital laryngismus stridulus	3301
334–025	Cricoid cartilage, abnormal union of, with thyroid cartilage	3301
33▲–064	Cyst of larynx, congenital. *Specify part*	3301
331–034	Epiglottis, fissure of, congenital	3301
331–016	Epiglottis, hypoplasia of	3301
3031–025	Larynx and trachea, abnormal union of	3301
331–013	Petiolus, elongation of	3301
333–025	Thyroid cartilage, abnormal union of, with hyoid bone	3301
333–037	Thyroid cartilage, total ventral cleft of, congenital	3301
330–023	Thyroid aberrant in larynx (laryngeal struma)	3301
337–027	Ventricular laryngocele, congenital	3301
337–026	Ventricular sacculation, intralaryngeal, congenital	3301
330–077	Web of larynx, congenital	3301

—I DISEASES DUE TO INFECTION WITH LOWER ORGANISM

330–100.2	Abscess of larynx. *Specify organism (page 57) when known*	3310
3381–100.4	Cricoarytenoid articulation, ankylosis of, ... *Specify organism (page 57) when known*	3310
3381–100	Cricoarytenoid articulation, arthritis of, ... *Specify organism (page 57) when known*	3310
330–125	Diphtheria, laryngeal	3311

332–100.8	Edema, obstructive, of glottis due to infection	*3310*
331–100	Epiglottitis. *Specify organism (page 57) when known*	*3310*
303▲–100.3	Fistula of larynx. *Specify site and organism (page 57) when known*	*3310*
33▲–100.6	Granuloma of . . . . *Specify site and organism when known*	*3310*
330–166	Herpes simplex of larynx	*3310*
330–100	Laryngitis, acute. *Specify organism (page 57) when known*	*3311*
330–100.0	Laryngitis, chronic, due to infection	*3311*
330–1x0.9	Atrophic laryngitis due to infection	*3311*
330–1x0.6	Infiltrative laryngitis due to infection	*3311*
330–1413	Laryngitis due to Borrelia vincenti	*3311*
3031–100	Laryngotracheitis, acute. *Specify organism (page 57) when known*	*3312*
3031–100.0	Laryngotracheitis, chronic, due to infection	*3312*
330–124	Leprosy of larynx	*3310*
335–100	Perichondritis of larynx. *Specify organism when known, e.g.*	*3310*
335–147	Syphilitic perichondritis of larynx	*3310*
330–1x0	Sarcoidosis of larynx	*3310*
330–100.4	Stenosis of larynx due to infection	*3310*
330–123	Tuberculosis of larynx	*3310*

—2 DISEASES DUE TO HIGHER PLANT OR ANIMAL PARASITE

330–29▲	Insects in larynx. *Specify (page 63)*	*3320*
33▲–2▲▲	Laryngitis due to parasitic infection. *Specify part of larynx and parasite (page 63)*	*3320*

—3 DISEASES DUE TO INTOXICATION

330–3▲▲	Chemical burn of larynx. *Specify poison (page 67)*	*3330*
330–300.0	Laryngitis, due to poison. *Specify poison (page 67) when known*	*3330*
332–300.8	Edema, obstructive, of glottis due to poison. *Specify poison (page 67) when known*	*3330*
336–3x0	Fibrinous chorditis due to poisonous gas or fumes	*3330*
339–3238.x	Paralysis of larynx due to lead poisoning	*3330*
330–3931	Serum diseases of larynx	*3330*
339–300.4	Spasm of larynx due to poison. *Specify poison when known*	*3330*

330–300.4	Stricture of larynx due to poison. *Specify poison when known*	*3330*
330–390	Urticaria of larynx; angioneurotic edema of larynx	*3330*

—4 DISEASES DUE TO TRAUMA OR PHYSICAL AGENT

330–441	Burn of larynx from heat	*3340*
330–472.0	Burn of larynx by radium	*3340*
330–471.0	Burn of larynx by roentgen rays (x-rays)	*3340*
336–43x	Chorditis, acute, due to overstrain	*3340*
338–406	Dislocation of articulation of larynx	*3340*
3381–406	Of cricoarytenoid	*3340*
3382–406	Of cricothyroid	*3340*
332–408	Edema, obstructive, of glottis due to trauma	*3340*
331–401	Epiglottis, abrasion of	*3340*
331–441	Epiglottis, burn of, from heat	*3340*
303▲–400.3	Fistula of larynx due to trauma	*3340*
303▲–415.3	Fistula of larynx following operation	*3340*
330–496	Foreign body in larynx	*3343*
330–414	Gunshot wound of larynx	*3340*
33▲–4x7	Hematoma of larynx. *Specify part*	*3340*
21x–416	Hyoid bone, fracture of	*3340*
336–430	Hyperkeratosis of vocal cord	*3340*
336–430.9	Contact ulcer due to hyperkeratosis of vocal cord	*3340*
33▲–4▲▲	Injury of larynx. *Specify part and injury (page 83)*	*3340*
336–43x.6	Laryngeal nodules	*3340*
337–4x9	Laryngeal ventricle, prolapse of, due to trauma or strain	*3340*
330–43x	Laryngitis, chronic, due to vocal overstrain	*3340*
335–4x0	Perichondritis due to trauma or following operation	*3340*
335–47▲	Radiation injury of laryngeal perichondrium. *Specify radioactive substance*	*3340*
339–438.4	Spasm of larynx due to foreign body	*3343*
330–411	Stab wound of larynx	*3340*
330–415.4	Stenosis of larynx, cicatricial, due to intubation or following operation	*3340*
330–4▲▲.4	Stenosis of larynx due to trauma. *Specify trauma*	*3340*
330–4702.4	Stenosis of larynx following radiation	*3340*
336–416	Thyroid cartilage, fracture of	*3340*

—50 DISEASES DUE TO CIRCULATORY DISTURBANCE
Record primary diagnosis when possible

332–505.8	Edema, obstructive, of glottis due to chemical changes in blood	*3350*
330–544.1	Necrosis of larynx in granulocytopenia	*3350*

—55 DISEASES DUE TO DISTURBANCE OF INNERVATION OR OF PSYCHIC CONTROL
Record primary diagnosis when possible

330–593	Hyperesthesia due to reflex action of larynx	*3355*
339–5631	Paralysis of larynx due to diphtheria toxin	*3355*
3391–5631	Abductor paralysis	*3355*
3392–5631	Adductor paralysis	*3355*
3393–5631	Bilateral paralysis	*3355*
3394–5631	Unilateral paralysis	*3355*
339–569	Paralysis of larynx due to pressure	*3355*
3391–569	Abductor paralysis	*3355*
3392–569	Adductor paralysis	*3355*
3393–569	Bilateral paralysis	*3355*
3394–569	Unilateral paralysis	*3355*
336–569	Paralysis of vocal cord due to lesion of nerve	*3355*
339–567	Spasm of glottis due to lesion of central nervous system	*3355*
339–590	Spasm of glottis, reflex, through recurrent laryngeal nerve	*3355*
330–567.4	Stenosis of larynx due to bilateral abductor paralysis from lesion of central nervous system	*3355*
330–560.4	Stenosis of larynx due to double abductor paralysis from peripheral lesion	*3355*

—6 DISEASES DUE TO OR CONSISTING OF STATIC MECHANICAL AB-NORMALITY

330–600.8	Cyst of larynx	*3360*
330–631	Laryngoptosis	*3360*
330–611	Obstruction of larynx due to foreign body	*3360*
337–631	Prolapse of laryngeal ventricle	*3360*
33x–641	Varix of vocal cord	*3360*

—7 DISEASES DUE TO DISORDER OF METABOLISM, GROWTH, OR NUTRITION
Record primary diagnosis when possible

330–776	Acromegaly affecting larynx	*3370*
330–776.4	Stricture of larynx due to acromegaly	*3370*

—8 NEW GROWTHS

337–8091	Adenocarcinoma of laryngeal ventricle. *Specify behavior*	*3380*
330–8091A	Adenoma of larynx	*3380*
330–873B	Chondroma of larynx	*3380*
33▲–814	Epidermoid carcinoma of larynx. *Specify behavior*	*3380*
330–870A	Fibroma of larynx	*3380*
330–872A	Lipoma of larynx	*3380*
330–8▲▲▲	Unlisted tumor of larynx. *Specify neoplasm and behavior*	*3380*

—9 DISEASES DUE TO UNKNOWN OR UNCERTAIN CAUSE WITH THE STRUCTURAL REACTION MANIFEST

330–913	Aphthous ulcer of larynx	*3390*
330–957	Atrophic laryngitis due to unknown cause	*3390*
330–923	Calcification of larynx	*3390*
330–940	Chronic laryngitis due to unknown cause	*3390*
330–900.8	Edema of larynx, cause unknown	*3390*
336–900.6	Hypertrophy of vocal cords, cause unknown	*3390*
330–954	Infiltrative laryngitis due to unknown cause	*3390*
336–941	Leukoplakia of vocal cord	*3390*
330–944	Polyp of larynx, simple	*3394*
336–944	Polyp of vocal cord, simple	*3394*
3301–940	Subglottic laryngitis due to unknown cause	*3390*

DISEASES OF THE TRACHEA

340– Trachea
341– Cartilages
342– Mucosa
343– Bifurcation

—0 DISEASES DUE TO GENETIC AND PRENATAL INFLUENCES

340–011	Absence of trachea, congenital	*3401*
341–076	Arrested development of tracheal rings	*3401*
340–036	Diverticulum of trachea, congenital	*3401*
304▲–029	Fistula of trachea, external or internal, congenital (tracheocele)	*3401*
3041–024	Fusion of bifurcation of trachea and esophagus with absence of trachea	*3401*
341–024	Incomplete separation of tracheal rings	*3401*
341–010	Malformation of tracheal rings	*3401*
340–017	Stenosis of trachea, congenital	*3401*
340–023	Thyroid aberrant in trachea	*3401*
3041–029	Tracheoesophageal fistula, congenital	*3401*

—I DISEASES DUE TO INFECTION WITH LOWER ORGANISM

340–100	Acute tracheitis due to infection. *Specify organism (page 57) when known*	*3411*
340–100.4	Stenosis of trachea due to infection	*3410*
340–147.4	Due to syphilis	*3410*
340–123	Tuberculosis of trachea	*3410*

—3 DISEASES DUE TO INTOXICATION

340–3▲▲	Acute tracheitis due to poison. *Specify (page 67)*	*3430*
340–300.4	Stenosis of trachea due to poison. *Specify (page 67) when known*	*3430*

—4 DISEASES DUE TO TRAUMA OR PHYSICAL AGENT

3041–400.3	Fistula, esophagotracheal due to trauma. *Specify trauma*	*3440*
340–496	Foreign body in trachea	*3440*
340–4▲▲	Injury of trachea. *Specify injury (page 83), e.g.*	*3440*
340–416	Fracture of trachea	*3440*
340–435	Stenosis of trachea due to pressure	*3440*
340–4▲▲.4	Stenosis of trachea due to trauma. *Specify trauma*	*3440*

340–415.4	Stenosis of tracheotomy wound	*3440*
340–438	Tracheitis acute due to foreign body (dust)	*3440*
340–438.0	Tracheitis chronic due to foreign body	*3440*
340–400.9	Ulceration of trachea due to trauma	*3440*
340–441.9	Due to burn from heat	*3440*
340–435.9	Due to pressure	*3440*
340–438.9	Due to foreign body	*3440*

—6 DISEASES DUE TO OR CONSISTING OF STATIC MECHANICAL AB-NORMALITY

34x–641	Varix of trachea	*3460*

—8 NEW GROWTHS

340–8091A	Adenoma of trachea	*3480*
340–873B	Chondroma of trachea	*3480*
340–814	Epidermoid carcinoma of trachea. *Specify behavior (page 99)*	*3480*
340–872A	Lipoma of trachea	*3480*
340–8▲▲▲	Unlisted tumor of trachea. *Specify neoplasm and behavior*	*3480*

—9 DISEASES DUE TO UNKNOWN OR UNCERTAIN CAUSE WITH THE STRUCTURAL REACTION MANIFEST

340–923	Calcification of trachea	*3490*

DISEASES OF THE BRONCHI

350 –   Bronchi
353 –   Bronchioles
3053–   Bronchi and skin of thorax
3051–   Bronchi and pleura

For detailed list of structures of bronchi, see page 35

—0 DISEASES DUE TO GENETIC AND PRENATAL INFLUENCES

350–011	Aplasia of bronchus (with aplasia of lung)	*3501*
350–018	Blind bronchus (with absence of lobe of lung)	*3501*
350–015	Bronchiectasis, congenital	*3501*
350–036	Diverticulum of bronchus	*3501*
350–077	Tracheal bronchus; rudimentary tracheal bronchus	*3501*

—I DISEASES DUE TO INFECTION WITH LOWER ORGANISM

350–100.6	Bronchiectasis due to infection. *Specify organism when known, e.g.*	*3514*
350–123.6	Bronchiectasis following tuberculosis	*3514*
353–100.6	Bronchiolectasis due to infection	*3514*
353–100	Bronchiolitis, acute. *Specify organism (page 57) when known*	*3511*
353–100.4	Bronchiolitis, obliterating, due to infection	*3511*
350–100	Bronchitis, acute. *Specify organism (page 57) when known*	*3511*
350–100.0	Bronchitis, chronic. *Specify organism (page 57) when known*	*3511*
350–108	Bronchitis, due to pertussis	*3513*
350–123.9	Broncholithiasis due to tuberculosis	*3512*
350–100.8	Edema of bronchus, localized, due to infection. *Specify organism (page 57) when known*	*3510*
3053–100.3	Fistula, bronchocutaneous, due to infection	*3510*
3053–123.3	Fistula, bronchocutaneous, due to tuberculosis	*3512*
3051–100.3	Fistula, bronchopleural, due to infection, *e.g.*	*3510*
3051–123.3	Fistula, bronchopleural, due to tuberculosis	*3512*
350–100.4	Stenosis of bronchus due to infection. *Specify organism (page 57) when known*	*3510*
350–147	Syphilis of bronchus. *Diagnose ordinarily as* Syphilis of lung	*3510*

350–123   Tuberculosis of bronchus. *Diagnose ordi-*
                     narily as Tuberculosis of lung, *page*
                     193   *3512*

—2 DISEASES DUE TO HIGHER PLANT OR ANIMAL PARASITE

350–220.9   Broncholithiasis due to histoplasmosis   *3520*
35▲–2▲▲   Myocitic or parasitic infection of bronchus.
                     Diagnose ordinarily as Mycotic or
                     parasitic disease of the lung. *Specify*
                     site and organism   *3520*

—3 DISEASES DUE TO INTOXICATION

350–390   Asthma   *3539*
350–3▲▲   Bronchitis due to poison. *Specify (page*
                     67)   *3530*
353–319   Bronchiolitis due to poisonous gas   *3530*
350–300.8   Edema of bronchus, localized, due to
                     poison. *Specify poison when known*
                     (page 67)   *3530*
353–300.4   Obliterating bronchiolitis due to poison.
                     Specify poison when known (page
                     67)   *3530*
350–300.4   Stenosis of bronchus due to poison. *Spec-*
                     ify poison when known (page 67)   *3530*

—4 DISEASES DUE TO TRAUMA OR PHYSICAL AGENT

350–438.6   Bronchiectasis due to foreign body   *3543*
350–430   Deformation of bronchus due to extra-
                     bronchial traction or mass   *3540*
350–400.8   Edema of bronchus, localized, due to
                     trauma   *3540*
305▲–415.3   Fistula of bronchus following operation.
                     Specify site   *3540*
350–496   Foreign body in bronchus   *3543*
350–4▲▲   Injury of bronchus. *Specify (page 83)*   *3540*
350–435   Stenosis of bronchus due to pressure   *3540*
350–400.9   Ulceration of bronchus due to trauma, *e.g.*   *3540*
  350–438.9   Due to foreign body   *3543*

—6 DISEASES DUE TO OR CONSISTING OF STATIC MECHANICAL AB-
NORMALITY

350–615   Broncholithiasis   *3560*
350–600.8   Edema of bronchus, localized, due to un-
                     known cause   *3560*

—8 NEW GROWTHS

350–8091	Adenocarcinoma of bronchus. *Specify behavior*	3580
350–8091A	Adenoma of bronchus	3580
350–814	Epidermoid carcinoma of bronchus. *Specify behavior (page 99)*	3580
350–870A	Fibroma of bronchus	3580
350–8191G	Undifferentiated carcinoma of bronchus	3580
350–8▲▲▲	Unlisted tumor of bronchus. *Specify neoplasm and behavior*	3580

—9 DISEASES DUE TO UNKNOWN OR UNCERTAIN CAUSE WITH THE STRUCTURAL REACTION MANIFEST

350–923	Calcification of bronchus	3590
350–956	Fibrinous bronchitis	3590
350–900.9	Ulcer of bronchus due to unknown cause	3590

—Y DISEASES DUE TO CAUSE NOT DETERMINABLE IN THE PARTICULAR CASE

Y signifies an incomplete diagnosis. It is to be replaced whenever possible by a code digit signifying the specific diagnosis

350–yx9	Broncholithiasis due to undetermined cause	0063

DISEASES OF THE LUNG

360–
361– } Lung
362–   Alveoli
368–   Interstitial tissue
36x–   Intrinsic vessels

For detailed list of lobes of lungs, see page 23

—0 DISEASES DUE TO GENETIC AND PRENATAL INFLUENCES

360–034	Abnormal division of lung; sequestration	*3601*
360–077	Absence of fissures of lung	*3601*
36▲–031	Accessory lobe of lung. *Specify lobe*	*3601*
361–031	Azygos lobe	*3601*
360–031	Accessory lung	*3601*
360–011	Agenesis or aplasia of lung, or both	*3601*
360–019	Atelectasis, congenital	*3601*
3071–029	Communication of pleural and pericardial sacs	*3601*
361–064	Cystic disease of lung, congenital	*3601*
360–034.8	Cystic disease of lung, congenital associated with introlobular sequestration	*3601*
300–032	Duplication of respiratory organs (in monsters)	*3601*
360–023	Ectopic bone and cartilage in lung	*3601*
36▲–015	Emphysema, congenital. *Specify site*	*3601*
360–064	Giant tension cyst of lung, congenital	*3601*
360–027	Hernia of lung, congenital	*3601*
360–016	Hypoplasia of lung; atrophy of lung	*3601*
300–075	Rudimentary respiratory organs (in thoracopagus)	*3601*

—I DISEASES DUE TO INFECTION WITH LOWER ORGANISM

360–100.2	Abscess of lung. *Specify organism (page 57) when known, e.g.*	*3613*
360–101.2	Due to Pneumococcus	*3613*
360–151	Amebiasis of lung; amebic abscess	*3613*
360–118	Anthrax of lung; anthrax pneumonia	*3611*
362–100.4	Atelectasis, due to infection. *Specify organism (page 57) when known, e.g.*	*3610*
362–123.4	Atelectasis due to bronchial tuberculosis	*3612*
361–190	Bronchopneumonia. *Specify organism (page 57) when known, e.g.*	*3614*
361–168	Influenzal pneumonia	*3614*
361–101	Pneumococcic bronchopneumonia	*3614*

361–173	Psittacosic bronchopneumonia	*3614*
361–102	Streptococcic bronchopneumonia	*3614*
361–123.0	Tuberculous bronchopneumonia	*3612*
361–107	Tularemic bronchopneumonia	*3614*
361–160	Virus bronchopneumonia	*3616*
361–100	Bronchopneumonia, suppurative. *Specify organism (page 57) when known, e.g.*	*3614*
361–100.0	Bronchopneumonia, unresolved	*3614*
360–100.9	Calcification of lung due to infection	*3610*
360–123.9	Calcification of lung following tuberculosis	*3610*
360–100.8	Edema, pulmonary, due to infection	*3610*
36x–1x0.4	Embolism, pulmonary, due to remote infection	*3610*
368–100.6	Emphysema, interstitial, due to infection	*3610*
360–123.0	Fibrosis of lung following tuberculosis *Do not use for active pulmonary tuberculosis*	*3610*
360–100.1	Gangrene of lung due to infection. *Specify organism (page 57) when known*	*3610*
360–100.6	Granuloma of lung. *Specify organism when known, e.g.*	*3610*
361–123.6	Granuloma of lungs due to tuberculosis	*3612*
3601–123	Infection of lung due to atypical mycobacterium	*3612*
368–100	Pneumonia, interstitial, acute. *Specify organism (page 57) when known*	*3611*
368–100.0	Pneumonia, interstitial, chronic; pulmonary fibrosis; chronic pneumonia; sclerosis of lung. *Specify organism (page 57) when known*	*3611*
360–100	Pneumonia, lobar. *Specify organism (page 57) when known, e.g.*	*3611*
360–101	Pneumococcic lobar pneumonia	*3611*
360–102	Streptococcic lobar pneumonia	*3611*
360–100.0	Pneumonia, lobar, unresolved	*3611*
360–160	Primary atypical pneumonia	*3616*
360–1x0	Pulmonary sarcoidosis	*3610*
360–147	Syphilis of lung	*3610*
360–123	Tuberculosis of lung (pulmonary tuberculosis) [1]	*3612*
360–1231	Minimal, active	*3612*
360–1232	Moderately advanced, active	*3612*
360–1233	Far advanced, active	*3612*
360–1234	Minimal, inactive	*3612*

[1] The digit 7 may be added to the etiologic code 123 to indicate tuberculosis, inactive, thus 1237. See statement in Introduction relative to coding an active tuberculosis in other areas of the body.

360–1235	Moderately advanced, inactive	*3612*
360–1236	Far advanced, inactive	*3612*
360–1237	Minimal, quiescent	*3612*
360–1238	Moderately advanced, quiescent	*3612*
360–1239	Far advanced, quiescent	*3612*
360–123x	Activity undetermined	*3612*
361–1233	Tuberculosis of lung, miliary, active	*3612*
361–1236	Tuberculosis of lung, miliary, inactive	*3612*
3063–123	Tuberculosis of lung, primary complex	*3612*
3063–1231	Predominantly pulmonary form	*3612*
3063–1232	Tracheobronchial form	*3612*
3063–1233	Combined form	*3612*

—2 DISEASES DUE TO HIGHER PLANT OR ANIMAL PARASITE

360–2▲▲.2	Abscess of lung due to fungus. *Specify (page 63)*	*3620*
360–2▲▲.6	Granuloma of lung due to fungus. *Specify fungus (page 63) when known*	*3620*
360–2▲▲	Parasitic infection of lung due to fungus, *e.g.*	*3620*
360–202	Actinomycosis of lung	*3621*
360–241	Ascariasis of lung	*3620*
360–217	Blastomycosis of lung	*3622*
360–219	Coccidioidomycosis of lung	*3620*
360–220	Histoplasmosis of lung	*3623*
360–201	Nocardiosis of lung	*3620*
360–2▲▲.8	Parasitic cyst of lung. *Specify parasite (page 63)*	*3620*
360–2▲▲	Parasitic infection of lung. *Specify parasite when known (page 63)*	*3620*
360–267	Pulmonary hydatid cyst (Echinococcosis)	*3620*
361–2▲▲.8	Infection of lung due to fungus with cavitation	*3620*

—3 DISEASES DUE TO INTOXICATION

360–3224	Acute berylliosis	*3630*
360–390	Allergic pneumonia; Loeffler's syndrome; pulmonary eosinophilia	*3630*
368–319	Chronic interstitial pneumonia due to poisonous gas	*3631*
368–3224	Chronic pulmonary granulomatosis in beryllium workers; chronic berylliosis	*3630*
360–3▲▲.8	Edema of lung due to poisoning. *Specify poison (page 67)*	*3630*

| 360–3▲▲ | Poisoning of lung by chemical (congestion). *Specify poison (page 67)* | *3630* |

—4 DISEASES DUE TO TRAUMA OR PHYSICAL AGENT

360–400.2	Abscess of lung due to trauma	*3640*
360–438.2	Due to foreign body	*3640*
360–496.2	Due to aspiration of foreign body	*3640*
362–435	Atelectasis due to compression	*3640*
362–415.4	Atelectasis following operation	*3640*
360–400.4	Atelectasis, massive, due to trauma	*3640*
361–496.0	Bronchopneumonia due to aspiration of foreign substance	*3640*
361–4961.0	Due to aspiration of oil (lipid pneumonia)	*3640*
361–415.0	Bronchopneumonia following operation	*3640*
360–428	Congestion of lung due to blast injury	*3640*
360–440	Congestion of lung due to hot or cold air	*3640*
360–400.8	Edema, pulmonary, acute, due to trauma or physical agent	*3640*
360–415.8	Edema, pulmonary following operation	*3640*
36x–429	Embolism, pulmonary, due to amniotic fluid	*3640*
36x–427	Embolism, pulmonary, air, due to remote trauma	*3640*
36x–426	Embolism, pulmonary, fat, due to remote trauma	*3640*
36x–425	Embolism, pulmonary, following operation (intrinsic vessels)	*3640*
362–434	Emphysema, postural	*3640*
368–427	Emphysema of lung, interstitial, due to trauma	*3640*
360–438.6	Fibrosis, pulmonary, due to foreign body	*3640*
360–4712.6	Fibrosis, pulmonary, due to roentgen rays	*3640*
360–496	Foreign body in lung; foreign body in lung aspirated	*3640*
360–400.1	Gangrene of lung due to trauma	*3640*
360–4x9	Hernia of lung, due to trauma	*3640*
360–406	Hernia of lung, subcutaneous, due to trauma	*3640*
360–424	Hernia of lung, transmediastinal	*3640*
360–4▲▲	Injury of lung. *Specify (page 83)*	*3640*
360–436	Laceration of lung by fractured rib. *Record primary diagnosis*	*3640*
360–415.3	Peripheral air leak from lung following operation (as distinguished from large bronchial fistula)	*3640*
360–471.0	Pneumonitis due to roentgen rays	*3640*

368–438▲	Pneumoconiosis. *Specify dust (page 84)*	*3643*
368–4382	Anthracosis	*3643*
368–4381	Asbestosis	*3643*
368–4384	Diatomite fibrosis	*3643*
368–4389	Siderosis	*3643*
368–4386	Silicosis	*3643*
362–438	Pneumonia due to aspiration of amniotic fluid	*3643*
368–498.0	Silicotuberculosis	*3643*

—50 DISEASES DUE TO CIRCULATORY DISTURBANCE

36x–500.4	Embolism, pulmonary, due to circulatory disturbance	*3653*
360–500.1	Gangrene of lung due to circulatory disturbance. *Specify, e.g.*	*3650*
360–512.1	Due to embolus	*3653*
360–520	Hypostatic congestion of lung	*3652*
360–510	Infarction of lung	*3651*
360–511	Due to thrombus	*3651*
360–512	Due to embolus	*3653*
360–522	Passive congestion of lung	*3652*
360–535.7	Pulmonary hemorrhage secondary to pulmonary hypertension	*3650*

—6 DISEASES DUE TO OR CONSISTING OF STATIC MECHANICAL ABNORMALITY

360–611.4	Atelectasis of lung due to foreign body in bronchus. *Record primary diagnosis*	*3660*
360–641	Emphysema, bullous	*3661*
362–600.6	Emphysema, compensatory	*3661*
362–610	Emphysema, obstructive	*3661*
362–600.8	Pulmonary cyst, acquired	*3660*
36x–618	Pulmonary embolism, due to unknown cause	*3660*

—7 DISEASES DUE TO DISORDER OF METABOLISM, GROWTH, OR NUTRITION
Record primary diagnosis when possible

362–797	Senile emphysema	*3670*

—8 NEW GROWTHS

360–8091	Adenocarcinoma of lung. *Specify behavior*	*3680*
360–8072	Alveolar cell (bronchiolar) carcinoma of lung. *Specify behavior*	*3680*
360–8191	Carcinoma of lung. *Specify behavior*	*3680*

360–814	Epidermoid carcinoma of lung. *Specify behavior* (*page 99*)	*3680*
360–8882	Hamartoma of lung. *Specify behavior*	*3680*
360–8191G	Undifferentiated carcinoma of lung	*3680*
360–8▲▲▲	Unlisted tumor of lung. *Specify neoplasm and behavior*	*3680*

—9 DISEASES DUE TO UNKNOWN OR UNCERTAIN CAUSE WITH THE STRUCTURAL REACTION MANIFEST

360–923	Calcification of lung due to unknown cause	*3690*
368–9xx1	Diffuse interstitial fibrosis of lung (Hamman-Rich syndrome)	*3691*
362–9x6	Emphysema, pulmonary, due to unknown cause	*3690*
368–9x6	Fibrosis, pulmonary, due to unknown cause	*3691*
360–9x0	Hyaline membrane of the lung	*3692*
360–932	Pneumonitis due to rheumatic fever	*3690*
362–923	Pulmonary alveolar microlithiasis	*3690*
362–941	Pulmonary alveolar proteinosis	*3690*

—Y DISEASES DUE TO CAUSE NOT DETERMINABLE IN THE PARTICULAR CASE

Y signifies an incomplete diagnosis. It is to be replaced whenever possible by a code digit signifying the specific diagnosis

360–yx2	Abscess of lung due to undetermined cause	*0063*
362–yx4	Atelectasis due to undetermined cause	*0063*
361–y10	Bronchopneumonia due to undetermined cause	*0063*
360–yx4	Collapse of lung, massive, due to undetermined cause	*0063*
360–y00.8	Edema, pulmonary, due to undetermined cause	*0063*
360–y00.6	Granuloma of lung; nodules of lung due to undetermined cause	*0063*
360–yx7	Pulmonary hemorrhage due to undetermined cause	*0063*

DISEASES OF THE PLEURA

370 –   Pleura
3074–   Pleura and thoracic wall
3051–   Bronchi and pleura

For detailed list of structures of pleura, see page 24

—0 DISEASES DUE TO GENETIC AND PRENATAL INFLUENCES

370–0▲▲	Anomaly of pleura. *Specify anomaly*	*3701*

—I DISEASES DUE TO INFECTION WITH LOWER ORGANISM

370–1x4	Adhesions of pleura due to infection	*3710*
370–100.9	Calcification of pleura due to infection. *Specify organism when known, e.g.*	*3710*
370–123.9	Calcification of pleura following tuberculosis	*3710*
370–100	Empyema, general. *Specify organism (page 57) when known*	*3715*
3074–100.3	Empyema perforating chest wall	*3715*
373–100	Interlobar empyema. *Specify organism (page 57) when known*	*3715*
375–100	Locculated empyema. *Specify organism (page 57) when known*	*3715*
370–1231	Tuberculous empyema, simple	*3716*
370–1232	Tuberculous empyema, mixed	*3716*
30754–1x4.5	Hemopneumothorax due to rupture of adhesion, due to infection	*3710*
370–100.7	Hemothorax due to infection	*3710*
30752–100	Hydropneumothorax due to infection	*3710*
30752–123	Hydropneumothorax due to tuberculosis	*3714*
370–190	Pleurisy, acute. *Specify organism (page 57) when known*	*3711*
370–190.8	Pleurisy with effusion	*3711*
370–123.8	Tuberculous pleurisy with effusion	*3712*
370–123.0	Tuberculous pleurisy, chronic	*3712*
370–1237	Tuberculous pleurisy, inactive	*3712*
370–190.0	Pleurisy, chronic. *Specify organism (page 57) when known*	*3711*
370–17x4	Pleurodynia, epidemic (Bornholm's disease) due to Coxsackie virus	*3710*
30751–100.5	Pneumothorax, spontaneous, due to infection. *Specify*	*3713*
30751–123.5	Pneumothorax, spontaneous, due to tuberculosis	*3714*

30751–100.4	Pneumothorax, tense valvular, due to infection	*3713*
30751–123.4	Pneumothorax, tense valvular, due to tuberculosis	*3714*
30753–100	Pyoneumothorax due to infection	*3713*
30753–123	Pyopneumothorax due to tuberculosis	*3714*
30753–100.5	Pyopneumothorax due to infection following injury to chest wall. *See also* Pyopneumothorax due to injury of chest wall (*page 200*)	*3713*

—2 DISEASES DUE TO HIGHER PLANT OR ANIMAL PARASITE

370–2▲▲.8	Chylothorax due to animal parasite. *Specify parasite* (*page 63*)	*3720*
370–2▲▲	Pleurisy due to fungus. *Specify*	*3720*
30571–2▲▲	Pneumothorax due to fungus. *Specify*	*3720*
30753–2▲▲	Pyopneumothorax due to fungus. *Specify*	*3720*

—4 DISEASES DUE TO TRAUMA OR PHYSICAL AGENT

370–400.4	Adhesions of pleura due to trauma	*3740*
	Chylothorax due to trauma. *See* Fistula of thoracic duct (*page 234*)	
370–438.2	Empyema due to foreign body. *If organism is known, record also as* Empyema due to infection, *page 198*	*3740*
370–415.2	Empyema following operation	*3740*
370–4x6	Fibrin, ball of, in pleural sac	*3740*
30751–415.8	Fluid of reexpansion	*3740*
30754–4x4.5	Hemopneumothorax produced by rupture of adhesion due to trauma	*3741*
370–400.7	Hemothorax due to trauma	*3740*
30752–400	Hydropneumothorax due to injury of chest wall	*3741*
30752–4001	Hydropneumothorax due to injury of lung	*3741*
30752–415	Hydropneumothorax following operation	*3741*
3075–415.4	Induced pneumothorax	*3741*
370–4▲▲	Injury of pleura. *Specify* (*page 83*)	*3740*
370–436	Laceration of pleura by fractured rib	*3740*
370–490	Oleothorax	*3740*
370–420	Pleural shock	*3740*
370–4x0	Pleurisy due to trauma. *Classify ordinarily as due to infection* (*page 198*)	*3740*
30751–43x.5	Pneumothorax spontaneous due to rupture of emphysematous or subpleural bleb	*3741*

30751–400	Pneumothorax due to injury of chest wall. *Not to be used for* Pneumothorax due to tuberculosis *or for allied conditions. Record both diagnoses when necessary*	*3741*
30751–4001	Pneumothorax due to injury of lung	*3741*
30751–415	Pneumothorax of chest wall, following operation	*3741*
30751–4151	Pneumothorax of lung following operation	*3741*
30751–400.4	Pneumothorax, tense valvular, due to trauma	*3741*
30753–400	Pyopneumothorax due to injury of chest wall	*3741*
30753–4001	Pyopneumothorax due to injury of lung. *Classify ordinarily as due to infection (page 199)*	*3741*
30753–415	Pyopneumothorax due to operative injury of chest wall	*3741*
30753–4151	Pyopneumothorax due to operative injury of lung	*3741*

—50 DISEASES DUE TO CIRCULATORY DISTURBANCE
Record primary diagnosis when possible

370–502	Chylothorax	*3750*
370–532	Hemothorax due to rupture of blood vessel	*3750*
370–522	Hydrothorax due to passive congestion	*3750*

—6 DISEASES DUE TO OR CONSISTING OF STATIC MECHANICAL AB-NORMALITY

30754–641.5	Hemopneumothorax, spontaneous	*3760*
376–641	Subpleural bleb	*3760*

—8 NEW GROWTHS

370–8▲▲.8	Hydrothorax due to neoplasm. *Specify*	*3780*
370–8772A	Mesothelioma of pleura	*3780*
370–8451	Neurofibroma of pleura. *Specify behavior*	*3780*
370–879	Sarcoma of pleura. *Specify behavior*	*3780*

—9 DISEASES DUE TO UNKNOWN OR UNCERTAIN CAUSE WITH THE STRUCTURAL REACTION MANIFEST

30754–900	Hemopneumothorax due to unknown cause	*3790*
30751–900	Spontaneous pneumothorax, due to unknown cause	*3790*
30752–9x5	Hydropneumothorax due to spontaneous pneumothorax	*3790*

4— DISEASES OF THE CARDIO VASCULAR SYSTEM

INTRODUCTION

Diseases of the cardiovascular system are classified in the same way as other diseases; the method is described in the general Introduction. The cardiovascular system is divided into its component parts, and the types of diseases affecting each are classified on an etiologic basis. This combination of site with etiologic factor defines the clinical process and gives the title to the basic diagnosis. In diseases of the heart and its structures, however, the list of Supplementary Terms (*page 491*) affords a further means for defining the symptomatic and physiologic manifestations and the degree of disability. As many of these may be recorded as the physician desires, and the code permits a considerable number to be entered on the code card. In all cases at least (1) the physiologic manifestations and (2) the degree of disability should be recorded in conformity with the list of Supplementary Terms (*page 491*). These follow the nomenclature of the American Heart Association.

Attention is directed to the explanatory notes in the general Introduction. A physiologic manifestation is not to be considered a diagnosis, except when it constitutes the sole evidence of disease; that is to say, when the etiologic factor is unknown and there is no evidence of any structural change. This concession is necessary because the disorder must be defined in some terms. It is to be understood, however, that such a diagnosis implies a belief that a no more complete diagnosis is possible. If the physician believes that there is organic disease or a determinable etiologic factor which he cannot identify, the diagnosis is then Heart Disease undiagnosed, and the physiologic (or other) manifestations are recorded according to the list of Supplementary Terms (*page 491*). The method of recording undiagnosed disease is described in the general Introduction.

4— DISEASES OF THE CARDIOVASCULAR SYSTEM

400— Cardiovascular System, generally

For detailed list of structures, see page 24

—0 DISEASES DUE TO GENETIC AND PRENATAL INFLUENCES

The principle to be followed in diagnosing these conditions is to enter each anomaly as an individual diagnostic title. An exception is made when certain anomalies commonly occur together so as to constitute a complex, e.g., Tetralogy of Fallot. The digits in the etiologic position are largely arbitrary.

ANOMALIES OF THE HEART AS A WHOLE

410–011	Acardia, hemicardia	*4101*
41▲–0▲▲	Anomalies of heart. *Specify site and anomaly*	*4101*

4151–0▲▲	Anomaly of Eustachian valve. *Specify anomaly*	*4101*
4195–0▲▲	Anomaly of valve of coronary sinus. *Specify anomaly*	*4101*
410–037	Bifid apex	*4101*
410–021	Dextrocardia, true	*4101*
410–0211	Dextrocardia with situs inversus	*4101*
410–022	Dextroversion; dextroposition; partial rotation	*4101*
410–026	Ectopy of heart	*4101*
410–0261	Abdominal	*4101*
410–0262	Cervical	*4101*
410–0263	Pectoral	*4101*
410–091	Fetal inflammatory disease of heart	*4101*
456–013	Fibroelastosis of mural endocardium, congenital	*4101*
410–0y0	Heart disease, congenital, incompletely diagnosed	*4101*
410–013	Hypertrophy of heart, congenital	*4101*

PERICARDIAL ABNORMALITIES

420–011	Absence of pericardium	*4201*
420–012	Defect of pericardium	*4201*
420–036	Diverticulum (or cyst) of pericardium	*4201*

ATRIAL SEPTAL DEFECTS AND ABNORMALITIES

412–0xx	Absence of atrial septum (cor triloculare biventricularis)	*4102*
412–030	Anomalous atrial septum	*4102*
412–0x9	Atrial septal defect with mitral stenosis and dilatation of pulmonary artery (Lutembacher syndrome)	*4102*
412–0x2	Patent foramen ovale (persistent ostium secundum)	*4102*
412–0x1	Persistent ostium primum	*4102*
411–0x6	Ostium primum with cleft mitral valve	*4102*
412–0▲▲	Other atrial septal abnormalities. *Specify abnormality*	*4102*

ATRIAL ABNORMALITIES

412–039	Anomalous atrial band (including network of Chiari)	*4101*
412–0391	Anomalous atrial fold	*4101*
430–01x	Anomalous muscle bundle between atrium and ventricle (Wolff-Parkinson-White syndrome)	*4101*
412–0▲▲	Other atrial abnormalities. *Specify abnormality*	*4102*

Ventricular Septal Defects and Abnormalities

413–0x8	Absence of ventricular septum (cor tri- loculare biatrium)	*4102*
413–030	Anomalous ventricular septum	*4102*
413–0x3	Ventricular septal defect with dextroposi- tion of aorta (Eisenmenger complex)	*4102*
413–0x4	Ventricular septal defect with levoposition of pulmonary artery	*4102*
413–0x5	Ventricular septal defect, localized	*4102*
413–0x0	Ventricular septal defect, pulmonary steno- sis or atresia, dextroposition of aorta, hypertrophy of right ventricle (Tetral- ogy of Fallot)	*4102*
413–0▲▲	Other ventricular septal abnormalities. *Specify abnormality*	*4102*

Ventricular Abnormalities

413–015	Aneurysm (dilatation) of ventricular septum	*4101*
457–030	Anomalous chordae tendineae	*4101*
437–030	Anomalous papillary muscle	*4101*
413–039	Anomalous ventricular band	*4101*
413–0391	Anomalous ventricular fold	*4101*
440–042	Heart block, congenital	*4101*
435–019	Infundibular stenosis (pulmonary conus)	*4101*
4443–042	Left bundle branch block, congenital	*4101*
413–0▲▲	Other ventricular abnormalities. *Specify abnormality*	*4101*
4442–042	Right bundle branch block, congenital	*4101*
436–019	Subaortic stenosis	*4101*

Combined Atrial and Ventricular Septal Defects

411–0x8	Absence of interatrial and interventricular septa (cor biloculare)	*4102*
411–0x5	Ostium primum with localized ventricular septal defect	*4102*
411–0xx	Other combined septal defects	*4102*

Valvular Abnormalities

454–031	Accessory leaflet of mitral valve	*4101*
452–031	Accessory leaflet of tricuspid valve	*4101*
455–018	Atresia of aortic valve	*4101*
455–0242	Bicuspid aortic valve	*4101*
453–0242	Bicuspid pulmonic valve	*4101*
454–032	Double orifice of mitral valve	*4101*
452–032	Double orifice of tricuspid valve	*4101*
452–021	Downward displacement of tricuspid valve (Ebstein's disease)	*4101*

455–038	Fenestration of aortic cusps	*4101*
453–038	Fenestration of pulmonic cusps, congenital	*4101*
455–024	Fusion or defect of aortic cusps, congenital	*4101*
453–024	Fusion or defect of pulmonic cusps, congenital	*4101*
454–017	Mitral stenosis or atresia, congenital	*4101*
454–015	Mitral insufficiency, congenital	*4101*
	Subaortic stenosis. (*See* Ventricular abnormalities)	
455–031	Supernumerary aortic cusps	*4101*
453–031	Supernumerary pulmonic cusps	*4101*
452–015	Tricuspid insufficiency, congenital	*4101*
452–017	Tricuspid stenosis or atresia, congenital	*4101*
451–0▲▲	Other valvular abnormalities. *Specify abnormality*	*4101*

Congenital Abnormalities of the Central Vessels

Ductus Arteriosus

40x–0x5	Absence of ductus arteriosus	*4101*
40x–0x0.6	Aneurysm (so-called) of patent ductus arteriosus	*4101*
40x–0x3	Aortic pulmonary septal defect	*4102*
40x–0x8	Bilateral ductus arteriosus	*4101*
40x–0x0	Patent ductus arteriosus	*4101*

Aorta

4612–015	Aneurysm of right aortic sinus (sinus of Valsalva)	*4601*
4612–015.5	Aneurysm of right aortic sinus, congenital ruptured	*4601*
461–0181	Coarctation of aorta, adult type	*4601*
461–0183	Coarctation of aorta, bicuspid aortic valve	*4601*
461–0181.6	Coarctation of aorta, dissecting aneurysm	*4601*
461–0181.5	Coarctation of aorta, dissecting aneurysm, rupture of aorta	*4601*
461–018	Coarctation of aorta, infantile type	*4601*
4611–0x3	Dextroposition of aorta	*4601*
	Dextroposition of aorta with ventricular septal defect. (*See* Ventricular abnormalities)	
461–016	Hypoplasia of aorta	*4601*
4611–016	Hypoplasia of ascending aorta	*4601*
461–019	Persistent double aortic arch	*4601*
4613–019	Persistent right aortic arch	*4601*

4613–0192	Persistent right aortic arch with left descending aorta	*4601*
4051–01x	Persistent truncus arteriosus	*4601*
	Subaortic stenosis. (*See* Ventricular abnormalities)	*4601*
4611–02x	Transposition of aorta	*4601*
4051–02x	Transposition of great vessels, complete	*4601*
4051–02x1	Transposition of great vessels, partial	*4601*

Pulmonary Artery

4711–031	Accessory pulmonary artery	*4701*
4711–021	Anomalous origin of pulmonary artery from aorta	*4701*
4711–018	Atresia of pulmonary artery	*4701*
471–015	Dilatation (aneurysm) of pulmonary arteries	*4701*
4711–015	Dilatation of main pulmonary artery	*4701*
	Levoposition of pulmonary artery with ventricular septal defect. (*See* Ventricular septal defect, *page 203*)	
471–016	Narrowing of pulmonary artery	*4701*
4711–02x	Transposition of pulmonary artery	*4701*

Other Central Vessels

4811–011	Absence of superior vena cava	*4801*
486–021	Anomalous entry of pulmonary veins into right atrium	*4701*
486–022	Anomalous entry of pulmonary veins into other vessels	*4701*
4621–021	Anomalous innominate artery	*4601*
4622–021	Anomalous left common carotid artery	*4601*
4623–021	Anomalous left subclavian artery	*4601*
4811–01x	Persistent left superior vena cava	*4801*

CONGENITAL ABNORMALITIES OF CORONARY ARTERIES

41x2–011	Absence of left coronary artery	*4101*
41x1–011	Absence of right coronary artery	*4101*
41x–031	Accessory coronary artery	*4101*
41x1–015	Aneurysm of right coronary artery, congenital	*4101*
41x–021	Anomalous distribution of coronary artery	*4101*
41x–026	Anomalous origin of coronary artery (one or both) from aorta	*4101*
41x–010	Anomalous origin of both coronary arteries from pulmonary artery	*4101*
41x2–010	Anomalous origin of left coronary artery from pulmonary artery	*4101*
41x1–010	Anomalous origin of right coronary artery from pulmonary artery	*4101*

400–535   Cardiovascular disease due to hyper-
                tension of lesser circulation   *4750*

> To be used for a disease manifested by hypertension of
> lesser circulation either with or without arteriosclerosis
> of the pulmonary arteries and affecting either the struc-
> ture or the function of the heart. Also record as separate
> diagnosis the cause of hypertension of the lesser circula-
> tion. Also record the effects upon the cardiovascular
> system; e.g., cardiac insufficiency.

400–533   Hypertensive cardiovascular disease   *4050*

> This term is to be used in the sense of a disease
> manifested by peripheral arterial hypertension either with
> or without arteriolar or arterial sclerosis and affecting
> either the structure or the function of the heart. It is not
> to be confused with Arteriosclerosis, general or with the
> effects of arteriosclerosis of the coronary arteries. If these
> diseases are present the appropriate additional diagnoses
> should be recorded.

**—55 DISEASES DUE TO DISTURBANCE OF INNERVATION OR OF PSYCHIC
CONTROL**

443–584.x   Carotid sinus syncope (syndrome)   *4455*

—7 DISEASE DUE TO DISORDER OF METABOLISM, GROWTH, OR NUTRITION

400–78x   Carcinoid cardiovascular disease. *Record
                primary neoplasm*   *4070*

DISEASES OF THE HEART

410– Heart
420– Pericardium, primarily or exclusively
430– Myocardium, primarily or exclusively
440– Conduction system, primarily or exclusively
450– Endocardium, primarily or exclusively
451– Valves generally; unspecified valve. Specify in each case by changing the last digit
452– Tricuspid valve
453– Pulmonary valve
454– Mitral valve
455– Aortic valve
456– Mural endocardium
457– Chordae tendineae
41x– Coronary arteries

For detailed list of structures of heart, see page 25

—0 DISEASES DUE TO GENETIC AND PRENATAL INFLUENCES
See under Cardiovascular System generally, page 201.

—I DISEASES DUE TO INFECTION WITH LOWER ORGANISM
If more than one valve is affected, use code 451

41x–147.6	Aneurysm of coronary artery due to syphilis	*4110*
410–100.6	Aneurysm of heart due to infection	*4110*
45▲–1x0.6	Aneurysm of valve due to subacute bacterial endocarditis. *Specify valve*	*4510*
41x–100	Bacterial coronary arteritis	*4110*
410–100	Carditis acute bacterial. *Specify organism (page 57) when known*	*4110*
410–100.0	Carditis subacute bacterial. *Specify organism (page 57) when known*	*4110*
41x–1x0.6	Coronary arteritis with embolic aneurysm	*4110*
450–100	Endocarditis acute bacterial. *Specify organism (page 57) when known*	*4511*
45▲–100.6	Aneurysm of valve due to acute bacterial endocarditis. *Specify valve*	*4510*
45▲–100.3	Perforation of valve due to acute bacterial endocarditis. *Specify valve*	*4510*
450–100.0	Endocarditis, subacute bacterial. *Specify organism when known*	*4511*
430–100	Myocarditis acute bacterial. *Specify organism (page 57) when known*	*4311*
430–168	Myocarditis due to influenza	*4311*

430–102	Myocarditis due to scarlet fever	*4311*
430–115	Myocarditis due to typhoid bacillus (Salmonella typhosa)	*4311*
430–160	Myocarditis due to virus, *unspecified*	*4311*
	Endocarditis, nonbacterial thrombotic. *See page 212*	
430–100.2	Abscess of myocardium. *Specify organism (page 57) when known*	*4310*
430–100.0	Myocarditis subacute bacterial. *Specify organism (page 57) when known*	*4311*
41x–147.4	Narrowing of coronary ostium due to syphilis	*4110*
45▲–1x0.3	Perforation of valve due to subacute bacterial endocarditis. *Specify valve*	*4510*
45▲–147.3	Perforation of valve due to syphilis. *Specify valve*	*4510*
420–102.8	Pericardial effusion due to scarlet fever	*4211*
420–115.8	Pericardial effusion due to typhoid	*4211*
420–100	Pericarditis acute bacterial. *Specify organism (page 57) when known*	*4211*
420–100.2	With purulent effusion	*4211*
420–100.8	With serous or seropurulent effusion	*4211*
420–100.0	Pericarditis subacute bacterial. *Specify organism (page 57) when known*	*4211*
420–100.3	Pneumopericardium due to infection	*4210*
420–1001.3	Pyopneumopericardium	*4210*
420–1002.3	Hydropneumopericardium	*4210*
	Purulent pericarditis. *See under* Acute bacterial pericarditis. *See above*	
410–100.5	Rupture of heart due to infection	*4110*
457–100.5	Rupture of chordae tendineae due to infection	*4510*
437–100.5	Rupture of papillary muscle due to infection	*4310*
430–1x0	Sarcoidosis of myocardium	*4310*
41▲–147	Syphilitic heart disease. *Specify site, e.g.*	*4110*
440–147	Syphilis of conduction system	*4410*
45▲–147.4	Syphilitic valvulitis, with deformity of valve. *Specify valve*	*4510*
430–123	Tuberculosis of myocardium	*4311*
404–123	Tuberculous mediastinopericarditis	*4210*
404–123	Tuberculous pericarditis	*4210*
420–123.4	Tuberculous pericarditis with adhesions	*4210*
420–123.9	Tuberculous pericarditis with calcification	*4210*
420–123.8	Tuberculous pericarditis with effusion	*4211*

—3 DISEASES DUE TO INTOXICATION

For toxic heart disease due to remote infection see under diseases due to infection

410–3▲▲	Poisoning of heart by drug. *Specify poison (page 67)*	*4130*
410–34819	Aconitine	*4130*
410–321	Arsenic	*4130*
410–33152	Chloroform	*4130*
410–33152.9	Chloroform (delayed poisoning)	*4130*
410–3471	Digitalis or related glucoside	*4130*
410–3185	Phosphorus	*4130*
410–34649	Pilocarpine	*4130*
410–34382	Quinine	*4130*
410–3844	Tobacco (nicotine)	*4130*
420–389	Uremic pericarditis	*4230*

—4 DISEASES DUE TO TRAUMA OR PHYSICAL AGENT

410–427	Air embolism of heart	*4140*
410–402.x	Cardiac arrest due to contusion	*4140*
410–435.x	Cardiac arrest due to traumatic interference with innervation. *Specify manifestations*	*4140*
410–4x4	Cardiac tamponade. Record primary diagnosis	*4140*
410–43x	Dilatation of heart due to overstrain	*4140*
451–43x	Valvular changes due to tension	*4540*
420–496	Foreign body in pericardium	*4240*
410–414	Gunshot wound of heart. *Specify structure when known*	*4140*
420–400.7	Hemopericardium due to trauma	*4240*
420–4001.7	With sanguinopurulent effusion	*4240*
420–4002.8	With serosanguineous effusion	*4240*
410–43x.6	Hypertrophy of heart due to overstrain	*4140*
420–400.4	Pericardial adhesions due to trauma	*4240*
420–400.3	Pneumopericardium due to trauma	*4240*
410–416	Rupture of heart due to trauma	*4140*
410–411	Stab wound of heart. *Specify structure when known*	*4140*

—50 DISEASES DUE TO DISTURBANCE OF NUTRIENT CIRCULATION

410–540	Anemia of heart due to blood disease. *Record primary diagnosis*	*4150*
41▲–516.6	Aneurysm of heart due to reduced coronary blood flow. *Specify site*	*4150*

410–516   Arteriosclerotic heart disease   *4151*

> This term is used in the presence of coronary arterio-sclerosis when the arterial disease has produced cardiac symptoms such as angina or arrhythmia or cardiac insufficiency. If there is evidence of gross damage of the heart such as infarction, fibrosis, aneurysm or rupture these should be used as additional diagnoses. In arteriosclerotic heart disease associated with arterial hypertension, diagnose (1) Arteriosclerotic heart disease (above) and (2) Essential vascular hypertension (page 219) or Hypertensive vascular disease (page 217), according to the stage of the hypertension.

444▲–516.x   Bundle branch block due to sclerosis of
                   nutrient artery. *Specify*   *4450*

416–535.6   Cor pulmonale due to pulmonary arterial
                   hypertension   *4150*

> This term is restricted to those cases with diseases of the heart secondary to pulmonary arterial hypertension. Pulmonary arterial hypertension the result of increased pulmonary venous pressure is excluded. *Record primary diagnosis of pulmonary hypertension.*

410–535.6   Enlargement of heart due to pulmonary
                   disease   *4150*

410–540.9   Fatty degeneration of heart due to anemia.
                   Record primary diagnosis   *4150*

430–5x9.6   Fibrosis of myocardium due to degenera-
                   tion and replacement fibrosis   *4350*

430–5x7.6   Fibrosis of myocardium due to infarction   *4350*

420–532   Hemopericardium due to rupture of ad-
                   jacent structure   *4250*

420–531.5   Hemopericardium due to ruptured
                   aneurysm   *4250*

420–522.8   Hydropericardium due to heart failure.
                   Record primary diagnosis   *4250*

430–516.7   Infarction of myocardium due to arterio-
                   sclerotic coronary thrombosis   *4351*

430–515.7   Infarction of myocardium from coronary
                   thrombosis due to arteritis   *4351*

430–512.7   Infarction of myocardium due to em-
                   bolism   *4351*

41▲–511.6   Aneurysm of heart due to infarction.
                   State exact site   *4150*

410–522   Passive congestion of heart. *Record
                   primary diagnosis*   *4150*

420–511.0   Pericarditis due to myocardial infarction   *4250*

410–5x7.5   Rupture of heart due to infarction   *4150*

DISEASES DUE TO DISTURBANCE OF INNERVATION OR OF PSYCHIC CONTROL
Record primary diagnosis when possible

430–563.0	Myocarditis due to diphtheria toxin	*4355*
440–580	Neurogenic arrhythmia	*4455*
440–590	Reflex arrhythmia	*4455*
41x–584	Spasm of coronary artery	*4155*
440–585	Vagal arrhythmia	*4455*
440–584	Vagal bradycardia	*4455*

—6 OBSTRUCTION DUE TO REMOTE CAUSE

41x–618	Embolism of coronary artery	*4161*
410–600.x	Heart disease due to deformity of chest.	
	Record primary diagnosis	*4160*
41▲–619	Thrombosis of heart chamber. *Specify*	*4160*

—7 DISEASES DUE TO DISORDER OF METABOLISM, GROWTH, OR NUTRITION
Record primary diagnosis when possible

410–701	Atrophy of heart due to inanition	*4170*
410–7621	Beriberi heart	*4170*
410–754	Fatty infiltration of heart	*4170*
430–751	Glycogen infiltration of myocardium	
	(in von Gierke's disease)	*4370*
430–748	Hemochromatosis of myocardium	*4370*
410–771	Hyperthyroid heart	*4170*
410–772	Myxedema heart	*4170*
410–798	Senile atrophy of heart	*4170*

—8 NEW GROWTHS

410–870A	Fibroma of heart	*4180*
410–850A	Hemangioma of heart	*4180*
410–8871	Mesenchymal mixed tumor. *Specify behavior (page 99)*	*4180*
430–871B	Myxoma of myocardium	*4380*
430–867A	Rhabdomyoma of myocardium	*4380*
430–867F	Rhabdomyosarcoma of myocardium	*4380*
410–879	Sarcoma of heart. *Specify behavior (page 99)*	*4180*
420–879	Sarcoma of pericardium. *Specify behavior (page 99)*	*4280*
410–882	Teratoma of heart. *Specify behavior (page 99)*	*4180*
410–8▲▲▲	Unlisted tumor of heart. *Specify neoplasm and behavior (page 99)*	*4180*

**—9 DISEASES DUE TO UNKNOWN OR UNCERTAIN CAUSE WITH THE
STRUCTURAL REACTION MANIFEST**

420–900.4	Adherent pericardium due to unknown cause	*4290*
410–922	Amyloidosis of heart due to unknown cause	*4190*
41x–942	Arteriosclerosis of coronary artery (without cardiac symptoms)	*4194*

If associated with cardiac symptoms, diagnose disease: (1) Arteriosclerotic heart disease, *page 210,* or (2) according to myocardial lesion produced if any exist (infarction, etc.), *page 210.*

41x–942.6	Aneurysm of coronary artery due to arteriosclerosis without cardiac symptoms	*4194*
41x–942.4	Arteriosclerosis with narrowing of coronary artery	*4194*

If associated with cardiac symptoms, diagnose (1) Arteriosclerotic heart disease, (2) according to myocardial lesion produced if any exists.

41x–942.7	Coronary thrombosis due to arteriosclerosis	*4194*

If associated with infarction, diagnose as infarction of myocardium due to arteriosclerotic coronary thrombosis, *page 210.*

410–911	Atrophy of heart due to unknown cause	*4190*
444▲–932.x	Bundle branch block due to rheumatic fever. *Specify*	*4490*
455–923	Calcification of aortic valve	*4590*
410–923	Calcification of heart due to unknown cause	*4190*
450–940.7	Endocarditis, nonbacterial thrombotic	*4590*
410–9x6	Enlargement of heart due to unknown cause. *See also* Glycogen infiltration of myocardium, *page 211*	*4190*
41x–956	Essential angiitis of coronary artery	*4190*
410–917	Fatty degeneration of heart due to unknown cause	*4190*
456–955	Fibroelastosis of endocardium, adult	*4590*
410–9x9	Fibrosis or calcification of heart due to unknown cause	*4190*
45▲.▲–941	Atherosclerosis of valve. *Specify valve*	*4590*
45▲–941.4	With deformity of valve	*4590*
420–923	Calcification of pericardium due to unknown cause	*4290*

45▲–9x9	Fibrosis or calcification of valve due to unknown cause. *Specify valve*	*4590*
430–932.6	Fibrosis of myocardium due to rheumatic fever	*4390*
430–955	Fibrosis of myocardium due to unknown cause	*4390*
410–925	Heart disease with atypical verrucous endocarditis	*4190*
450–925	Endocarditis atypical verrucous	*4590*
456–925	Endocarditis mural atypical verrucous	*4590*
420–900.8	Hydropericardium due to unknown cause	*4290*
430–9x7	Infarction of myocardium due to unknown cause	*4390*
404–900.4	Mediastinopericarditis due to unknown cause	*4290*
430–930	Myocarditis, acute, isolated due to unknown cause	*4390*
430–950	Myocarditis of unknown cause (Fiedler)	*4395*
420–930	Pericarditis acute benign	*4290*
41x–932	Rheumatic coronary arteritis	*4190*
410–932	Rheumatic heart disease, active	*4193*
450–932	Rheumatic endocarditis, active	*4590*
456–932	Rheumatic mural endocarditis, active	*4590*
45▲–932.4	Rheumatic valvulitis, active, with deformity of valve. *Specify valve*	*4590*
404–932	Rheumatic mediastinopericarditis, active	*4290*
430–932	Rheumatic myocarditis, active	*4390*
420–932	Rheumatic pericarditis, active	*4290*
420–932.4	With adherent pericardium	*4290*
420–932.8	With effusion or exudate	*4290*
410–932.0	Rheumatic heart disease, inactive	*4193*
450–932.0	Rheumatic endocarditis, inactive	*4590*
430–932.0	Rheumatic myocarditis, inactive	*4390*
420–932.0	Rheumatic pericarditis, inactive	*4290*
45▲–932.6	Rheumatic valvulitis, inactive with deformity of valve. *Specify valve*	*4590*

—X DISEASES DUE TO UNKNOWN CAUSE WITH THE FUNCTIONAL RE-ACTION ALONE MANIFEST [1]

Etiologic digits in this section are used arbitrarily

444▲–x31	Aberrant ventricular conduction	*4490*
431–x26	Atrial fibrillation chronic due to unknown cause	*4390*
431–x25	Atrial fibrillation paroxysmal due to unknown cause	*4390*
431–x24	Atrial flutter chronic due to unknown cause	*4390*

[1] If the cause is known, these physiologic disturbances are not to be diagnosed under this section. The appropriate etiologic factor codes should be used, and these titles should be recorded according to the list of Supplementary Terms, page 491.

431–x23	Atrial flutter paroxysmal due to unknown cause	*4390*
431–x22	Atrial paroxysmal tachycardia due to unknown cause	*4390*
431–x21	Atrial premature contractions due to unknown cause	*4390*
444–x36	Atrioventricular block, complete, due to unknown cause	*4490*
444–x35	Atrioventricular block, incomplete, due to unknown cause	*4490*
444–x34	Atrioventricular block with prolonged conduction time due to unknown cause	*4490*
443–x33	Atrioventricular nodal rhythm due to unknown cause	*4490*
4443–x37	Branch block, left bundle, due to unknown cause	*4490*
4442–x37	Branch block, right bundle, due to unknown cause	*4490*
443–x32	Paroxysmal tachycardia, atrioventricular nodal due to unknown cause	*4490*
443–x31	Premature contractions, atrioventricular nodal due to unknown cause	*4490*
441–x16	Sino-atrial block due to unknown cause	*4490*
441–x11	Sinus arrest due to unknown cause	*4490*
441–x12	Sinus arrhythmia due to unknown cause	*4490*
441–x13	Sinus bradycardia due to unknown cause	*4490*
441–x14	Sinus tachycardia due to unknown cause	*4490*
434–x43	Ventricular escape due to unknown cause	*4390*
434–x45	Ventricular fibrillation due to unknown cause	*4390*
4441–x37	Intraventricular block due to unknown cause. *See* Bundle branch block due to unknown cause, *above*	*4490*
434–x42	Ventricular paroxysmal tachycardia due to unknown cause [1]	*4390*
434–x41	Ventricular premature contractions due to unknown cause	*4390*
434–x44	Ventricular standstill due to unknown cause [1]	*4390*
441–x15	Wandering pacemaker due to unknown cause [1]	*4490*

[1] The phrase "due to unknown cause" means that the condition is not the result of a demonstrable congenital, infectious, toxic, nutritional, or nervous cause or of structural disease. None of the terms given is to be considered the diagnosis if any underlying disease is discovered. If an underlying disease is known, the appropriate etiologic digits should be substituted in the proper place and the arrhythmia recorded according to the list of Supplementary Terms, page 491.

—Y UNDIAGNOSED DISEASES OF THE HEART

Y signifies an incomplete diagnosis. It is to be replaced whenever possible by a code digit signifying the specific diagnosis

410–y00   Heart disease, undiagnosed   *0064*

451–y00   Valvular disease undiagnosed   *0064*

This diagnosis is to be used when it is believed that the murmur is due to an undiagnosed or undiagnosable valvular disease. When the source of the murmur is not known, the title "Murmur of unknown origin" is to be used. See Supplementary Terms (*page 491*).

DISEASES OF THE ARTERIES

460–
470– } Arteries
402–   Arteries and veins
47x–   Peripheral arterioles

*For detailed list of arteries, see page 26.   If intrinsic artery
(of organ) is involved, see under organ affected*

—0 DISEASES DUE TO GENETIC AND PRENATAL INFLUENCES

See also under Cardiovascular System, generally, *page 201*

46▲–015	Aneurysm of artery, congenital. *Specify artery*	*4601*
46▲–010	Anomaly of artery. *Specify artery*	*4601*
463–010	Anomalous origin of subclavian artery, right	*4601*
4623–010	Anomalous origin of subclavian artery, left	*4601*
402–029	Arteriovenous fistula, congenital	*4601*

—1 DISEASES DUE TO INFECTION WITH LOWER ORGANISM

46▲–100.2	Abscess of wall of artery. *Specify artery and organism (page 57) when known*	*4610*
46▲–1x0.6	Aneurysm embolic of artery. *Specify artery when known*	*4610*
46▲–147.6	Aneurysm of artery due to syphilis. *Specify artery*	*4610*
46▲–100.6	Aneurysm of . . . artery due to infection. *Specify artery and infection when known*	*4610*
402▲–100.6	Arteriovenous aneurysm due to infection	*4610*
46▲–100	Arteritis, acute. *Specify artery and organism (page 57) when known*	*4611*
46▲–100.0	Arteritis, chronic. *Specify artery and organism (page 57) when known*	*4611*
46▲–1x0.4	Embolism of artery due to remote infection. *Specify artery*	*4610*
46▲–100.5	Hemorrhage from artery due to infection. *Specify artery*	*4610*
46▲–147.5	Rupture of artery due to syphilis. *Specify artery*	*4610*
4602–147	Syphilitic mesarteritis.	*4611*
46▲–100.7	Thrombosis of artery due to infection. *Specify artery and organism (page 57) when known*	*4610*

| 46▲–123 | Tuberculosis of artery. *Specify artery* | *4611* |

| 460–3▲▲ | Poisoning of artery. *Specify poison (page 67), e.g.* | *4630* |
| 460–3238 | Lead arteriosclerosis | *4630* |

46▲–427	Air embolism of artery	*4640*
46▲–400.6	Aneurysm of artery due to trauma	*4640*
402▲–400.6	Arteriovenous aneurysm due to trauma	*4640*
402–400.3	Arteriovenous fistula due to trauma	*4640*
46▲–420.4	Embolism of artery due to remote trauma	*4640*
46▲–425	Embolism of artery following operation	*4640*
46▲–426	Fat embolism of artery	*4640*
46▲–4▲▲	Injury of artery. *Specify artery and injury (page 83)*	*4640*
46▲–416	Rupture of artery due to trauma	*4640*
46▲–415.5	Rupture of artery following operation	*4640*
46▲–400.7	Thrombosis of artery due to trauma	*4640*
46▲–415.7	Thrombosis of artery following operation	*4640*

47x–513	Angiospasm of arteries of leg and foot	*4650*
460–534	Constitutional arterial hypotension	*4650*
460–533	Hypertensive vascular disease	*4653*

> This term is to be used in the sense of a disease manifested by arterial hypertension accompanied by arteriolar sclerosis without evidence of structural or functional abnormality of the heart. It is not to be confused with Arteriosclerosis, general (*page 218*). If both diseases are present, both are to be diagnosed. In the presence of cardiac manifestations, such as angina arrhythmia or hypertrophy, diagnose Hypertensive cardiovascular disease (*page 206*).

| 46▲–547 | Thrombosis of . . . due to thrombocytosis. *Specify artery* | *4650* |

402x–564	Circulatory disturbance in foot due to previous poliomyelitis	*4655*
46▲–5x7.4	Embolism of . . . from thrombus. *Specify artery*	*4650*
47x–581	Erythromalalgia	*4655*
47x–582	Raynaud's disease	*4655*

—6 DISEASES DUE TO OR CONSISTING OF STATIC MECHANICAL AB-NORMALITY

46▲–615.6	Aneurysm of artery due to calcareous particle. *Specify artery*	*4663*
46▲–618	Embolism of artery. *Specify artery*	*4661*
46▲–618.6	Embolic aneurysm of artery. *Specify artery*	*4663*
46▲–619	Thrombosis of artery due to unknown cause. *Specify artery*	*4662*

—7 DISEASES DUE TO DISORDER OF METABOLISM, GROWTH, OR NUTRITION
Record primary diagnosis

460–781	Arterial hypertension due to disease of adrenal glands	*4670*
460–776	Arterial hypertension due to disease of pituitary gland	*4670*
460–782	Arterial hypotension due to disease of adrenal glands	*4670*

—9 DISEASES DUE TO UNKNOWN OR UNCERTAIN CAUSE WITH THE STRUCTURAL REACTION MANIFEST

46▲–9x6	Aneurysm of . . . due to unknown cause. *Specify artery*	*4690*
460–942	Arteriosclerosis, general. Or specify artery. *To be diagnosed whenever present*	*4694*
46▲–942.6	Aneurysm of artery due to arteriosclerosis. *Specify artery*	*4690*
46▲–942.5	Rupture of artery due to arteriosclerosis. *Specify artery*	*4690*
4602–955	Arteriosclerosis, medial, especially with calcification	*4694*
46x.2–955	Of iliac arteries	*4694*
460–952	Arteriosclerosis obliterans	*4694*
46▲–941	Atherosclerosis of . . . *Specify artery*	*4694*
460–923	Calcification of arteries due to unknown cause	*4690*
402–931	Periarteritis nodosa. *Specify artery and vein when known*	*4690*
46▲–931.6	Aneurysm of artery due to periarteritis nodosa. *Specify artery*	*4690*
46▲–931.5	Hemorrhage from artery due to periarteritis nodosa. *Specify artery*	*4690*
46▲–931.7	Thrombosis of artery due to periarteritis nodosa. *Specify artery*	*4690*
46▲–932	Rheumatic arteritis. *Specify artery*	*4690*

401–992	Telangiectasia hemorrhagica (Osler-Rendu-Weber syndrome)	*4690*
402–930	Thromboangiitis obliterans	*4690*
46▲–942.7	Thrombosis of artery secondary to arteriosclerosis. *Specify artery or see under organ affected. Record primary diagnosis*	*4690*
47x–943	Arteriolar sclerosis, generalized	4694

This term refers to a more or less wide-spread sclerosis of the arterioles which may or may not be accompanied by arterial hypertension. It is to be distinguished from Arteriosclerosis, general. If arterial hypertension is present, diagnose (1) Hypertensive vascular disease (*page 217*) or (2) Hypertensive cardiovascular disease (*page 206*) depending on the stage of the disease.

—X DISEASES DUE TO UNKNOWN OR UNCERTAIN CAUSE WITH THE FUNCTIONAL REACTION ALONE MANIFEST; HEREDITARY AND FAMILIAL DISEASES OF THIS NATURE

47x–x30	Essential vascular hypertension	*4699*

This term is used in a sense of a disease manifested by arterial hypertension without anatomical changes in the arterioles and without structural or functional abnormality of the heart. If structural arteriolar changes are present, diagnose Hypertensive vascular disease (*page 217*). If the heart is affected in structure or function, diagnose Hypertensive cardiovascular disease (*page 206*).

460–x10	Orthostatic hypotension	*4690*

DISEASES OF THE AORTA

461– Aorta
4616– Abdominal aorta
40▲– Combined structures

—0 DISEASES DUE TO GENETIC AND PRENATAL INFLUENCES

See also under Cardiovascular System, generally, *page 201*

—I DISEASES DUE TO INFECTION WITH LOWER ORGANISM

461–100.6	Aneurysm of aorta due to infection. *Specify organism (page 57) when known, e.g.*	4610
461–147.6	Due to syphilis	4610
461–100	Aortitis acute bacterial. *Specify organism (page 57) when known*	4611
461–190	Aortitis subacute bacterial.	4611
461–100.9	Dilatation of aorta due to infection. *Specify organism (page 57) when known*	4610
461–100.5	Rupture of aorta due to infection. *Specify organism (page 57) when known*	4610
4034–100.5	Into esophagus	4610
4032–100.5	Into great vein	4610
4051–100.5	Into pulmonary artery	4610
4033–100.5	Into trachea	4610
4051–147.5	Rupture of syphilitic aneurysm of aorta into pulmonary artery	4610
46▲–147	Syphilitic arteritis	4611

—4 DISEASES DUE TO TRAUMA

461–4▲▲	Injury of aorta. *Specify injury (page 83)*	4640
461–416	Rupture of aorta due to trauma	4640

—50 DISEASES DUE TO CIRCULATORY DISTURBANCE

461–533.9	Dynamic dilatation of aorta	4650

—6 DISEASES DUE TO OR CONSISTING OF STATIC MECHANICAL ABNORMALITY

4616–618	Saddle embolus of aorta. *Record primary diagnosis*	4665

—7 DISEASE DUE TO DISORDER OF METABOLISM, GROWTH, OR NUTRITION

461–754	Fatty infiltration of aorta	4670

—9 DISEASES DUE TO UNKNOWN OR UNCERTAIN CAUSE WITH THE STRUCTURAL REACTION MANIFEST

461–932	Acute rheumatic aortitis	*4690*
461.2–915.6	Aneurysm of aorta due to medial necrosis	*4690*
461–942	Arteriosclerosis of aorta	*4694*
461–942.6	Aneurysm (dilatation) of aorta due to arteriosclerosis	*4690*
4616–942.6	Abdominal	*4690*
4615–942.6	Thoracic	*4690*
4616–942	Arteriosclerosis of abdominal aorta	*4694*
461–942.5	Rupture of aorta due to arteriosclerosis	*4694*
461–942.4	Obstruction of aorta due to arteriosclerosis	*4694*
461–941.6	Dissecting aneurysm of aorta due to unknown cause	*4690*
461–915.6	Due to cystic medial necrosis	*4690*
461.2–955	Medial degeneration of aorta (not due to syphilis)	*4690*
461.2–955.5	Rupture of aorta due to medial degeneration	*4690*
461–942.7	Thrombosis of aorta due to arteriosclerosis	*4694*
4051–942.5	Rupture of arteriosclerotic aneurysm of aorta into pulmonary artery	*4690*

DISEASES OF LESSER CIRCULATION

471– Pulmonary arteries generally
4711– Pulmonary artery
486– Pulmonary veins

—0 DISEASES DUE TO GENETIC AND PRENATAL INFLUENCES

See also under Cardiovascular System, generally, *page 201*

—I DISEASES DUE TO INFECTION WITH LOWER ORGANISM

471–100.6	Aneurysm of pulmonary artery due to infection. *Specify organism (page 57) when known*	4710
471–123	Tuberculosis of pulmonary artery	4710

—4 DISEASES DUE TO TRAUMA OR PHYSICAL AGENT

471–425	Embolism of pulmonary arteries due to operative trauma	4740
4711–4▲▲	Injury of pulmonary artery. *Specify injury (page 83)*	4740

—50 DISEASES DUE TO CIRCULATORY DISTURBANCE

471–522.4	Embolism of pulmonary arteries due to venous stasis and thrombosis	4750
471–533	Hypertension of lesser circulation due to obstruction of blood flow as by pulmonary disease, mitral stenosis, failure of left ventricle, etc. *Record primary diagnosis. If cardiac symptoms or signs have resulted from the hypertension, diagnose* Cardiovascular disease due to Hypertension of lesser circulation *(page 206)*	4750
471–533.3	Hypertension of lesser circulation due to arteriovenous shunt as patent ductus arteriosus, patent interventricular septum, etc.	4750
471–522.7	Thrombosis of pulmonary arteries due to venous stasis. *Record primary diagnosis*	4750
486–522.7	Thrombosis of pulmonary veins due to venous stasis. *Record primary diagnosis*	4750

**—6 DISEASES DUE TO OR CONSISTING OF STATIC MECHANICAL AB-
NORMALITY**

4711–610.9	Dilatation of pulmonary artery due to stenosis of mitral valve	*4760*
4711–641	Dilatation of pulmonary artery, due to unknown cause	*4760*
471–618	Embolism of pulmonary arteries due to unknown cause	*4761*
4711–619	Thrombosis of pulmonary artery, due to unknown cause	*4762*
486–619	Thrombosis of pulmonary vein due to unknown cause	*4760*

**—9 DISEASES DUE TO UNKNOWN OR UNCERTAIN CAUSE WITH THE
STRUCTURAL REACTION ALONE MANIFEST**

471–942	Arteriosclerosis of lesser circulation. *If coronary arteriosclerosis is present and if cardiac symptoms are present, such as angina or arrythmia, diagnose as under* Arteriosclerotic heart disease, *page 210*	*4694*
4711–942.6	Aneurysm of pulmonary artery due to arteriosclerosis	*4694*

DISEASES OF THE VEINS

480– Veins

For detailed list of veins, see page 27. If intrinsic vein (of organ) is involved, see under organ affected

—0 DISEASES DUE TO GENETIC AND PRENATAL INFLUENCES

48▲–010	Anomaly of vein. *Specify vein*	*4801*
482–010	Anomaly of portal vein (in situs transversus)	*4801*
480–015	Phlebectasia, congenital	*4801*

See also under Cardiovascular System, generally, *page 201*

—1 DISEASES DUE TO INFECTION WITH LOWER ORGANISM

487–100	Acute septic phlebitis of jugular vein. *Specify organism when known*	*4811*
48▲–190	Phlebitis. *Specify vein and organism (page 57) when known*	*4811*
48▲–115	Due to Eberthella typhosa	*4811*
48▲–124	Due to Mycobacterium leprae	*4811*
48▲–184	Due to typhus	*4811*
482–190	Phlebitis of portal vein. *Specify organism (page 57) when known*	*4811*
48▲–1901	Phlebitis, puerperal. *Specify vein*	*5750*
482–100	Suppurative pylephlebitis. *Specify organism (page 57) when known*	*4811*
487–100.7	Thrombosis of jugular vein due to infection. *Specify organism when known*	*4810*
482–100.7	Thrombosis of portal vein due to infection. *Specify organism when known*	*4810*
48▲–100.7	Thrombophlebitis. *Specify vein and organism (page 57) when known*	*4812*
48▲–123	Tuberculosis of vein. *Specify vein*	*4810*

—3 DISEASES DUE TO INTOXICATION

48▲–3▲▲	Poisoning of vein. *Specify vein and poison (page 67)*	*4830*

—4 DISEASES DUE TO TRAUMA OR PHYSICAL AGENT

48▲–4▲▲	Injury of vein. *Specify vein and trauma (page 83)*	*4840*
	Arteriovenous aneurysm. *See under* Arteries, *page 217*	

48▲–415.0	Phlebitis, following operation. *Specify vein*	*4840*
48▲–400.0	Phlebitis due to trauma. *Specify vein and trauma (page 83)*	*4840*
48▲–4x6.5	Rupture of varix. *Specify vein*	*4840*
48▲–415.7	Thrombosis of vein following operation	*4840*
48▲–400.7	Thrombosis of vein due to trauma	*4840*
48▲–430.6	Varix due to constant or intermittent trauma. *Specify vein*	*4840*
48▲–433.6	Due to clothing	*4840*
48▲–432.6	Due to occupation	*4840*
48▲–431.6	Due to posture	*4840*
48▲–434.6	Due to pressure of abnormal structure	*4840*
48▲–435.4	Due to pressure of gravid uterus	*4840*

—50 DISEASES DUE TO CIRCULATORY DISTURBANCE
Record primary diagnosis when possible

480–520	Distension collateral of veins	*4850*
48▲–547	Thrombosis of . . . due to thrombocytosis	*4850*
48▲–541.7	Thrombosis of vein due to polycythemia	*4850*
48▲–522	Varix due to passive congestion	*4850*

—6 DISEASES DUE TO OR CONSISTING OF STATIC MECHANICAL AB-
NORMALITY

481–610	Obstruction of . . . veins. *Specify vein*	*4860*
48▲–615	Phlebolith of . . . . *Specify vein*	*4860*
48▲–619.0	Phlebothrombosis with secondary infection	*4860*
48▲–619	Thrombosis of vein due to unspecified cause	*4860*
48▲–641	Varix of . . . . *Specify vein, e.g.*	*4864*
48x–641	Varicose veins of leg	*4864*
48x–641.0	Varicose veins with infection	*4864*

—9 DISEASES DUE TO UNKNOWN OR UNCERTAIN CAUSE WITH THE
STRUCTURAL REACTION MANIFEST

480–930	Idiopathic recurrent thrombophlebitis	*4890*
480–952	Phlebosclerosis	*4890*
	Thromboangiitis obliterans. *See under Arteries, page 219*	
48▲–931.7	Thrombosis of vein due to periarteritis nodosa. *Specify vein*	*4890*
48▲–9x6	Varicose veins due to unknown cause. *Specify vein*	*4890*

DISEASES OF THE CAPILLARIES

490– Capillaries

—I DUE TO INFECTION WITH LOWER ORGANISM

490–100.5   Capillary purpura due to infection   *4910*

—3 DISEASES DUE TO INTOXICATION

490–300.5   Capillary purpura due to allergy or drug
reaction   *4930*

—4 DISEASES DUE TO TRAUMA

490–400.5   Capillary purpura due to mechanical cause;
trauma   *4940*

—50 DISEASES DUE TO CIRCULATORY DISTURBANCE

490–5x5.5   Capillary purpura, generally   *4950*
490–512.5   Due to embolism   *4950*

—7 DISEASE DUE TO DISORDER OF METABOLISM, GROWTH, OR NUTRITION

490–700.5   Capillary purpura due to metabolic disturbance (purpura simplex)   *4970*

—8 NEW GROWTHS

See under Regions and Organs

**—9 DISEASES DUE TO UNKNOWN OR UNCERTAIN CAUSE WITH THE
STRUCTURAL REACTION MANIFEST; HEREDITARY AND FAMILIAL
DISEASES OF THIS NATURE**

490–991   Hemophilia, vascular (prolonged bleeding
time with deficiency of a coagulation
factor)   *4990*
490–992.5   Hereditary capillary fragility   *4990*
490–955   Pseudohemophilia "A"   *4990*
490–993.5   Pseudohemophilia "B"   *4990*

5- DISEASES OF THE HEMIC AND LYMPHATIC SYSTEMS

INTRODUCTION

The great majority of diagnoses in this section are secondary conditions and when possible should be accompanied by a primary diagnosis. For example, 501–736.7 Hypochromic microcytic anemia, from chronic blood loss. There are many causes of chronic blood loss and if the etiologic numbers were given for each of these, such anemias would be widely scattered in the diagnostic file. The primary diagnosis will always indicate the site and cause of the bleeding.

DISEASES OF THE BLOOD AND BLOOD-FORMING ORGANS

500–   Blood and blood-forming organs
501–   Erythrocytic tissue (Erythropoietic)
502–   Granulocytic tissue (Myeloid)
  5021–   Neutrophilic granulocytic tissue
  5022–   Eosinophilic granulocytic tissue
  5023–   Basophilic granulocytic tissue
503–   Lymphocytic tissue (Lymphoid)
504–   Plasmocytic tissue
505–   Reticuloendothelial system tissue
506–   Monocytic tissue (Parent tissue of monocytes)
507–   Thrombocytic tissue

—0 DISEASES DUE TO GENETIC AND PRENATAL INFLUENCES

500–016	Anemia, normocytic hypoplastic (pancytopenia), congenital	*5001*
501–016	Anemia, normocytic due to erythrocytic hypoplasia, congenital	*5001*
507–076	Thrombocytopenia, congenital	*5001*

—I DISEASES DUE TO INFECTION WITH LOWER ORGANISM
Record primary diagnosis

500–100.9	Anemia, normocytic hypoplastic (pancytopenia) due to infection	*5010*
501–100.9	Anemia, normocytic due to erythrocytic hypoplasia from infection	*5010*
501–100	Anemia, normocytic hemolytic due to infection. *Specify organism when known, e.g.*	*5010*

227

501–157	Anemia due to malaria	*5010*
507–1▲▲	Thrombocytopenic purpura due to infection. *Specify organism*	*5010*

—2 DISEASES DUE TO HIGHER PLANT OR ANIMAL PARASITE

501–200	Anemia, normocytic hemolytic due to parasite. *Specify parasite when known*	*5020*

—3 DISEASES DUE TO INTOXICATION
Record primary diagnosis

501–3▲▲	Acquired hemolytic anemia. *Specify drug or poison when known*	*5030*
501–397	Due to cold agglutinins	*5030*
501–3432	Due to sulfonamide	*5030*
501–399	Due to sensitization to Rh-Hr or other erythrocytic agglutinogens	*5030*
501–3991	Hemolytic disease of the (fetus and) newborn	*5030*
501–3992	Transfusion hemolysis	*5030*
502–300	Agranulocytosis due to intoxication or drug reaction	*5030*
500–3▲▲.9	Anemia, normocytic, hypoplastic (pancytopenia) due to poison. *Specify*	*5030*
500–33131	Due to benzene (benzol)	*5030*
507–3▲▲	Thrombocytopenic purpura due to drugs or toxic agents. *Specify*	*5030*

—4 DISEASES DUE TO TRAUMA OR PHYSICAL AGENT

501–400.7	Anemia, normocytic, due to acute blood loss, due to trauma. *Specify trauma when known*	*5041*
500–470.9	Anemia, normocytic hypoplastic due to radiation generally or unspecified	*5040*
500–471.9	Due to roentgen rays	*5040*
500–47▲.9	Anemia, normocytic hypoplastic due to radioactive substance. *Specify radioactive substance*	*5040*

—50 DISEASES DUE TO CIRCULATORY DISTURBANCE

502–536	Agranulocytosis due to splenic diseases	*5050*
500–536	Anemia, normocytic, due to congestive splenomegaly	*5050*
500–5361	Congestive splenomegaly	*5050*
501–5x7.5	Anemia, normocytic, due to erythrocytic destruction, generally	*5050*

501–5x6	Hyperplasia, erythroid, secondary to anemia. *Record primary diagnosis*	*5050*
501–5x9	Hypoplasia, erythroid, secondary to anemia. *Record primary diagnosis*	*5050*

—7 DISEASES DUE TO DISORDER OF METABOLISM, GROWTH, OR NUTRITION
Record primary diagnosis

502–790	Agranulocytosis, generally and unspecified (granulocytopenia)	*5070*
501–736	Anemia, hypochromic microcytic, generally and unspecified	*5073*
501–736.7	Due to chronic blood loss	*5073*
501–736.x	Due to deficient intake, absorption or metabolism of iron; prematurity; pregnancy	*5073*
501–794	Anemia, macrocytic, not pernicious anemia type	*5070*
501–703	Anemia, megaloblastic	*5070*
501–7031	Due to pregnancy	*5070*
501–7032	Due to sprue	*5070*
501–7033	Infantile	*5070*
501–7034	Due to intestinal stasis	*5070*
501–7035	Pernicious anemia	*5071*
501–790.9	Anemia, normocytic due to erythrocytic hypoplasia, generally and unspecified	*5070*
500–790.9	Anemia, normocytic, hypoplastic (pancytopenia), generally and unspecified	*5070*
500–7901.9	Idiopathic hypoplastic anemia (aplastic anemia)	*5070*
501–700	Anemia, normocytic metabolic	*5070*
501–715	Due to protein deficiency	*5070*
501–709	Due to sprue	*5070*
501–772	Due to hypothyroidism	*5070*
501–704.6	Erythrocytoses due to arterial anoxemia	*5070*
505–755	Histiocytosis due to lipids, generally and unspecified	*5070*
505–756	Lipid histiocytosis of kerasin type (Gaucher's disease)	*5070*
505–758	Lipid histiocytosis of phosphatide type (Niemann-Pick disease)	*5070*
507–792.6	Thrombocytosis, generally and unspecified	*5079*
507–7921.6	Idiopathic thrombocythemia	*5079*
507–791	Thrombocytopenic purpura, generally and unspecified	*5079*
507–7911	Idiopathic thrombocytopenic purpura	*5079*
507–790.9	Thrombocytic hypoplasia	*5079*

—8 NEW GROWTHS

503–834	Giant follicular lymphoma.[1] *Specify behavior*	5080
502▲–822▲	Granulocytic leukemia.[2] *Specify site when known and behavior*	5080
505–832	Hodgkin's disease.[1] *Specify behavior*	5080
500–829	Leukemia, type unspecified.[2] *Specify behavior*	5080
503–820	Lymphocytic leukemia.[2] *Specify behavior*	5080
500–839	Lymphoma, type not specified.[1] *Specify behavior*	5080
503–830	Lymphosarcoma.[1] *Specify behavior*	5080
507–8281	Megakaryocytic leukemia.[2] *Specify behavior*	5080
506–821	Monocytic leukemia.[2] *Specify behavior*	5080
504–833	Plasma cell myeloma.[1] *Specify behavior*	5080
504–8282	Plasmacytic leukemia.[2] *Specify behavior*	5080
501–8271	Polycythemia vera. *Specify behavior*	5080
505–831	Reticulum cell sarcoma.[1] *Specify behavior*	5080
500–8283	Stem cell (Blast cell) leukemia.[2] *Specify behavior*	5080
5▲▲–8▲▲▲	Unlisted tumor of blood and blood-forming organs. *Specify site, neoplasm, and behavior (page 99)*	5080

—9 DISEASES DUE TO UNKNOWN OR UNCERTAIN CAUSE WITH THE STRUCTURAL REACTION MANIFEST; HEREDITARY AND FAMILIAL DISEASES OF THIS NATURE

501–991.5	Anemia, hemolytic hereditary	5090
501–9x0	Anemia, normocytic, cause unknown	5091
501–920.1	Anemia, normocytic myelophthisic	5091
500–995	Familial hypercholesteremia	5090
501–991	Hemoglobinopathy, type not specified	5090
501–9915	Hemoglobin "C" disease	5090
501–9916	Hemoglobin "C" trait	5090
501–9913	Hemoglobin "C" thalassemia disease	5090
501–9914	Hemoglobin "S" thalassemia disease	5090
501–9912.5	Hemoglobin (Sickle cell disease)	5090
501–9912.4	Hemoglobin S-A (Sickle cell trait)	5090
501–991.4	Hereditary ovalocytosis	5090
501–9911.5	Hereditary spherocytosis	5090
501–9911.4	Hereditary nonspherocytosis anemia	5090
501–9x6	Hyperplasia, erythroid, due to unknown cause	5090
502–9x6	Hyperplasia, myeloid, due to unknown cause	5090

[1] Use lymphoma behavior code (page 99).
[2] Use leukemia behavior code (page 99).

501–9x9	Hypoplasia, erythroid, due to unknown cause	*5090*
501–9913.5	Thalassemia major (Cooley's anemia)	*5090*
501–9913.4	Thalassemia minor (trait)	*5090*
507–920	Thrombocytopenic purpura due to myelophthisis	*5090*
507–9x7	Thrombotic thrombocytopenia	*5090*

—X DISEASES DUE TO UNKNOWN CAUSE WITH THE FUNCTIONAL REACTION ALONE MANIFEST; HEREDITARY AND FAMILIAL DISEASES OF THIS NATURE

507–x90.5	Thrombocytopathic purpura (pseudohemophilia)	*5090*

—Y DISEASES DUE TO CAUSE NOT DETERMINABLE OR NOT INDICATED IN THE PARTICULAR CASE

501–y00.1	Normocytic anemia, cause undetermined	*0065*

DISEASES OF THE SPLEEN

520–   Spleen (Fixed cells)

—0 DISEASES DUE TO GENETIC AND PRENATAL INFLUENCES

520–011	Absence of spleen	*5201*
520–031	Accessory spleen	*5201*
520–021	Displacement of spleen, congenital	*5201*
520–027	Hernia of spleen (through diaphragm), congenital	*5201*
520–010	Lobulation of spleen	*5201*

—I DISEASES DUE TO INFECTION WITH LOWER ORGANISM

520–100.2	Abscess of spleen. *Specify organism (page 57) when known*	*5210*
520–1x0	Sarcoidosis of spleen	*5210*
520–100	Splenitis	*5210*
520–100.6	Splenomegaly due to infection. *Specify organism when known*	*5210*
520–157.6	Splenomegaly due to malaria	*5210*

—4 DISEASES DUE TO TRAUMA OR PHYSICAL AGENT

520–4▲▲	Injury of spleen. *Specify injury (page 83), e.g.*	*5240*
520–416	Rupture of spleen	*5240*

—50 DISEASES DUE TO CIRCULATORY DISTURBANCE

520–511	Infarction of spleen due to arterial thrombosis	*5250*
520–512	Infarction of spleen due to embolism	*5250*
520–536	Passive congestion of spleen (splenomegaly) due to portal obstruction	*5250*

—6 DISEASES DUE TO OR CONSISTING OF STATIC MECHANICAL ABNORMALITY

520–630	Floating spleen	*5260*
520–631	Splenoptosis	*5260*
520–637	Torsion of spleen	*5260*

—7 DISEASES DUE TO DISORDER OF METABOLISM, GROWTH, OR NUTRITION

520–796	Atrophy of spleen, functional or secondary to sicklemia	*5270*
520–798 ·	Senile atrophy of spleen	*5270*
520–700.6	Splenomegaly due to metabolic disturbance	*5270*

—8 NEW GROWTHS

520–870A	Fibroma of spleen	*5280*
520–850A	Hemangioma of spleen	*5280*
520–832	Hodgkin's disease of spleen.[1] *Specify behavior*	*5280*
520–830	Lymphosarcoma of spleen.[1] *Specify behavior*	*5280*
520–831	Reticulum cell sarcoma of spleen.[1] *Specify behavior*	*5280*
520–8▲▲▲	Unlisted tumor of spleen.[1] *Specify neoplasm and behavior*	*5280*

—9 DISEASES DUE TO UNKNOWN OR UNCERTAIN CAUSE WITH THE STRUCTURAL REACTION MANIFEST

520–922	Amyloidosis of spleen due to unknown cause	*5290*
520–958	Myeloid metaplasia of the spleen	*5290*
520–958.4	Due to osteopetrosis	*5290*
520–958.9	Due to myelofibrosis	*5290*

—Y DISEASES DUE TO CAUSE NOT DETERMINABLE IN THE PARTICULAR CASE

520–yx6	Splenomegaly of undetermined origin	*0065*

[1] Use lymphoma behavior code (page 99).

DISEASES OF THE LYMPHATIC CHANNELS

540– Lymphatic channels
541– Thoracic duct

For detailed list of lymphatic channels, see page 29

—0 DISEASES DUE TO GENETIC AND PRENATAL INFLUENCES

542–019.8	Hygroma of neck	*5401*

—I DISEASES DUE TO INFECTION WITH LOWER ORGANISM

541–100.3   Fistula of thoracic duct due to infection   *5410*

54▲–100.6   Lymphangiectasis due to infection. *Specify channel*   *5410*

54▲–100   Lymphangitis, acute. *Specify channel*   *5411*

54▲–100.0   Lymphangitis, chronic. *Specify channel*   *5411*

54▲–123   Lymphangitis due to tuberculosis. *Specify channel*   *5411*

54▲–100.4   Occlusion of lymphatic channel due to infection. *Specify channel*   *5410*

54▲–100.5   Rupture of lymphatic channel, due to infection. *Specify channel*   *5410*

—2 DISEASES DUE TO HIGHER PLANT OR ANIMAL PARASITE

54▲–257   Filariasis of lymphatic channels. *Specify channels*   *5420*

—4 DISEASES DUE TO TRAUMA OR PHYSICAL AGENT

541–400.3   Fistula of thoracic duct due to trauma   *5440*

54▲–4▲▲   Injury of lymphatic channel. *Specify channel and injury*   *5440*

54▲–400.4   Occlusion of lymphatic channel due to trauma. *Specify channel*   *5440*

54▲–415.4   Occlusion of lymphatic channel following operation. *Specify channel*   *5440*

—8 NEW GROWTHS

54▲–854A   Lymphangioma. *Specify site*   *5480*

54▲–854G   Lymphangiosarcoma. *Specify site*   *5480*

54▲–854B   Lymphendothelioma. *Specify site*   *5480*

—9 DISEASES DUE TO UNKNOWN OR UNCERTAIN CAUSE WITH THE STRUCTURAL REACTION MANIFEST; HEREDITARY AND FAMILIAL DISEASES OF THIS NATURE

546–900.8   Lymphedema precox of leg   *5490*

DISEASES OF THE LYMPH NODES

550– Lymph nodes (Fixed cells)

For detailed list of lymph nodes, see page 29

—I DISEASES DUE TO INFECTION WITH LOWER ORGANISM

55▲–100.2	Abscess of lymph node. *Specify lymph node*	5512
558–190.8	Bubo, inguinal	5512
558–10x.8	Due to Hemophilus ducreyi	5512
558–103.8	Due to Neisseria gonorrheae	5512
558–147.8	Due to Treponema pallidum	5512
55▲–100.9	Calcification of lymph node due to infection. *Specify lymph node*	5510
55.–123.9	Calcification of lymph node due to tuberculosis. *Specify lymph node*	5510
55▲–100	Lymphadenitis, acute, due to infection. *Specify lymph node and organism when known*	5511
55▲–100.0	Lymphadenitis, chronic, due to infection. *Specify lymph node and organism when known*	5511
55▲–100.1	Lymphadenitis, purulent. *Specify lymph node and organism when known*	5511
55▲–198	Lymphopathia, venereum. *Specify lymph node*	5510
55▲–130	Nonbacterial regional lymphadenitis (cat scratch fever)	5513

—3 DISEASES DUE TO INTOXICATION

55▲–3▲▲	Toxic lymphadenitis due to exogenous poison. *Specify*	5530

—4 DISEASES DUE TO TRAUMA OR PHYSICAL AGENT

55▲–496	Foreign body of lymph node. *Specify lymph node*	5540
55▲–438	Lymphadenitis due to irritation by foreign body (anthracosis, silicosis). *Specify lymph node*	5540
55▲–400.0	Lymphadenitis due to trauma. *Specify lymph node*	5540

—8 NEW GROWTHS

55▲–838A	Benign lymphoid polyp. *Specify site*	*5580*
55▲–834	Giant follicular lymphoma. *Specify site and behavior*	*5580*
55▲–832	Hodgkin's disease.[1] *Specify site and behavior*	*5580*
55▲–839	Lymphoma.[1] *Specify site and behavior*	*5580*
55▲–830	Lymphosarcoma.[1] *Specify site and behavior*	*5580*
55▲–833	Plasma cell myeloma. *Specify site and behavior*	*5580*
55▲–831	Reticulum cell sarcoma.[1] *Specify site and behavior*	*5580*
55▲–8▲▲▲	Unlisted tumor of lymph nodes. *Specify site and neoplasm*	*5580*

—9 DISEASES DUE TO UNKNOWN OR UNCERTAIN CAUSE WITH THE STRUCTURAL REACTION MANIFEST; HEREDITARY AND FAMILIAL DISEASES OF THIS NATURE

55▲–959	Endometriosis of lymph node. *Specify lymph node*	*5590*
55▲–943	Hyperplasia of lymph node due to unknown cause. *Specify lymph node*	*5594*

—Y DISEASES DUE TO CAUSE NOT DETERMINABLE IN THE PARTICULAR CASE

550–y10	Lymphadenopathy due to undetermined cause	*0065*

1 Use lymphoma behavior code (page 99).

DISEASES OF PLASMA CONSTITUENTS

510–   Plasma or serum, generally
511–   Electrolytes
512–   Proteins
  5121–   Albumin
  5122–   Globulins
513–   Plasma components affecting coagulation, generally
    For detailed list of plasma components, see page 28
514–   Hemoglobin pigments
    For detailed list of hemoglobin pigments, see page 29
515–   Porphyrins
519–   Other organic constituents

—0 DISEASES DUE TO GENETIC AND PRENATAL INFLUENCES

5122–011   Agammaglobulinemia, congenital   *5101*

—3 DISEASES DUE TO INTOXICATION

514▲–3▲▲   Hemoglobin pigment disturbance due to poison. *Specify pigment and poison*   *5130*
5132–3▲▲   Hypoprothrombinemia due to drugs. *Specify drug*   *5130*
515–3▲▲   Porphyria due to drugs. *Specify drug*   *5130*

—4 DISEASES DUE TO TRAUMA OR PHYSICAL AGENT

5145–404   Myoglobinuria due to crush syndrone   *5140*
5141–44x   Paroxysmal hemoglobinuria due to cold   *5140*
515–450   Photosensitive porphyria   *5140*

—50 DISEASES DUE TO CIRCULATORY DISTURBANCE

513▲–549   Plasma defects affecting coagulation. *Specify plasma constituent if possible*   *5150*

—7 DISEASES DUE TO DISORDER OF METABOLISM, GROWTH, OR NUTRITION

5142–7671   Methemoglobinemia, hereditary   *5170*
5141–712   Paroxysmal hemoglobinuria due to exertion   *5170*
515–749   Porphyria, generally   *5170*

—X DISEASES DUE TO UNKNOWN OR UNCERTAIN CAUSE WITH THE FUNCTIONAL REACTION ALONE MANIFEST; HEREDITARY AND FAMILIAL DISEASES OF THIS NATURE

5122–x80   Agammaglobulinemia, acquired   *5190*
519–x80   Constitutional hyperbilirubinemia   *5190*

DISEASES OF THE MARROW

530– Marrow (Fixed cells)

—I DISEASES DUE TO INFECTION WITH LOWER ORGANISM

530–123	Tuberculosis of bone marrow	*5310*

—8 NEW GROWTHS

530–875G	Ewing's sarcoma of bone marrow	*5380*
530–832	Hodgkin's disease of bone marrow.[1] *Specify behavior*	*5380*
530–831	Reticulum cell sarcoma of bone marrow	*5380*
530–8▲▲▲	Unlisted tumor of bone marrow. *Specify neoplasm and behavior*	*5380*

—9 DISEASES DUE TO UNKNOWN OR UNCERTAIN CAUSE WITH THE STRUCTURAL REACTION MANIFEST

530–941	Agnogenic myeloid metaplasia	*5390*
530–922	Amyloidosis of bone marrow	*5390*
530–942	Myelofibrosis, idiopathic	*5390*

1 Use lymphoma behavior code (page 99).

6– DISEASES OF THE DIGESTIVE SYSTEM

600–   Alimentary tract

—0   DISEASES DUE TO GENETIC AND PRENATAL INFLUENCES

600–011	Complete absence of alimentary tract, congenital (only in marked fetal malformations, such as acardiacus amorphus)	6001
600–012	Partial absence of alimentary tract, congenital (in marked fetal malformations)	6001
600–026	Ectopia of abdominal viscera due to defect in anterior abdominal wall	6001

—7   DISEASES DUE TO DISORDER OF METABOLISM, GROWTH, OR NUTRITION

600–716	Celiac disease	6070

DISEASES OF THE MOUTH

610–   Mouth
618–   Cheek
122–   Mucous membrane of mouth

—1 DISEASES DUE TO INFECTION WITH LOWER ORGANISM

610–100.2	Abscess of mouth. *Specify organism (page 57) when known*	6110
122–1x1	Aphthous stomatitis	1200
6102–100	Cellulitis of floor of mouth. *Specify organism when known*	6110
6101–100.3	Fistula, buccal pharyngeal due to infection	6110
610–190.1	Gangrenous stomatitis (noma)	6110
610–166	Herpes of mouth	6110
610–100.3	Sinus of mouth due to infection	6110
610–190	Stomatitis. *Specify organism (page 57) when known*	6110
610–1413	Vincent's infection of mouth	6110

—2 DISEASES DUE TO HIGHER PLANT OR ANIMAL PARASITE

610–209	Thrush of mouth	6120

—3 DISEASES DUE TO INTOXICATION

610–3▲▲	Stomatitis due to poison. *Specify poison (page 67)*	6130

—4 DISEASES DUE TO TRAUMA OR PHYSICAL AGENT

6101–415.3	Fistula buccal cavity postoperative	6140
6101–400.3	Fistula, buccal pharyngeal due to trauma	6140
610–4▲▲	Injury of mouth. *Specify injury (page 83), e.g.*	6140
610–414	Gunshot wound of mouth	6140
610–411	Stab wound of mouth	6140
610–400.3	Sinus of mouth due to trauma	6140

—6 DISEASES DUE TO OR CONSISTING OF STATIC MECHANICAL ABNORMALITY

610–600.8	Buccal cyst	6160
61x–641	Varix of mouth	6160

—8 NEW GROWTHS

618–814	Epidermoid carcinoma of cheek. *Specify behavior (page 99)*	6180

122–8032A	Epithelioma adenoides cysticum of mucous membrane of mouth (acanthoma)	*6180*
610–870A	Fibroma of mouth	*6180*
610–870F	Fibrosarcoma of mouth	*6180*
610–854A	Lymphangioma of mouth	*6180*
610–8852	Mixed tumor salivary gland type of mouth. *Specify behavior (page 99)*	*6180*
610–8▲▲▲	Unlisted tumor of mouth. *Specify neoplasm and behavior*	*6180*

—9 DISEASES DUE TO UNKNOWN OR UNCERTAIN CAUSE WITH THE STRUCTURAL REACTION MANIFEST

122–943	Cutaneous horn of mouth (cheek)	*1200*
122–951	Ulcer of mouth due to unknown cause	*1200*

DISEASES OF THE LIPS

611– Lips
123– Mucous membrane of lips
134– Skin of lips
156– Mucous glands of lips

—0 DISEASES DUE TO GENETIC AND PRENATAL INFLUENCES

6111–0▲▲	Abnormality of labium frenum, congenital. *Specify anomaly*	6101
6112–037	Cleft of upper lip congenital; unilateral; median or bilateral; complete or incomplete	6102
6112–0371	Complete, bilateral	6102
6112–0372	Complete, unilateral	6102
6112–0373	Incomplete, bilateral	6102
6112–0374	Incomplete, unilateral	6102
611–022	Deformity of lip, congenital	6101
611–029	Fistula in lip, congenital	6101
611–013	Macrocheilia; congenital hypertrophy of lip	6101
611–034	Macrostomia; congenital split lips	6101
611–017	Microstomia	6101
1231–023	Sebaceous glands of mucocutaneous junction of lips, aberrant	1200

—I DISEASES DUE TO INFECTION WITH LOWER ORGANISM

611–100.2	Abscess of lip. *Specify organism (page 57) when known*	6110
611–190	Cheilitis due to infection. *Specify organism (page 57) when known. See also* under Skin, *page 140*	6110
611–166	Herpes of lip	6110

—3 DISEASES DUE TO INTOXICATION

611–3▲▲	Chemical burn of lip. *Specify poison (page 67)*	6130

—4 DISEASES DUE TO TRAUMA OR PHYSICAL AGENT

611–415.4	Cicatricial deformity of lip following operation	6140
611–451	Cheilitis, actinic	6140
611–400.4	Deformity of lip due to trauma. *Specify trauma (page 83) when known*	6140
611–4▲▲	Injury of lip. *Specify (page 83)*	6140

—6 DISEASES DUE TO OR CONSISTING OF STATIC MECHANICAL ABNOR-MALITY

156–600.8	Cyst of glands of lip	*6160*
611–640	Deformity of lip due to unknown cause	*6160*

—7 DISEASES DUE TO DISORDER OF METABOLISM, GROWTH, OR NUTRITION

611–7622	Cheilosis due to riboflavin deficiency	*6170*

—8 NEW GROWTHS

611▲–8091	Adenocarcinoma of lip. *Specify site and behavior (page 99)*	*6180*
611▲–812	Basal cell carcinoma of lip. *Specify site and behavior (page 99)*	*6180*
611▲–873B	Chondroma of lip. *Specify site*	*6180*
611▲–814	Epidermoid carcinoma of lip. *Specify site and behavior (page 99)*	*6180*
611▲–870A	Fibroma of lip. *Specify site*	*6180*
611▲–868A	Granular cell myoblastoma of lip. *Specify site*	*6180*
611▲–850A	Hemangioma of lip. *Specify site*	*6180*
611▲–872A	Lipoma of lip. *Specify site*	*6180*
611▲–854A	Lymphangioma of lip. *Specify site*	*6180*
611▲–8852	Mixed tumor salivary gland type of lip. *Specify site and behavior (page 99)*	*6180*
611▲–8451	Neurofibroma of lip. *Specify site and behavior (page 99)*	*6180*
611▲–8▲▲▲	Unlisted tumor of lip. *Specify site, neoplasm and behavior*	*6180*

—9 DISEASES DUE TO UNKNOWN OR UNCERTAIN CAUSE WITH THE STRUCTURAL REACTION MANIFEST

611–9x5	Fissure of lip due to unknown cause	*6190*
611–951	Ulcer of lip due to unknown cause	*6190*

DISEASES OF THE TONGUE

612–   Tongue
6121–   Frenum linguae
124–   Mucous membrane of tongue

—0 DISEASES DUE TO GENETIC AND PRENATAL INFLUENCES

612–025	Adhesion of tongue to gum or roof of mouth, congenital	*6101*
612–011	Aglossia; congenital absence of tongue	*6101*
6121–017	Ankyloglossia; tongue-tie (shortening of frenum linguae)	*6101*
612–035	Bifurcation of tongue, congenital	*6101*
612–064	Cyst of tongue, congenital	*6101*
612–021	Displacement of tongue downward, congenital	*6101*
612–032	Double tongue, congenital	*6101*
6121–013	Elongated frenum linguae	*6101*
612–010	Fissured tongue, congenital (deep furrows)	*6101*
612–013	Macroglossia; congenital hypertrophy of tongue (often associated with idiocy, mongolism, and cretinism)	*6101*
612–016	Microglossia; hypoplasia of tongue	*6101*

—I DISEASES DUE TO INFECTION WITH LOWER ORGANISM

612–100.2	Abscess of tongue. *Specify organism (page 57) when known*	*6110*
612–100	Acute glossitis. *Specify organism (page 57) when known*	*6110*
612–100.0	Chronic glossitis due to infection. *Specify organism (page 57) when known*	*6110*
124–147.6	Leukoplakia of tongue following syphilis	*6110*
612–1413	Vincent's infection of tongue	*6110*

—3 DISEASES DUE TO INTOXICATION

612–3▲▲	Chemical burn of tongue. *Specify poison (page 67)*	*6130*
124–300.6	Leukoplakia of tongue due to poison. *Specify poison (page 67)*	*6130*

—4 DISEASES DUE TO TRAUMA OR PHYSICAL AGENT

612–4▲▲	Injury of tongue. *Specify injury (page 83)*	*6140*
124–400.6	Leukoplakia of tongue due to trauma	*6140*

—55 DISEASES DUE TO DISTURBANCE OF INNERVATION OR OF PSYCHIC CONTROL

Record primary diagnosis when possible

612–565	Atrophy of tongue, neurogenic	*6155*

—6 DISEASES DUE TO OR CONSISTING OF STATIC MECHANICAL ABNORMALITY

612–600.8	Cyst of tongue	*6160*
612–640	Deformity of tongue due to unknown cause	*6160*

—7 DISEASES DUE TO DISORDER OF METABOLISM, GROWTH, OR NUTRITION

612–760	Atrophy of tongue due to avitaminosis	*6170*
612–798	Senile atrophy of tongue	*6170*

—8 NEW GROWTHS

612–8091	Adenocarcinoma of tongue. *Specify behavior (page 99)*	*6180*
612–873B	Chondroma of tongue	*6180*
612–814	Epidermoid carcinoma of tongue. *Specify behavior (page 99)*	*6180*
612–868A	Granular cell myoblastoma of tongue	*6180*
612–850A	Hemangioma of tongue	*6180*
612–872A	Lipoma of tongue	*6180*
612–854A	Lymphangioma of tongue	*6180*
612–8▲▲▲	Unlisted tumor of tongue. *Specify neoplasm and behavior*	*6180*

—9 DISEASES DUE TO UNKNOWN OR UNCERTAIN CAUSE WITH THE STRUCTURAL REACTION MANIFEST

124–960	Acanthosis of tongue	*1200*
124–910	Atrophy of mucous membrane of tongue (in pernicious anemia and achylia gastrica)	*1200*
124–944	Black, hairy tongue	*1200*
612–9x5	Fissure of tongue	*6190*
124–957	Geographic tongue	*1200*
124–941	Leukoplakia of tongue due to unknown cause	*1200*
612–9x6	Macroglossia, acquired	*6190*
612–940	Median rhomboidal glossitis	*6190*
612–951	Ulcer of tongue due to unknown cause	*6190*

DISEASES OF TEETH AND GINGIVA

613– Teeth
614– Supporting structures, tooth
218– Maxilla
219– Mandible

For detailed list of supporting structures, see page 33

—0 DISEASES DUE TO GENETIC AND PRENATAL INFLUENCES

6145–010	Abnormal alveolar ridge, congenital	*6101*
6135–011	Anodontia	*6101*
61431–037	Cleft of upper alveolus, congenital, unilateral; median; median or bilateral; complete (to incisive foramen), or incomplete	*6101*
6142–064	Cyst of gingiva, congenital	*6101*
6134–077	Dentinogenesis imperfecta (opalescent dentin)	*6101*
613–077	Fusion of teeth, congenital	*6101*
613–024	Gemination of teeth	*6101*
613–051	Hutchinson's teeth	*6101*
6135–012	Oligodontia	*6101*
613–075	Precocious dentition, congenital	*6101*
613–031	Supernumerary tooth	*6101*

—I DISEASES DUE TO INFECTION WITH LOWER ORGANISM

6142–100.2	Abscess of gingiva. *Specify organism (page 57) when known*	*6110*
6142–100	Gingivitis. *Specify organism when known as:*	*6110*
6142–102	Acute streptococcal	*6110*
6143–100	Apical infection	*6111*
6143–100.6	Apical granuloma	*6110*
6143–100.8	Apical cyst	*6110*
613–100.1	Caries of teeth	*6114*
6132–100.0	Exposed pulp, due to infection	*6110*
614–100.3	Dental fistula	*6110*
6142–166	Herpetic gingivitis	*6110*
6132–100.1	Necrotic pulp	*6110*
6142–1413	Necrotizing ulcerating gingivitis (Vincent's gingivitis)	*6110*
614–100.2	Periodontal abscess	*6112*
6132–100	Pulpitis	*6110*
6132–100.9	Putrescent pulp	*6110*

6145–100.9	Sequestrum formation of alveolar arches, due to infection	*6110*

—3 DISEASES DUE TO INTOXICATION

6142–3116	Bismuth line of gingiva	*6130*
613–3▲▲▲.1	Chemical delcalcification of teeth. *Specify chemical (page 67) when known*	*6130*
6142–33731	Dilantin hyperplasia of gingiva	*6130*
6142–3112	Lead line of gingiva	*6130*
6142–3111	Mercurial gingivitis	*6130*
6133–3195	Mottled enamel due to fluorine (endemic fluorosis)	*6130*

—4 DISEASES DUE TO TRAUMA OR PHYSICAL AGENT

61353–415.1	Absence of teeth, acquired, mandibular, complete	*6140*
61354–415.1	Absence of teeth, acquired, mandibular, partial	*6140*
61351–415.1	Absence of teeth, acquired, maxillary, complete	*6140*
61352–415.1	Absence of teeth, acquired, maxillary, partial	*6140*
6143–415.0	Alveolitis; alveolar osteitis	*6140*
613–438.1	Dental abrasion (not attrition)	*6140*
613–437.1	Dental attrition	*6140*
6132–415	Exposed pulp due to operation	*6140*
6143–415	Extraction wound	*6141*
613▲–418	Fracture of tooth. *Specify site*	*6140*
6143–400.7	Hemorrhage from alveolus due to trauma. *Specify trauma as:*	*6140*
6143–415.7	Hemorrhage from alveolus following extraction	*6140*
6142–415.0	Infection following extraction of tooth	*6140*
6142–4▲▲	Injury of gingiva. *Specify injury*	*6140*
6136–415.3	Perforated root	*6140*
614–495	Periodontitis, due to filth	*6140*
614–434	Periodontal traumatism	*6140*
6132–496	Pulp capped tooth	*6140*
613–415.1	Pulpless tooth	*6140*
6145–430	Resorbed alveolar ridge	*6140*
6136–416.0	Retained root fragment	*6140*
613–405.1	Tooth with resected root	*6140*

—6 DISEASES DUE TO OR CONSISTING OF STATIC MECHANICAL ABNORMALITY

613–615	Calculus on teeth	*6160*
613–63▲	Faulty position of tooth; malposed teeth. *Specify abnormality*	*6160*
6135–63▲	Malocclusion. *Specify abnormality*	*6160*
6142–610.0	Pericoronitis of eruption	*6160*

—7 DISEASES DUE TO DISORDER OF METABOLISM, GROWTH, NUTRITION, OR DEVELOPMENT

613–7x4	Dens in dente	*6170*
6142–770	Gingivitis, due to metabolic disturbance	*6170*
6142–700.9	Gingivosis (desquamative gingivitis)	*6170*
6131–793	Hypercementosis	*6170*
6142–793	Hyperplasia of gingiva	*6170*
6132–793	Hyperplasia of pulp	*6170*
6133–793	Hyperplastic enamel	*6170*
6133–791	Hypoplastic enamel	*6170*
613–794	Impacted tooth	*6179*
614–798	Periodontosis	*6170*
6135–793	Precocious deciduous dentition	*6170*
6135–7931	Precocious permanent dentition	*6170*
6132–700.6	Pulp nodule	*6170*
6135–791	Retarded deciduous dentition	*6170*
6135–7911	Retarded permanent dentition	*6170*
6142–763	Scorbutic gingivitis	*6170*

—8 NEW GROWTHS

6133–886E	Ameloblastoma	*6180*
6131–886A	Cementoma	*6180*
6142–814	Epidermoid carcinoma of gingiva. *Specify behavior*	*6180*
614–8741	Giant cell tumor (epulis). *Specify behavior*	*6180*
613–886A	Odontogenic tumor excluding ameloblastoma	*6180*
6▲▲▲–8▲▲	Unlisted tumor of teeth and gums. *Specify site, neoplasm and behavior*	*6180*

—9 DISEASES DUE TO UNKNOWN OR UNCERTAIN CAUSE WITH THE STRUCTURAL REACTION MANIFEST

6131–900.4	Concrescence (fusion of cementum)	*6190*
613–9x1	Dental erosion	*6190*
6143–900.8	Dentigerous cyst	*6190*
6136–900.1	Idiopathic resorption of tooth root	*6190*
219▲–900.6	Torus mandibularis	*6190*
218▲–900.6	Torus palatinus	*6190*

DISEASES OF THE PALATE AND UVULA

616–   Palate
617–   Uvula
218–   Superior maxilla

—0 DISEASES DUE TO GENETIC AND PRENATAL INFLUENCES

617–011	Absence of uvula, congenital	*6101*
616–064	Anterior nasopalatine cyst	*6101*
616–037	Cleft palate, congenital, complete (to incisive foramen) or incomplete	*6102*
616–0371	Cleft of soft palate	*6102*
616–0372	Cleft of soft and hard palate	*6102*
617–037	Duplication of uvula (bifid uvula)	*6101*
617–013	Elongation of uvula, congenital	*6101*
617–016	Shortening of uvula, congenital	*6101*
616–016	Shortening of palate, congenital	*6101*

—I DISEASES DUE TO INFECTION WITH LOWER ORGANISM

616–100.2	Abscess of palate. *Specify organism (page 57) when known*	*6110*
617–100.2	Abscess of uvula. *Specify organism (page 57) when known*	*6110*
617–100.4	Deformity of uvula due to infection	*6110*
617–125.x	Paralysis of uvula following diphtheria	*6110*
616–147	Syphilis of palate (mucous patches, gumma)	*6110*
616–147.3	Syphilitic perforation of palate	*6110*
617–190	Uvulitis. *Specify organism (page 57) when known*	*6110*

—3 DISEASES DUE TO INTOXICATION

616–3▲▲	Chemical burn of palate	*6130*
617–3238.x	Paralysis of uvula due to lead	*6130*

—4 DISEASES DUE TO TRAUMA OR PHYSICAL AGENT

616–415.4	Deformity of palate following operation	*6140*
616–4▲▲	Injury of palate. *Specify injury (page 83)*	*6140*

—55 DISEASES DUE TO DISTURBANCE OF INNERVATION OR OF PSYCHIC CONTROL
Record primary diagnosis when possible

617–569	Paralysis of uvula due to pressure on nerves	*6155*

—6 DISEASES DUE TO OR CONSISTING OF STATIC MECHANICAL ABNOR-MALITY

616–640	Deformity of palate due to unknown cause	*6160*
617–649	Elongation of uvula, acquired	*6160*

—8 NEW GROWTHS

61▲–812	Basal cell carcinoma of . . . . *Specify site and behavior*	*6180*
616–873B	Chondroma of palate	*6180*
616–8887	Craniopharyngioma of palate. *Specify behavior (page 99)*	*6180*
61▲–814	Epidermoid carcinoma. *Specify site and behavior (page 99)*	*6180*
616–870A	Fibroma of palate	*6180*
616–850A	Hemangioma of palate	*6180*
61▲–830	Lymphosarcoma of . . . . *Specify site and behavior*	*6180*
616–8852	Mixed tumor, salivary gland type, of palate. *Specify behavior*	*6180*
218–876A	Osteoma of palate	*6180*
616–8170	Pigmented nevus of palate. *Specify behavior (page 99)*	*6180*
616–833	Plasma cell myeloma of palate. *Specify behavior*	*6180*
61▲–879	Sarcoma of . . . . *Specify site and behavior*	*6180*
61▲–811	Transitional cell carcinoma of . . . . *Specify site and behavior (page 99)*	*6180*
6▲▲–8▲▲▲	Unlisted tumor of . . . . *Specify site, neoplasm and behavior*	*6180*

—9 DISEASES DUE TO UNKNOWN OR UNCERTAIN CAUSE WITH THE STRUCTURAL REACTION MANIFEST

616–951	Ulcer of palate due to unknown cause	*6190*

DISEASES OF THE SALIVARY GLANDS AND DUCTS

620– Salivary glands and ducts
621– Parotid gland and duct
622– Sublingual gland and duct
623– Submaxillary gland and duct

—0 DISEASES DUE TO GENETIC AND PRENATAL INFLUENCES

620–011	Absence of all salivary glands, complete, congenital	6201
621–011	Absence of one parotid gland, complete, congenital	6201
623–011	Absence of both submaxillary glands, complete	6201
621–031	Accessory parotid glands and ducts	6201
622–018	Atresia of sublingual duct, congenital	6201
623–018	Atresia of submaxillary gland or duct, unilateral or bilateral, congenital	6201
623–064	Cyst of submaxillary gland, congenital	6201
622–064	Cyst, sublingual, congenital; ranula, congenital	6201
6231–021	Displacement of opening of Wharton's duct in mouth	6201
621–021	Displacement of parotid gland over masseter or buccinator muscle	6201
622–021	Displacement of sublingual duct downward, congenital	6201
6231–063	Dilatation of Wharton's duct due to closure of opening in mouth, congenital	6201
622–029	Fistula of sublingual gland, congenital	6201
623–029	Fistula of submaxillary gland, congenital	6201
620–024	Fusion of submaxillary and sublingual glands, congenital	6201
6201–024	Fusion of sublingual duct with submaxillary (Wharton's) duct at opening in mouth, congenital	6201
622–013	Hypertrophy of sublingual gland, congenital	6201
621–016	Hypoplasia of both parotid glands	6201
623–026	Islands of submaxillary glands in neck muscles, fascia or lymph nodes	6201
621–026	Islands of parotid tissue in neck structures or lymph nodes	6201
6211–021	Stensen's duct, opening of, in neck	6201
622–061	Stone in sublingual duct, congenital	6201

—1 DISEASES DUE TO INFECTION WITH LOWER ORGANISM

62▲–100	Acute sialadenitis. *Specify gland and organism (page 57) when known*	6210
62▲–100.2	Abscess of salivary gland or duct. *Specify gland or duct and organism (page 57) when known*	6210
62▲–190	Chronic sialadenitis. *Specify gland or duct and organism (page 57) when known*	6210
	Epidemic parotitis (mumps). *See page 57*	
62▲–100.3	Fistula of salivary gland or duct due to infection. *Specify gland or duct and organism (page 57) when known*	6210
62▲–100.4	Stenosis of salivary duct due to infection. *Specify duct*	6210

—3 DISEASES DUE TO INTOXICATION

62▲–3197	Poisoning of salivary gland by iodide. *Specify gland*	6230
62▲–3▲▲	Sialadenitis due to poison. *Specify poison (page 67)*	6230

—4 DISEASES DUE TO TRAUMA OR PHYSICAL AGENT

62▲–400.3	Fistula of salivary gland or duct due to trauma. *Specify gland or duct*	6240
62▲–4▲▲	Injury of salivary gland or duct. *Specify gland or duct and injury (page 83)*	6240
621–415.0	Parotitis following operation	6240

—6 DISEASES DUE TO OR CONSISTING OF STATIC MECHANICAL ABNORMALITY

62▲–615	Calculus of salivary gland. *Specify gland*	6260
62▲–600.8	Cyst of salivary gland. *Specify gland*	6260
622–600.8	Ranula	6260

—8 NEW GROWTHS

62▲–8091	Adenocarcinoma of . . . . *Specify site and behavior (page 99)*	6280
62▲–8091A	Adenoma of . . . . *Specify site*	6280
621–8842	Adenolymphoma. *Specify behavior*	6280
62▲–8852	Mixed tumor salivary gland type of . . . . *Specify site and behavior*	6280
62▲–8851A	Myoepithelial tumor. *Specify site*	6280
62▲–8▲▲▲	Unlisted tumor of . . . . *Specify site, neoplasm, and behavior*	6280

—9 DISEASES DUE TO UNKNOWN OR UNCERTAIN CAUSE WITH THE
      STRUCTURAL REACTION MANIFEST

62▲–943   Hypertrophy of salivary gland. *Specify*
                            gland   *6280*

DISEASES OF THE PHARYNX

631– Pharynx
6311– Branchial vestiges
639– Retropharyngeal lymphadenoid tissue

For detailed list of structures, see page 33

—0 DISEASES DUE TO GENETIC AND PRENATAL INFLUENCES

6311–064	Branchial cyst, congenital	6301
6311–01x	Branchial vestige	6301
6311–019	Fistula into pharynx (branchial cleft)	6301
6311–01x.3	Sinus, branchial vestige	6301

—1 DISEASES DUE TO INFECTION WITH LOWER ORGANISM

631–100.2	Abscess of pharynx. *Specify organism (page 57) when known*	6310
631–100	Acute pharyngitis. *Specify organism (page 57) when known*	6311
631–100.4	Adhesion; contracture; distortion of pharynx due to infection. *Specify organism when known*	6310
631–100.0	Chronic pharyngitis. *Specify organism (page 57) when known*	6311
639–100.2	Retropharyngeal abscess. *Specify organism (page 57) when known*	6310
639–123.2	Retropharyngeal abscess due to tuberculosis	6310
631–102	Streptococcic sore throat	6313

—2 DISEASES DUE TO HIGHER PLANT OR ANIMAL PARASITE

631–209	Thrush of pharynx	6320

—3 DISEASES DUE TO INTOXICATION

631–3▲▲	Acute pharyngitis due to poison. *Specify poison (page 67)*	6330
631–3▲▲	Chemical burn of pharynx. *Specify poison (page 67)*	6330
631–300.0	Chronic pharyngitis due to poison. *Specify poison (page 83)*	6330
631–319▲	Pharyngitis due to irritant gas. *Specify gas (page 83)*	6330
631–300.4	Stricture of pharynx due to poison. *Specify poison (page 83) when known*	6330

256 DIGESTIVE SYSTEM

—4 DISEASES DUE TO TRAUMA

631–4▲▲	Injury of pharynx. *Specify injury (page 83)*	6340
631–438	Pharyngitis due to foreign body	6340
631–444	Pharyngitis due to scald	6340
630–430	Pharyngoesophageal pulsion diverticulum	6340
631–400.4	Stricture of pharynx due to trauma	6340

—50 DISEASES DUE TO CIRCULATORY DISTURBANCE
Record primary diagnosis when possible

631–544.1	Necrosis of pharynx in granulocytopenia	6350

—55 DISEASES DUE TO DISTURBANCE OF INNERVATION OR OF PSYCHIC CONTROL
Record primary diagnosis when possible

631–590	Spasm of pharynx, reflex	6355

—6 DISEASES DUE TO OR CONSISTING OF STATIC MECHANICAL ABNORMALITY

631–611	Obstruction of pharynx due to foreign body	6360

—8 NEW GROWTHS

631–812	Basal cell carcinoma of pharynx. *Specify behavior*	6380
631–873B	Chondroma of pharynx	6380
631–8887	Craniopharyngioma of pharynx. *Specify behavior (page 99)*	6380
631–814	Epidermoid carcinoma of pharynx. *Specify behavior (page 99)*	6380
631–870A	Fibroma of pharynx	6380
631–850A	Hemangioma of pharynx	6380
631–872A	Lipoma of pharynx	6380
631–830	Lymphosarcoma of pharynx. *Specify behavior*	6380
631–8852	Mixed tumor salivary gland type of pharynx. *Specify behavior*	6380
631–8170	Pigmented nevus of pharynx. *Specify behavior (page 99)*	6380
631–833	Plasma cell myeloma. *Specify behavior*	6380
631–879	Sarcoma of pharynx. *Specify behavior*	6380
631–811	Transitional cell carcinoma of pharynx. *Specify behavior (page 99)*	6380
631–8▲▲	Unlisted tumor of pharynx. *Specify neoplasm and behavior*	6380

—9 DISEASES DUE TO UNKNOWN OR UNCERTAIN CAUSE WITH THE STRUCTURAL REACTION MANIFEST

DISEASES OF THE ADENOIDS AND TONSILS

632–   Pharyngeal lymphadenoid tissue
633–   Adenoids
634–   Faucial tonsil
635–   Lingual tonsil
636–   Peritonsillar tissue

—I DISEASES DUE TO INFECTION WITH LOWER ORGANISM

635–100.2	Abscess of lingual tonsil. *Specify organism when known*	6310
634–100.2	Abscess of tonsil. *Specify organism (page 57) when known*	6310
636–100.2	Abscess of peritonsillar tissue. *Specify organism when known*	6310
633–100	Adenoiditis, acute	6314
633–100.0	Adenoiditis, chronic	6314
636–100	Cellulitis of peritonsillar tissue	6310
636–100.7	Hemorrhage of peritonsillar tissue due to infection	6310
633–100.6	Hypertrophy of adenoids due to infection	6314
635–100.6	Hypertrophy of lingual tonsil due to infection	6315
634–100.6	Hypertrophy of tonsil due to infection	6315
632–100.6	Hypertrophy of tonsils and adenoids due to infection	6315
634–100	Tonsillitis, acute. *Specify organism (page 57) when known*	6312
634–100.0	Tonsillitis, chronic	6312
635–100	Tonsillitis, lingual, acute	6312
6340–100	Tonsils, resected, infection of	6312
634–100.9	Ulcer of tonsil. *Specify organism (page 57) when known*	6310
635–1413	Vincent's infection of lingual tonsil	6312
634–1413	Vincent's infection of tonsil	6312

—4 DISEASES DUE TO TRAUMA OR PHYSICAL AGENT

635–496	Foreign body in lingual tonsil	6340
636–496	Foreign body in peritonsillar tissue	6340
634–496	Foreign body in tonsil	6340
634–415.7	Hemorrhage after operation on tonsils	6340
633–415.7	Hemorrhage after operation on adenoids	6340

—50 DISEASES DUE TO CIRCULATORY DISTURBANCE

634–544.1   Necrosis of tonsil in granulocytopenia.
             Record primary diagnosis   *6350*

**—6 DISEASES DUE TO OR CONSISTING OF STATIC MECHANICAL ABNOR-
MALITY**

634–615   Calculus in tonsil   *6360*

—8 NEW GROWTHS

634–814   Epidermoid carcinoma of tonsil. *Specify
             behavior (page 99)*   *6380*
634–830   Lymphosarcoma of tonsil. *Specify be-
             havior*   *6380*
634–831   Reticulum cell sarcoma of tonsil. *Specify
             behavior*   *6380*
634–814A   Squamous cell papilloma of tonsil   *6380*
634–8▲▲   Unlisted tumor of tonsil. *Specify neo-
             plasm and behavior*   *6380*

**—9 DISEASES DUE TO UNKNOWN OR UNCERTAIN CAUSE WITH THE
STRUCTURAL REACTION MANIFEST**

632–940   Hypertrophy of adenoids and tonsils due
             to unknown cause   *6391*
633–940   Hypertrophy of adenoids due to unknown
             cause   *6391*
635–940   Hypertrophy of lingual tonsil due to un-
             known cause   *6391*
634–940   Hypertrophy of tonsil due to unknown
             cause   *6391*
632–943   Keratosis pharyngeus   *6390*

DISEASES OF THE ESOPHAGUS

637–   Esophagus
6371–   Cervical portion of esophagus
6372–   Thoracic portion of esophagus
6373–   Cardiac sphincter

—0 DISEASES DUE TO GENETIC AND PRENATAL INFLUENCES

637–011	Absence of esophagus, congenital	*6301*
637–018	Atresia of esophagus, congenital	*6301*
637–064	Cysts, esophageal, congenital	*6301*
637–012	Defect of esophagus, congenital	*6301*
637–015	Dilatation of esophagus, congenital	*6301*
638–023	Displacement of gastric mucosa into esophagus	*6301*
637–036	Diverticulum, esophageal, congenital	*6301*
637–032	Duplication of esophagus, congenital	*6301*
3054–029	Fistula, bronchoesophageal, congenital	*6301*
637–013	Giant esophagus, congenital	*6301*
637–016	Short esophagus, congenital	*6301*
637–017	Stricture of esophagus, congenital	*6301*
63x–015	Varix, esophageal, congenital	*6301*

—I DISEASES DUE TO INFECTION WITH LOWER ORGANISM

637–100.2	Abscess of esophagus. *Specify organism (page 57) when known*	*6310*
637–100	Esophagitis due to infection. *Specify organism (page 57) when known*	*6310*
637–100.3	Perforation of esophagus due to infection	*6310*
637–100.4	Stricture of esophagus due to infection	*6310*
637–100.9	Ulcer of esophagus due to infection	*6310*

—3 DISEASES DUE TO INTOXICATION

637–3▲▲	Esophagitis due to poison. *Specify poison (page 67)*	*6330*
637–382x	Esophagitis, peptic	*6330*
637–300.3	Fistula of esophagus due to poison. *Specify poison (page 67) when known*	*6330*
637–300.5	Rupture of esophagus due to poison. *Specify poison (page 67) when known*	*6330*
637–300.4	Stricture of esophagus due to poison. *Specify poison (page 67) when known*	*6330*
637–300.9	Ulcer of esophagus due to poison. *Specify poison (page 67) when known*	*6330*

—4 DISEASES DUE TO TRAUMA OR PHYSICAL AGENT

637–430	Diverticulum of esophagus due to traction or pulsion. *See also* Pharyngoesophageal pulsion diverticulum, *page 256*	*6340*
637–4x0	Esophagitis due to trauma	*6340*
6004–400.3	Esophagocutaneous fistula due to trauma	*6340*
637–400.3	Fistula of esophagus due to trauma	*6340*
637–438.3	Fistula of esophagus due to foreign body	*6340*
637–496	Foreign body in esophagus	*6340*
637–4▲▲	Injury of esophagus. *Specify (page 83)*	*6340*
637–438.5	Perforation of esophagus due to foreign body	*6340*
637–43x.5	Rupture of esophagus due to overstrain	*6340*
637–400.4	Stricture of esophagus due to trauma. *Specify trauma when known (page 83)*	*6340*
637–438.9	Ulcer of esophagus due to foreign body	*6340*

—50 DISEASES DUE TO CIRCULATORY DISTURBANCE
Record primary diagnosis when possible

637–500.9	Ulcer of esophagus (circulatory origin)	*6350*

—55 DISEASES DUE TO DISTURBANCE OF INNERVATION
Record primary diagnosis when possible

6373–580	Achalasia (cardiospasm)	*6355*
6376–599	Cardiochalasia	*6355*
6373–590	Cardiospasm reflex	*6355*
6375–580.6	Dilatation of esophagus due to achalasia	*6355*
637–586	Spasm of esophagus	*6355*

—6 DISEASES DUE TO OR CONSISTING OF STATIC MECHANICAL ABNORMALITY

637–641	Dilatation of esophagus due to unknown cause	*6360*
637–642	Diverticulum of esophagus due to unknown cause	*6360*
637–630.5	Spontaneous rupture of esophagus	*6360*
63x–641	Varix of esophagus	*6360*

—8 NEW GROWTHS

637–8091	Adenocarcinoma of esophagus. *Specify behavior (page 99)*	*6380*
637–814	Epidermoid carcinoma of esophagus. *Specify behavior (page 99)*	*6380*

**—9 DISEASES DUE TO UNKNOWN OR UNCERTAIN CAUSE WITH THE
STRUCTURAL REACTION MANIFEST**

DISEASES OF THE STOMACH

640– Stomach
641– Region of cardia
642– Acid-secreting structures
60▲– Combined structures
6011– Stomach and abdominal wall

For detailed list of structures of stomach, see page 34

—0 DISEASES DUE TO GENETIC AND PRENATAL INFLUENCES

641–043	Cardiospasm, congenital	*6401*
640–026	Displacement of stomach into thorax, congenital; congenital hernia of stomach	*6401*
640–036	Diverticulum of stomach, congenital	*6401*
640–017	Hourglass stomach, congenital; cascade stomach	
640–023	Inclusion of islands of pancreatic tissue in wall of stomach, congenital	*6401*
640–013	Megalogastria, congenital	*6401*
640–016	Microgastria, congenital	*6401*
647–023	Prolapse of esophageal mucosa into cardia of stomach, congenital	*6401*
645–043	Pylorospasm, congenital	*6401*
645–093	Pylorus, hypertrophic stenosis of, congenital	*6402*
647–075	Redundancy of gastric mucosa, congenital	*6401*
640–02x	Transposition of stomach, congenital (alone or with general transposition of viscera)	*6401*

—I DISEASES DUE TO INFECTION WITH LOWER ORGANISM

640–100.2	Abscess of stomach wall. *Specify organism (page 57) when known*	*6410*
640–190	Gastritis, acute infectious. *Specify organism (page 57) when known*	*6411*
640–190.9	Gastritis, acute, ulcerative	*6411*
640–190.0	Gastritis, chronic	*6411*
640–100.3	Perforation of stomach due to infection	*6410*
649–100	Perigastritis. *Specify organism (page 57) when known*	*6410*
649–100.2	Perigastric abscess. *Specify organism (page 57) when known*	*6410*

264 DIGESTIVE SYSTEM

—3 DISEASES DUE TO INTOXICATION

642–300.x	Achlorhydria due to poison. *Specify poison (page 57) when known*	*6430*
640–300.4	Deformity of stomach due to poison. *Specify poison (page 57) when known*	*6430*
640–3▲▲	Gastritis, acute corrosive. *Specify agent (page 57)*	*6430*
640–300.3	Perforation of stomach due to poison. *Specify poison (page 57)*	*6430*
640–389.9	Ulcer of stomach due to uremia	*6430*

—4 DISEASES DUE TO TRAUMA OR PHYSICAL AGENT

640–400.4	Deformity of stomach due to trauma	*6440*
640–415.6	Dilatation, acute, of stomach, following operation	*6440*
640–430	Diverticulum of stomach due to traction or pulsion	*6440*
6011–400.3	Fistula of stomach due to trauma	*6440*
6011–414.3	Fistula into stomach following gunshot wound	*6440*
640–415.0	Gastritis, chronic, following operation	*6440*
6011–415	Gastrostomy opening	*6440*
640–415.7	Hemorrhage of stomach following operation	*6440*
640–424	Hernia of stomach, traumatic, transdiaphragmatic	*6440*
640–4▲▲	Injury of stomach. *Specify injury (page 83), e.g.*	*6440*
640–414	Gunshot wound of stomach	*6440*
645–415.4	Stenosis of pylorus following operation	*6440*

—50 DISEASES DUE TO CIRCULATORY DISTURBANCE
Record primary diagnosis when possible

640–522	Passive congestion of stomach	*6450*
640–514	Strangulation of stomach due to hernia. *Record diagnosis of hernia*	*6450*

—55 DISEASES DUE TO DISTURBANCE OF INNERVATION OR OF PSYCHIC CONTROL
Record primary diagnosis when possible

640–599	Acute dilatation of stomach, reflex	*6455*
640–586	Atony of stomach	*6455*
645–590	Pylorospasm, reflex	*6459*

**—6 DISEASES DUE TO OR CONSISTING OF STATIC MECHANICAL ABNOR-
MALITY**

640–642	Diverticulum of stomach	*6460*
640–611	Foreign body in stomach, nontraumatic	*6460*
64x–641	Gastric varix	*6460*
640–631	Gastroptosis	*6460*
640–612	Hair ball in stomach	*6460*
647–639	Herniation of gastric mucosa	*6460*
640–617	Phytobezoar	*6460*
647–631	Prolapse of gastric mucosa	*6460*
640–637	Volvulus of stomach	*6460*

—8 NEW GROWTHS

640–8091	Adenocarcinoma of stomach. *Specify behavior (page 99)*	*6480*
640–8881A	Adenomyoma of stomach (adenomyosis)	*6480*
640–8191	Carcinoma of stomach. *Specify behavior*	*6480*
640–870A	Fibroma of stomach	*6480*
640–866A	Leiomyoma of stomach	*6480*
640–872A	Lipoma of stomach	*6480*
640–830	Lymphosarcoma of stomach. *Specify behavior*	*6480*
640–8451	Neurofibroma of stomach. *Specify behavior (page 99)*	*6480*
640–8023A	Polyp of stomach, neoplastic	*6480*
640–8023F	Polypoid carcinoma of stomach	*6480*
640–8076G	Scirrhous carcinoma of stomach	*6480*
640–8▲▲▲	Unlisted tumor of stomach. *Specify neoplasm and behavior*	*6480*

**—9 DISEASES DUE TO UNKNOWN OR UNCERTAIN CAUSE WITH THE
STRUCTURAL REACTION MANIFEST**

640–940	Gastritis, chronic, nonspecific	*6490*
640–940.6	Gastritis, chronic, hypertrophic	*6490*
640–940.9	Gastritis, chronic, atrophic	*6490*
642–940.9	Achlorhydria due to chronic atrophic gastritis	*6490*
647–951	Gastritis, erosive	*6495*
649–951.4	Perigastric adhesions due to ulcer	*6490*
641–954	Stenosis of cardia	*6490*
645–954	Stenosis of pylorus, acquired	*6490*
640–951	Ulcer of stomach	*6495*
640–951.4	Deformity of stomach due to ulcer (hourglass contracture)	*6495*
640–951.7	Hemorrhage of stomach due to ulcer	*6495*
640–951.3	Perforation of stomach due to ulcer	*6495*

—Y   DISEASES DUE TO CAUSE NOT DETERMINABLE IN THE PARTICULAR CASE

Y signifies an incomplete diagnosis. It is to be replaced whenever possible by a code digit signifying the specific diagnosis

640–xy7   Hematemesis due to undetermined cause   *0066*

DISEASES OF THE STOMACH AND INTESTINE COMBINED

601– Stomach combined
  6012– Stomach and duodenum
  6013– Stomach and jejunum
  6014– Stomach and colon
  6015– Stomach, jejunum, and colon

For detailed list of structures, see page 31

601–190	Gastroenteritis due to infection. *Specify organism (page 57) when known*	6012
601–105	Gastroenteritis due to staphylococcus toxin	6012
601–1142	Gastroenteritis due to Salmonella paratyphi B (food poisoning)	6012
6012–190	Gastroduodenitis due to infection. *Specify organism (page 57) when known*	6012
6014–123.3	Gastrocolic fistula due to tuberculosis	6010
6012–300	Gastroduodenitis due to poison. *Specify poison (page 57) when known*	6030
601–300	Gastroenteritis due to poison. *Specify poison (page 57) when known*	6030
601–384	Gastroenteritis due to naturally toxic foods	6030
601–390	Gastrointestinal allergy. *Specify allergen when known*	6030
601–930	Gastroenteritis due to unknown cause	6090
6013–951	Gastrojejunal ulcer	6092
6014–951.3	Gastrocolic fistula due to ulcer	6092
6015–951.3	Gastrojejunocolic fistula due to ulcer	6092
601▲–415	Gastroileostomy. *Specify site*	6040
601▲–415.x	Malfunction of gastroenteric stoma. *Specify site*	6040
601▲–415.4	Stenosis of gastroenteric stoma. *Specify site*	6040

DISEASES OF THE INTESTINES

604–   Small and large intestine combined
6049– Intestines and abdominal wall
656–   Lymphatic structures
60▲▲– Combined structures

For detailed list of structures, see page 34

—1 DISEASES DUE TO INFECTION WITH LOWER ORGANISM

604–100	Acute enterocolitis. *Specify organism (page 57) when known*	*6011*
60▲–100.4	Adhesions due to infection. *Specify site*	*6010*
604–156	Chilomastix infection of intestine	*6010*
604–100.0	Chronic enterocolitis	*6011*
604–105	Enterocolitis, staphylococcic	*6011*
604–155	Giardia infection of intestine (giardiasis)	*6010*
6048–100.3	Ileorectal fistula	*6010*
604–1x0	Parenteral diarrhea	*6010*
604–1231	Tuberculosis of intestine, primary; hyperplastic ileocecal tuberculosis	*6011*
604–1232	Tuberculosis of intestine, secondary; tuberculous enterocolitis	*6011*

—2 DISEASES DUE TO HIGHER PLANT OR ANIMAL PARASITE

604–242	Oxyuriasis of intestine	*6020*
604–246	Strongyloidiasis	*6020*

—3 DISEASES DUE TO INTOXICATION

604–3▲▲	Acute enterocolitis due to poison. *Specify poison (page 67)*	*6030*
604–3▲▲.0	Chronic enterocolitis due to poison. *Specify poison (page 67)*	*6030*

—4 DISEASES DUE TO TRAUMA OR PHYSICAL AGENT

60▲–415.4	Adhesions postoperative. *Specify site*	*6041*
604–4x9	Enterocele	*6040*
6049–400.9	Eventration	*6040*
60▲▲–415.3	Fecal fistula following operation. *Specify site*	*6040*
60▲▲–400.3	Fecal fistula due to trauma. *Specify site*	*6040*
604–4▲▲	Injury of intestine. *Specify injury (page 83)*	*6040*
6049–415.4	Stenosis of stoma after enterostomy	*6040*

—50 DISEASES DUE TO CIRCULATORY DISTURBANCE
Record primary diagnosis when possible

604–510	Infarction of intestine	*6050*
604–510.4	Obstruction of intestine due to infarction	*6050*
604–522	Passive congestion of intestine	*6050*

—6 DISEASES DUE TO OR CONSISTING OF STATIC MECHANICAL ABNORMALITY

604–642	Diverticulosis, general intestinal	*6061*
604–631	Enteroptosis	*6060*
604–611	Foreign body in intestine not due to trauma	*6060*
604–611.4	Acute intestinal obstruction due to foreign body	*6060*
604–611.6	Chronic intestinal obstruction due to foreign body	*6060*
604–630	Intussusception	*6563*
6036–630	Intussusception, rectosigmoid (internal procidentia)	*6563*
6▲▲–637	Volvulus of intestine. *Specify*	*6564*
604–637.3	Volvulus of intestine with perforation	*6564*

—7 DISEASES DUE TO DISORDER OF METABOLISM, GROWTH, OR NUTRITION

604–714	Fermentative diarrhea	*6070*
6024–753.6	Intestinal lipodystrophy	*6070*
604–716	Nontropical sprue; steatorrhea; fat indigestion	*6070*
604–715	Putrefactive diarrhea	*6070*

—8 NEW GROWTHS

604–830	Lymphosarcoma of intestine. *Specify behavior (See also under Small intestine, page 274)*	*6080*

—9 DISEASES DUE TO UNKNOWN OR UNCERTAIN CAUSE WITH THE STRUCTURAL REACTION MANIFEST

604–930	Pseudomembranous enterocolitis, acute	*6090*

—X DISEASES DUE TO UNKNOWN OR UNCERTAIN CAUSE WITH THE FUNCTIONAL REACTION ALONE MANIFEST

604–x11	Constipation	*6091*

—Y   DISEASES DUE TO CAUSE NOT DETERMINABLE IN THE PARTICULAR CASE

Y signifies an incomplete diagnosis. It is to be replaced whenever possible by a code digit signifying the specific diagnosis

604–yx9	Diarrhea due to undetermined cause	*0066*
604–yx7	Intestinal hemorrhage due to undetermined cause	*0066*
604–yx4	Intestinal obstruction due to undetermined cause	*0066*

DISEASES OF THE SMALL INTESTINE
AND MESENTERY

650– Small intestine
657– Serosa
658– Meckel's diverticulum
659– Mesentery

For detailed list of structures of small intestine, see page 34

—0 DISEASES DUE TO GENETIC AND PRENATAL INFLUENCES

650–018	Atresia and stenosis of small intestine, single or multiple, congenital	*6501*
650–036	Diverticulosis of small intestine, congenital	*6501*
651–036	Diverticulum of duodenum, congenital	*6501*
658–091	Diverticulitis (Meckel's), congenital	*6502*
	Hernia of small intestine, congenital. *See* Femoral hernia, congenital, etc. (*page 298*)	
650–047.4	Ileus due to meconium	*6501*
650–023	Inclusion of pancreatic tissue in wall of small intestine	*6501*
658–019	Meckel's diverticulum	*6502*
658–063	Meckel's diverticulum, dilatation of, congenital	*6502*
658–023	Meckel's diverticulum, displacement of gastric mucosa into, congenital	*6502*
658–027	Meckel's diverticulum, hernia of, congenital	*6502*
658–013	Meckel's diverticulum, hypertrophy of, congenital	*6502*
658–067	Meckel's diverticulum, incarceration of, congenital	*6502*
658–036	Meckel's diverticulum, small diverticulations on end of, congenital	*6502*
658–065	Meckel's diverticulum, torsion of, congenital	*6502*
651–023	Prolapse of gastric mucosa into duodenum	*6501*
65▲–075	Redundancy of small intestine, congenital. *Specify site*	*6501*
65▲–066	Strangulation of small intestine, congenital. *Specify site*	*6501*
650–065	Volvulus of small intestine, congenital	*6501*

—I DISEASES DUE TO INFECTION WITH LOWER ORGANISM

650–100.2	Abscess of small intestine. *Specify organism (page 57) when known*	6510
657–100.4	Adhesions, intestinal, due to infection	6510
650–100.9	Amyloid degeneration of small intestine due to infection	6510
650–118	Anthrax of small intestine	6510
658–190	Diverticulitis (Meckel's)	6512
658–190.3	Diverticulitis (Meckel's) with perforation	6512
651–190	Duodenitis. *Specify organism (page 57) when known*	6511
650–100	Enteritis, acute. *Specify organism (page 57) when known*	6511
650–100.0	Enteritis, chronic. *Specify organism (page 57) when known*	6511
650–100.x	Ileus, paralytic, due to remote infection. *Specify organism (page 57) when known*	6510
650–101.x	Due to pneumococcus	6510
659–100.4	Mesenteric adhesions due to infection	6510
65▲–100.3	Perforation of small intestine due to infection. *Specify site*	6510
650–130.6	Pneumatosis intestinalis	6510
65▲–100.4	Stricture of small intestine due to infection. *Specify site*	6510

—2 DISEASES DUE TO HIGHER PLANT OR ANIMAL PARASITE

650–243	Ancylostomiasis, intestinal	6520
650–241	Ascariasis, intestinal	6520
650–270	Distomiasis, intestinal. *Specify trematode (page 65) when known*	6520
650–240.4	Obstruction of small intestine due to helminthiasis	6520
650–246	Strongyloidiasis	6520
650–2▲▲	Unlisted parasitic infection. *Specify parasite*	6520

—3 DISEASES DUE TO INTOXICATION

650–3▲▲	Acute enteritis due to poison. *Specify poison (page 67)*	6530
650–300.0	Chronic enteritis due to poison. *Specify poison (page 67) when known*	6530
659–382	Fat necrosis of mesentery	6530

650–300.3	Perforation of small intestine due to poison. *Specify poison (page 67) when known*	*6530*

651–449.9	Duodenal ulcer due to burns	*6540*
650–415.3	Fecal fistula following operation	*6540*
650–400.3	Fecal fistula due to trauma	*6540*
659–4x7	Hematoma of mesentery	*6540*
650–415.x	Ileus, paralytic, following operation	*6540*
659–4▲▲	Injury of mesentery. *Specify (page 83)*	*6540*
65▲–4▲▲	Injury of small intestine. *Specify site and injury (page 83)*	*6540*
657–415.4	Intestinal adhesions following operation	*6540*
657–400.4	Intestinal adhesions due to trauma	*6540*
650–400.7	Intestinal hemorrhage due to trauma	*6540*
650–415.4	Intestinal obstruction due to postoperative adhesions. *See also* Obstruction of colon following operation, *page 277*	*6540*
6013–415.9	Marginal ulcer; stoma ulcer; jejunal ulcer, due to trauma	*6540*
658–417.5	Meckel's diverticulum, rupture of, during birth	*6502*
659–415.4	Mesenteric adhesions following operation	*6540*
65▲–416	Rupture of small intestine due to trauma. *Specify site*	*6540*
654–415.x	Stenosis of ileostomy	*6540*
65▲–415.4	Stricture of small intestine following operation	*6540*

Record primary diagnosis when possible

651–500.x	Duodenal stasis due to circulatory disturbance	*6550*
659–502	Extravasation of chyle into mesentery	*6550*
650–510.1	Gangrene of small intestine due to circulatory disturbance	*6550*
650–544	Granulocytopenic ulcer of small intestine	*6550*
65▲–510	Infarction of small intestine. *Specify site*	*6550*
65▲–511	Due to thrombosis of mesenteric artery	*6550*
65▲–512	Due to embolism of mesenteric artery	*6550*
650–514	Strangulation of intestine. *Record primary diagnosis*	*6550*

651–560	Duodenal stasis	*6555*

| 650–560 | Paralytic ileus, neurogenic | *6555* |
| 6511–590 | Spasm of sphincter of Oddi | *6555* |

—6 DISEASES DUE TO OR CONSISTING OF STATIC MECHANICAL ABNORMALITY

659–600.8	Cyst of mesentery, simple	*6560*
65▲–642	Diverticulosis of small intestine. *Specify site*	*6561*
65▲–642.0	Diverticulitis of small intestine. *Specify site*	*6561*
651–6x3	Duodenal fistula	*6560*
6021–646	Duodenojejunal obstruction due to bands	*6560*
650–600.8	Enteric cyst	*6560*
650–615	Gallstone obstruction of small intestine	*6560*
	Hernia of small intestine into omental sac or fossae. *See* Internal hernia, *page 300*	
650–639.4	Intestinal obstruction due to hernia. *Record diagnosis of hernia*	*6560*
659–637	Torsion of mesentery	*6560*

—8 NEW GROWTHS

650–8091	Adenocarcinoma of intestine. *Specify behavior (page 99)*	*6580*
650–844	Argentaffinoma of intestine. *Specify behavior*	*6580*
650–814	Epidermoid carcinoma of intestine. *Specify behavior*	*6580*
650–870A	Fibroma of intestine	*6580*
659–870A	Fibroma of mesentery	*6580*
650–850A	Hemangioma of intestine	*6580*
659–850A	Hemangioma of mesentery	*6580*
659–866A	Leiomyoma of mesentery	*6580*
650–872A	Lipoma of intestine	*6580*
659–872A	Lipoma of mesentery	*6580*
659–854A	Lymphangioma of mesentery	*6580*
650–830	Lymphosarcoma of intestine. *Specify behavior*	*6580*
650–8023	Polyp of intestine, neoplastic. *Specify behavior*	*6580*
650–831	Reticulum cell sarcoma of intestine. *Specify behavior*	*6580*
650–879	Sarcoma of intestine. *Specify behavior*	*6580*
659–879	Sarcoma of mesentery. *Specify behavior*	*6580*
650–8▲▲▲	Unlisted tumor of intestine. *Specify neoplasm and behavior*	*6580*

—9 DISEASES DUE TO UNKNOWN OR UNCERTAIN CAUSE WITH THE STRUCTURAL REACTION MANIFEST

651–930	Duodenitis due to unknown cause	*6590*
651–951	Duodenal ulcer	*6595*
651–951.3	Duodenal ulcer with perforation	*6595*
651–951.4	Duodenal ulcer with constriction	*6595*
651–951.7	Duodenal ulcer with hemorrhage	*6595*
650–930	Enteritis due to unknown cause	*6590*
659–9x8	Gas cysts of mesentery	*6590*
650–945	Granuloma of small intestine due to unknown cause	*6590*
654–952	Ileitis, regional	*6590*
650–951.4	Intestinal obstruction due to ulcer	*6595*
653–951	Jejunal ulcer	*6595*
653–951.3	Jejunal ulcer with perforation	*6595*
651–944	Polyp, simple, of the duodenum due to unknown cause	*6590*

DISEASES OF COLON

660–   Colon
662–   Cecum
666–   Sigmoid colon

For detailed list of structures of colon, see page 35

—0 DISEASES DUE TO GENETIC AND PRENATAL INFLUENCES

662–026	Cecum mobile	*6601*
660–063	Dilatation of colon, congenital, due to mechanical obstruction	*6601*
660–015	Dilatation of colon, congenital; megacolon, congenital	*6602*
660–036	Diverticulum of colon, congenital	*6601*
662–032	Duplication of cecum, congenital, with · duplication of appendix	*6601*
660–032	Duplication of colon, congenital	*6601*
660–027	Hernia of colon, congenital	*6601*
660–016	Microcolon, congenital	*6601*
662–028	Nondescent of cecum	*6601*
660–028	Nondescent of colon; rotation, incomplete of colon	*6601*
660–075	Redundancy of colon, congenital	*6601*
662–050	Rupture of cecum, spontaneous, during birth, associated with imperforate anus or rectum	*6601*
660–02x	Transposition of colon, congenital, alone or associated with general transposition of viscera	*6601*
660–033	Triplication of colon, congenital	*6601*
660–062	Valve formation of colon, congenital (usually in sigmoid colon and rectum)	*6601*

—1 DISEASES DUE TO INFECTION WITH LOWER ORGANISM

660–100.2	Abscess of wall of colon. *Specify organism (page 57) when known*	*6610*
66▲–1x4	Adhesions of colon due to infection. *Specify site*	*6610*
660–100	Colitis acute. *Specify organism (page 57) when known*	*6615*
660–151	Colitis, amebic	*6615*
660–159	Colitis, balantidial	*6615*
660–100.0	Colitis, chronic. *Specify organism (page 57) when known*	*6615*
660–116▲	Dysentery, bacillary. *Specify (page 57)*	*6615*

66▲–100.3	Fistula of colon due to infection. *Specify site*	*6610*
66▲–100.5	Rupture of colon due to infection. *Specify site*	*6610*
666–190	Sigmoiditis. *Specify organism (page 57) when known*	*6615*
66▲–100.4	Stricture of colon due to infection. *Specify site*	*6610*
662–100	Typhlitis. *Specify organism (page 57) when known*	*6615*

—2 DISEASES DUE TO HIGHER PLANT OR ANIMAL PARASITE

660–2▲▲	Parasitic colitis. *Specify parasite (page 63), e.g.*	*6620*
660–209	Moniliasis	*6620*
660–242	Oxyuriasis of colon	*6620*
660–254	Trichuriasis of colon	*6620*

—3 DISEASES DUE TO INTOXICATION

660–3▲▲	Acute colitis due to poison. *Specify poison (page 67)*	*6630*
660–3▲▲.0	Chronic colitis due to poison. *Specify poison (page 67) when known*	*6630*

—4 DISEASES DUE TO TRAUMA OR PHYSICAL AGENT

6038–415	Artificial anus (colostomy)	*6641*
660–415.3	Fistula of colon, postoperative	*6640*
660–4▲▲	Injury of colon. *Specify injury (page 83)*	*6640*
660–415.4	Obstruction of colon following operation	*6640*
6038–415.x	Stenosis of colostomy (malfunctioning colostomy)	*6641*

—50 DISEASES DUE TO CIRCULATORY DISTURBANCE
Record primary diagnosis when possible

667–510.1	Gangrene of appendices epiploicae	*6650*
660–510.1	Gangrene of colon due to disturbance of circulation. *Record primary diagnosis*	*6650*
660–544	Granulocytopenic ulcer of colon	*6650*
667–511	Infarction of appendices epiploicae	*6650*
660–514	Strangulation of colon due to hernia. *Record diagnosis of hernia*	*6650*

—55 DISEASES DUE TO DISTURBANCE OF INNERVATION OR OF PSYCHIC CONTROL

660–586	Atony of colon	*6655*
660–580	Irritability of colon	*6655*
660–585	Ulcerative colitis, sacro-parasympathetic	*6655*

—6 DISEASES DUE TO OR CONSISTING OF STATIC MECHANICAL ABNORMALITY

660–600.8	Cyst of colon	*6660*
660–641	Dilatation of colon	*6660*
660–642.0	Diverticulitis of colon	*6664*
660–642	Diverticulosis of colon	*6664*
66▲–642.3	Diverticulosis of colon with perforation	*6664*
66▲–642.4	Diverticulosis of colon with obstruction	*6664*
660–615	Enterolith	*6660*
6055–615.3	Fistula between colon and gall bladder due to calculus	*6660*
660–611	Impacted feces	*6661*
660–630	Intussusception of colon	*6660*
66▲–631	Ptosis of colon. *Specify site*	*6660*
660–616.9	Stercoraceous ulcer	*6660*
66x–641	Varix of intrinsic vessels of large intestine	*6660*
66.–637	Volvulus of colon. *Specify site*	*6660*

—8 NEW GROWTHS

660–8091	Adenocarcinoma of colon. *Specify behavior (page 99)*	*6680*
660–8023	Polyp of colon, neoplastic. *Specify behavior*	*6680*
660–8▲▲▲	Unlisted tumor of colon. *Specify neoplasm and behavior. (See also under* Intestines and Mesentery, *page 271)*	*6680*

—9 DISEASES DUE TO UNKNOWN OR UNCERTAIN CAUSE WITH THE STRUCTURAL REACTION MANIFEST

66▲–952	Colitis, regional. *Specify segment*	*6695*
660–945	Granuloma of colon due to unknown cause	*6690*
6045–951	Ileocolitis, progressive caudal	*6695*
6046–951	Ileocolitis, progressive cephalic	*6695*
660–951.3	Simple ulcer of colon with perforation	*6695*
660–951.4	Stricture of colon due to simple ulcer	*6690*
66▲–951	Ulcerative colitis. *Specify site*	*6695*
660–951	Ulcerative colitis, left-sided or universal	*6695*
663–951	Ulcerative colitis, right-sided or regional	*6695*
6035–951	Ulcerative rectocolitis	*6695*

DISEASES OF THE APPENDIX

661–   Appendix
6611– Lymphatic tissue of appendix
6612– Nerves of appendix

—0 DISEASES DUE TO GENETIC AND PRENATAL INFLUENCES

661–011	Absence of appendix, congenital	*6601*
661–021	Displacement of appendix, retrocecal	*6601*
661–013	Excessively long appendix, congenital	*6601*
661–016	Excessively short appendix, congenital	*6601*
661–02x	Transposition of appendix (in situs transversus)	*6601*

—I DISEASES DUE TO INFECTION WITH LOWER ORGANISM

661–100	Acute appendicitis. *Specify organism (page 57) when known*	*6611*
661–100.2	Acute appendicitis with abscess. *Specify organism (page 57) when known*	*6611*
661–100.1	Acute appendicitis with gangrene. *Specify organism (page 57) when known*	*6611*
661–100.3	Acute appendicitis with perforation. *Specify organism (page 57) when known*	*6611*
661–100.0	Chronic recurrent appendicitis	*6611*
661–190.3	Fistula of appendix due to infection	*6611*
6613–100	Periappendicitis. *Specify organism (page 57) when known*	*6611*

—2 DISEASES DUE TO HIGHER PLANT OR ANIMAL PARASITE

661–240.4	Obstruction of appendix due to helminthiasis	*6620*

—4 DISEASES DUE TO TRAUMA OR PHYSICAL AGENT

661–4▲▲	Injury of appendix. *Specify injury (page 83)*	*6640*

—50 DISEASES DUE TO CIRCULATORY DISTURBANCE
Record primary diagnosis when possible

661–514	Strangulation of appendix. *Record primary diagnosis*	*6650*

**—6 DISEASES DUE TO OR CONSISTING OF STATIC MECHANICAL ABNOR-
MALITY**

661–642	Diverticulum in appendix due to unknown cause	*6660*
661–616	Fecalith in appendix	*6660*
661–611	Foreign body in appendix	*6660*
661–630	Intussusception of appendix	*6660*
661–643	Kinking of appendix	*6660*
661–610.8	Mucocele of appendix due to obstruction	*6660*

—7 DISEASES DUE TO DISORDER OF METABOLISM, GROWTH, OR NUTRITION
Record primary diagnosis when possible

661–796	Appendical fibrosis, noninflammatory	*6670*

—8 NEW GROWTHS

661–8091	Adenocarcinoma of appendix. *Specify behavior (page 99)*	*6680*
661–844	Argentaffinoma of appendix. *Specify behavior*	*6680*
661–8▲▲▲	Unlisted tumor of appendix. *Specify neoplasm and behavior*	*6680*

**—9 DISEASES DUE TO UNKNOWN OR UNCERTAIN CAUSE WITH THE
STRUCTURAL REACTION MANIFEST**

6611–943	Lymphoid hyperplasia of appendix	*6690*

DISEASES OF THE RECTUM

668–   Rectum
669–   Perirectal tissue
66x–   Intrinsic vessels

—0 DISEASES DUE TO GENETIC AND PRENATAL INFLUENCES

668–018	Atresia of rectum, congenital	*6601*
668–028	Undescended rectum	*6601*

—I DISEASES DUE TO INFECTION WITH LOWER ORGANISM

669–100.2	Abscess of perirectal tissue	*6610*
669–105.2	Staphylococcic perirectal abscess	*6610*
6691–100.2	Superior pelvirectal abscess	*6610*
6692–100.2	Submucous abscess	*6610*
6693–100.2	Retrorectal abscess	*6610*
668–151	Amebic proctitis	*6613*
668–10x	Chancroid of rectum	*6610*
668–100.3	Fistula of rectum due to infection	*6610*
668–123.3	Tuberculous fistula of rectum	*6610*
669–100.3	Fistula, perirectal. *Diagnose as* Fistula of rectum *when this exists*	*6610*
669–123.3	Tuberculous perirectal fistula	*6610*
66x–100	Phlebitis of rectum, suppurative	*6610*
668–100	Proctitis, acute. *Specify organism (page 57) when known*	*6613*
668–100.0	Proctitis, chronic. *Specify organism (page 57) when known*	*6613*
668–103	Proctitis, gonococcic	*6613*
668–103.4	Stricture of rectum due to gonococcic proctitis	*6610*
668–100.5	Rupture of rectum due to infection	*6610*
668–100.4	Stricture of rectum due to infection	*6610*
668–1732.4	Stricture of rectum due to lymphopathia venereum	*6610*
668–100.9	Ulcer of rectum due to infection	*6610*

—3 DISEASES DUE TO INTOXICATION

668–3▲▲	Chemical burn of rectum. *Specify poison (page 67)*	*6630*
668–3▲▲.4	Stricture of rectum due to chemical burn. *Specify poison (page 67) when known*	*6630*

668–300.9   Ulceration of rectum due to poison.
                   *Specify poison (page 67) when
                   known*   *6630*

—4 DISEASES DUE TO TRAUMA OR PHYSICAL AGENT

668–441   Burn of rectum   *6640*
668–4▲▲   Injury of rectum. *Specify injury (page
                   83)*   *6640*
668–435   Obstruction of rectum due to compression *6640*
668–415   Perforation of rectum by an instrument   *6640*
668–438.3   Perforation of rectum due to foreign body *6640*
668–4111   Puncture of rectum by foreign body   *6640*
668–47▲▲.0   Radiation proctitis   *6640*
668–416   Rupture of rectum   *6640*
668–415.4   Stricture of rectum following operation *6640*
668–400.4   Stricture of rectum due to trauma   *6640*
668–400.9   Ulceration of rectum due to trauma   *6640*

—50 DISEASES DUE TO CIRCULATORY DISTURBANCE

668–522.9   Varicose ulceration of rectum   *6650*

—6 DISEASES DUE TO OR CONSISTING OF STATIC MECHANICAL ABNORMALITY

668–631   External procidentia of rectum   *6660*
668–611   Foreign body in rectal lumen   *6660*
6682–631   External prolapse of rectum, mucosal   *6660*
668–616.9   Stercoraceous ulceration of rectum   *6660*

—8 NEW GROWTHS

668–8091   Adenocarcinoma of rectum. *Specify be-
                   havior (page 99)*   *6680*
668–8091A   Adenoma of rectum   *6680*
668–844   Carcinoid of rectum (argentaffinoma).
                   Specify behavior   *6680*
668–814   Epidermoid carcinoma of rectum. *Specify
                   behavior (page 99)*   *6680*
668–872A   Lipoma of rectum   *6680*
668–838A   Lymphoma, benign of rectum
668–830   Lymphosarcoma of rectum. *Specify be-
                   havior*   *6680*
668–8173   Melanoma of rectum. *Specify behavior*   *6680*
668–8023   Polyp of rectum, neoplastic. *Specify be-
                   havior*   *6680*
668–8▲▲▲   Unlisted tumor of rectum. *Specify
                   neoplasm and behavior*   *6680*

—9 DISEASES DUE TO UNKNOWN OR UNCERTAIN CAUSE WITH THE STRUCTURAL REACTION MANIFEST

668–945   Granuloma of rectum due to unknown
                            cause   *6690*
668–944   Polyp, simple, of rectum due to unknown
                            cause   *6694*
668–951   Ulcer of rectum due to unknown cause   *6690*

—X DISEASES DUE TO UNKNOWN OR UNCERTAIN CAUSE WITH THE FUNCTIONAL REACTION ALONE MANIFEST; HEREDITARY AND FAMILIAL DISEASES OF THIS NATURE

668–x00   Proctalgia fugax   *6690*

DISEASES OF THE ANUS

670– Anus
672– External sphincter
675– Crypts of Morgagni
67x– Intrinsic vessels of anus
143– Perianal skin

For detailed list of structures of anus, see page 35

—0 DISEASES DUE TO GENETIC AND PRENATAL INFLUENCES

670–011	Absence of anus, entire, congenital	*6701*
670–012	Absence of anus, partial, congenital	*6701*
70x5–018	Atresia ani perinealis	*6701*
70x2–018	Atresia ani vaginalis	*6701*
709–018	Atresia ani urethralia	*6701*
7085–018	Atresia ani vesicalis	*6701*
670–018	Atresia of anus, complete (imperforate anus) or partial, congenital	*6701*
670–0182	Fibrous	*6701*
670–0181	Membranous	*6701*
670–029	Fistula of anus, congenital	*6701*
1271–023	Sebaceous glands of mucocutaneous junction of anus, aberrant	*6701*

—1 DISEASES DUE TO INFECTION WITH LOWER ORGANISM

677–100.2	Abscess of perianal tissue. *Specify organism (page 57) when known*	*6712*
6771–100.2	Ischiorectal abscess	*6712*
6773–100.2	Posterior anal triangle tissue	*6712*
6772–100.2	Subcutaneous abscess	*6712*
6731–100	Anusitis	*6710*
670–10x	Chancroid of anus	*6710*
670–100.4	Cicatrix of anus due to infection	*6710*
670–100.6	Condyloma acuminatum of anus. *Specify organism (page 57) when known*	*6710*
675–100	Cryptitis. *Specify organism (page 57) when known*	*6710*
670–100.3	Fistula of anus due to infection	*6711*
676–100	Infected anal papillae. *Specify organism (page 57) when known*	*6710*
670–100.2	Marginal abscess of anus	*6710*
670–1x4.4	Stenosis of anus due to infection (pectinosis)	*6710*
670–147.6	Syphilitic condyloma lata	*6710*

| 67x–100.7 | Thrombophlebitis of hemorrhoidal vein. *Specify organism (page 57) when known* | 6710 |

—2 DISEASES DUE TO HIGHER PLANT OR ANIMAL PARASITE

| 6731–209 | Moniliasis of anoderm | 6720 |

—3 DISEASES DUE TO INTOXICATION

670–3▲▲	Chemical burn of anus. *Specify poison (page 67)*	6730
670–300.4	Stricture of anus due to poison. *Specify (page 67)*	6730
670–300.9	Ulceration of anus due to poison. *Specify (page 67)*	6730

—4 DISEASES DUE TO TRAUMA OR PHYSICAL AGENT

670–415.2	Abscess of anus following operation	6740
143–430	Decubitus ulcer of sacrococcygeal region	6740
670–400.1	Fissure of anus	6745
670–496	Foreign body in anus	6740
675–496	Foreign body in anal crypt	6740
672–400.x	Incontinence of sphincter ani due to trauma	6740
672–415.x	Incontinence of sphincter ani following operation	6740
670–4▲▲	Injury of anus. *Specify (page 83), e.g.*	6740
670–412	Laceration of anus	6740
672–412	Laceration of sphincter ani	6740
670–415.4	Stricture (stenosis) of anus due to operation	6740

—55 DISEASES DUE TO DISTURBANCE OF INNERVATION OR OF PSYCHIC CONTROL
Record primary diagnosis when possible

672–560	Incontinence of sphincter ani due to paralysis	6755
2747–551	Irritability of levator ani muscle	6755
143–573	Pruritus ani	6755
672–586	Relaxation of sphincter ani	6755
672–588	Relaxation of sphincter ani due to central lesion	6755
672–561	Spasm of sphincter ani due to paralysis	6755
672–590	Spasm of sphincter ani due to reflex action	6755

**—6 DISEASES DUE TO OR CONSISTING OF STATIC MECHANICAL ABNOR-
MALITY**

67x–641.6	Fibrous anal tags	*6760*
67x–641	Hemorrhoids, internal and/or external	*6764*
67x–631	Hemorrhoids, internal and/or external pro- lapsed	*6764*
67x–619	Hemorrhoids, thrombosed	*6764*
673–631	Prolapse of anal canal	*6760*

—8 NEW GROWTHS

670–8091	Adenocarcinoma of anus. *Specify be- havior (page 99)*	*6780*
670–814	Epidermoid carcinoma of anus. *Specify behavior (page 99)*	*6780*
670–870A	Fibroma of anus	*6780*
670–8170	Pigmented nevus of anus. *Specify be- havior (page 99)*	*6780*
670–8▲▲▲	Unlisted tumor of anus. *Specify neoplasm and behavior*	*6780*

**—9 DISEASES DUE TO UNKNOWN OR UNCERTAIN CAUSE WITH THE
STRUCTURAL REACTION MANIFEST**

675–9401	Enlarged anal crypt	*6790*
676–940	Hypertrophy of anal papillae	*6790*
143–943	Hypertrophy of anal skin ; skin tabs	*6790*
670–951	Ulcer of anus due to unknown cause	*6790*

DISEASES OF THE LIVER

680–   Liver
68x–   Intrinsic vessels
30▲–   Combined structures (*see page 22*)

—0 DISEASES DUE TO GENETIC AND PRENATAL INFLUENCES

680–011	Absence of liver, entire, congenital (only in monsters)	6801
680–031	Accessory livers	6801
682–091	Cirrhosis of liver with obliterative cholangitis, congenital	6801
680–091	Cirrhosis of liver, congenital	6801
680–064	Cystic disease of liver, congenital (polycystic)	6801
680–027	Hernia of liver, congenital (into cord, into thorax or through anterior abdominal wall)	6801
680–016	Hypoplasia of one lobe of liver, congenital, with compensatory hyperplasia of the others	6801
680–023	Inclusion of gallbladder in liver, congenital	6801
680–010	Lobulation of liver, abnormal, congenital (absence of lobulation; excessive lobulation; Reidel's lobe)	6801

—I DISEASES DUE TO INFECTION WITH LOWER ORGANISM

680–100.2	Abscess of liver. *Specify organism (page 57) when known*	6810
680–1x2.3	Fistula due to abscess of liver	6810
680–100	Acute hepatitis due to infection. *Specify organism (page 57) when known*	6811
680–151.2	Amebic abscess of liver	6810
680–151	Amebic hepatitis	6811
680–100.9	Amyloid degeneration of liver due to infection	6810
680–100.0	Chronic hepatitis	6811
680–158	Coccidiosis of liver	6811
680–100.6	Granuloma of liver due to infection	6810
680–160	Hepatitis following serum or blood transfusion (homologous serum jaundice)	6811
6095–100.3	Hepatoabdominal wall fistula	6810
3056–100.3	Hepatobronchial fistula	6810
3073–100.3	Hepatopleural fistula	6810
3062–100.3	Hepatopulmonary fistula	6810
680–1891	Infectious hepatitis (epidemic)	6811

681–100	Perihepatitis	6811
680–1x0	Sarcoidosis of liver	6810
680–147.0	Syphilitic hepatitis, secondary stage; syphilitic cirrhosis of liver (heparlobatum)	6810

—2 DISEASES DUE TO HIGHER PLANT OR ANIMAL PARASITE

680–266	Cysticercosis of liver	6820
680–270	Distomiasis of liver. *Specify trematode when known (page 65)*	6820
680–267	Echinococcosis of liver	6820
680–285	Porocephaliasis of liver	6820

—3 DISEASES DUE TO INTOXICATION

	Alcoholic cirrhosis. *See* Laennec's cirrhosis, *page 289*	
680–3▲▲	Diffuse degeneration of liver (hepatitis) due to poison. *Specify poison (page 67)*	6830
680–3222	Due to antimony	6830
680–321	Due to arsenic	6830
680–3151	Due to carbon monoxide	6830
680–33154	Due to carbon tetrachloride	6830
680–34850	Due to chloral	6830
680–3231	Due to copper	6830
680–3154	Due to cyanides	6830
680–3313	Due to derivative of benzene	6830
680–33152	Due to chloroform (delayed chloroform poisoning)	6830
680–3185	Due to phosphorus	6830
680–33212	Fatty liver due to alcohol poisoning	6830

—4 DISEASES DUE TO TRAUMA OR PHYSICAL AGENT

| 680–400.2 | Abscess of liver due to trauma | 6840 |
| 680–4▲▲ | Injury of liver. *Specify (page 83)* | 6840 |

—50 DISEASES DUE TO CIRCULATORY DISTURBANCE
Record primary diagnosis when possible

680–522.6	Cirrhosis of liver due to passive congestion	6850
680–512	Infarction of liver due to embolism	6850
680–511	Infarction of liver due to thrombosis	6850
680–515	Infarction of liver due to periarteritis nodosa	6850
680–522	Passive congestion of liver	6850
68x–533	Portal hypertension	6850

—55 DISEASES DUE TO DISTURBANCE OF INNERVATION OR OF PSYCHIC CONTROL

680–563	Hepatitis due to diphtheria	*6855*

—6 DISEASES DUE TO OR CONSISTING OF STATIC MECHANICAL ABNORMALITY

680–6x8.0	Cysts, inflammatory of, falciform ligament of liver	*6860*
680–615.8	Cyst of liver due to calculus	*6860*
680–615	Intrahepatic calculosis	*6860*
680–6x6	Obstructive biliary cirrhosis	*6860*
680–631	Ptosis of liver	*6860*

—7 DISEASES DUE TO DISORDER OF METABOLISM, GROWTH, OR NUTRITION
Record primary diagnosis when possible

680–701	Fatty liver associated with malnutrition	*6870*
680–753	Fatty liver associated with obesity	*6870*
680–748	Hemochromatosis of liver	*6870*
680–751	Hepatic glycogenosis (in von Gierke's disease)	*6870*

—8 NEW GROWTHS

680–8091	Adenocarcinoma of liver. *Specify behavior* (*page 99*)	*6880*
680–8091A	Adenoma of liver	*6880*
680–8073	Cholangioma of liver. *Specify behavior*	*6880*
680–870A	Fibroma of liver	*6880*
680–850A	Hemangioma of liver	*6880*
680–8063	Hepatoma. *Specify behavior*	*6880*
680–8833	Hepatoblastoma. *Specify behavior*	*6880*
680–8▲▲▲	Unlisted tumor of liver. *Specify neoplasm and behavior*	*6880*

—9 DISEASES DUE TO UNKNOWN OR UNCERTAIN CAUSE WITH THE STRUCTURAL REACTION MANIFEST
Record primary diagnosis when possible

680–911	Acute or subacute yellow atrophy	*6890*
680–915	Acute diffuse hepatic necrosis	*6890*
680–922	Amyloidosis of liver due to unknown cause	*6890*
680–953	Cirrhosis in lenticular nuclear degeneration	*6891*
680–952	Coarse nodular cirrhosis (following acute degeneration of liver)	*6891*
680–9x6	Hypertrophic cirrhosis (Hanot's)	*6891*
680–956	Laennec's cirrhosis	*6891*

**—X DISEASES DUE TO UNKNOWN OR UNCERTAIN CAUSE WITH THE FUNC-
TIONAL REACTION ALONE MANIFEST; HEREDITARY AND FAMILIAL
DISEASES OF THIS NATURE**

680–x71	Chronic idiopathic jaundice (Dubin-Johnson syndrome)	*6890*
680–x72	Familial nonhemolytic jaundice (Crigler-Najjer disease)	*6890*
680–x70	Physiologic jaundice of the newborn	*6890*

**—Y DISEASES DUE TO CAUSE NOT DETERMINABLE IN THE PARTICULAR
CASE**

Y signifies an incomplete diagnosis. It is to be replaced whenever possible
by a code digit signifying the specific diagnosis

680–yx0	Acute catarrhal jaundice due to undetermined cause	*0066*
680–yx6	Hepatomegaly of undetermined origin	*0066*
680–yx7	Hepatorenal syndrome	*0066*

DISEASES OF THE BILE PASSAGES

682– Bile passages
683– Intrahepatic biliary passages
684– Hepatic ducts
685– Common bile duct
686– Cystic duct
687– Gallbladder .
688– Ampulla of Vater
60▲– Combined structures (*page 32*)

For detailed list of structures of liver and biliary tract, see page 36

—0 DISEASES DUE TO GENETIC AND PRENATAL INFLUENCES

686–023	Aberrant cystic duct	6801
684–023	Aberrant hepatic duct	6801
682–011	Absence of bile passages, congenital	6801
687–011	Absence of gallbladder (usually associated with imperfect development of pancreas, also with imperforate anus), congenital	6801
684–031	Accessory hepatic ducts	6801
687–035	Bifurcation of gallbladder, congenital	6801
687–061	Calculus of gallbladder, congenital	6801
685–015	Dilatation of common bile duct (associated with congenital absence of gallbladder), congenital	6801
687–021	Displacement of gallbladder (upward, downward, to right or left), congenital	6801
685–032	Duplication of common bile duct, congenital	6801
686–032	Duplication of cystic duct (and gallbladder), congenital	6801
687–032	Duplication of gallbladder (and cystic duct), congenital	6801
685–013	Elongation of common bile duct, congenital	6801
686–013	Elongation of cystic duct, congenital	6801
687–029	Fistula between gallbladder and cystic duct, congenital	6801
687–027	Hernia of gallbladder in femoral ring, congenital	6801
687–017	Hourglass gallbladder, congenital	6801
687–091	Inflammation of gallbladder, congenital	6801
686–065	Kinking of cystic duct, congenital	6801
682–018	Obliteration (atresia) of bile ducts (in congenital hepatic cirrhosis)	6801

685–016	Shortening of common bile duct, congenital	*6801*
686–016	Shortening of cystic duct, congenital	*6801*
687–065	Torsion of gallbladder associated with long mesentery, congenital	*6801*
688–021	Variations of common bile duct and pancreatic duct openings into ampulla of Vater	*6801*

—I DISEASES DUE TO INFECTION WITH LOWER ORGANISM

6871–100.2	Abscess, pericholecystic. *Specify organism (page 57) when known*	*6810*
687–100.6	Adhesions, pericholecystic, due to infection	*6810*
683–100	Cholangiolitis. *Specify organism (page 57) when known*	*6812*
682–100	Cholangitis. *Specify organism (page 57) when known*	*6812*
687–100	Cholecystitis, acute. *Specify organism (page 57) when known*	*6812*
687–114	Paratyphoidal cholecystitis	*6812*
687–115	Typhoidal cholecystitis	*6812*
687–100.0	Cholecystitis, chronic. *Specify organism (page 57) when known*	*6812*
687–100.5	Cholecystitis with perforation, acute. *Specify organism (page 57) when known*	*6812*
687–100.1	Cholecystitis, gangrenous. *Specify organism (page 57) when known*	*6812*
687–100.2	Empyema of gallbladder. *Specify organism (page 57) when known*	*6812*
6052–100.3	Cholecystointestinal fistula	*6810*
68▲–100.3	Fistula of . . . due to infection. *Specify passage*	*6810*
687–100.3	Fistula of gallbladder due to infection	*6810*
68▲–100.4	Stenosis of . . . due to infection. *Specify passage*	*6810*

—2 DISEASES DUE TO HIGHER PLANT OR ANIMAL PARASITE

682–270	Distomiasis of bile passages. *Specify parasite (page 63) when known*	*6820*
68▲–2▲▲.4	Parasitic obstruction of . . . . *Specify passage and parasite (page 63)*	*6820*

—4 DISEASES DUE TO TRAUMA OR PHYSICAL AGENT

68▲–415.6	Adhesions about . . . following operation. *Specify passage*	*6840*
687–415.6	Adhesions pericholecystic, following operation	*6840*

687–400.6	Adhesions, pericholecystic, due to trauma	*6840*
687–4x0	Cholecystitis due to trauma	*6840*
6051–415.3	Cholecystogastric fistula following operation	*6840*
68▲–415.3	Fistula of . . . following operation. *Specify passage*	*6840*
687–415.3	Fistula of gallbladder following operation	*6840*
68▲–4▲▲	Injury of . . . . *Specify injury (page 83) and passage*	*6840*
687–4▲▲	Injury of gallbladder. *Specify injury (page 83)*	*6840*
68▲–415.4	Stenosis of . . . following operation. *Specify passage*	*6840*
68▲–435	Stenosis of . . . due to adhesions. *Specify passage*	*6840*
68▲–400.4	Stenosis of . . . due to trauma. *Specify passage*	*6840*
685–430	Stenosis of common bile duct due to pressure	*6840*

—55 DISEASES DUE TO DISTURBANCE OF INNERVATION OR OF PSYCHIC CONTROL

687–580	Biliary dyskinesia	*6855*

—6 DISEASES DUE TO OR CONSISTING OF STATIC MECHANICAL ABNORMALITY

68▲–615	Calculus, biliary; cholelithiasis. *Specify passage*	*6861*
687–615	In gallbladder	*6861*
687–615.x	Cholelithiasis, no dye visualized	*6861*
6051–615.3	Fistula, cholecystogastric, due to calculus	*6861*
6052–615.3	Fistula, cholecystointestinal, due to calculus	*6861*
68▲–615.3	Fistula of . . . due to calculus. *Specify passage*	*6861*
687–600.8	Hydrops of gallbladder	*6860*
68▲–615.0	Inflammation of bile passage due to calculus. *Specify duct*	*6861*
682–6xx	Jaundice, catarrhal, due to acute gastroduodenitis	*6860*
68▲–611	Obstruction due to foreign body in bile passage. *Specify passage*	*6860*
68▲–615.4	Stenosis of . . . due to calculus	*6861*
687–637	Torsion of gallbladder due to unknown cause	*6860*
685–615.9	Ulceration of common bile duct due to calculus	*6861*
687–615.9	Ulceration of gallbladder due to calculus	*6861*

—8 NEW GROWTHS

**—9 DISEASES DUE TO UNKNOWN OR UNCERTAIN CAUSE WITH THE
STRUCTURAL REACTION MANIFEST**

DISEASES OF THE PANCREAS

See also Diseases of the Insular Tissue, *page 398*

690– Pancreas
692– Pancreatic ducts
69x– Intrinsic vessels of pancreas

—0 DISEASES DUE TO GENETIC AND PRENATAL INFLUENCES

690–021	Aberrant pancreas	*6901*
690–031	Accessory pancreas (with separate ducts), congenital	*6901*
690–010	Annular pancreas	*6901*
690–035	Bifurcation of part of pancreas, congenital	*6901*
690–010.6	Fibrocystic disease of the pancreas (mucoviscidosis)	*6901*
690–045	Pancreatic infantilism	*6901*
692–017	Stricture of pancreatic duct, congenital	*6901*

—I DISEASES DUE TO INFECTION WITH LOWER ORGANISM

690–100.2	Abscess of pancreas	*6910*
690–190	Acute pancreatitis. *Specify organism (page 57) when known*	*6910*
690–190.7	Acute hemorrhagic pancreatitis. *Specify organism (page 57) when known*	*6910*
690–100	Acute suppurative pancreatitis. *Specify organism (page 57) when known*	*6910*
690–190.0	Chronic pancreatitis due to infection	*6910*
690–100.1	Pancreatic necrosis due to infection	*6910*
690–1x0.6	Pseudocyst due to infection	*6910*

—2 DISEASES DUE TO HIGHER PLANT OR ANIMAL PARASITE

692–2▲▲▲.4	Parasitic obstruction of pancreatic duct. *Specify parasite (page 63)*	*6920*

—3 DISEASES DUE TO INTOXICATION

690–3▲▲	Acute pancreatitis due to poison. *Specify poison (page 67)*	*6930*
690–3▲▲.0	Chronic pancreatitis due to poison. *Specify poison (page 67)*	*6930*

—4 DISEASES DUE TO TRAUMA OR PHYSICAL AGENT

690–400.3	Fistula of pancreas	*6940*
690–4▲▲	Injury of pancreas. *Specify (page 83)*	*6940*

690–400.1	Necrosis of pancreas due to trauma	6940
690–4x1.6	Pseudocyst of pancreas due to traumatic necrosis	6940
690–416	Rupture of pancreas due to trauma	6940

—50 DISEASES DUE TO CIRCULATORY DISTURBANCE
Record primary diagnosis when possible

690–512.7	Hemorrhage of pancreas due to embolism	6950
690–540.7	Hemorrhage of pancreas due to blood dyscrasia	6950
690–510.1	Ischemic necrosis of pancreas	6950
690–516	Due to arteriosclerosis of pancreatic artery	6950

—6 DISEASES DUE TO OR CONSISTING OF STATIC MECHANICAL ABNORMALITY

690–600.9	Atrophy of pancreas due to obstruction of duct	6960
692–615	Calculus of pancreatic duct	6960
690–6x0	Chronic pancreatitis due to obstruction	6960
690–600.8	Cyst and pseudocyst of pancreas due to obstruction	6960
69x–618	Embolism of pancreatic artery	6960

—7 DISEASES DUE TO DISORDER OF METABOLISM, GROWTH, OR NUTRITION
Record primary diagnosis when possible

690–763	Hemorrhage of pancreas due to scurvy	6970
690–713	Pancreatic atrophy due to malnutrition	6970
690–716	Pancreatic dysfunction (steatorrhea)	6970
690–798	Senile atrophy of pancreas	6970

—8 NEW GROWTHS

690–8091	Adenocarcinoma of pancreas. *Specify behavior (page 99)*	6980
690–8091A	Adenoma of pancreas	6980
690–8044	Functioning islet cell tumor of pancreas. *Specify behavior*	6980
690–8074	Nonfunctioning islet cell tumor of pancreas. *Specify behavior*	6980
690–8▲▲▲	Unlisted tumor of pancreas. *Specify neoplasm and behavior*	6980

—9 DISEASES DUE TO UNKNOWN OR UNCERTAIN CAUSE WITH THE STRUCTURAL REACTION MANIFEST

690–930	Acute interstitial pancreatitis due to unknown cause	6990

69x–942.6	Aneurysm of pancreatic artery due to arteriosclerosis	6990
69x–942	Arteriosclerosis of pancreatic artery	6990
690–923	Calcification of pancreas due to unknown cause	6990
690–956	Chronic interstitial pancreatitis	6990
690–926	Fibrosis of pancreas due to unknown cause	6990

DISEASES OF THE ABDOMEN AND PERITONEUM

040–   Abdomen
060–   Peritoneum
067–   Omentum
068–   Serous sacs
069–   Abdominal contents

*For detailed list of regions of abdomen and peritoneum
see page 4*

—0 DISEASES DUE TO GENETIC AND PRENATAL INFLUENCES

067–025	Anomalous omental adhesions	*0601*
0602–027	Femoral hernia, congenital	*0602*
0601–027	Inguinal hernia,[1] congenital	*0602*
06.–025	Peritoneal adhesions and bands, congenital. *Specify region*	*0601*
06.–025.4	Intestinal obstruction due to congenital peritoneal adhesions and bands. *Specify region*	*0401*
069–02x	Transposition of abdominal viscera	*0401*
044–027	Umbilical hernia, congenital; omphalocele	*0402*
042–027	Ventral hernia, congenital	*0402*

—I DISEASES DUE TO INFECTION WITH LOWER ORGANISM

042–100.2	Abscess of abdominal wall. *Specify organism (page 57) when known*	*0412*
067–100.2	Abscess of omentum. *Specify organism (page 57) when known*	*0612*
041–100.2	Abscess, pelvic. *Specify organism (page 57) when known*	*0412*
06.–100.2	Abscess, peritoneal. *Specify region and organism (page 57) when known*	*0612*
063–100.2	Subdiaphragmatic abscess	*0612*
064–100.2	Subhepatic abscess	*0612*
065–100.2	Retroperitoneal abscess	*0612*
0651–100.2	Retrocecal abscess	*0612*
066–100.2	Pelvic peritoneal abscess	*0612*
06.–1x4	Adhesions, peritoneal, due to infection. *Specify region*	*0610*
060–158	Coccidiosis of peritoneum	*0610*
042–100.3	Fistula, abdominal, due to infection	*0410*
060–1x7	Hemoperitoneum due to infection	*0610*

1 For irreducible, nonstrangulated hernia, or incarcerated hernia, change the second part of the code to –639.0. In case of incarcerated hernia inguinal, direct, add .0 to the etiologic code –4x9. When the hernial sac is strangulated, change the second part of the code to –639.4 (this does not refer to strangulation of contents of the sac).

044–100	Omphalitis, acute	*0410*
044–100.0	Omphalitis, chronic	*0410*
060–100	Peritonitis, acute. *Specify organism (page 57) when known*	*0611*
060–101	Due to Pneumococcus	*0611*
060–102	Due to Streptococcus	*0611*
060–105	Due to Staphylococcus	*0611*
060–112	Due to coliform organism	*0611*
063–100	Subdiaphragmatic peritonitis	*0611*
066–100	Peritonitis, pelvic. *Specify organism (page 57) when known*	*0611*
0661–100	Pelvic peritonitis during pregnancy	*0611*
0662–100	Puerperal pelvic peritonitis	*5750*
060–100.0	Peritonitis, chronic. *Specify organism (page 57) when known*	*0611*
065–100	Retroperitoneal cellulitis. *Specify organism (page 57) when known*	*0610*
060–123	Tuberculous peritonitis	*0611*
060–123.8	Ascites due to tuberculous peritonitis	*0611*

—2 DISEASES DUE TO HIGHER PLANT OR ANIMAL PARASITE

060–240.6	Granuloma of peritoneum due to nematodes	*0620*
060–260.6	Granuloma of peritoneum due to ova of cestodes	*0620*

—3 DISEASES DUE TO INTOXICATION

060–382	Fat necrosis of peritoneum	*0630*
060–3▲▲	Peritonitis, chemical. *Specify agent (page 67)*	*0630*
060–380	Peritonitis due to extravasated contents of viscera	*0630*

—4 DISEASES DUE TO TRAUMA OR PHYSICAL AGENT

042–415.3	Abdominal fistula following operation	*0440*
042–400.3	Abdominal fistula due to trauma	*0440*
06.–415.4	Adhesions, peritoneal, following operation. *Specify region*	*0640*
06.–4x4	Adhesions, peritoneal, due to trauma. *Specify region*	*0640*
042–496	Foreign body in abdominal wall, due to trauma or following operation	*0440*
060–438.6	Granuloma of peritoneum due to foreign body	*0640*
060–415.7	Hemoperitoneum following operation	*0640*

060–4x7	Hemoperitoneum due to trauma	0640
0601–4x9	Hernia, inguinal, direct.[1] *For* Hernia, inguinal, indirect, *see following*	0645
060–4▲▲	Injury of peritoneum. *Specify (page 83)*	0640
060–420	Peritonitis due to remote injury	0640
042–4x9	Ventral hernia due to trauma	0445
	Strangulated [2] ventral hernia	
042–415.9	Postoperative ventral hernia (including hernia in scar)	0445
042–4x9.5	Recurrent ventral hernia, due to trauma	0445
0421–4x9	Spigelian hernia	0445

—50 DISEASES DUE TO CIRCULATORY DISTURBANCE
Record primary diagnosis when possible

060–522.8	Ascites due to venous congestion (portal stasis)	0650
060–502	Chylous ascites (nonfilarial)	0650
060–501	Chylous cyst of peritoneum	0650
067–514	Strangulation of omentum. *Record primary diagnosis*	0650
044–514	Strangulation of umbilicus. *Record primary diagnosis*	0450

—6 DISEASES DUE TO OR CONSISTING OF STATIC MECHANICAL ABNOR-
MALITY

	Hernia, diaphragmatic. *See page 171*	
043–639	Hernia, epigastric	0463
	Strangulated [2] epigastric hernia	
043–639.5	Recurrent epigastric hernia	0463
0602–639	Hernia,[1] femoral	0663
0602–639.5	Recurrent femoral hernia	0663
0601–639	Hernia,[1] inguinal	0663
0601–6393	Hernia, inguinal, indirect. For hernia, inguinal, direct, *see above*	0663
0601–6392	Interstitial inguinal hernia	0663
	Strangulated [2] inguinal hernia	
0601–639.5	Recurrent inguinal hernia	0663
0601–639.6	Sliding inguinal hernia	0663
650–639	Hernia, internal [3]	

1 For irreducible, nonstrangulated hernia, or incarcerated hernia change the second part of the code to –639.0.   In case of incarcerated hernia inguinal, direct add .0 to the etiologic code –4x9.   When the hernial sac is strangulated, change the second part of the code to –639.4 (this does not refer to strangulation of contents of the sac).
2 Instead of Strangulated hernia, diagnose Strangulation of . . . (intestine, omentum, appendix, ovary, etc.).
3 If small intestine is not involved, specify viscus (omentum, appendix, ovary, etc.).

650–639.5	Recurrent internal hernia	*0663*
	Strangulated [1] internal hernia	
057–639	Hernia, ischiatic	*0563*
057–639.5	Recurrent ischiatic hernia	*0563*
066–639	Hernia, ischiorectal	*0663*
066–639.5	Recurrent ischiorectal hernia	*0663*
056–639	Hernia, lumbar	*0563*
056–639.5	Recurrent lumbar hernia	*0563*
091–639	Hernia, obturator	*0963*
044–639	Hernia, umbilical	*0463*
044–639.5	Recurrent umbilical hernia	*0463*
067–639	Omentum, hernia of	*0663*
067–637	Omentum, torsion of	*0663*
048–641	Relaxation of inguinal ring	*0463*

—7 DISEASES DUE TO DISORDER OF METABOLISM, GROWTH, OR NUTRITION

060–794	Cyst of peritoneum. Developmental abdominal pregnancy. *See page 380*	*0670*

—8 NEW GROWTHS

060–850A	Hemangioma of peritoneum	*0680*
060–850F	Hemangiosarcoma of peritoneum	*0680*
067–830	Lymphosarcoma of omentum. *Specify behavior*	*0680*
060–830	Lymphosarcoma of peritoneum. *Specify behavior*	*0680*
060–8772A	Mesothelioma of peritoneum	*0680*
065–840A	Ganglioneuroma, retroperitoneal	*0680*
065–866A	Leiomyoma, retroperitoneal	*0680*
065–872A	Lipoma, retroperitoneal	*0680*
065–872F	Liposarcoma, retroperitoneal	*0680*
065–830	Lymphosarcoma, retroperitoneal. *Specify behavior*	*0680*
065–8431	Pheochromocytoma, retroperitoneal. *Specify behavior*	*0680*
065–841F	Sympathicoblastoma, retroperitoneal	*0680*
065–882	Teratoma, retroperitoneal. *Specify behavior*	*0680*
06▲–879	Sarcoma of . . . . *Specify site and behavior (page 99)*	*0680*
06▲–8▲▲▲	Unlisted tumor of . . . . *Specify site, neoplasm, and behavior*	*0680*

[1] Instead of Strangulated hernia, diagnose Strangulation of . . . (intestine, omentum, appendix, ovary, etc.).

—9 DISEASES DUE TO UNKNOWN OR UNCERTAIN CAUSE WITH THE STRUCTURAL REACTION MANIFEST

040–941	Chronic adhesive peritonitis due to unknown cause	*0490*
040–9x1	Fatty necrosis of abdomen due to unknown cause	*0490*
067–9x7	Idiopathic spontaneous infarction of omentum	*0690*
068–9x8	Polyserositis	*0690*

—Y DISEASES DUE TO CAUSE NOT DETERMINABLE IN THE PARTICULAR CASE

Y signifies an incomplete diagnosis. It is to be replaced whenever possible by a code digit signifying the specific diagnosis

060–yx7	Hemoperitoneum due to undetermined cause	*0066*

DISEASES OF PORTAL AND HEPATIC VESSELS

482– Portal vein
466– Hepatic artery
689– Intrahepatic vessels, generally
68x– Hepatic veins

—I DISEASES DUE TO INFECTION WITH LOWER ORGANISM

466–100.6	Aneurysm of hepatic artery, embolic. *Specify organism (page 57) when known*	4610
68x–190	Phlebitis of hepatic veins. *Specify organism (page 57) when known*	6810
68x–100	Suppurative phlebitis of hepatic veins. *Specify organism (page 57) when known*	6810
482–1x7.3	Recanalized thrombus of portal vein	4810
68x–147	Syphilitic endophlebitis of hepatic veins	6810
68x–100.7	Thrombosis of hepatic veins due to infection	6810
482–100.7	Thrombosis of portal vein. *Specify organism (page 57) when known*	4812

—4 DISEASES DUE TO TRAUMA OR PHYSICAL AGENT

466–400.6	Aneurysm of hepatic artery due to trauma	4640
466–400.4	Embolism of hepatic artery due to trauma	4640
466–425	Embolism of hepatic artery following operation	4640
482–4▲▲	Injury of portal vein. *Specify (page 83)*	4840
482–435	Thrombosis of portal vein due to compression	4840

—50 DISEASES DUE TO CIRCULATORY DISTURBANCE
Record primary diagnosis when possible

482–547.7	Thrombosis of portal vein due to thrombocytosis	4850

—6 DISEASES DUE TO OR CONSISTING OF STATIC MECHANICAL ABNORMALITY

466–618	Embolism of hepatic artery due to unspecified cause	4661
68x–600.7	Thrombosis of hepatic veins due to obstruction	6860

—9 DISEASES DUE TO UNKNOWN OR UNCERTAIN CAUSE WITH THE STRUCTURAL REACTION ALONE MANIFEST

466–942	Arteriosclerosis of hepatic artery	*4694*
68x–930	Endophlebitis of hepatic veins due to unknown cause	*6890*
466–931	Periarteritis nodosa of hepatic artery	*4690*
482–952	Phlebosclerosis of portal vein	*4890*
482–952.7	Thrombosis of portal vein due to phlebosclerosis	*4890*
482–900.7	Thrombosis of portal vein due to unknown cause	*4890*
466–900.7	Thrombosis of hepatic artery due to unknown cause	*4662*
68x–900.7	Thrombosis of hepatic veins due to unknown cause	*6890*

DISEASES OF MESENTERIC VESSELS

469–   Mesenteric arteries
485–   Mesenteric veins

—I DISEASES DUE TO INFECTION WITH LOWER ORGANISM

485–190   Phlebitis of mesenteric veins due to infec-
                 tion   *4811*
485–100.7   Thrombosis of mesenteric veins due to
                 infection   *4812*

—4 DISEASES DUE TO TRAUMA OR PHYSICAL AGENT

469–400.4   Embolism of mesenteric artery due to
                 trauma   *4640*
469–425   Embolism of mesenteric artery following
                 operation   *4640*
469–4▲▲   Injury of mesenteric artery. *Specify*
                 (*page 83*)   *4640*

—6 DISEASES DUE TO OR CONSISTING OF STATIC MECHANICAL ABNOR-
MALITY

469–618   Embolism of mesenteric artery due to un-
                 specified cause   *4661*
469–619   Thrombosis of mesenteric artery due to un-
                 specified cause   *4662*
485–619   Thrombosis of mesenteric veins due to un-
                 specified cause   *4860*

—9 DISEASES DUE TO UNKNOWN OR UNCERTAIN CAUSE WITH THE
STRUCTURAL REACTION MANIFEST

469–942   Arteriosclerosis of mesenteric artery   *4694*
469–942.7   Mesenteric thrombosis due to arterio-
                 sclerosis   *4694*
469–942.4   Narrowing of mesenteric artery due to
                 arteriosclerosis   *4694*
469–931   Periarteritis nodosa of mesenteric artery *4690*
469–931.7   Thrombosis of mesenteric artery due to
                 periarteritis nodosa   *4690*
485–952   Phlebosclerosis of mesenteric veins   *4890*
485–900.7   Thrombosis of mesenteric veins due to un-
                 known cause   *4890*

7- DISEASES OF THE UROGENITAL SYSTEM

70▲- Urogenital system combined
See also under name of specific organ

—0 DISEASES DUE TO GENETIC AND PRENATAL INFLUENCES

70x7–029	Abnormal communication between uterus and anterior abdominal wall	*7001*
7032–029	Abnormal communication between uterus and bladder	*7001*
7061–019	Persistence of cloaca (common cavity for rectum, vagina, and bladder)	*7001*
704–019	Persistence of sinus urogenitalis	*7001*
700–01x	Wolffian duct, vestigial cyst	*7001*

71– DISEASES OF THE URINARY SYSTEM

DISEASES OF THE KIDNEY

710– Kidney

For details of structures of kidney, see page 37

—0 DISEASES DUE TO GENETIC AND PRENATAL INFLUENCES

710–011	Absence of kidney, one or both	*7101*
710–012	Absence of kidney, partial, one or both	*7101*
71x–031	Accessory blood vessels of kidney	*7101*
71x–026	Anomalous connection of renal vessels with kidney	*7101*
71x–021	Anomalous origin of renal vessels	*7101*
722–034	Bifurcation of renal pelvis; ramifying renal pelvis	*7201*
719–061	Calculi, renal, congenital	*7101*
710–010	Cystic kidney, congenital; polycystic kidney	*7103*
710–064	Cyst of kidney, congenital	*7103*
721–036	Diverticulum of calyx, congenital	*7201*
719–032	Double kidney with double renal pelvis	*7102*
710–028	Ectopic kidney	*7101*
710–0281	Crossed ectopia of kidney	*7101*
710–024	Fused kidney; shield kidney	*7102*
710–025	Incomplete fusion of kidney; horseshoe kidney	*7102*
719–063	Hydronephrosis, congenital (due to phimosis, congenital valve in vesical part of ureter, congenital valve of ureter at ureteropelvic junction or kink in ureter over abnormal branch of renal vessels). *See also* Hydronephrosis due to pressure of aberrant vessel, *page 309*	*7101*
710–014	Hyperplasia of kidney (giant kidney) one or both	*7101*
710–013	Hypertrophy of kidney, one or both	*7101*
710–016	Hypoplasia of kidney, one or both	*7101*
710–022	Insufficient rotation of kidney	*7101*
710–027	Intrathoracic kidney with defect in diaphragm	*7101*
710–019	Lobulation of kidney, fetal	*7101*
710–091	Nephritis, congenital	*7101*
710–072	Renal rickets	*7101*

710–050	Rupture of kidney during delivery	*7101*
710–031	Supernumerary kidney	*7101*
710–1471	Syphilis of kidney, congenital; congenital interstitial nephritis; congenital gumma of kidney	*7101*
710–033	Triple kidneys	*7101*
710–021	Wandering kidney, congenital; renmobilis	*7101*

—I DISEASES DUE TO INFECTION WITH LOWER ORGANISM

710–100.2	Abscess of kidney. *Specify organism (page 57) when known, e.g.*	*7110*
710–105.2	Due to Staphylococcus	*7110*
716–100.2	Abscess, perirenal. *Specify organism (page 57) when known*	*7110*
716–1x4	Adhesions, perirenal, due to infection	*7110*
710–100.9	Amyloid degeneration of kidney due to infection	*7110*
710–100.4	Contracted kidney due to pyelonephritis	*7110*
710–100.3	Fistula of kidney due to infection	*7110*
712–100	Glomerulonephritis, acute (acute hemorrhagic nephritis). *Specify organism (page 57) when known, e.g.*	*7111*
712–103	Due to Gonococcus (remote infection)	*7111*
712–100.0	Glomerulonephritis, chronic or subacute	*7111*
712–1x4	Glomerulonephritis; embolic	*7111*
712–190	Glomerulonephritis, focal (including non-suppurative excretory nephritis)	*7111*
722–1x6	Leukoplakia of pelvis of kidney due to infection	*7210*
722–1x9	Malacoplakia of pelvis of kidney	*7210*
714–100	Nephritis, interstitial, acute (acute exudative nephritis)	*7111*
710–100	Nephritis, suppurative, acute. *Specify organism (page 57) when known*	*7111*
714–100.0	Nephritis, chronic, interstitial	*7111*
713–100.0	Nephrosis due to remote infection	*7111*
713–123.0	Due to tuberculosis	*7111*
713–147.0	Due to syphilis	*7111*
716–100	Perinephritis, acute. *Specify organism (page 57) when known*	*7110*
716–100.0	Perinephritis, chronic	*7110*
484–190	Phlebitis of renal vein due to infection	*4811*
722–100	Pyelitis. *Specify organism (page 57) when known, e.g.*	*7211*
722–103	Due to Gonococcus	*7211*

719–100	Pyelonephritis. *Specify organism (page 57) when known, e.g.*	*7111*
719–112	Due to Coliform organisms	*7111*
719–100.1	Pyelonephritis, acute, necrotizing	*7111*
719–1x0.1	Pyelonephritis, chronic, necrotizing	*7111*
722–100.2	Pyonephrosis. *Specify organism (page 57) when known*	*7210*
468–100.7	Thrombosis of renal artery due to infection	*4610*

—3 DISEASES DUE TO INTOXICATION

713–300.9	Nephrosis due to exogenous poison. *Specify poison (page 67) when known, e.g.*	*7130*
713–38x.9	Due to hemoglobinemia following blood transfusion	*7130*
719–3▲▲	Poisoning of kidney due to . . . . *Specify drug*	*7130*
722–3▲▲	Pyelitis due to poison (as injected chemical). *Specify (page 67)*	*7230*

—4 DISEASES DUE TO TRAUMA OR PHYSICAL AGENT

710–435	Atrophy of kidney due to pressure	*7140*
710–400.8	Cyst of kidney due to trauma	*7140*
710–415.3	Fistula of kidney following operation	*7140*
710–400.3	Fistula of kidney due to trauma	*7140*
710–496	Foreign body in kidney due to trauma	*7140*
722–496	Foreign body (exogenous) in pelvis of kidney	*7240*
716–4x7	Hematoma, perirenal, due to trauma	*7140*
710–4x7	Hematoma of kidney due to trauma	*7140*
710–415.7	Hemorrhage of kidney following operation	*7140*
710–415.9	Herniation of kidney following operation	*7140*
719–435.8	Hydronephrosis due to pressure of aberrant vessel	*7140*
710–420.5	Indirect rupture of kidney	*7140*
710–4x0	Infection of kidney due to trauma	*7140*
710–4▲▲	Injury of kidney. *Specify (page 83)*	*7140*
710–406	Luxation of kidney due to trauma	*7140*
713–449	Nephrosis, toxic, due to burn	*7140*
710–4▲▲.5	Rupture of kidney due to trauma. *Specify trauma*	*7140*
468–400.7	Thrombosis of renal artery due to trauma	*4640*

—50 DISEASES DUE TO CIRCULATORY DISTURBANCE
Record primary diagnosis when possible

710–517	Arteriolar nephrosclerosis	*7150*
710–5171	Arteriolar nephrosclerosis, advanced stage; malignant nephrosclerosis	*7150*
710–511	Infarction of kidney due to thrombosis	*7150*
710–512	Infarction of kidney due to embolism	*7150*
710–5x7	Necrosis of cortex of kidney due to ischemia (bilateral cortical necrosis)	*7150*
710–522	Passive congestion of kidney	*7150*
710–516	Senile arteriosclerotic nephrosclerosis	*7150*

—55 DISEASES DUE TO DISTURBANCE OR INNERVATION OF PSYCHIC CONTROL

710–563	Nephrosis due to diphtheria	*7155*

—6 DISEASES DUE TO OR CONSISTING OF STATIC MECHANICAL ABNORMALITY

710–6xx	Albuminuria, orthostatic	*7160*
722–615	Calculus in pelvis of kidney	*7161*
721–615.8	Calculus encysted in calyx	*7161*
710–600.8	Cyst of kidney, solitary	*7160*
710–6x8	Cysts of kidney, multiple	*7160*
721–641	Dilatation of calyx due to obstruction	*7260*
710–630	Displacement of kidney	*7160*
71x–618	Embolism, renal, due to unspecified cause	*7160*
719–639	Herniation of kidney due to unknown cause	*7160*
719–6▲▲.8	Hydronephrosis. *Specify abnormality (page 89)*	*7169*
719–6x8.0	Hydronephrosis, infected. If infectious agent is identified, make secondary diagnosis accordingly	*7169*
719–6x8.4	Hydronephronic contracted kidney	*7169*
710–631	Nephroptosis	*7160*
710–610	Nephrosis due to obstruction	*7160*
71x–619	Thrombosis, renal, due to unspecified cause	*7160*
718–637	Torsion of pedicle of kidney	*7160*
71x–641	Varix of renal papilla	*7160*

—7 DISEASES DUE TO DISORDER OF METABOLISM, GROWTH, OR NUTRITION
Record primary diagnosis when possible

710–741.7	Infarction of kidney due to uric acid	*7170*
712–7x9	Intercapillary glomerulosclerosis	*7170*

713–700.9	Nephrosis due to disorders of metabolism	*7170*
713–785.9	Nephrosis due to diabetes	*7170*
713–720.9	Nephrosis due to disturbance of acid-base balance; nephrosis of alkalosis	*7170*
710–798	Senile atrophy of kidney	*7170*

—8 NEW GROWTHS

710–8091	Adenocarcinoma of kidney. *Specify behavior (page 99)*	*7180*
710–8091A	Adenoma of kidney	*7180*
710–812	Basal cell carcinoma of kidney. *Specify behavior (page 99)*	*7180*
710–8191	Carcinoma of kidney	*7180*
710–8831F	Carcinosarcoma of kidney	*7180*
710–8034	Cholesteatoma of kidney	*7180*
722–814	Epidermoid carcinoma of renal pelvis. *Specify behavior (page 99)*	*7280*
710–870A	Fibroma of kidney	*7180*
710–870F	Fibrosarcoma of kidney	*7180*
710–850G	Hemangiosarcoma of kidney	*7180*
710–850A	Hemangioma of kidney	*7180*
710–866A	Leiomyoma of kidney	*7180*
710–866F	Leiomyosarcoma of kidney	*7180*
718–872A	Lipoma of hilus	*7180*
710–872A	Lipoma of kidney	*7180*
716–872A	Lipoma, perirenal	*7180*
716–872F	Liposarcoma, perirenal	*7180*
722–872F	Liposarcoma of renal pelvis	*7280*
722–8690A	Myoma of kidney pelvis	*7280*
718–871B	Myxoma of hilus	*7180*
718–871G	Myxosarcoma of hilus	*7180*
710–8834	Nephroblastoma. *Specify behavior (page 99)*	*7180*
722–8023	Papillary carcinoma of kidney pelvis. *Specify behavior*	*7280*
710–8021	Serous papillary cystic tumor. *Specify behavior (page 99)*	*7180*
710–879	Sarcoma of kidney. *Specify behavior (page 99)*	*7180*
710–882	Teratoma of kidney. *Specify behavior (page 99)*	*7180*
721–811	Transitional cell carcinoma of renal calyx. *Specify behavior (page 99)*	*7280*
7▲▲–8▲▲▲	Unlisted tumor of kidney. *Specify site, neoplasm, and behavior*	*7180*

—9 DISEASES DUE TO UNKNOWN OR UNCERTAIN CAUSE WITH THE STRUCTURAL REACTION MANIFEST

710–922	Amyloidosis of kidney due to unknown cause	7190
468–942	Arteriosclerosis of renal artery	4694
468–942.7	Thrombosis of renal artery due to arteriosclerosis	4694
710–923	Calcification of kidney	7190
710–959	Endometriosis of kidney	7190
71x–931	Periarteritis nodosa of kidney	7190
722–9x8	Pyelitis cystica	7290
710–900.5	Rupture of kidney, spontaneous	7190
715–955	Sclerotic capsulitis of kidney	7190

—X DISEASES DUE TO UNKNOWN OR UNCERTAIN CAUSE WITH THE FUNCTIONAL REACTION ALONE MANIFEST

713–x40.9	Lower nephron nephrosis	7190
713–x40	Nephrotic syndrome due to unknown cause	7190
710–x10	Renal glycosuria	7190
71x–x30	Renal hematuria due to unknown cause	7190

DISEASES OF THE URETER

723– Ureter
70▲– Combined structures
724– Ureteropelvic junction
725– Periureteral tissue
726– Ureterovesical junction
727– Ureterovesical orifice

For detailed list of structures of ureter, see page 37

—0 DISEASES DUE TO GENETIC AND PRENATAL INFLUENCES

723–011	Absence of ureter, congenital	*7201*
723–012	Absence of ureter, partial, congenital	*7201*
723–035	Bifurcation of ureter, congenital	*7201*
727–064	Cyst at ureterovesical orifice, congenital	*7201*
723–015	Dilatation of ureter, congenital; megalo-ureter	*7201*
727–036	Diverticulum at ureterovesical orifice, congenital	*7201*
723–036	Diverticulum of ureter, congenital	*7201*
720–032	Double pelvis with double ureter	*7201*
723–032	Double ureter (one or both sides)	*7201*
723–063	Hydroureter, congenital (with hydro-nephrosis)	*7201*
723–021	Implantation, anomalous, of ureter	*7201*
723–018	Occlusion of ureter, complete, congenital	*7201*
723–017	Occlusion of ureter, partial, congenital	*7201*
727–021	Opening of ureter, displacement of, con-genital (into seminal vesicles, ejacula-tory ducts, vulva, vagina, rectum or uterus)	*7201*
723–075	Redundancy of ureter, congenital	*7201*
723–0211	Retrocaval ureter	*7201*
724–017	Stricture at ureteropelvic junction, con-genital	*7201*
727–017	Stricture of ureterovesical orifice, con-genital	*7201*
723–033	Triplication of ureter	*7201*
726–027	Ureterocele, congenital	*7201*
724–062	Valve formation at ureteropelvic junction, congenital	*7201*
727–062	Valve formation at ureterovesical orifice, congenital	*7201*

—I DISEASES DUE TO INFECTION WITH LOWER ORGANISM

725–100.2	Abscess, periureteral. *Specify organism (page 57) when known*	7210
727–100.4	Contracture of ureterovesical orifice due to infection	7210
7023–100.3	Fistula of ureter and common iliac artery due to infection	7210
723–1x6	Leukoplakia of ureter due to infection	7210
723–1x9	Malacoplakia of ureter	7210
725–100	Periureteritis. *Specify organism (page 57) when known*	7212
723–100.2	Pyoureter. *Specify organism (page 57) when known*	7212
723–100.4	Stricture of ureter due to infection	7210
724–100.4	Stricture of ureteropelvic junction due to infection	7210
723–100	Ureteritis, acute. *Specify organism (page 57) when known, e.g.*	7212
723–103	Due to gonococcus	7212
723–100.0	Ureteritis, chronic	7212
7071–100.3	Ureteroduodenal fistula due to infection	7210

—3 DISEASES DUE TO INTOXICATION

723–3432	Calculi in ureter due to sulfonamide	7230
723–3▲▲	Ureteritis due to poison. *Specify (page 67)*	7230

—4 DISEASES DUE TO TRAUMA OR PHYSICAL AGENT

723–43x.6	Diverticulum of ureter due to stress	7240
723–400.3	Fistula of ureter due to trauma	7240
7075–400.3	Fistula, ureterorectal, due to trauma	7240
7022–400.3	Fistula, ureterovaginal, due to trauma	7240
7022–415.3	Fistula, ureterovaginal, following operation	7240
723–496	Foreign body (exogenous) in ureter	7240
723–4▲▲	Injury of ureter. *Specify (page 83), e.g.*	7240
723–416	Rupture of ureter due to trauma	7240
723–415	Injury of ureter, operative	7240
723–435	Occlusion of ureter by pressure	7240
723–435.4	Obstruction of ureter by pressure	7240
723–400.4	Stricture of ureter due to trauma	7240
723–415.4	Stricture of ureter following operation	7240
723–401.0	Ureteritis due to passage of catheter	7240
723–449	Ureteritis due to diathermy	7240
723–472	Ureteritis due to radium	7240

—55 DISEASES DUE TO DISTURBANCE OF INNERVATION
Record primary diagnosis when possible

723–584	Spastic constriction of ureter	*7255*

**—6 DISEASES DUE TO OR CONSISTING OF STATIC MECHANICAL ABNOR-
MALITY**

723–643	Angulation of ureter	*7260*
723–615	Calculus in ureter	*7261*
723–642	Diverticulum of ureter (acquired) due to unknown cause	*7260*
7071–6x3	Fistula, ureteroduodenal	*7260*
7074–6x3	Fistula, ureterosigmoid	*7260*
723–641	Hydroureter due to unknown cause	*7260*
723–600.8	Hydroureter due to obstruction	*7260*
723–630	Intussusception, ureter	*7260*
723–650	Megaloureter due to unknown cause	*7260*
723–631	Prolapse of ureter	*7260*
723–615.0	Ureteritis due to calculus	*7260*
726–645	Ureterocele (acquired)	*7260*
723–644	Valve formation in ureter	*7260*

—8 NEW GROWTHS

723–8091	Adenocarcinoma of ureter. *Specify behavior*	*7280*
723–814	Epidermoid carcinoma of ureter. *Specify behavior*	*7280*
723–870A	Fibroma of ureter	*7280*
723–850G	Hemangiosarcoma of ureter	*7280*
723–866F	Leiomyosarcoma of ureter	*7280*
723–872F	Liposarcoma of ureter	*7280*
723–854A	Lymphangioma of ureter	*7280*
723–854G	Lymphangiosarcoma of ureter	*7280*
723–8451	Neurofibroma of ureter. *Specify behavior (page 99)*	*7280*
723–8023	Papillary carcinoma of ureter. *Specify behavior*	*7280*
723–8023A	Polyp of ureter	*7280*
723–879	Sarcoma of ureter. *Specify behavior (page 99)*	*7280*
723–814A	Squamous cell papilloma of ureter	*7280*
723–882	Teratoma of ureter. *Specify behavior (page 99)*	*7280*
723–811	Transitional cell carcinoma of ureter. *Specify behavior (page 99)*	*7280*

723–8▲▲▲   Unlisted tumor of ureter. *Specify neo-*
                    plasm and behavior (*page 99*)   *7280*

—9 DISEASES DUE TO UNKNOWN OR UNCERTAIN CAUSE WITH THE
STRUCTURAL REACTION MANIFEST

723–923   Calcification of ureter due to unknown
                      cause   *7290*
723–959   Endometriosis of ureter   *7290*
720–941   Leukoplakia of pelvis and ureter due to
                      unknown cause   *7290*
723–9x8   Ureteritis cystica   *7290*

DISEASES OF THE BLADDER

730– Bladder
70▲– Combined structures
732– Neck of bladder
749– External sphincter
7301– Urachus

For detailed list of structures of bladder, see page 37

—0 DISEASES DUE TO GENETIC AND PRENATAL INFLUENCES

730–011	Absence, complete, of bladder	7301
730–015	Dilatation of bladder, congenital	7301
730–036	Diverticulum of bladder, congenital	7301
730–032	Double bladder	7301
730–026	Ectopia of bladder	7301
730–012	Exstrophy of bladder	7301
730–027	Hernia of bladder, congenital	7301
7311–013	Hypertrophy of interureteral ridge, congenital	7301
733–021	Paramedial vesicourethral orifice	7301
7301–046	Patent urachus	7301
736–021	Prolapse of mucosa of bladder (into urethral opening), congenital	7301
733–017	Stricture of vesicourethral orifice, congenital	7301

—1 DISEASES DUE TO INFECTION WITH LOWER ORGANISM

730–100.2	Abscess of wall of bladder. *Specify organism (page 57) when known*	7310
7301–100.2	Abscess of urachus. *Specify organism (page 57) when known*	7310
739–100.2	Abscess, perivesical. *Specify organism (page 57) when known*	7310
739–100.4	Adhesions, perivesical, due to infection	7310
730–151	Amebiasis of bladder	7310
733–100.4	Contracture of vesicourethral orifice due to infection	7310
730–100	Cystitis, acute. *Specify organism (page 57) when known, e.g.*	7310
730–103	Due to Gonococcus	7311
730–100.8	Cystitis, acute, exudative	7311
730–100.7	Cystitis, acute, hemorrhagic	7311
730–100.0	Cystitis, chronic. *Specify organism (page 57) when known*	7311
736–100.0	Cystitis, chronic, glandularis	7311

736–100.8	Cystitis cystica due to infection	*7311*
730–100.1	Cystitis, gangrenous	*7311*
730–100.3	Fistula of bladder, due to infection	*7310*
7033–100.3	Fistula, vesical, into seminal vesicle	*7310*
708▲–100.3	Fistula, vesicoenteric, due to infection. *Specify organism (page 57) when known, e.g.*	*7310*
7084–100.3	Fistula between bladder and sigmoid due to infection	*7310*
7083–100.3	Fistula between bladder and colon due to infection	*7310*
7011–100.3	Fistula, vesicoureteral, due to infection	*7310*
7032–100.3	Fistula, vesicouterine, due to infection	*7310*
7031–100.3	Fistula, vesicovaginal, due to infection	*7310*
736–1x6	Leukoplakia of bladder due to infection	*7310*
737–1x9	Malacoplakia of bladder	*7310*
739–100	Pericystitis. *Specify organism (page 57) when known*	*7311*
731–100	Trigonitis. *Specify organism (page 57) when known*	*7311*
730–1764	Zoster of bladder	*7311*

—2 DISEASES DUE TO HIGHER PLANT OR ANIMAL PARASITE

730–2▲▲	Infestation of bladder. *Specify parasite (page 63), e.g.*	*7320*
730–2952	Myiasis of bladder	*7320*

—3 DISEASES DUE TO INTOXICATION

730–3▲▲.9	Calculi in bladder due to drug. *Specify (page 67)*	*7330*
730–3▲▲	Cystitis, chemical. *Specify poison (page 67)*	*7330*
730–390	Cystitis, allergic. *Specify allergen (page 67) when known*	*7330*

—4 DISEASES DUE TO TRAUMA OR PHYSICAL AGENT

732–415.4	Contracture of neck of bladder following operation	*7340*
733–400.4	Contracture of vesicourethral orifice due to trauma	*7340*
730–4x0	Cystitis due to trauma	*7340*
730–4x9	Cystocele	*7341*
7086–415	Cystostomy, opening	*7340*
730–43x	Diverticulum of bladder due to stress	*7340*
7083–400.3	Fistula between colon and bladder due to trauma	*7340*

7083–415.3	Fistula between colon and bladder following operation	*7340*
730–400.3	Fistula of bladder due to trauma	*7340*
7302–415.3	Fistula, vesicoabdominal, following operation	*7340*
7303–415.3	Fistula, vesicoperineal, following operation	*7340*
730–496	Foreign body in bladder due to trauma	*7340*
730–400.7	Hemorrhage of bladder due to trauma	*7340*
730–415.7	Hemorrhage of bladder following operation	*7340*
730–4▲▲	Injury of bladder. *Specify (page 83), e.g.*	*7340*
730–416	Rupture of bladder due to trauma	*7340*
730–415	Puncture of bladder by an instrument	*7340*
736–415.9	Prolapse of mucosa of bladder into urethra following operation	*7340*
7085–415.3	Rectovesical fistula following operation	*7340*
7085–400.3	Rectovesical fistula due to trauma	*7340*
730–43x.6	Sacculation of bladder due to stress	*7340*
730–472.9	Ulcer of bladder due to radium burn	*7340*
730–400.x	Urine stress incontinence	*7340*

—50 DISEASES DUE TO CIRCULATORY DISTURBANCE
Record primary diagnosis when possible

730–512	Embolism of bladder	*7350*
730–512.0	Infected embolus of bladder	*7350*
730–514	Strangulation of bladder. *Record primary diagnosis*	*7350*

—55 DISEASES DUE TO DISTURBANCE OF INNERVATION OR OF PSYCHIC CONTROL
Record primary diagnosis when possible

730–589	Paralysis of bladder due to injury of cord	*7355*
730–560	Paralysis of bladder, flaccid	*7355*
730–591	Paralysis of bladder due to trauma; inhibition of bladder following operation	*7355*
730–569	Paralysis of bladder, postpartum	*7355*
730–561	Paralysis of bladder, spastic	*7355*
749–591	Paralysis of external sphincter of bladder due to trauma	*7355*
749–560	Paralysis of external sphincter, flaccid	*7355*
749–561	Paralysis of external sphincter, spastic	*7355*
733–560	Paralysis of internal sphincter, flaccid	*7355*
733–591	Paralysis of internal sphincter due to trauma	*7355*
733–561	Paralysis of internal sphincter, spastic	*7355*

| 730–566 | Paresis of bladder, tabetic | 7355 |
| 749–580 | Spasm of external sphincter of bladder, neurogenic | 7355 |

—6 DISEASES DUE TO OR CONSISTING OF STATIC MECHANICAL ABNORMALITY

730–615	Calculus of bladder	7361
730–600.8	Cyst (mucous) of bladder	7360
7301–600.8	Cyst of urachus	7360
730–600.0	Cystitis, acute, due to obstruction	7360
730–615.0	Acute cystitis due to calculus	7361
730–640	Deformity of bladder (acquired) due to unknown cause	7360
730–641	Dilatation of bladder due to unknown cause	7360
730–630	Displacement of bladder	7360
730–642	Diverticulum of bladder (acquired) due to unknown cause	7360
730–642.0	Diverticulitis of bladder	7360
739–613	Extravasation of urine	7360
730–611	Foreign body in bladder due to cause other than trauma	7360
730–639	Hernia of bladder (displacement into hernial sac)	7360
739–639	Hernia, prevesical	7360
730–638	Inversion of bladder	7360
730–631	Prolapse of bladder	7360
733–615.4	Stricture of vesicourethral orifice due to calculus	7360
73x–641	Varix of bladder	7360

—7 DISEASES DUE TO DISORDER OF METABOLISM, GROWTH, OR NUTRITION

| 730–7xx | Atony of bladder | 7370 |

—8 NEW GROWTHS

730–8091	Adenocarcinoma of bladder. *Specify behavior (page 99)*	7380
730–8091A	Adenoma of bladder	7380
730–873F	Chondrosarcoma of bladder	7380
730–814	Epidermoid carcinoma of bladder. *Specify behavior (page 99)*	7380
730–870A	Fibroma of bladder	7380
730–850A	Hemangioma of bladder	7380
730–866A	Leiomyoma of bladder	7380
730–866F	Leiomyosarcoma of bladder	7380
730–872A	Lipoma of bladder	7380

730–854A	Lymphangioma of bladder	*7380*
730–854G	Lymphangiosarcoma of bladder	*7380*
730–8871	Mesenchymal mixed tumor, malignant of bladder. *Specify behavior*	*7380*
730–8772A	Mesothelioma of bladder	*7380*
730–8012	Mucinous carcinoma of bladder. *Specify behavior (page 99)*	*7380*
730–871B	Myxoma of bladder	*7380*
730–871G	Myxosarcoma of bladder	*7380*
730–8451	Neurofibroma of bladder. *Specify behavior (page 99)*	*7380*
730–876A	Osteoma of bladder	*7380*
730–8023	Papillary carcinoma of bladder. *Specify behavior*	*7380*
730–8023A	Polyp of bladder	*7380*
730–867A	Rhabdomyoma of bladder	*7380*
730–867F	Rhabdomyosarcoma of bladder	*7380*
730–879	Sarcoma of bladder. *Specify behavior (page 99)*	*7380*
730–882	Teratoma of bladder. *Specify behavior (page 99)*	*7380*
730–811	Transitional cell carcinoma of bladder (papillary carcinoma). *Specify behavior (page 99)*	*7380*
730–8▲▲▲	Unlisted tumor of urinary bladder. *Specify neoplasm and behavior*	*7380*

—9 DISEASES DUE TO UNKNOWN OR UNCERTAIN CAUSE WITH THE STRUCTURAL REACTION MANIFEST

730–922	Amyloidosis of bladder	*7390*
730–9x8	Cystitis cystica	*7390*
736–9x8	Cystitis follicularis	*7390*
730–959	Endometriosis of bladder	*7390*
730–957	Interstitial cystitis	*7390*
730–957.9	Interstitial cystitis with ulceration	*7390*
730–941	Leukoplakia of bladder due to unknown cause	*7390*
736–965	Lichen planus of bladder	*7390*
730–944	Polyp, simple, of bladder	*7390*
730–900.5	Rupture of bladder due to unknown cause	*7390*
730–951	Solitary ulcer of bladder due to unknown cause	*7390*

DISEASES OF THE URETHRA

740–   Urethra
7471– Urethral glands (Littre's)
70▲– Combined structures
7401– Submucous tissue
7402– Utriculus masculinus
7403– Paraurethral ducts (anomalous)

For detailed list of structures of urethra, see page 38

—0 DISEASES DUE TO GENETIC AND PRENATAL INFLUENCES

740–011	Absence of urethra, congenital	*7401*
740–018	Atresia of urethra, congenital	*7401*
740–036	Diverticulum of urethra, congenital	*7401*
746–032	Double meatus urinarius	*7401*
740–032	Double urethra (bifurcation of single urethra)	*7401*
740–0121	Epispadias	*7401*
740–029	Fistula of urethra, congenital	*7401*
740–0122	Hypospadias	*7401*
740–01221	Glandular hypospadias	*7401*
740–01222	Frenular hypospadias	*7401*
740–01223	Penile hypospadias	*7401*
740–01224	Penoscrotal hypospadias	*7401*
740–01225	Scrotal hypospadias	*7401*
740–01226	Perineal hypospadias	*7401*
740–027	Prolapse of urethra, congenital	*7401*
740–016	Shortening of urethra, congenital	*7401*
746–017	Stricture of meatus urinarius, congenital	*7401*
740–017	Stricture of urethra, congenital	*7401*
709–037	Urethrorectal fistula, congenital	*7401*
740–062	Valve formation of urethra, congenital	*7401*

—I DISEASES DUE TO INFECTION WITH LOWER ORGANISM

747–100.2	Abscess of bulbourethral gland (Cowper's). *Specify organism (page 57) when known, e.g.*	*7410*
747–103.2	Due to Gonococcus	*7410*
748–100.2	Abscess, periurethral. *Specify organism (page 57) when known, e.g.*	*7410*
748–103.2	Due to Gonococcus	*7410*
7471–100.2	Abscess of urethral gland. *Specify organism (page 57) when known, e.g.*	*7410*
7471–103.2	Due to Gonococcus	*7410*
747–100	Adenitis of bulbourethral gland (Cowper's), acute. *Specify organism (page 57) when known, e.g.*	*7410*

747–103	Due to Gonococcus	*7410*
747–100.0	Adenitis of bulbourethral gland Cowper's), chronic. *Specify organism (page 57) when known, e.g.*	*7410*
747–103.0	Due to Gonococcus	*7410*
7461–100	Adenitis of Skene's glands, acute	*7410*
748–100	Cellulitis, periurethral. *Specify organism (page 57) when known*	*7410*
740–10x	Chancroid of urethra (Ducrey's bacillus)	*7410*
745–100	Colliculitis. *Specify organism (page 57) when known*	*7410*
7471–100.8	Cyst of urethral gland. *Specify organism (page 57) when known*	*7410*
744–100.3	Fistula, penile, due to infection. *Specify organism (page 57) when known*	*7410*
7044–100.3	Fistula, urethroperineal, due to infection. *Specify organism (page 57) when known*	*7410*
7042–100.3	Fistula, urethrovaginal (or urethroscrotal), due to infection. *Specify organism (page 57) when known*	*7410*
709–100.3	Fistula, urethrorectal, due to infection	*7410*
7403–100	Infection of paraurethral ducts. *Specify organism (page 57) when known*	*7411*
740–1x6	Leukoplakia of urethra due to infection	*7410*
7401–1x9	Malacoplakia of urethra	*7410*
746–100	Meatitis, urethral. *Specify organism (page 57) when known, e.g.*	*7411*
746–100.4	Stricture of meatus urinarius due to infection	*7410*
740–100.5	Rupture of urethra due to infection	*7410*
740–100.4	Stricture of urethra due to infection. *Specify organism (page 57) when known, e.g.*	*7410*
740–103.4	Due to Gonococcus	*7410*
740–147	Syphilis (including chancre) of urethra	*7410*
747–123	Tuberculosis of bulbourethral gland (Cowper's)	*7410*
740–100	Urethritis, acute. *Specify organism (page 57) when known*	*7411*
740–103	Due to Gonococcus	*7411*
744–100.0	Urethritis, anterior, chronic	*7411*
740–100.0	Urethritis, chronic. *Specify organism (page 57) when known*	*7411*
740–1x0	Urethritis due to remote infection	*7411*
740–103.0	Urethritis following gonococcic infection	*7411*
740–100.6	Urethritis, granular	*7411*
741–100.0	Urethritis, posterior, chronic	*7411*

740–100.8	Urethritis, chronic, polypoid	*7411*
7402–100	Utriculus masculinus, infection of. *Specify organism (page 57) when known, e.g.*	*7410*
7402–100.8	Cyst of utriculus masculinus due to infection	*7410*

—3 DISEASES DUE TO INTOXICATION

745–3▲▲	Colliculitis due to poison. *Specify (page 67)*	*7430*
740–300.4	Stricture of urethra due to medication. *Specify medication when known (page 67)*	*7430*
740–390	Urethritis, allergic. *Specify allergen (page 67) when known*	*7430*
740–3▲▲	Urethritis due to medication. *Specify (page 67)*	*7430*

—4 DISEASES DUE TO TRAUMA OR PHYSICAL AGENT

741–415.4	Adhesions of prostatic portion of urethra following operation	*7440*
740–420	Chill and fever, urethral due to trauma	*7440*
740–400.6	Diverticulum of urethra due to trauma	*7440*
740–415.6	Diverticulum of urethra following operation	*7440*
740–461	Electric burn of urethra	*7440*
740–400.3	Fistula of urethra due to trauma; false passage	*7440*
7044–415.3	Fistula, urethroperineal, following operation	*7440*
709–400.3	Fistula, urethrorectal, due to trauma	*7440*
709–415.3	Fistula, urethrorectal, following operation	*7440*
7042–415.3	Fistula, urethrovaginal, following operation	*7440*
7042–412.3	Fistula, urethrovaginal, following parturition	*7440*
740–496	Foreign body in urethra (exogenous)	*7440*
740–4x0	Infection of urethra due to trauma	*7440*
740–4▲▲	Injury of urethra. *Specify (page 83), e.g.*	*7440*
740–412	Laceration of urethra following parturition	*7440*
740–472.0	Radium burn of urethra	*7440*
740–416	Rupture of urethra due to trauma	*7440*
740–415	Wound of urethra caused by instrument	*7440*
740–412.9	Prolapse of urethra following parturition	*7440*
740–415.4	Stricture of urethra following operation	*7440*

740–400.4	Stricture of urethra due to trauma	*7440*
749–400.4	Stricture of urethra, spasmodic, due to trauma	*7440*
740–4x9	Urethrocele	*7440*

—6 DISEASES DUE TO OR CONSISTING OF STATIC MECHANICAL ABNOR-MALITY

740–615	Calculus in urethra	*7460*
747–6x8	Cyst of bulbourethral gland (Cowper's)	*7460*
745–6x8	Cyst of verumontanum	*7460*
740–640	Deformity of urethra (acquired) due to unknown cause	*7460*
740–641	Dilatation of urethra (acquired) due to unknown cause	*7460*
128–631	Prolapse of meatus urinarius (acquired)	*7460*
74x–641	Varix of urethra	*7460*

—8 NEW GROWTHS

747–8091	Adenocarcinoma of bulbourethral glands (Cowper's). *Specify behavior (page 99)*	*7480*
740–8091	Adenocarcinoma of urethra. *Specify behavior (page 99)*	*7480*
740–814	Epidermoid carcinoma of urethra. *Specify behavior (page 99)*	*7480*
740–870A	Fibroma of urethra	*7480*
740–850A	Hemangioma of urethra	*7480*
740–8173	Melanoma of urethra. *Specify behavior (page 99)*	*7480*
740–8023	Papillary carcinoma of urethra. *Specify behavior*	*7480*
740–8023A	Polyp of urethra	*7480*
740–879	Sarcoma of urethra. *Specify behavior (page 99)*	*7480*
740–814A	Squamous cell papilloma of urethra.	*7480*
740–882	Teratoma of urethra. *Specify behavior (page 99)*	*7480*
740–8▲▲▲	Unlisted tumor of urethra. *Specify neoplasm and behavior*	*7480*

—9 DISEASES DUE TO UNKNOWN OR UNCERTAIN CAUSE WITH THE STRUCTURAL REACTION MANIFEST

740–930	Caruncle of urethra	*7490*
74x–900.7	Hemorrhage of urethra due to unknown cause	*7490*

75– DISEASES OF THE GENITAL SYSTEM

For Diseases of the Urogenital System, *see page 306*

705– Genital system generally

For Diseases of the Urogenital System, *see page 306*

—0 DISEASES DUE TO GENETIC AND PRENATAL INFLUENCES

70x3–029	Abnormal communication between uterus and rectum	7001
705–011	Absence, complete, of internal and external genitalia	7001
705–010	Combined anomalies of genital system (associated with anomalies of other organs)	7001
705–01x	Hermaphroditism, true; both ovaries and testes present	7001
750–019	Pseudohermaphroditism; male with testes present with incomplete masculinization of internal or external genital organs	7001
770–019	Pseudohermaphroditism; female with ovaries present	7001
705–019	Pseudohermaphroditism; sex undetermined	7001
760–01x	Rudimentary uterus (in male)	7001
7052–019	Urogenital sinus with vagina communicating	7001

—7 DISEASES DUE TO DISORDER OF METABOLISM, GROWTH, OR NUTRITION
Record primary diagnosis when possible

705–791	Infantile genitalia	7070
705–7862	Pseudohermaphroditism, female, due to increase in progesterone	7070
705–7872	Pseudohermaphroditism, male, due to decrease in progesterone	7070

DISEASES OF THE MALE GENITAL SYSTEM

705–   Male genital system

—I DISEASES DUE TO INFECTION WITH LOWER ORGANISM

041–100   Pelvic cellulitis in male. *Specify organism
(page 57) when known*   *0410*

—55 DISEASES DUE TO DISTURBANCE OF INNERVATION OR OF PSYCHIC CONTROL
Record primary diagnosis when possible

705–588   Neurogenic sexual impotence   *7055*

—X DISEASES DUE TO UNKNOWN OR UNCERTAIN CAUSE WITH THE FUNCTIONAL REACTION ALONE MANIFEST

705–x11   Sexual impotence due to unknown cause   *7090*

DISEASES OF THE PENIS

751–   Penis
752–   Glans penis
753–   Prepuce
754–   Corpora cavernosa (including fascia and septa)
75x–   Intrinsic vessels
545–   Lymphatic channels
145–   Skin of penis

—0 DISEASES DUE TO GENETIC AND PRENATAL INFLUENCES

751–011	Absence of penis	7501
751–025	Adhesion of penis to scrotum	7501
751–034	Cleft penis	7501
751–021	Concealed penis	7501
753–064	Cyst of prepuce, congenital	7501
752–032	Double glans penis	7501
751–032	Double penis	7501
753–017	Phimosis, congenital	7502
1281–023	Sebaceous glands of mucocutaneous junction of penis, aberrant	7501
751–022	Torsion of penis, congenital	7501

—I DISEASES DUE TO INFECTION WITH LOWER ORGANISM

754–100.2	Abscess of corpora cavernosa. *Specify organism (page 57) when known*	7510
751–100.2	Abscess of penis. *Specify organism (page 57) when known*	7510
753–100.4	Adhesions, preputial, due to infection	7510
753–100	Balanitis, due to infection. *Specify organism (page 57) when known, e.g.*	7510
753–103	Due to Gonococcus	7510
145–100	Cellulitis of penis. *Specify organism (page 57) when known*	7510
751–10x	Chancroid of penis (Ducrey's bacillus)	7510
754–100.4	Chordee. *Specify organism (page 57) when known*	7510
754–103.4	Due to Gonococcus	7510
751–1792	Condyloma accuminatum of penis	7510
754–100	Corpora cavernosa, inflammation of. *Specify organism (page 57) when known*	7510
145–166	Herpes simplex of penis or prepuce	7510
145–1x6	Leukoplakia of penis due to infection	7510
545–100	Lymphangitis of penis, acute. *Specify organism (page 57) when known, e.g.*	5411
545–103	Due to Gonococcus	5411

545–100.0	Lymphangitis of penis, chronic	*5411*
751–1732	Lymphopathia venereum of penis	*7510*
753–100.6	Phimosis due to infection. *Specify organism (page 57) when known*	*7510*
751–147	Syphilis of penis (chancre)	*7510*

—2 DISEASES DUE TO HIGHER PLANT OR ANIMAL PARASITE

| 145–2831 | Scabies of penis | *1320* |

—4 DISEASES DUE TO TRAUMA OR PHYSICAL AGENT

753–495	Balanoposthitis due to filth	*7540*
751–448	Frostbite of penis	*7540*
751–400.1	Gangrene of penis due to trauma	*7540*
751–402.7	Hematoma of penis due to trauma	*7540*
751–400.7	Hemorrhage of penis due to trauma	*7540*
751–4▲▲	Injury of penis. *Specify (page 83)*	*7540*
145–4x6	Leukoplakia of penis due to trauma	*1340*
751–406	Luxation of penis	*7540*
751–400.9	Ossification of penis due to trauma	*7540*
753–415.6	Phimosis following operation	*7540*
751–416	Rupture of penis	*7540*
751–422	Strangulation of penis	*7540*

—50 DISEASES DUE TO CIRCULATORY DISTURBANCE

| 750–501 | Lymphangiectatic elephantiasis of external genitalia | *7550* |

—55 DISEASES DUE TO DISTURBANCE OF INNERVATION OR OF PSYCHIC CONTROL
Record primary diagnosis when possible

| 751–584 | Priapism | *7555* |

—6 DISEASES DUE TO OR CONSISTING OF STATIC MECHANICAL ABNORMALITY

753–615	Concretion in prepuce	*7560*
751–640	Deformity of penis (acquired) due to unknown cause	*7560*
75x–618	Embolism of penile vessels due to unknown cause	*7560*
753–600.4	Paraphimosis	*7560*
75x–619	Thrombosis of penile vessels due to unknown cause	*7560*
751–637	Torsion of penis due to cause other than trauma	*7560*

—7 DISEASES DUE TO DISORDER OF METABOLISM, GROWTH, OR NUTRITION

753–794	Phimosis due to unknown cause	*7570*
753–792	Redundant prepuce	*7579*

—8 NEW GROWTHS

751–812	Basal cell carcinoma of penis. *Specify behavior*	*7580*
752–814	Epidermoid carcinoma of glans. *Specify behavior (page 99)*	*7580*
751–814	Epidermoid carcinoma of penis. *Specify behavior (page 99)*	*7580*
753–814	Epidermoid carcinoma of prepuce. *Specify behavior (page 99)*	*7580*
751–870A	Fibroma of penis	*7580*
751–850A	Hemangioma of penis	*7580*
751–866A	Leiomyoma of penis	*7580*
751–872A	Lipoma of penis	*7580*
751–8173	Malignant melanoma of penis. *Specify behavior*	*7580*
751–876A	Osteoma of penis	*7580*
751–8170	Pigmented nevus of penis. *Specify behavior (page 99)*	*7580*
751–879	Sarcoma of penis. *Specify behavior (page 99)*	*7580*
751–8▲▲▲	Unlisted tumor of penis. *Specify neoplasm and behavior*	*7580*

—9 DISEASES DUE TO UNKNOWN OR UNCERTAIN CAUSE WITH THE STRUCTURAL REACTION MANIFEST

754–923	Calcification of corpora cavernosa due to unknown cause	*7590*
754–942	Induration of corpora cavernosa; dorsal fibrosis of penis	*7590*
752–943	Kraurosis of penis (balanitis xerotica obliterans)	*7590*

DISEASES OF THE TESTIS

For Spermatozoa, *see Supplementary Terms, page 499*

755–   Testis
7551– Appendix of testis

—0 DISEASES DUE TO GENETIC AND PRENATAL INFLUENCES

755–011	Anorchism (absence of testes)	7501
755–028	Cryptorchism	7503
755–026	Ectopia of testis	7501
755–1471	Gumma of testis, congenital	7501
755–013	Hypertrophy of testis, congenital	7501
755–016	Hypoplasia of testis, congenital	7501
755–0161	Congenital defect of development; sclerosis of tubules (Klinefelter's syndrome)	7501
755–0162	Congenital defect of development, germinal aplasia	7501
755–0163	Congenital defect of development, tubular sclerosis and germinal aplasia combined	7501
755–022	Inversion or retroversion of testis	7501
755–031	Polyorchism (three testes)	7501
755–023	Rest, infantile, testis	7501
755–012	Rudimentary testes	7501
755–064	Spermatocele, congenital	7501
755–024	Synorchism (fusion of both testes)	7501
755–0281	Undescended testis, unilateral	7503

—I DISEASES DUE TO INFECTION WITH LOWER ORGANISM

755–100.2	Abscess of testis. *Specify organism (page 57) when known*	7510
755–100.9	Degeneration of testis due to infection. *Specify organism (page 57) when known*	7510
755–147.6	Fibrosis of testis following syphilis	7510
755–100.1	Gangrene of testis due to infection	7510
755–124	Leprosy of testis	7510
755–190	Orchitis, acute. *Specify organism (page 57) when known, e.g.*	7510
755–170	Due to mumps	7510
755–100.0	Orchitis, chronic. *Specify organism (page 57) when known*	7510
755–100	Orchitis, suppurative, acute (including epididymo-orchitis. *Specify organism (page 57) when known*	7510

755–1x3	Sinus of testis due to infection	*7510*
755–1xx	Sterility, male, due to infection	*7510*

—4 DISEASES DUE TO TRAUMA OR PHYSICAL AGENT

755–4x7	Hematoma of testis due to trauma	*7540*
755–4▲▲	Injury of testis. *Specify (page 83), e.g.*	*7540*
755–406	Luxation of testis	*7540*
755–416	Rupture of testis due to trauma	*7540*
755–400.1	Necrosis of testis due to trauma	*7540*
755–4x0	Orchitis due to trauma	*7540*

—50 DISEASES DUE TO CIRCULATORY DISTURBANCE
Record primary diagnosis when possible

755–510	Atrophy of testis, circulatory	*7550*
755–514.1	Gangrene of testis due to constriction of spermatic cord	*7550*
755–511	Infarction of testicle, due to thrombosis	*7550*

—6 DISEASES DUE TO OR CONSISTING OF STATIC MECHANICAL ABNOR-MALITY

755–637	Torsion of testis due to unknown cause	*7560*
7551–637	Torsion of appendix testis due to un-known cause	*7560*

—7 DISEASES DUE TO DISORDER OF METABOLISM, GROWTH, OR NUTRITION

755–786	Testicular hypergonadism (testicular disease undetermined)	*7570*
755–787	Testicular hypogonadism (testicular disease undetermined)	*7570*

—8 NEW GROWTHS

755–8091	Adenocarcinoma of testis. *Specify behavior (page 99)*	*7580*
755–8091A	Adenoma of testis	*7580*
755–880F	Choriocarcinoma of testis	*7580*
755–881	Disgerminoma of testis. *Specify behavior*	*7580*
755–8835	Embryonal carcinoma of testis. *Specify behavior*	*7580*
755–870A	Fibroma of testis	*7580*
755–850A	Hemangioma of testis	*7580*
755–8043	Interstitial cell tumor of testis. *Specify behavior (page 99)*	*7580*
755–872A	Lipoma of testis	*7580*
755–830	Lymphosarcoma of testis. *Specify behavior*	*7580*

755–8690A	Myoma of testis	*7580*
755–871B	Myxoma of testis	*7580*
755–867A	Rhabdomyoma of testis	*7580*
755–879	Sarcoma of testis. *Specify behavior (page 99)*	*7580*
755–8068	Sertoli cell tumor of testis. *Specify behavior (page 99)*	*7580*
755–882	Teratoma of testis. *Specify behavior (page 99)*	*7580*
755–8▲▲	Unlisted tumor of testis. *Specify neoplasm and behavior (page 99)*	*7580*

—9 DISEASES DUE TO UNKNOWN OR UNCERTAIN CAUSE WITH THE STRUCTURAL REACTION MANIFEST

| 755–911 | Atrophy of testis due to unknown cause | *7590* |

DISEASES OF THE EPIDIDYMIS

756– Epididymis
7561– Appendix of epididymis

—1 DISEASES DUE TO INFECTION WITH LOWER ORGANISM

756–100.2	Abscess of epididymis. *Specify organism (page 57) when known*	7511
756–100.8	Cyst of epididymis due to infection	7510
756–100	Epididymitis, acute. *Specify organism (page 57) when known, e.g.*	7511
756–103	Due to Gonococcus	7511
756–170	Due to mumps	7511
756–100.0	Epididymitis, chronic	7511
756–100.6	Fibrosis of epididymis due to infection	7510
756–100.3	Fistula of epididymis due to infection	7510
756–100.1	Gangrene of epididymis due to infection	7511
756–123.3	Tuberculous fistula of epididymis	7511

—3 DISEASES DUE TO INTOXICATION

756–3▲▲	Epididymitis due to poison. *Specify (page 67)*	7530

—4 DISEASES DUE TO TRAUMA OR PHYSICAL AGENT

756–4x7	Hematoma of epididymis due to trauma	7540
756–4▲▲	Injury of epididymis. *Specify (page 83)*	7540
756–4x0	Traumatic epididymitis	7540

—50 DISEASES DUE TO CIRCULATORY DISTURBANCE
Record primary diagnosis when possible

756–510	Atrophy of epididymis, circulatory	7550
756–514.1	Gangrene of epididymis due to constriction of spermatic cord	7550

—6 DISEASES DUE TO OR CONSISTING OF STATIC MECHANICAL ABNORMALITY

756–615	Calculus in epididymis	7560
756–600.8	Spermatocele	7560
7561–637	Torsion of appendix epididymis due to unknown cause	7560

—8 NEW GROWTHS

756–8091A	Adenoma of epididymis	7580
756–8091	Adenocarcinoma of epididymis. *Specify behavior (page 99)*	7580

756–870A	Fibroma of epididymis	*7580*
756–850A	Hemangioma of epididymis	*7580*
756–872A	Lipoma of epididymis	*7580*
756–8871	Mesenchymal mixed tumor of epididymis. *Specify behavior*	*7580*
756–8772A	Mesothelioma of epididymis	*7580*
756–8451	Neurofibroma of epididymis. *Specify behavior*	*7580*
756–8077	Rete cell tumor of epididymis. *Specify behavior*	*7580*
756–879	Sarcoma of epididymis. *Specify behavior (page 99)*	*7580*
756–882	Teratoma of epididymis. *Specify behavior (page 99)*	*7580*
756–8▲▲▲	Unlisted tumor of epididymis. *Specify neoplasm and behavior*	*7580*

—9 DISEASES DUE TO UNKNOWN OR UNCERTAIN CAUSE WITH THE STRUCTURAL REACTION MANIFEST

756–900.8	Cyst of epididymis due to unknown cause	*7590*

DISEASES OF THE TUNICA VAGINALIS

757– Tunica vaginalis

—0 DISEASES DUE TO GENETIC AND PRENATAL INFLUENCES

757–095	Congenital hydrocele or hematocele of tunica vaginalis	7501
757–050	Hematocele of tunica vaginalis induced during delivery	7501

—I DISEASES DUE TO INFECTION WITH LOWER ORGANISM

757–100	Acute infection of tunica vaginalis. *Specify organism (page 57) when known*	7510
757–100.8	Acute hydrocele of tunica vaginalis due to infection	7510
757–100.2	Acute suppurative hydrocele of tunica vaginalis	7510
757–1x8.0	Chronic hydrocele of tunica vaginalis due to infection	7510

—2 DISEASES DUE TO HIGHER PLANT OR ANIMAL PARASITE

757–257	Chylocele of tunica vaginalis, filarial	7520

—4 DISEASES DUE TO TRAUMA OR PHYSICAL AGENT

757–4x7	Hematocele of tunica vaginalis due to trauma	7540
757–400.8	Hydrocele of tunica vaginalis due to trauma	7540
757–4▲▲	Injury of tunica vaginalis. *Specify (page 83)*	7540

—50 DISEASES DUE TO CIRCULATORY DISTURBANCE
Record primary diagnosis when possible

757–502	Chylocele of tunica vaginalis (nonfilarial)	7550

—6 DISEASES DUE TO OR CONSISTING OF STATIC MECHANICAL ABNOR-MALITY

757–615	Calculus of tunica vaginalis	7560

—7 DISEASES DUE TO DISORDER OF METABOLISM, GROWTH, OR NUTRITION

757–797.8	Senile hydrocele of tunica vaginalis	7570

—8 NEW GROWTHS

757–870A	Fibroma of tunica vaginalis	*7580*
757–850A	Hemangioma of tunica vaginalis	*7580*
757–872A	Lipoma of tunica vaginalis	*7580*
757–8871	Mesenchymal mixed tumor of tunica vaginalis. *Specify behavior*	*7580*
757–8772A	Mesothelioma of tunica vaginalis	*7580*
757–871B	Myxoma of tunica vaginalis	*7580*
757–8451	Neurofibroma of tunica vaginalis. *Specify behavior*	*7580*
757–867A	Rhabdomyoma of tunica vaginalis	*7580*
757–879	Sarcoma of tunica vaginalis. *Specify behavior (page 99)*	*7580*
757–882	Teratoma of tunica vaginalis. *Specify behavior (page 99)*	*7580*
757–8▲▲▲	Unlisted tumor of tunica vaginalis. *Specify neoplasm and behavior (page 99)*	*7580*

—9 DISEASES DUE TO UNKNOWN OR UNCERTAIN CAUSE WITH THE STRUCTURAL REACTION MANIFEST

757–930.8	Acute inflammatory hydrocele of tunica vaginalis due to unknown cause	*7591*
757–923	Calcification of the tunica vaginalis	*7590*
757–9x7	Hematocele of tunica vaginalis due to unknown cause	*7590*
757–900.8	Hydrocele of tunica vaginalis due to unknown cause	*7591*

SCROTUM 339

DISEASES OF THE SCROTUM

758– Scrotum

—0 DISEASES DUE TO GENETIC AND PRENATAL INFLUENCES

758–074	Abnormal pigmentation of scrotum	*7501*
758–012	Absence of one half of scrotum (corresponding to undescended testis)	*7501*
758–019	Cleft scrotum (in pseudohermaphroditism)	*7501*

—I DISEASES DUE TO INFECTION WITH LOWER ORGANISM

758–100.2	Abscess of scrotum. *Specify organism (page 57) when known*	*7510*
758–100	Cellulitis of scrotum. *Specify organism (page 57) when known*	*7510*
758–10x	Chancroid of scrotum	*7510*
758–102	Erysipelas of scrotum	*7510*
758–100.3	Fistula of scrotum. *Specify organism (page 57) when known*	*7510*
758–100.1	Gangrene of scrotum. *Specify organism (page 57) when known*	*7510*
758–166	Herpes simplex of scrotum	*7510*
758–190	Infection of scrotum, acute. *Specify organism (page 57) when known*	*7510*
758–190.0	Infection of scrotum, chronic. *Specify organism (page 57) when known*	*7510*

—2 DISEASES DUE TO HIGHER PLANT OR ANIMAL PARASITE

758–215	Epidermophytosis of scrotum	*7520*

—3 DISEASES DUE TO INTOXICATION

758–390	Eczema of scrotum, allergic	*7530*

—4 DISEASES DUE TO TRAUMA OR PHYSICAL AGENT

758–448	Frostbite of scrotum	*7540*
758–400.7	Hemorrhage of scrotum due to trauma	*7540*
758–4▲▲	Injury of scrotum. *Specify (page 83)*	*7540*

—50 DISEASES DUE TO CIRCULATORY DISTURBANCE

758–501	Lymphangiectatic elephantiasis of scrotum, nonfilarial	*7550*

MALE GENITAL SYSTEM

—55 DISEASES DUE TO DISTURBANCE OF INNERVATION OR OF PSYCHIC CONTROL
Record primary diagnosis when possible

| 758–573 | Pruritus of scrotum, neurogenic | *7555* |

—7 DISEASES DUE TO DISORDER OF METABOLISM, GROWTH, OR NUTRITION

| 758–792 | Redundant scrotum | *7570* |

—8 NEW GROWTHS

758–812	Basal cell carcinoma of scrotum. *Specify behavior*	*7580*
758–814	Epidermoid carcinoma of scrotum. *Specify behavior (page 99)*	*7580*
758–870A	Fibroma of scrotum	*7580*
758–850A	Hemangioma of scrotum	*7580*
758–866A	Leiomyoma of scrotum	*7580*
758–872A	Lipoma of scrotum	*7580*
758–854A	Lymphangioma of scrotum	*7580*
758–8173	Melanoma malignant of scrotum. *Specify behavior*	*7580*
758–8170	Pigmented nevus of scrotum. *Specify behavior (page 99)*	*7580*
758–879	Sarcoma of scrotum. *Specify behavior (page 99)*	*7580*
758–814A	Squamous cell papilloma of scrotum	*7580*
758–882	Teratoma of scrotum. *Specify behavior (page 99)*	*7580*
758–8▲▲▲	Unlisted tumor of scrotum. *Specify neoplasm and behavior (page 99)*	*7580*

DISEASES OF THE VAS DEFERENS

761– Vas deferens

—0 DISEASES DUE TO GENETIC AND PRENATAL INFLUENCES

761–011	Absence of vas deferens, congenital	*7501*
761–018	Atresia of vas deferens, congenital	*7501*

—1 DISEASES DUE TO INFECTION WITH LOWER ORGANISM

761–100	Acute infection of vas deferens; vasitis. *Specify organism (page 57) when known*	*7510*
761–100.0	Chronic infection of vas deferens. *Specify organism (page 57) when known*	*7510*
761–100.4	Stricture of vas deferens due to infection	*7510*

—3 DISEASES DUE TO INTOXICATION

761–3▲▲	Inflammation of vas deferens (vasitis) due to poison. *Specify (page 67)*	*7530*

—4 DISEASES DUE TO TRAUMA OR PHYSICAL AGENT

761–4▲▲	Injury of vas deferens. *Specify (page 83)*	*7540*
761–416	Rupture of vas deferens	*7540*
761–400.4	Stricture of vas deferens due to trauma	*7540*

DISEASES OF THE SPERMATIC CORD

762–   Spermatic cord
76x–   Intrinsic vessels

—0 DISEASES DUE TO GENETIC AND PRENATAL INFLUENCES

762–011	Absence of spermatic cord	*7601*
762–095	Hydrocele of spermatic cord, congenital	*7601*

—1 DISEASES DUE TO INFECTION WITH LOWER ORGANISM

762–100.2	Abscess of spermatic cord. *Specify organism (page 57) when known*	*7610*
762–100	Acute funiculitis. *Specify organism (page 57) when known*	*7610*
762–100.0	Chronic funiculitis. *Specify organism (page 57) when known*	*7610*
762–130	Endemic funiculitis	*7610*

—4 DISEASES DUE TO TRAUMA OR PHYSICAL AGENT

762–4x7	Hematoma of spermatic cord due to trauma	*7640*
762–415.7	Hematoma of spermatic cord following operation	*7640*
762–4▲▲	Injury of spermatic cord. *Specify (page 83)*	*7640*
762–4x4	Torsion of spermatic cord due to trauma	*7640*
762–415	Traumatism of spermatic cord due to operation	*7640*

—6 DISEASES DUE TO OR CONSISTING OF STATIC MECHANICAL ABNORMALITY

76x–619	Thrombosed varicocele	*7660*
762–637	Torsion of spermatic cord due to cause other than trauma	*7660*
76x–6x6	Varicocele	*7660*

—8 NEW GROWTHS

762–870A	Fibroma of spermatic cord	*7680*
762–872A	Lipoma of spermatic cord	*7680*
762–8772A	Mesothelioma of spermatic cord	*7680*
762–871B	Myxoma of spermatic cord	*7680*
762–867A	Rhabdomyoma of spermatic cord	*7680*
762–867F	Rhabdomyosarcoma of spermatic cord	*7680*

| 762–879 | Sarcoma of spermatic cord. *Specify behavior (page 99)* | *7680* |
| 762–8▲▲▲ | Unlisted tumor of spermatic cord. *Specify neoplasm and behavior (page 99)* | *7680* |

—9 DISEASES DUE TO UNKNOWN OR UNCERTAIN CAUSE WITH THE STRUCTURAL REACTION MANIFEST

| 762–9x7 | Hematocele of spermatic cord due to unknown cause | *7690* |
| 762–900.8 | Hydrocele of spermatic cord due to unknown cause | *7690* |

DISEASES OF THE SEMINAL VESICLES

763–   Seminal vesicle
7631– Perivesicular tissue

—I DISEASES DUE TO INFECTION WITH LOWER ORGANISM

763–100.2	Abscess of seminal vesicle. *Specify organism (page 57) when known, e.g.*	7610
763–103.2	Due to Gonococcus	7610
763–100.4	Adhesions of seminal vesicle due to infection	7610
763–151	Ambiasis of seminal vesicle	7610
763–100.6	Fibrosis of seminal vesicle due to infection	7610
7631–100	Perivesiculitis. *Specify organism (page 57) when known*	7610
7631–100.4	Perivesicular adhesions due to infection	7610
763–100	Seminal vesiculitis, acute. *Specify organism (page 57) when known*	7610
763–100.0	Seminal vesiculitis, chronic	7610

—3 DISEASES DUE TO INTOXICATION

763–300.0	Seminal vesiculitis due to chemical poison. *Specify (page 67)*	7630

—55 DISEASES DUE TO DISTURBANCE OF INNERVATION OR OF PSYCHIC CONTROL
Record primary diagnosis when possible

763–580	Spermatorrhea	7655

—6 DISEASES DUE TO OR CONSISTING OF STATIC MECHANICAL ABNORMALITY

763–615	Calculus in seminal vesicle	7660
763–600.8	Cyst of seminal vesicle	7660
763–610.6	Distention of seminal vesicle due to obstruction	7660

—8 NEW GROWTHS

763–8091	Adenocarcinoma of seminal vesicle. *Specify behavior (page 99)*	7680
763–8091A	Adenoma of seminal vesicle	7680
763–814	Epidermoid carcinoma of seminal vesicles. *Specify behavior (page 99)*	7680
763–870A	Fibroma of seminal vesicles	7680

DISEASES OF THE PROSTATE

764–   Prostate
765–   Ejaculatory ducts
766–   Periprostatic tissue

—0 DISEASES DUE TO GENETIC AND PRENATAL INFLUENCES

765–011	Absence of ejaculatory ducts, congenital	7601
764–011	Absence of prostate, congenital	7601
765–018	Atresia of ejaculatory ducts, congenital	7601
764–076	Lack of development of prostate, congenital	7601
764–075	Overdevelopment of prostate, congenital	7601

—I DISEASES DUE TO INFECTION WITH LOWER ORGANISM

766–100.2	Abscess, periprostatic. *Specify organism (page 57) when known*	7611
764–100.2	Abscess of prostate due to infection. *Specify organism (page 57) when known, e.g.*	7611
766–100.4	Adhesions, periprostatic, due to infection	7610
764–151	Amebiasis of prostate	7611
765–100.6	Fibrosis of ejaculatory ducts. *Specify organism (page 57) when known*	7610
764–100.6	Fibrosis of prostate due to infection. *Specify organism (page 57) when known*	7610
764–100.3	Fistula of prostate due to infection. *Specify organism (page 57) when known*	7610
764–1x0.6	Granuloma of prostate	7610
764–100	Prostatitis, acute. *Specify organism (page 57) when known, e.g.*	7611
764–117	Brucellosis of prostate	7611
764–103	Prostatitis, gonococcic	7611
764–100.0	Prostatitis, chronic. *Specify organism (page 57) when known*	7611
765–100.4	Stricture of ejaculatory ducts. *Specify organism (page 57) when known*	7610
764–154	Trichomonas infection of prostate	7611

—2 DISEASES DUE TO HIGHER PLANT OR ANIMAL PARASITE

764–219	Prostatitis due to coccidioides	7620

—4 DISEASES DUE TO TRAUMA OR PHYSICAL AGENT

764–400.3	Fistula of prostate due to trauma	7640
764–415.7	Hemorrhage of prostate following operation	7640

764–4▲▲	Injury of prostate. *Specify* (*page 83*), e.g.	*7640*
764–410	Puncture of prostate	*7640*
764–416	Rupture of prostate	*7640*
764–4x0	Prostatitis due to trauma	*7640*

—50 DISEASES DUE TO CIRCULATORY DISTURBANCE
Record primary diagnosis when possible

764–521	Active congestion of prostate	*7650*
764–511	Infarction of prostate due to thrombus	*7650*
764–512	Infarction of prostate due to embolus	*7650*
764–522	Passive congestion of prostate	*7650*

—55 DISEASES DUE TO DISTURBANCE OF INNERVATION OR OF PSYCHIC CONTROL
Record primary diagnosis when possible

764–580	Prostatorrhea	*7655*

—6 DISEASES DUE TO OR CONSISTING OF STATIC MECHANICAL ABNORMALITY

764–616	Accumulation of secretion in prostate	*7660*
764–615	Calculus in prostate	*7660*
764–600.8	Cyst of prostate, simple	*7660*
767–641	Varix of prostate	*7660*

—7 DISEASES DUE TO DISORDER OF METABOLISM, GROWTH, OR NUTRITION

764–799	Prostate hypertrophy, benign	*7679*

—8 NEW GROWTHS

764–8091	Adenocarcinoma of prostate. *Specify behavior* (*page 99*)	*7680*
764–8831A	Adenofibroma of prostate	*7680*
764–8091A	Adenoma of prostate	*7680*
764–873F	Chondrosarcoma of prostate	*7680*
764–870A	Fibroma of prostate	*7680*
764–866A	Leiomyoma of prostate	*7680*
764–866F	Leiomyosarcoma of prostate	*7680*
764–830	Lymphosarcoma of prostate. *Specify behavior* (*page 99*)	*7680*
764–8871	Mesenchymal mixed tumor of prostate. *Specify behavior*	*7680*
764–8012	Mucinous carcinoma of prostate. *Specify behavior* (*page 99*)	*7680*
764–867F	Rhabdomyosarcoma of prostate	*7680*

764–879   Sarcoma of prostate. *Specify behavior*
                      (*page 99*)   *7680*
764–8▲▲▲   Unlisted tumor of prostate. *Specify neo-*
                      plasm and behavior (*page 99*)   *7680*

**—9 DISEASES DUE TO UNKNOWN OR UNCERTAIN CAUSE WITH THE
STRUCTURAL REACTION MANIFEST**

764–911   Atrophy of prostate due to unknown cause   *7690*
764–942   Median bar   *7690*

DISEASES OF THE FEMALE GENITAL SYSTEM

See also Diseases of Genital System, *page 327*

705– Female genital system
780– Internal female organs

—I DISEASES DUE TO INFECTION WITH LOWER ORGANISM

780–100	Acute diffuse inflammation of internal female genital organs. Salpingo-oophoritis. *Specify organism (page 57) when known*	7810
780–100.0	Chronic diffuse inflammation of internal female genital organs. *Specify organism (page 57) when known*	7810
705–1xx	Sterility due to obstruction following infection. *Record primary diagnosis when possible*	7010

—4 DISEASES DUE TO TRAUMA OR PHYSICAL AGENT

705–4xx	Sterility due to trauma or operation	7040

—6 DISEASES DUE TO OR CONSISTING OF STATIC MECHANICAL ABNORMALITY

705–6xx	Sterility due to distortion or displacement of pelvic organs of unknown cause. *Record primary diagnosis when possible*	7070

—7 DISEASES DUE TO DISORDER OF METABOLISM, GROWTH, OR NUTRITION

705–787	Premature menopause due to unknown cause	7070
705–777	Sterility due to hypopituitarism	7070
705–7871	Sterility, functional, due to decrease in estrogenic substance	7070
705–7872	Sterility, functional, due to decrease in progesterone	7070
705–7xx	Sterility due to absence or destruction of ovary. *Record primary diagnosis when possible*	7070

—X DISEASES DUE TO UNKNOWN OR UNCERTAIN CAUSE WITH THE FUNCTIONAL REACTION ALONE MANIFEST

705–x12	Delayed menstruation due to unknown cause	7090

705–x31	Infrequent menstruation due to unknown cause	7090
705–x32	Leukorrhea due to unknown cause	7090
705–x10	Sterility due to unknown cause	7090

DISEASES OF THE VULVA

774– Vulva
740– Urethra
129– Mucous membrane
144– Skin of vulva

For detailed structures of external female organs, see page 39

—0 DISEASES DUE TO GENETIC AND PRENATAL INFLUENCES

774–011	Absence of vulva, complete	*7701*
774–018	Atresia of vulva, superficial, congenital (usually incomplete)	*7701*
779–019	Canal of Nuck, patent	*7701*
775–011	Clitoris, absence of, congenital	*7701*
775–034	Clitoris, bifid	*7701*
775–013	Clitoris, hypertrophy of, congenital	*7701*
776–011	Hymen, absence of	*7701*
776–024	Hymen, atresia of, congenital	*7701*
776–064	Hymen, cyst of, embryonal	*7701*
776–021	Hymen, displacement of, upward	*7701*
776–034	Hymen, division of, into two parts	*7701*
776–077	Hymen, excessive blood supply of	*7701*
776–013	Hymen, hypertrophy of, congenital	*7701*
776–010	Hymen, variations in form of: circular, septate, labiate, punctiform fimbriate, falciform, fenestrate, cribriform	*7701*
776–030	Hymens, supernumerary	*7701*
772–011	Labia majora, absence of (associated with ectopia vesicae)	*7701*
740–012	Hypospadias in female	*7701*
772–025	Labia majora, adhesion of	*7701*
772–013	Labia majora, congenital hypertrophy of	*7701*
772–024	Labia majora, fusion of, congenital with urogenital sinus	*7701*
773–011	Labia minora, absence of (with epispadias)	*7701*
773–025	Labia minora, adhesion of, congenital	*7701*
7812–023	Sebaceous glands at junction of vagina and vulva, aberrant	*7701*
774–064	Vulva, cyst of, embryonal	*7701*
774–019	Vulva, infantile	*7701*
774–091	Vulvitis, adhesive, congenital	*7701*
70x1–037	Vulvorectal fistula, congenital	*7701*

—I   DISEASES DUE TO INFECTION WITH LOWER ORGANISM

777–100.2	Abscess of Bartholin's gland. *Specify organism (page 57) when known*	7712
772–100.2	Abscess of labium majus. *Specify organism (page 57) when known*	7710
774–100.2	Abscess of vulva. *Specify organism (page 57) when known*	7710
777–100	Adenitis of Bartholin's gland. *Specify organism (page 57) when known, e.g.*	7712
777–103	Due to Gonococcus	7710
776–100.4	Atresia of hymen due to infection	7710
129–100	Cellulitis of vulva. *Specify organism (page 57) when known*	1811
774–10x	Chancroid of vulva (due to Ducrey's bacillus)	7710
774–103.6	Condyloma acuminatum of vulva, gonococcic	7710
774–125	Diphtheria of vulva	7710
70x4–100.3	Fistula, rectolabial, due to infection	7710
70x1–100.3	Fistula, vulvorectal, due to infection	7710
774–100.1	Gangrene of vulva due to infection	7710
144–166	Herpes of vulva	1310
777–100.8	Retention cyst of Bartholin's gland, due to infection. *Specify organism (page 57) when known*	7710
774–147.6	Syphiloma of vulva; syphilitic condyloma acuminatum	7710
774–100.9	Ulcer of vulva due to infection. *Specify organism (page 57) when known*	7710
144–100.9	Ulcus vulvae acutum	1310
774–100	Vulvitis, acute. *Specify organism (page 57) when known, e.g.*	7710
774–103	Vulvitis, gonococcic	7710
774–100.0	Vulvitis, chronic. *Specify organism (page 57) when known*	7710
705–100	Vulvovaginitis. *Specify organism (page 57) when known*	7711

—2   DISEASES DUE TO HIGHER PLANT OR ANIMAL PARASITE

774–215	Epidermophytosis of vulva	7720
144–292	Pediculosis of vulva (Phthirus pubis)	1320
144–2831	Scabies of vulva	1320
774–209	Thrush of vulva	7720

—4 DISEASES DUE TO TRAUMA OR PHYSICAL AGENT

774–495.6	Condyloma acuminatum of vulva due to filth	*7740*
776–412.8	Cyst of hymen due to lacerations	*7740*
774–412.8	Cyst of vulva due to lacerations	*7740*
773–43x	Elongation of labia minora	*7740*
774–400.1	Gangrene of vulva due to trauma	*7740*
774–4x7	Hematoma of vulva, nonpuerperal	*7740*
776–4▲▲	Injury of hymen. *Specify (page 83)*	*7740*
774–4▲▲	Injury of vulva. *Specify (page 83)*	*7740*
774–495	Vulvitis, acute, due primarily to uncleanliness	*7740*
774–437	Vulvitis, intertriginous	*7740*
70x1–400.3	Vulvorectal fistula due to trauma	*7740*
70x1–415.3	Vulvorectal fistula following operation	*7740*

—50 DISEASES DUE TO CIRCULATORY DISTURBANCE

774–501	Elephantiasis of vulva, nonfilarial	*7750*
774–500.7	Hemorrhage of vulva due to cause other than trauma	*7750*

—55 DISEASES DUE TO DISTURBANCE OF INNERVATION OR OF PSYCHIC CONTROL
Record primary diagnosis when possible

774–570	Pruritus vulvae, neurogenic	*7755*

—6 DISEASES DUE TO OR CONSISTING OF STATIC MECHANICAL ABNORMALITY

775–615	Concretion in clitoris	*7760*
777–600.8	Cyst of Bartholin's gland due to unspecified cause	*7763*
779–600.8	Cyst of canal of Nuck	*7760*
775–600.8	Cyst of clitoris	*7760*
776–600.8	Cyst of hymen	*7760*
772–600.8	Cyst of labium majus	*7760*
77x–641	Varix of vulva	*7760*

—7 DISEASES DUE TO DISORDER OF METABOLISM, GROWTH, OR NUTRITION
Record primary diagnosis when possible

16x–792	Abnormal growth of pubic hair	*1600*
774–785	Diabetic vulvitis	*7770*
774–798	Senile atrophy of vulva	*7770*
129–747	Vitiligo of vulva	*1200*

—8 NEW GROWTHS

774–8091	Adenocarcinoma of vulva. *Specify behavior (page 99)*	*7780*
774–8091A	Adenoma of vulva	*7780*
774–812	Basal cell carcinoma of vulva. *Specify behavior*	*7780*
775–814	Epidermoid carcinoma of clitoris. *Specify behavior (page 99)*	*7780*
774–814E	Epidermoid carcinoma in situ	*7780*
774–814	Epidermoid carcinoma of vulva. *Specify behavior (page 99)*	*7780*
774–870A	Fibroma of vulva	*7780*
774–850A	Hemangioma of vulva	*7780*
774–866A	Leiomyoma of vulva	*7780*
774–872A	Lipoma of vulva	*7780*
774–8173F	Malignant melanoma of vulva	*7780*
774–8173	Melanoma of vulva	*7780*
774–8871	Mesenchymal mixed tumor malignant of vulva. *Specify behavior*	*7780*
774–8451	Neurofibroma of vulva. *Specify behavior (page 99)*	*7780*
774–8170	Pigmented nevus of vulva. *Specify behavior (page 99)*	*7780*
774–8023	Polyp of vulva. *Specify behavior*	*7780*
774–879	Sarcoma of vulva. *Specify behavior (page 99)*	*7780* *7780*
774–8075	Sebaceous cyst of vulva. *Specify behavior (page 99)*	*7780*
774–8061	Sweat gland tumor of vulva. *Specify behavior*	*7780*
774–8▲▲▲	Unlisted tumor of vulva. *Specify neoplasm and behavior (page 99)*	*7780*

—9 DISEASES DUE TO UNKNOWN OR UNCERTAIN CAUSE WITH THE STRUCTURAL REACTION MANIFEST

779–900.8	Hydrocele of canal of Nuck	*7790*
775–9x6	Hypertrophy of clitoris	*7790*
774–9x6	Hypertrophy of vulva due to unknown cause	*7790*
129–943	Kraurosis of vulva (leukoplakia)	*1200*
776–940	Thickening of hymen	*7790*
774–951	Ulcer of vulva due to unknown cause	*7790*

—Y DISEASES DUE TO CAUSE NOT DETERMINABLE IN THE PARTICULAR CASE

Y signifies an incomplete diagnosis. It is to be replaced whenever possible by a code digit signifying the specific diagnosis

776–yx4	Atresia of hymen due to undetermined cause	*7790*

DISEASES OF THE VAGINA

781–   Vagina
70▲–   Combined structures

—0 DISEASES DUE TO GENETIC AND PRENATAL INFLUENCES

781–012	Unilateral vagina (associated with uterus unicornis)	*7801*
781–011	Absence of vagina, congenital, associated with absence of uterus	*7801*
781–018	Atresia of vagina, congenital, complete or partial, associated with normal, rudimentary, or absent uterus (including atresia of unilateral vagina)	*7801*
781–091	Colpitis, adhesive, congenital	*7801*
781–064	Cyst of vagina, embryonal	*7801*
781–032	Double vagina, complete or in part (usually associated with uterus bicornis)	*7801*
781–030	Double vagina; two distinct vaginas	*7801*
70x2–037	Rectovaginal fistula, congenital	*7801*
781–016	Rudimentary vagina	*7801*
781–034	Septum of vagina, congenital	*7801*
781–017	Stenosis of vagina, congenital, complete, or in certain parts	*7801*
7031–029	Vesicovaginal fistula	*7801*

—I DISEASES DUE TO INFECTION WITH LOWER ORGANISM

781–100.2	Abscess of vaginal wall. *Specify organism (page 57) when known*	*7810*
7811–100.2	Abscess, paravaginal. *Specify organism (page 57) when known*	*7810*
781–125	Diphtheria of vagina	*7811*
781–100.x	Dyspareunia due to infection	*7810*
70x2–100.3	Fistula, rectovaginal, due to infection	*7810*
781–1732	Lymphopathia venereum, of vagina	*7810*
7811–190	Paravaginitis. *Specify organism (page 57) when known*	*7811*
781–100.8	Pyocolpos	*7810*
781–100.4	Stricture of vagina due to infection	*7810*
781–103.4	Stricture of vagina following gonococcic infection	*7810*
781–154	Trichomonas infection of vagina	*7811*
781–100	Vaginitis. *Specify organism (page 57) when known*	*7811*
781–190	Vaginitis, emphysematous	*7811*

—2 DISEASES DUE TO HIGHER PLANT OR ANIMAL PARASITE

781–209	Moniliasis (candidiasis) of vagina	7820
781–2▲▲	Parasitic infection of vagina. *Specify* (*page 63*)	7280

—3 DISEASES DUE TO INTOXICATION

781–3▲▲	Chemical burn of vagina. *Specify (page 67)*	7830

—4 DISEASES DUE TO TRAUMA OR PHYSICAL AGENT

70x2–412.3	Anovaginal fistula following parturition	7840
781–415.x	Dyspareunia due to plastic operation	7840
781–400.x	Dyspareunia due to trauma	7840
781–400.1	Exfoliative vaginitis due to trauma, *e.g.*	7840
781–441.1	Due to burn	7840
781–415.8	Inclusion cyst of vagina following operation	7840
781–4▲▲	Injury of vagina (not obstetric). *Specify* (*page 83*)	7840
70x2–415.3	Rectovaginal fistula following operation	7840
70x2–400.3	Rectovaginal fistula due to trauma	7840
70x2–472.3	Rectovaginal fistula due to radium	7840
781–400.4	Stricture of vagina due to trauma	7840
70x21–412	Tear of rectovaginal septum	7840
781–412	Vaginal tear	7840
781–438	Vaginitis due to foreign body	7840
781–439	Vaginitis due to pressure	7840
7053–412.3	Vaginocutaneous fistula following parturition	7840
7031–400.3	Vesicovaginal fistula due to trauma. *Specify trauma, e.g.*	7840
7031–415.3	Vesicovaginal fistula, postoperative	7840

—50 DISEASES DUE TO CIRCULATORY DISTURBANCE
Record primary diagnosis when possible

781–544.1	Necrosis of vagina in granulocytopenia	7850

—55 DISEASES DUE TO DISTURBANCE OF INNERVATION OR OF PSYCHIC CONTROL
Record primary diagnosis when possible

781–594	Vaginismus	7855

—6 DISEASES DUE TO OR CONSISTING OF STATIC MECHANICAL ABNORMALITY

781–600.8	Cyst of vagina	7860
781–610.x	Dyspareunia due to obstruction	7860

781–611	Foreign body in vagina	*7860*
781–61x	Hematocolpos	*7860*
781–631	Prolapse of vagina	*7860*
781–631.9	Ulceration of vagina due to prolapse	*7860*
781–6x0	Vaginitis due to obstruction (atresia)	*7860*

—7 DISEASES DUE TO DISORDER OF METABOLISM, GROWTH, OR NUTRITION

781–797.4	Senile atresia of vagina	*7870*
781–798	Senile atrophy of vagina	*7870*
781–797	Senile vaginitis	*7870*

—8 NEW GROWTHS

781–814	Epidermoid carcinoma of vagina. *Specify behavior (page 99)*	*7880*
781–870A	Fibroma of vagina	*7880*
781–8173	Malignant melanoma of vagina. *Specify behavior*	*7880*
781–8871	Mesenchymal mixed tumor, malignant, of vagina. *Specify behavior*	*7880*
781–8▲▲▲	Unlisted tumor of vagina. *Specify neoplasm and behavior (page 99)*	*7880*

—9 DISEASES DUE TO UNKNOWN OR UNCERTAIN CAUSE WITH THE STRUCTURAL REACTION MANIFEST

| 781–943 | Kraurosis of vagina | *7890* |

—X DISEASES DUE TO UNKNOWN OR UNCERTAIN CAUSE WITH THE FUNCTIONAL REACTION ALONE MANIFEST

| 781–x30 | Dyspareunia due to unknown cause | *7890* |

DISEASES OF THE CERVIX UTERI

783–   Cervix uteri

—0 DISEASES DUE TO GENETIC AND PRENATAL INFLUENCES

783–011	Absence, complete of cervix	7801
783–012	Absence, partial, of cervix	7801
7051–025	Adhesions, cervicovaginal, congenital	7801
783–018	Atresia of cervix (solid, complete, or partial), congenital	7801
785–021	Displacement of cuboidal epithelium beyond limits of external os; congenital pseudoerosion of cervix	7801
783–036	Diverticulum, congenital, cervix	7801
783–034	Division of external os into two openings by frenum	7801
783–064	Embryonal cyst of cervix	7801
783–013	Hypertrophy of cervix, congenital	7801
783–016	Hypoplasia of cervix, congenital	7801
783–015	Incompetent cervical os, congenital	7801
783–019	Persistence of fetal form of cervix	7801
783–021	Prolapse of hypertrophied cervix, congenital	7801
783–023	Squamous epithelium in cervical canal	7801

—I DISEASES DUE TO INFECTION WITH LOWER ORGANISM

783–100.2	Abscess of cervical stump. *Specify organism (page 57) when known*	7810
783–100	Acute cervicitis. *Specify organism (page 57) when known, e.g.*	7810
783–103	Due to Gonococcus	7810
783–100.0	Chronic cervicitis primarily due to infection. *Specify organism (page 57) when known*	7810
783–100.9	Erosion of cervix due to infection	7810
783–100.6	Eversion of cervix (ectropion) due to infection	7810
783–1x6	Polyp of cervix, due to infection	7810
783–100.4	Stricture of cervix due to infection	7810
783–154	Trichomonas infection of cervix	7810

—3 DISEASES DUE TO INTOXICATION

783–3▲▲.9	Erosion of cervix due to chemicals. *Specify (page 67)*	7830

—4 DISEASES DUE TO TRAUMA OR PHYSICAL AGENT

7051–412.4	Adhesions, cervicovaginal, following parturition	*7840*
783–400.0	Cervicitis, chronic, primarily due to trauma	*7840*
783–438	Cervicitis due to foreign body	*7840*
783–400.4	Cicatrix of cervix due to trauma	*7840*
783–412.4	Cicatrix of cervix following parturition	*7840*
783–415.4	Cicatrix of cervix following operation	*7840*
783–400.8	Cyst of cervix due to trauma	*7840*
783–409	Detachment of cervix, annular	*7840*
783–400.9	Erosion of cervix, primarily due to trauma	*7840*
783–412.6	Eversion of cervix (ectropion) due to lacerations	*7840*
783–415.7	Hemorrhage of cervix following operation	*7840*
783–4x6	Hypertrophy of cervix, primarily due to trauma	*7840*
783–400.6	Incompetent cervical os	*7840*
783–4▲▲	Injury of cervix. *Specify injury*	*7840*
783–412	Lacerations of cervix	*7840*
783–415.9	Prolapse of cervical stump due to operation	*7840*
7832–400.4	Stricture of cervix due to trauma	*7840*
7832–415.4	Stricture of cervix following operation	*7840*
7832–412.4	Stricture of cervix following parturition	*7840*

—6 DISEASES DUE TO OR CONSISTING OF STATIC MECHANICAL ABNOR-MALITY

783–600.8	Nabothian cyst	*7865*

—7 DISEASES DUE TO DISORDER OF METABOLISM, GROWTH, OR NUTRITION
Record primary diagnosis when possible

783–787	Atrophy of cervix at menopause	*7870*
783–798	Senile atrophy of cervix	*7870*
783–797	Senile cervicitis	*7870*

—8 NEW GROWTHS

See under Uterus, *page 364*

—9 DISEASES DUE TO UNKNOWN OR UNCERTAIN CAUSE WITH THE STRUCTURAL REACTION MANIFEST

783–954	Basal cell hyperplasia of cervix	*7890*
783–923	Calcification of cervix	*7890*
783–951	Erosion of cervix, cause unknown	*7895*
783–941	Leukoplakia of cervix	*7890*
783–944	Polyp, simple of cervix	*7894*
783–958	Squamous metaplasia of cervix	*7890*

DISEASES OF THE UTERUS

782– Uterus
70▲– Combined structures
78x– Uterine vessels

For detailed structures of internal female organs, see page 39

—0 DISEASES DUE TO GENETIC AND PRENATAL INFLUENCES

780–011	Absence of uterus and adnexa, complete, congenital	*7801*
782–018	Atresia of uterus, congenital	*7801*
782–064	Cyst, embryonal, of uterus	*7801*
782–0212	Congenital prolapse of uterus	*7801*
782–022	Congenital retroflexion or retroversion of uterus	*7801*
782–016	Rudimentary uterus	*7801*
782–023	Squamous epithelium in uterine mucosa	*7801*
782–032	Two distinct uteri, one in front of the other	*7801*
782–037	Uterus didelphys, complete or partial (uterus bicornis, uterus arcuatus, uterus septus, uterus subseptus, uterus uniforis, uterus unicollis, uterus unicorporeus, uterus biforis supra simplex, etc.)	*7801*
782–019	Uterus fetalis	*7801*
782–012	Uterus unicornis (second horn may be absent or rudimentary)	*7801*

—I DISEASES DUE TO INFECTION WITH LOWER ORGANISM

784–100.2	Abscess, parauterine. *Specify organism (page 57) when known*	*7810*
784–100.4	Adhesions, parauterine. *Specify organism (page 57) when known*	*7810*
782–100.4	Displacement of uterus due to infection. *Specify organism (page 57) when known*	*7810*
782–1x41	Retroflexion of uterus	*7810*
782–1x42	Retroversion of uterus	*7810*
782–1x43	Anteflexion of uterus	*7810*
782–1x44	Lateral flexion of uterus	*7810*
785–190	Endometritis, acute. *Specify organism (page 57) when known*	*7813*
785–103	Gonococcic endometritis	*7813*

785–190.0	Endometritis, chronic. *Specify organism* (*page 57*) *when known*	*7813*
785–100	Endometritis, septic. *Specify organism* (*page 57*) *when known*	*7813*
782–100.3	Fistula of uterus due to infection	*7810*
70x3–100.3	Fistula, uterorectal due to infection	*7810*
785–1xx	Menorrhagia due to acute infectious general disease	*7810*
782–190	Metritis, acute. *Specify organism* (*page 57*) *when known*	*7813*
782–190.0	Metritis, chronic. *Specify organism* (*page 57*) *when known*	*7813*
782–100.7	Metrorrhagia due to infection. *Specify organism* (*page 57*) *when known*	*7810*
785–100.9	Obliteration of endometrium due to infection	*7810*
784–100	Parametritis. *Specify organism* (*page 57*) *when known*	*7813*
785–1x6	Polyp of endometrium due to infection	*7810*
782–100.2	Pyometra. *Specify organism* (*page 57*) *when known*	*7810*
785–100.4	Stricture (atresia) of uterus due to infection. *Specify organism* (*page 57*) *when known*	*7810*

—3 DISEASES DUE TO INTOXICATION

| 785–3▲▲.9 | Atrophy of endometrium due to poison. *Specify* (*page 67*) | *7830* |

—4 DISEASES DUE TO TRAUMA OR PHYSICAL AGENT

782–415.x	Amenorrhea due to surgery	*7840*
785–470	Atrophy of endometrium due to irradiation	*7840*
782–415.4	Displacement of uterus following operation	*7841*
782–4x4	Displacement of uterus following previous parturition	*7841*
782–4x43	Anteflexion of uterus	*7841*
782–4x47	Inversion of uterus	*7841*
782–4x44	Lateral flexion of uterus	*7841*
782–4x45	Lateral version of uterus	*7841*
782–4x46	Prolapse of uterus	*7841*
782–4x41	Retroflexion of uterus	*7841*
782–4x42	Retroversion of uterus	*7841*
782–4▲▲	Injury of uterus. *Specify* (*page 83*)	*7840*
782–415	Instrumentation wound of uterus	*7840*
782–43x	Inversion of uterus due to traction	*7840*
784–4x4	Parauterine adhesions due to trauma	*7840*

784–412.4	Parauterine adhesions following parturi-tion	7840
785–415.4	Stricture of uterus following operation	7840
786–415.4	Scar of uterus following operation	7840

—50 DISEASES DUE TO CIRCULATORY DISTURBANCE
Record primary diagnosis when possible

Amenorrhea due to anemia. *Diagnose the anemia and record amenorrhea as a symptom, page 498*

Menorrhagia due to anemia or other blood disease. *Diagnose the blood disease and record menorrhagia as a symptom, page 499*

—55 DISEASES DUE TO DISTURBANCE OF INNERVATION
Record primary diagnosis when possible

| 782–580 | Disturbance of sympathetic and para-sympathetic innervation of uterus | 7855 |

—6 DISEASES DUE TO OR CONSISTING OF STATIC MECHANICAL ABNOR-MALITY

782–6431	Anteflexion of uterus due to unknown or uncertain cause	7864
780–6x7	Dysmenorrhea due to mechanical cause	7860
782–61x	Hematometra	7860
782–6432	Lateral flexion of uterus due to unknown or uncertain cause	7864
782–6371	Lateral version of uterus due to unknown or uncertain cause	7864
782–633	Laterocession of uterus due to unknown or uncertain cause	7864
785–630.7	Menorrhagia due to distortion or displacement of uterus	7864
782–630.7	Metrorrhagia due to distortion or displacement of uterus	7864
782–631	Prolapse of uterus due to unknown or uncertain cause	7864
782–643	Retroflexion of uterus due to unknown or uncertain cause	7864
782–63x	Retroversion of uterus due to unknown or uncertain cause	7864
782–636	Retrodisplacement of uterus due to unknown or uncertain cause	7864

—7 DISEASES DUE TO DISORDER OF METABOLISM, GROWTH, OR NUTRITION

Record primary diagnosis when possible

785–712	Amenorrhea due to debility	7870
785–70x	Amenorrhea due to obesity	7870
785–7862	Amenorrhea due to persistence of corpus luteum	7870
785–787	Atrophy of endometrium due to absence, destruction or atrophy of ovary. *Record ovarian disease, page 368*	7870
785–771	Endometrial dysfunction (without morphologic change) secondary to hyperthyroidism. *Record thyroid disease, page 388*	7875
	With amenorrhea. *See page 498*	
	With menorrhagia. *See page 499*	
785–772	Endometrial dysfunction (without morphologic change) secondary to hypothyroidism. *Record thyroid disease, page 388*	7875
	With amenorrhea. *See page 498*	
	With menorrhagia. *See page 499*	
785–781	Endometrial dysfunction (without morphologic change) secondary to hyperadrenalism. *Record adrenal disease, page 396*	7875
	With amenorrhea. *See page 498*	
	With menorrhagia. *See page 499*	
785–782	Endometrial dysfunction (without morphologic change) secondary to hypoadrenalism. *Record adrenal disease, page 396*	7875
	With amenorrhea. *See page 498*	
	With menorrhagia. *See page 499*	
785–7761	Endometrial dysfunction (without morphologic change) secondary to eosinophilic hyperpituitarism. *Record pituitary disease, page 393*	7875
785–777	Endometrial dysfunction (without morphologic change) secondary to hypopituitarism. *Record pituitary disease, page 393*	7875
	With amenorrhea. *See page 498*	
	With menorrhagia. *See page 499*	
785–7861	Endometrial dysfunction due to excessive administration of estrogenic substance	7875
	With menorrhagia. *See page 499*	

785–7871	Endometrial dysfunction (amenorrhea or dysmenorrhea) due to decrease in estrogenic substance	7875
	With amenorrhea. *See page 498*	
	With dysmenorrhea. *See page 498*	
785–7763	Endometrial hyperplasia secondary to basophilic hyperpituitarism. *Record pituitary disease, page 393*	7875
782–787	Hypoplasia of uterus due to ovarian hypofunction. *Record ovarian disease, page 368*	7870
782–791	Infantile uterus	7870
002–7861	Premenstrual tension	0007
	Hyperhormonal amenorrhea. *See* Endometrial hyperplasia secondary to basophilic hyperpituitarism	
782–798	Senile atrophy of uterus	7870
785–786.6	Static endometrial hyperplasia due to continuous ovarian stimulation	7875
786–786.6	Static myometrial hyperplasia due to continuous ovarian stimulation (fibrosis uteri)	7875

—8 NEW GROWTHS

782–8091	Adenocarcinoma of uterus. *Specify behavior (page 99)*	7880
782–8881A	Adenomyosis of uterus	7880
782–8831F	Carcinosarcoma of uterus	7880
783–814E	Epidermoid carcinoma in situ of cervix	7880
783–814	Epidermoid carcinoma of cervix. *Specify behavior (page 99)*	7880
782–866F	Leiomyosarcoma of uterus	7880
782–866A	Myoma of uterus (fibroid)	7880
782–8023	Polyp of uterus (neoplastic). *Specify behavior*	7880
783–879	Sarcoma of cervix. *Specify behavior (page 99)*	7880
785–879	Sarcoma of endometrium. *Specify behavior (page 99)*	7880
782–8▲▲▲	Unlisted tumor of uterus. *Specify neoplasm and behavior (page 99)*	7880

—9 DISEASES DUE TO UNKNOWN OR UNCERTAIN CAUSE WITH THE STRUCTURAL REACTION MANIFEST

78x.2–955	Arteriosclerosis, medial, of uterine vessels	7890
78x–942	Arteriosclerosis of uterine vessels	7890
782–959	Endometriosis of uterus	7893

785–943	Hyperplasia of endometrium due to unknown cause	7894
786–956	Hyperplasia of myometrium due to unknown cause	7894
785–995	Membranous dysmenorrhea	7890
785–944	Polyp, simple of uterus	7891
785–911	Spontaneous atrophy of endometrium	7890

—X DISEASES DUE TO UNKNOWN OR UNCERTAIN CAUSE WITH THE FUNCTIONAL REACTION ALONE MANIFEST

785–x10	Primary amenorrhea	7896
785–x20	Menorrhagia (functional)	7896
782–x30	Metrorrhagia (functional)	7896
780–x32	Dysmenorrhea (functional)	7896

DISEASES OF THE FALLOPIAN TUBES

787–   Fallopian tubes (Oviducts)
7871– Serous coat of Fallopian tube (Oviduct)

—0 DISEASES DUE TO GENETIC AND PRENATAL INFLUENCES

787–0111	Absence of one tube (associated with uterus unicornis)	7801
787–011	Absence, bilateral, of tubes (associated with absence of uterus)	7801
787–012	Absence of tubes, partial	7801
787–019	Convolutions of tubes, persistence of	7801
787–064	Cyst of tube, congenital; hydatid of Morgagni	7801
787–021	Displacement of uterine opening of tubes (downward or posteriorly)	7801
787–032	Duplication of tubes and ostiums; accessory fimbriae	7801
787–013	Length, abnormal, of tubes (alone or with ovarian hernia)	7801
787–018	Occlusion of tubes (blind sacs), congenital	7801
787–023	Ovarian rest in tube	7801
787–031	Supernumerary tubes (may be associated with supernumerary ovaries)	7801
787–033	Triplication of ostiums	7801

—I DISEASES DUE TO INFECTION WITH LOWER ORGANISM

787–100	Acute salpingitis. *Specify organism (page 57) when known, e.g.*	7814
787–103	Gonococcic salpingitis	7814
787–100.4	Atresia of tube due to infection	7810
787–100.0	Chronic salpingitis. *Specify organism (page 57) when known*	7814
787–100.7	Hematosalpinx due to infection	7814
7871–100	Perisalpingitis	7814
787–100.2	Pyosalpinx. *Specify organism (page 57) when known, e.g.*	7814
787–103.2	Gonococcic pyosalpinx	7814
787–1x2.5	Ruptured pyosalpinx	7814
7803–100.2	Tubo-ovarian abscess. *Specify organism (page 57) when known*	7810

—4 DISEASES DUE TO TRAUMA OR PHYSICAL AGENT

7804–415.3	External fistula of tube following operation	7840
787–400.7	Hemorrhage of tube due to trauma	7840

| 787–4▲▲ | Injury of tube. *Specify (page 57)* | *7840* |
| 787–415.4 | Occlusion of tube following operation | *7840* |

—6 DISEASES DUE TO OR CONSISTING OF STATIC MECHANICAL ABNOR-MALITY

787–630	Displacement of tube	*7860*
787–6x8	Hydrosalpinx	*7860*
787–61x	Hematosalpinx	*7860*
787–637	Volvulus of tube	*7860*

—7 DISEASES DUE TO DISORDER OF METABOLISM, GROWTH, OR NUTRITION

| 787–796 | Fibrosis of tube | *7870* |
| 787–798 | Senile atrophy of tube | *7870* |

—8 NEW GROWTHS

787–8091	Adenocarcinoma of tube. *Specify behavior (page 99)*	*7880*
787–8772A	Mesothelioma of tube (adenomatoid tumor)	*7880*
787–8▲▲▲	Unlisted tumor of tube. *Specify neoplasm and behavior (page 99)*	*7880*

—9 DISEASES DUE TO UNKNOWN OR UNCERTAIN CAUSE WITH THE STRUCTURAL REACTION MANIFEST

787–959	Endometriosis of tube	*7893*
787–941	Nodular salpingitis	*7890*
787–944	Polyp of tube, simple	*7891*

DISEASES OF THE OVARY

788–   Ovary

For detailed list of structures of ovary, see page 39

—0 DISEASES DUE TO GENETIC AND PRENATAL INFLUENCES

788–011	Absence, complete, of ovaries	7801
788–032	Accesory ovaries, (formed by constriction)	7801
788–025	Adhesions of ovary (to sigmoid, cecum or omentum)	7801
788–064	Cystic ovaries, congenital	7801
788–021	Displacement of ovary (free in peritoneal cavity)	7801
788–091	Fetal oophoritis	7801
788–027	Hernia of ovary (into inguinal canal, unilateral or bilateral, into labium majus or into canal of Nuck)	7801
788–013	Hypertrophy of one or both ovaries	7801
788–016	Hypoplasia of normal or ectopic ovary	7801
788–01x	Ovotestis	7801
788–031	Supernumerary ovaries (three)	7801
788–065	Torsion of ovarian pedicle, congenital	7801

—I DISEASES DUE TO INFECTION WITH LOWER ORGANISM

788–100.2	Abscess of ovary. *Specify organism (page 57) when known, e.g.*	7810
788–103.2	Gonococcic abscess of ovary	7810
788–100	Acute oophoritis. *Specify organism (page 57) when known, e.g.*	7815
788–170	Oophoritis of mumps	7815
788–100.0	Chronic oophoritis due to infection. *Specify organism (page 57) when known*	7815
788–100.7	Hemorrhage of ovary due to remote infection	7810
7886–100	Perioophoritis. *Specify organism (page 57) when known*	7815
788–1x6	Sclerosis of ovary due to infection	7810

—4 DISEASES DUE TO TRAUMA OR PHYSICAL AGENT

788–400.7	Hemorrhage of ovary due to trauma	7840
788–4▲▲	Injury of ovary. *Specify (page 83)*	7840
788–471	Ovarian hypofunction due to roentgen rays (x-rays); artificial menopause due to roentgen rays	7840

788–472	Ovarian hypofunction due to radium; artificial menopause due to radium	*7840*
788–415	Ovarian transplants	*7840*
788–415.x	Dysfunction due to surgery (indicate supplementary term)	*7840*

—50 DISEASES DUE TO CIRCULATORY DISTURBANCE
Record primary diagnosis when possible

788–532	Hematoma of ovary due to cause other than trauma	*7850*
788–522	Hemorrhage of ovary due to venous obstruction	*7850*
788–510.1	Necrosis of ovary due to circulatory disturbance	*7850*
788–514	Strangulation of ovary. *Record primary diagnosis*	*7850*

—6 DISEASES DUE TO OR CONSISTING OF STATIC MECHANICAL ABNORMALITY
Record primary diagnosis when possible

788–630	Displacement of ovary	*7860*
788–639	Displacement of ovary into hernial sac	*7860*
788–637	Torsion of ovarian pedicle	*7860*

—7 DISEASES DUE TO DISORDER OF METABOLISM, GROWTH, OR NUTRITION

788–777	Decreased function of ovary in hypopituitarism. *Record pituitary disease, page 393*	*7870*
788–796.7	Hemorrhage of ovary from rupture of graafian follicle	*7870*
788–795	Ovarian cyst due to failure of involution	*7877*
7888–795	Corpus albicans cyst	*7877*
7881–795	Cyst of graafian follicle	*7877*
7882–795	Corpus luteum cyst	*7877*
7881–7701	Ovarian cystic disease with hirsutism	*7877*
788–786	Ovarian hypergonadism (ovarian disease undetermined)	*7870*
788–787	Ovarian hypogonadism, primary (ovarian disease undetermined)	*7870*
	Ovarian pregnancy. *See page 380*	
7881–770	Polycystic ovaries (Stein-Leventhal syndrome)	*7877*
788–798	Senile involution of ovary	*7870*

—8 NEW GROWTHS

7887–8042	Arrhenoblastoma of ovary. *Specify behavior (page 99)*	*7880*
788–8836	Brenner tumor of ovary. *Specify behavior*	*7880*
788–8033	Cystadenoma of ovary. *Specify behavior*	*7880*
788–8033F	Cystadenocarcinoma of ovary	*7880*
788–881	Disgerminoma of ovary. *Specify behavior*	*7880*
788–870A	Fibroma of ovary	*7880*
788–8053	Granulosa cell tumor of ovary. *Specify behavior (page 99)*	*7880*
788–8013	Krukenberg tumor of ovary. *Specify behavior (page 99)*	*7880*
788–8884	Mesonephroma of ovary. *Specify behavior*	*7880*
788–8011	Pseudomucinous cystadenoma of ovary. *Specify behavior*	*7880*
788–8012	Pseudomucinous cystadenocarcinoma of ovary. *Specify behavior*	*7880*
788–8021F	Serous papillary cystadenocarcinoma of ovary	*7880*
788–8021B	Serous papillary cystadenoma of ovary	*7880*
788–882	Teratoma of ovary. *Specify behavior (page 99)*	*7880*
788–882.8	Teratoma of ovary, cystic. *Specify behavior*	*7880*
788–8052	Thecoma of ovary. *Specify behavior (page 99)*	*7880*
788–8▲▲▲	Unlisted tumor of ovary. *Specify neoplasm and behavior (page 99)*	*7880*

—9 DISEASES DUE TO UNKNOWN OR UNCERTAIN CAUSE WITH THE STRUCTURAL REACTION MANIFEST

788–923	Calcification of ovary	*7890*
788–952	Chronic interstitial oophoritis	*7890*
788–911	Cystic degeneration of ovary	*7890*
788–959	Endometriosis of ovary	*7890*
7883–9x8	Epoophoron cyst	*7890*
7884–9x8	Paroophoron cyst	*7890*

—X DISEASES DUE TO UNKNOWN OR UNCERTAIN CAUSE WITH THE FUNCTIONAL REACTION ALONE MANIFEST

788–x10	Hypofunction of ovary due to unknown cause	*7890*
	Sterility, ovarian, due to unknown cause. *See* Sterility, functional, due to decrease in estrogenic substance, *page 349*	

DISEASES OF THE PELVIC SUPPORTING STRUCTURES

789– Pelvic supporting structures
066– Pelvic peritoneum
047– Pelvic floor
074– Perineum
78x– Intrinsic vessels
142– Perineal skin and cellular tissue

—0 DISEASES DUE TO GENETIC AND PRENATAL INFLUENCES

074–017	Contracture of perineum, congenital	*0701*

—I DISEASES DUE TO INFECTION WITH LOWER ORGANISM

7892–100.2	Abscess of broad ligament. *Specify organism (page 57) when known*	*7810*
789–100.2	Abscess of pelvic cellular tissue. *Specify organism (page 57) when known*	*7810*
074–100.2	Abscess of perineum. *Specify organism (page 57) when known*	*0710*
066–100.4	Adhesions of pelvic peritoneum due to infection	*0611*
7892–100	Cellulitis of broad ligament. *Specify organism (page 57) when known as:*	*7810*
789–100	Cellulitis of pelvis. *Specify organism (page 57) when known*	*7810*
142–100	Cellulitis of perineum. *Specify organism (page 57) when known*	*1310*
074–100.3	Fistula of perineum due to infection	*0710*
559–198	Lymphopathia venereum of pelvis	*5510*

—4 DISEASES DUE TO TRAUMA OR PHYSICAL AGENT

066–415.4	Adhesions of pelvic peritoneum following operation	*0640*
074–415.3	Fistula of perineum following operation	*0740*
7892–435.7	Hematoma of broad ligament due to hemorrhage from adjacent structures	*7840*
066–4x9	Hernia of cul-de-sac of Douglas	*0645*
047–4123	Lacerations of pelvic floor (old), incomplete. *See also page 374*	*0442*
047–4122	Lacerations of pelvic floor (old), complete. *See also page 374*	*0442*
70x6–4x9	Posterior vaginal hernia (vaginal enterocele)	*7840*
668–4x9	Rectocele	*6642*

047–43x	Relaxation of pelvic floor due to cause other than parturition	*0442*
047–4x9	Relaxation of pelvic floor due to parturition	*0442*
074–410	Wound of perineum	*0741*

—50 DISEASES DUE TO CIRCULATORY DISTURBANCE

789–532	Pelvic hematocele	*7850*

—6 DISEASES DUE TO OR CONSISTING OF STATIC MECHANICAL ABNORMALITY

78x–641	Varix of broad ligament	*7860*

—7 DISEASES DUE TO DISORDER OF METABOLISM, GROWTH, OR NUTRITION

Intraligamentous pregnancy. *See page 380*

—8 NEW GROWTHS

7892–870A	Fibromyoma of broad ligament	*7880*
7892–866A	Leiomyoma of broad ligament	*7880*
784–866A	Leiomyoma of parametrium	*7880*
7891–866A	Leiomyoma of round ligament	*7880*
7893–866A	Leiomyoma of sacrouterine ligament	*7880*
789▲–8772A	Mesothelioma. *Specify site*	*7880*
789–8▲▲▲	Unlisted tumor of pelvic supporting structures. *Specify neoplasm and behavior (page 99)*	*7880*

—9 DISEASES DUE TO UNKNOWN OR UNCERTAIN CAUSE WITH THE STRUCTURAL REACTION MANIFEST

7892–959	Endometriosis of broad ligament	*7890*
7891–900.8	Hydrocele of round ligament	*7890*

OBSTETRIC CONDITIONS AND DISEASES

See also pages 349 to 372 for diseases occurring in the nonpregnant state. Any of them which occurs during pregnancy may be transferred to the present section with appropriate changes in the code, e.g., change 782 nonpregnant uterus to 7x2 pregnant uterus.

The record of every live birth demands two principal diagnoses on two separate cards, e.g., every case of terminated uterine pregnancy is recorded as 7x2–00▲▲ the time of termination and the multiplicity being indicated by the appropriate second and third digits to the right of the hyphen. Every living child is recorded as 790–0▲▲, the second and third digits to the right of the hyphen, similarly indicating time and multiplicity of birth (*See page* 378).

Stillbirths of any kind including immature delivery and abortions are of course recorded only on the mother's card.

The pregnancy is recorded on the mother's card and the living birth on the infant's card, a separate card with appropriate headings being used for each of the several pregnancy diagnoses and each type of birth diagnoses.

All codes beginning with 7x2 are for the mother's card; all codes beginning with 790 are for the infant's card.

7x0– Female genital organs during pregnancy, parturition, and
      puerperium
7x1– Vagina
7x2– Uterus
7x3– Cervix
7x4– Vulva
7x5– Endometrium
7x7– Fallopian tube
7x8– Ovary
7x9– Supporting structures
7xx– Pelvic floor
78x– Pelvic veins

—I DISEASES DUE TO INFECTION WITH LOWER ORGANISM

7x9–100.2	Abscess of pelvis during pregnancy. *Specify organism (page 57) when known*	5610
7x94–100	Cellulitis of pelvis during pregnancy. *Specify organism (page 57) when known*	5610
7x9–100	Cellulitis of pelvis during puerperium. *Specify organism (page 57) when known*	5610
7x3–100.4	Cicatrix of cervix during pregnancy due to infection	5610
7x52–100	Deciduitis, acute. *Specify organism (page 57) when known*	5610

7x51–100	Endometritis during pregnancy, acute. *Specify organism (page 57) when known*	5610
7x5–100	Puerperal endometritis, acute. *Specify organism (page 57) when known*	5610
7x21–100	Metritis during pregnancy, acute. *Specify organism (page 57) when known*	5610
7x2–100	Puerperal metritis, acute. *Specify organism (page 57) when known*	5610
78x–100.7	Thrombophlebitis of pelvis. *Specify organism (page 57) when known*	5610

—3 DISEASES DUE TO INTOXICATION

7x2–34637	Abnormal contraction of pregnant uterus due to ergot	5630
7x2–3824	Abnormal contraction of pregnant uterus due to pituitary extract	5630
7x2–33▲▲	Atony of pregnant uterus due to anesthetic. *Specify agent*	5630

—4 DISEASES DUE TO TRAUMA OR PHYSICAL AGENT

7x3–409	Annular detachment of cervix, obstetric	5640
7x3–415.4	Cicatrix of cervix following operation	5640
7x3–412.4	Cicatrix of cervix following parturition	5640
7x3–400.4	Cicatrix of cervix due to trauma	5640
7x3–430	Edema of cervix, obstetric, acute	5640
7x4–435	Edema of vulva, obstetric, acute	5640
7x4–4x7	Hematoma of vulva during pregnancy	5640
7x2–400	Injury of pregnant uterus. *Specify (page 83)*	5640
7x2–43x	Inversion of puerperal uterus due to traction	5640
7x2–400.9	Inversion of puerperal uterus due to trauma	5640
7x3–412	Laceration[1] of cervix, obstetric	5640
7x41–412	Laceration[1] of fourchet, obstetric	5640
7xx–400.5	Laceration[1] of pelvic floor, obstetric, involving sphincter ani (complete tear)	5640
7xx–412	Laceration[1] of pelvic floor, obstetric, not involving sphincter ani	5640
7x1–412	Laceration[1] of vagina, obstetric, not involving pelvic floor	5640
7x4–412	Laceration[1] of vulva, obstetric	5640
7x2–415	Penetration of pregnant uterus by instrument	5640

[1] If infected, add .0 to code as: 7x3–412.0 Infected laceration of cervix.

70x2–412.3	Rectovaginal fistula, obstetric	*5640*
7x2–416	Rupture of pregnant uterus	*5640*
7x2–416.4	Rupture of pregnant uterus due to uterine scar	*5640*
7x2–400.7	Uterine hemorrhage due to trauma	*5640*
7x2–412.7	Hemorrhage, uterine, due to lacerations	*5640*
77x–435.6	Varix of vulva due to pregnancy	*5640*
7031–412.3	Vesicovaginal fistula, obstetric	*5640*

—55 DISEASES DUE TO DISTURBANCE OF INNERVATION

7x3–561	Abnormal contraction of cervix, obstetric	*5655*
7x2–560.7	Postpartum hemorrhage due to uterine inertia	*5655*
7x2–561	Abnormal contraction of pregnant uterus	*5655*
7x21–561	Contraction or constriction ring	*5655*
7x2–560	Uterine inertia intrapartum	*5655*

—6 DISEASES DUE TO OR CONSISTING OF STATIC MECHANICAL ABNOR-MALITY

7x2–600.7	Hemorrhage, uterine, due to partial separation of placenta	*5660*
7x2–614.7	Hemorrhage, uterine, due to retained secundines	*5660*
7x2–639	Hernia of pregnant uterus	*5660*
7x2–638	Inversion of pregnant uterus due to unknown cause	*5660*
7x2–631	Prolapse of pregnant uterus	*5660*
7x2–636	Retrodisplacement of pregnant uterus	*5660*
7x2–643	Retroflexion of pregnant uterus	*5660*
7x2–63x	Retroversion of pregnant uterus	*5660*
7x3–646	Rigidity of cervix during labor; conglutination	*5660*
7xx–646	Rigidity of perineum during labor	*5660*
7x2–610.5	Rupture of uterus due to obstructed labor	*5660*
7x2–6x6	Sacculation of pregnant uterus	*5660*
7x2–6x4	Abnormal contraction of uterus due to obstructed labor	*5660*
7x2–637	Torsion of pregnant uterus	*5660*

—7 DISEASES DUE TO DISORDER OF METABOLISM, GROWTH, OR NUTRITION

7x2–796	Hyperinvolution of uterus	*5670*
7x2–7x9	Puerperal lactation atrophy of uterus	*5670*
7x2–795	Subinvolution of uterus	*5670*

—8 NEW GROWTHS

7x2–8▲▲▲   Tumor of pregnant uterus. *Specify neo-*
plasm and behavior (page 99). See
also under Uterus and Placenta   5680

**—X DISEASES DUE TO UNKNOWN OR UNCERTAIN CAUSE WITH THE
STRUCTURAL REACTION MANIFEST**

7x2–x90   Atony of uterus due to unknown cause   5690

**—Y DISEASES DUE TO CAUSE NOT DETERMINABLE IN THE PARTICULAR
CASE**

Y signifies an incomplete diagnosis. It is to be replaced whenever possible
by a code digit signifying the specific diagnosis

7x2–yx7   Hemorrhage, uterine, due to undetermined cause   0067

PREGNANCY AND LABOR
FETUS AND BIRTH

In this section etiologic digits beginning 0 are used arbitrarily.

7x2–   Uterus (in pregnancy)
7x7–   Fallopian tube (in pregnancy)
060–   Peritoneum; peritoneal cavity
789–   Pelvic supporting structures
794–   Placenta
799–   Umbilical cord

SINGLE FETATION

7x2–000	Pregnancy delivered. *To be diagnosed in all cases of uterine pregnancy in which patient is admitted to hospital as having such, provided live birth occurs.*	5710
7x2–001	Pregnancy delivered, antepartum death	5710
7x2–002	Pregnancy delivered, intrapartum death	5710
7x2–004	Pregnancy delivered, prematurely [1]	5713
7x2–0041	Pregnancy delivered, prematurely, threatened [1]	5713
7x2–005	Pregnancy delivered, prematurely, antepartum death [1]	5713
7x2–006	Pregnancy delivered, prematurely, intrapartum death [1]	5713
7x2–007	Pregnancy delivered, immaturely, living child [2]	5715
7x2–008	Pregnancy delivered, immaturely, ante- or intrapartum death [2]	5715
7x2–0085	Accidental following operation	5715
7x2–0082	Complete	5715
7x2–0083	Incomplete	5715
7x2–0081	Inevitable	5715
7x2–0084	Missed	5715
7x2–0086	Threatened	5715
7x2–00x	Pregnancy delivered, postmaturely	5716
7x2–00x1	Pregnancy delivered, postmaturely, antepartum death	5716
7x2–00x2	Pregnancy delivered, postmaturely, intrapartum death	5716

---

[1] Premature delivery is to be diagnosed if the following criteria are present:
(1) The size of the infant is between 1,000 and 2,499 grams
(2) The length of the infant is from 35 to 47 centimeters
[2] Immature delivery is to be diagnosed if the following criteria are present:
(1) The size of the infant is between 500 and 999 grams
(2) The length of the infant is from 28 to 35 centimeters

7x2–009	Abortion [1]	*5720*
7x2–0095	Accidental following operation	*5720*
7x2–0092	Complete	*5720*
7x2–0093	Incomplete	*5720*
7x2–0091	Inevitable	*5720*
7x2–0094	Missed	*5720*
7x2–0096	Threatened	*5720*

MULTIPLE FETATION

7x2–050	Pregnancy delivered, twins	*5712*
7x2–0501	Pregnancy delivered, single ovum twins	*5712*
7x2–0502	Pregnancy delivered, double ovum twins	*5712*
7x2–051	Pregnancy delivered, twins, antepartum death	*5712*
7x2–0511	Pregnancy delivered, twins, antepartum death, single ovum	*5712*
7x2–0512	Pregnancy delivered, twins, antepartum death, double ovum	*5712*
7x2–052	Pregnancy delivered, twins, intrapartum death	*5712*
7x2–0521	Pregnancy delivered, twins, intrapartum death, single ovum	*5712*
7x2–0522	Pregnancy delivered, twins, intrapartum death, double ovum	*5712*
7x2–053	Pregnancy delivered, twins, one living child	*5712*
7x2–0531	Pregnancy delivered, twins, one living child, single ovum	*5712*
7x2–0532	Pregnancy delivered, twins, one living child, double ovum	*5712*
7x2–054	Pregnancy delivered, twins, prematurely [2]	*5714*
7x2–0541	Pregnancy delivered, twins, prematurely, single ovum [2]	*5714*
7x2–0542	Pregnancy delivered, twins, prematurely, double ovum [2]	*5714*
7x2–0543	Pregnancy delivered, twins, prematurely, antepartum or intrapartum death [2]	*5714*
7x2–0544	Pregnancy delivered, twins, prematurely, antepartum or intrapartum death, single ovum [2]	*5714*

[1] Abortion is presumed to have occurred if the following criteria are present:
(1) The fetal size is less than 500 grams
(2) The fetal length is less than 28 centimeters
[2] Premature delivery is to be diagnosed if the following criteria are present:
(1) The size of the infant is between 1,000 and 2,499 **grams**
(2) The length of the infant is from 35 to 47 centimeters

7x2–0545	Pregnancy delivered, twins, prematurely, antepartum or intrapartum death,[1] double ovum	*5714*
7x2–0546	Pregnancy delivered, twins prematurely, one living child [1]	*5714*
7x2–0547	Pregnancy delivered, twins, prematurely, one living child, single ovum [1]	*5714*
7x2–0548	Pregnancy delivered, twins, prematurely, one living child, double ovum [1]	*5714*
7x2–055	Pregnancy delivered, triplets	*5712*
7x2–0551	Pregnancy delivered, triplets, prematurely	*5714*
7x2–056	Pregnancy delivered, triplets, ante or intrapartum death	*5712*
7x2–0561	Pregnancy delivered, triplets, ante or intrapartum death, prematurely [1]	*5714*
7x2–057	Pregnancy delivered, triplets one (or two) living child	*5712*
7x2–0571	Pregnancy delivered, triplets one (or two) living child, prematurely [1]	*5714*
7x2–058	Pregnancy delivered, multiple birth	*5712*
7x2–0581	Pregnancy delivered, multiple birth, prematurely [1]	*5714*
7x2–059	Pregnancy delivered, multiple birth, ante or intrapartum death	*5712*
7x2–0591	Pregnancy delivered, multiple birth, ante or intrapartum death, prematurely [1]	*5714*
7x2–05x	Pregnancy delivered, multiple birth, one (or more) living child	*5712*
7x2–05x1	Pregnancy delivered, multiple birth, one (or more) living child, prematurely [1]	*5714*

[1] Premature delivery is to be diagnosed if the following criteria are present:
  (1) The size of the infant is between 1,000 and 2,499 grams
  (2) The length of the infant is from 35 to 47 centimeters
Abortuses: fetuses at birth weighing less than 500 grams (17 oz). No chance of survival.
Immature infants: fetuses at birth weighing 500 to 999 grams (17 oz–2 lb). Chances of survival range from poor to good depending on weight.
Premature infants: babies at birth weighing from 1,000 to 2,499 grams (2–5½ lb). Chances of survival range from poor to good depending on weight.
Mature infants: babies of 2,500 grams (5½ lb or more). Chances of survival optimal.
Twin birth is defined as immature, premature, or term by weight of heaviest infant.

ABNORMAL PREGNANCIES AND CONDITIONS

7x2–789	Pregnancy not delivered. *To be diagnosed when condition is incidental and not cause of admission to hospital or when patient is admitted to the hospital and the diagnosis of pregnancy is made.*	5602
7x2–7891	False labor	5700
7x2–7892	Missed labor	5700
060–789	Abdominal pregnancy	5702
060–789.5	Abdominal pregnancy, ruptured	5702
7x2–147.9	Abortion, habitual, due to syphilis	5720
7x2–y00.9	Abortion, due to undetermined cause	5720
7x3–789	Cervical pregnancy	5702
7x21–789	Cornual pregnancy	5702
7x2–9x9	Fetus papyraceous	5690
7892–789	Intraligamentous pregnancy	5702
7x2–911	Lithopedion	5690
7x8–789	Ovarian pregnancy	5702
7x22–789	Pregnancy in rudimentary horn	5702
7x7–789	Tubal pregnancy	5702
7x7–789.6	Tubal pregnancy with abortion	5702
7x7–789.5	Tubal pregnancy with rupture	5702

INFANTS (live births)

790–007	Immature birth [1]	5732
790–004	Premature birth [2]	5732
790–00x	Postmature birth	5733
790–000	Term birth	5730
790–050	Twin birth	5734
790–0501	Twin birth, single ovum	5734
790–0502	Twin birth, double ovum	5734
790–054	Twin birth, premature [2]	5734
790–0541	Twin birth, premature, single ovum [2]	5734
790–0542	Twin birth, premature, double ovum [2]	5734
790–005	Triplets	5734
790–0551	Triplets, premature	5734
790–058	Multiple births	5734
790–0581	Multiple births, premature	5734

[1] Immature delivery is to be diagnosed if the following criteria are present:
(1) The size of the infant is between 500 and 999 grams
(2) The length of the infant is from 28 to 35 centimeters
[2] Premature delivery is to be diagnosed if the following criteria are present:
(1) The size of the infant is between 1,000 and 2,499 grams
(2) The length of the infant is from 35 to 47 centimeters

CONDITIONS OF INFANT

790–514	Asphyxia due to interference with fetal circulation	*5760*
790–430	Caput succedaneum	*5760*
790–421	Fetal asphyxia due to trauma	*5760*
7991–019	Patent vitelline duct (omphalomesenteric duct)	*5760*
790–165	Rubella, congenital	*5760*
790–1577	Toxoplasmosis infection, congenital	*5760*

PRESENTATION

790–650	Cephalopelvic disproportion	*5770*
790–660	Vertex	*5770*
790–661	Left occipitoanterior (L.O.A.)	*5770*
790–662	Right occipitoanterior (R.O.A.)	*5770*
790–663	Left occipitoposterior (L.O.P.)	*5770*
790–664	Right occipitoposterior (R.O.P.)	*5770*
790–665	Left occipitotransverse (L.O.T.)	*5770*
790–666	Right occipitotransverse (R.O.T.)	*5770*
790–670	Breech	*5770*
790–676	Double footling	*5770*
790–675	Footling	*5770*
790–671	Left sacroanterior (L.S.A.)	*5770*
790–673	Left sacroposterior (L.S.P.)	*5770*
790–672	Right sacroanterior (R.S.A.)	*5770*
790–674	Right sacroposterior (R.S.P.)	*5770*
790–677	Frank (or single)	*5770*
790–678	Complete (or double)	*5770*
790–679	Incomplete	*5770*
790–690	Brow	*5770*
790–691	Left frontoanterior (L.F.A.)	*5770*
790–692	Right frontoanterior (R.F.A.)	*5770*
790–693	Left frontoposterior (L.F.P.)	*5770*
790–694	Right frontoposterior (R.F.P.)	*5770*
790–680	Face	*5770*
790–681	Left mentoanterior (L.M.A.)	*5770*
790–682	Right mentoanterior (R.M.A.)	*5770*
790–683	Left mentoposterior (L.M.P.)	*5770*
790–684	Right mentoposterior (R.M.P.)	*5770*
790–695	Shoulder position	*5770*
790–696	Left scapuloanterior (L.Sc.A.)	*5770*
790–697	Right scapuloanterior (R.Sc.A)	*5770*
790–698	Left scapuloposterior (L.Sc.P.)	*5770*
790–699	Right scapuloposterior (R.Sc.P.)	*5770*
790–699	Compound (position unspecified)	*5770*
790–6y0	Undetermined	*5770*

PLACENTA

794– Placenta
795– Amnion; membranes generally
796– Chorion
797– Chorionic villi
798– Syncytium
79x– Placental vessels

—I DISEASES DUE TO INFECTION WITH LOWER ORGANISM

795–100   Acute inflammation of membranes   *7910*
794–100   Placentitis. *Specify organism (page 57)*
                  when known   *7910*

—4 DISEASES DUE TO TRAUMA OR PHYSICAL AGENT

794–4x5   Premature separation of placenta (abruptio
                  placentae)   *7940*

—50 DISEASES DUE TO CIRCULATORY DISTURBANCE

794–5x7   Hematoma of placenta   *7955*
794–511   Infarction of placenta   *7955*

—6 DISEASES DUE TO OR CONSISTING OF STATIC MECHANICAL ABNORMALITY

794–6x4   Adherent placenta   *7960*
794–631   Placenta previa   *7960*
794–6311   Total placenta previa   *7960*
794–6312   Partial placenta previa   *7960*
794–6313   Low insertion of placenta   *7960*
795–600.5   Premature rupture of membranes   *7960*
7x52–614   Retention of decidual fragment   *7960*
795–614   Retention of membranes   *7960*
794–614   Retention of placenta   *7960*
7941–614   Retention of placenta and membranes   *7960*
7942–614   Retention of placental fragment   *7960*
7951–614   Retention of portion of membranes   *7960*
79x–631   Vasa previa   *7960*

—7 DISEASES DUE TO DISORDER OF METABOLISM, GROWTH, OR NUTRITION

795–794   Amniotic adhesions of fetus   *7970*
794–794   Placenta duplex   *7970*
794–7941   Placenta tripartita   *7970*
794–7942   Placenta multipartita   *7970*
794–7943   Placenta fenestrata   *7970*

794–7944	Placenta circumvallata	*7970*
794–7945	Placenta membranacea	*7970*
794–791	Placenta spuria	*7970*
794–7911	Placenta succenturiata	*7970*

—8 NEW GROWTHS

796–880E	Chorioadenoma	*7980*
796–880F	Choriocarcinoma (chorioepithelioma)	*7980*
797–880B	Hydatidiform mole	*7980*
79▲–8▲▲▲	Unlisted tumor of placenta. *Specify site, neoplasm, and behavior (page 99)*	*7980*

—9 DISEASES DUE TO UNKNOWN OR UNCERTAIN CAUSE WITH THE STRUCTURAL REACTION MANIFEST

795–900.8	Amniotic cyst	*7990*
794–900.8	Cyst of placenta	*7990*
794–940	Fibrosis of placenta	*7990*
794–9x4	Placenta accreta	*7990*
794–900.5	Premature separation of placenta due to unknown cause (abruptio placentae)	*7990*

—X DISEASES DUE TO UNKNOWN OR UNCERTAIN CAUSES WITH THE FUNCTIONAL REACTION ALONE MANIFEST

795–x30	Hydrorrhea gravidarum	*7990*
795–x10	Oligohydramnios	*7990*
795–x20	Polyhydramnios	*7990*

UMBILICAL CORD

799–638	Cord around neck	*5752*
799–792	Excessively long cord	*5752*
799–790	Excessively short cord	*5752*
799–400.7	Hemorrhage from cord	*5752*
799–639	Hernia into cord	*5752*
799–100	Inflammation of cord, acute	*5752*
799–6301	Lateral insertion of cord; battledore placenta	*5752*
799–190	Phlebitis of umbilical vein	*5752*
799–631	Prolapse of cord	*5752*
799–6311	Cord presentation	*5752*
799–416	Rupture of cord due to trauma	*5752*
799–794	Skin navel	*5752*
799–422	Strangulation of cord	*5752*
799–643	True knots in cord	*5752*
799–630	Velamentous insertion of cord	*5752*

22x–	Bony pelvis
246–	Symphysis pubis

See also under Joints, *page 156*

—0 DISEASES DUE TO GENETIC AND PRENATAL INFLUENCES

22x–021	Assimilation pelvis	*5741*

—I DISEASES DUE TO INFECTION WITH LOWER ORGANISM

22x–123.4	Deformity of pelvis due to tuberculosis; tuberculous funnel pelvis; kyphotic pelvis; scoliotic pelvis	*5741*

—4 DISEASES DUE TO TRAUMA OR PHYSICAL AGENT

22x–435	Deformity of pelvis due to congenital dislocation of hip. Use as secondary diagnosis only	*5741*
22x–436	Deformity of pelvis due to fracture	*5741*
22x–43x	Deformity of pelvis due to unequal strain: coxalgic pelvis, Nagele's pelvis (obliquely contracted pelvis)	*5741*
246–408	Separation of symphysis pubis	*5741*
22x–434	Spondylolisthetic pelvis	*5741*

—55 DISEASES DUE TO DISTURBANCE OF INNERVATION

22x–564	Scoliotic pelvis following poliomyelitis	*5741*

—6 DISEASES DUE TO OR CONSISTING OF STATIC MECHANICAL ABNOR-MALITY

22x–651	Flat pelvis due to unknown or unspecified cause (platypelloid pelvis)	5741
22x–6510	Simple flat pelvis	5741
22x–6511	Generally contracted flat pelvis	5741
22x–646	Funnel pelvis due to unspecified cause	5741
22x–640	Generally contracted pelvis due to unknown or unspecified cause	5741
22x–6408	Due to asymmetrical contraction	5741
22x–6401	Due to contracted inlet	5741
22x–6402	Due to contracted midplane	5741
22x–6403	Due to contracted outlet	5741
22x–6409	Due to inlet and midplane contraction	5741
22x–6404	Due to inlet and outlet contraction	5741
22x–6407	Due to inlet, outlet, and midplane con-traction	5741
22x–6405	Due to midplane contraction	5741
22x–6406	Due to midplane and outlet contraction	5741
22x–650	Infantile pelvis (generally contracted) due to unknown cause	5741
22x–657	Obliquely contracted pelvis due to unspeci-fied cause	5741
22x–652	Transversely contracted pelvis due to un-specified cause (anthropoid pelvis)	5741

—7 DISEASES DUE TO DISORDER OF METABOLISM, GROWTH, OR NUTRITION

22x–771	Cretin pelvis, dwarf type	5741
22x–787	Masculine pelvis (generally contracted) (android pelvis)	5741
22x–764	Rachitic pelvis, dwarf type, flat type, scoliotic type	5741
	Osteomalacic pelvis	5741

—9 DISEASES DUE TO UNKNOWN OR UNCERTAIN CAUSE WITH THE STRUCTURAL REACTION MANIFEST

22x–940	Robert's pelvis	5741

8- DISEASES OF THE ENDOCRINE SYSTEM

800– Endocrine glands, generally

—9 DISEASES DUE TO UNKNOWN OR UNCERTAIN CAUSE WITH THE STRUCTURAL REACTION MANIFEST

800–953   Pluriglandular atrophy or sclerosis   *8090*

DISEASES OF THE THYROID GLAND

810– Thyroid gland

For detailed list of structures of thyroid gland, see page 40

—0 DISEASES DUE TO GENETIC AND PRENATAL INFLUENCES

810–016	Absence or congenital defect of thyroid gland (athyrotic cretinism)	*8102*
810–031	Accessory thyroid gland	*8101*
810–1471	Congenital syphilis of thyroid gland	*8101*
810–070	Enzymatic defect of hormone synthesis (familial, goitrous cretinism)	*8102*
810–093	Goiter, congenital	*8101*
815–019	Thyroglossal duct, persistent	*8101*
815–064	Thyroglossal cyst	*8101*
815–064.0	Thyroglossal cyst, infected	*8101*

—I DISEASES DUE TO INFECTION WITH LOWER ORGANISM

810–100.2	Abscess of thyroid gland. *Specify organism (page 57) when known*	*8110*
810–100	Suppurative thyroiditis. *Specify organism (page 57) when known*	*8110*
810–190	Thyroiditis. *Specify organism (page 57) when known*	*8110*

—3 DISEASES DUE TO INTOXICATION

810–300	Hyperthyroidism (factitious) due to chronic ingestion of thyroid hormone	*8130*
810–38214	Hypothyroidism due to action of goitrogens thiouracil, etc.)	*8130*

—4 DISEASES DUE TO TRAUMA OR PHYSICAL AGENT

810–4▲▲	Injury of thyroid gland. *Specify (page 83)*	*8140*
810–415	Due to operation	*8140*
810–415.6	Athyrea following operation	*8140*
810–471	Roentgen ray (x-ray) injury of thyroid gland	*8140*
810–471.6	With hypothyroidism	*8140*

—6 DISEASES DUE TO OR CONSISTING OF STATIC MECHANICAL ABNORMALITY

814–600.8	Cyst of lateral aberrant thyroid	*8160*
810–600.8	Cyst of thyroid gland	*8160*

Record primary diagnosis when possible

810–739	Goiter, juvenile or adolescent, due to iodine deficiency	8170
810–771	Hyperthyroidism without evident goiter. If goiter is present, use appropriate diagnosis. *See following*	8177
810–776	Hyperthyroidism secondary to hyperpituitarism	8177
	Hypothyroidism, congenital (cretinism). *See page 388*	
	Athyrotic	
	Enzymatic	
810–7721	Hypothyroidism, juvenile, due to unknown cause	8178
810–7722	Hypothyroidism, adult, due to unknown cause	8178
810–777	Hypothyroidism secondary to hypopituitarism	8178

—8 NEW GROWTHS

810–8091	Adenocarcinoma of thyroid gland. *Specify behavior*	8180
810–8091A	Adenoma of thyroid gland	8180
810–870F	Fibrosarcoma of thyroid gland	8180
810–8047A	Functionally hyperactive adenoma of thyroid gland	8180
810–8047F	Functionally active adenocarcinoma of thyroid gland	8180
810–8066	Giant cell carcinoma of thyroid gland. *Specify behavior (page 99)*	8180
810–8065A	Hürthle cell adenoma of thyroid gland	8180
810–8065F	Hürthle cell carcinoma of thyroid gland	8180
810–830	Lymphosarcoma of thyroid gland. *Specify behavior*	8180
810–8▲▲▲	Unlisted tumor of thyroid gland. *Specify neoplasm and behavior (page 99)*	

—9 DISEASES DUE TO UNKNOWN OR UNCERTAIN CAUSE WITH THE STRUCTURAL REACTION MANIFEST

810–911	Atrophy of thyroid gland with myxedema	8190
810–942	Chronic thyroiditis	8190
810–941	Chronic thyroiditis, granulomatous	8190
810–942.1	Chronic thyroiditis, lymphomatous	8190
810–943	Nontoxic diffuse goiter [1]	8194

[1] To indicate the substernal extension of any goiter, add the digit 1 at the end of the topographic code.

810–952	Nontoxic nodular goiter [1]	*8194*
810–943.6	Toxic diffuse goiter;[1] diffuse goiter with hyperthyroidism	*8194*
810–952.6	Toxic nodular goiter;[1] nodular goiter with hyperthyroidism	*8194*

[1] To indicate the substernal extension of any goiter, add the digit 1 at the end of the topographic code.

DISEASES OF THE PARATHYROID GLANDS

820– Parathyroid glands

—4 DISEASES DUE TO TRAUMA OR PHYSICAL AGENT

820–4▲▲	Injury of parathyroid gland. *Specify* (*page 83*)	8240
820–415	Due to operation	8240
820–415.x	With hypoparathyroidism	8240
820–47▲.x	Radiation injury of parathyroid gland with hypoparathyroidism. *Specify*	8240

—50 DISEASES DUE TO CIRCULATORY DISTURBANCE

820–5x7	Spontaneous hemorrhage into parathyroid gland	8250

—7 DISEASES DUE TO DISORDER OF METABOLISM, GROWTH, OR NUTRITION

820–773	Parathyroid hyperplasia, secondary	8200

—8 NEW GROWTHS

820–8091	Adenocarcinoma of parathyroid gland. *Specify behavior* (*page 99*)	8280
820–8091A	Adenoma of parathyroid gland	8280
820–8046A	Functionally hyperactive adenoma of parathyroid gland	8280
820–8046F	Functionally hyperactive adenocarcinoma of parathyroid gland	8280
820–8▲▲▲	Unlisted tumor of parathyroid gland. *Specify neoplasm and behavior*	8280

—9 DISEASES DUE TO UNKNOWN OR UNCERTAIN CAUSE WITH THE STRUCTURAL REACTION MANIFEST

820–943	Parathyroid hyperplasia	8290
820–943.6	With hyperparathyroidism. *See also* Osteitis fibrosa cystica (*page 153*)	8290
820–940	Parathyroid hyperplasia, adenomatous	8290

—X DISEASES DUE TO UNKNOWN OR UNCERTAIN CAUSE WITH THE FUNCTIONAL REACTION ALONE MANIFEST

820–x10	Pseudohypoparathyroidism	8290

DISEASES OF THE THYMUS

830–   Thymus

—0 DISEASES DUE TO GENETIC AND PRENATAL INFLUENCES

830–064	Cyst of thymus, congenital	*8301*
830–013	Hypertrophy of thymus, congenital	*8301*

—I DISEASES DUE TO INFECTION WITH LOWER ORGANISM

830–100.2	Abscess of thymus. *Specify organism (page 57) when known*	*8310*
830–100	Inflammation of thymus. *Specify organism (page 57) when known*	*8310*

—4 DISEASES DUE TO TRAUMA OR PHYSICAL AGENT

830–4x7	Hemorrhage into thymus due to trauma	*8340*

—7 DISEASES DUE TO DISORDER OF METABOLISM, GROWTH, OR NUTRITION

830–795	Failure of involution of thymus	*8370*

—8 NEW GROWTHS

830–8841A	Thymoma, benign	*8380*
830–8841F	Thymoma, malignant [1]	*8380*
830–8▲▲▲	Unlisted tumor of thymus. *Specify neoplasm and behavior*	*8380*

—9 DISEASES DUE TO UNKNOWN OR UNCERTAIN CAUSE WITH THE STRUCTURAL REACTION MANIFEST

830–921	Fatty atrophy of thymus	*8390*
830–943	Hyperplasia of thymus	*8390*

[1] If myasthenia gravis is present, change malignancy code F to G and record additional diagnosis.

DISEASES OF THE PITUITARY GLAND

840– Pituitary gland
841– Anterior lobe
842– Posterior lobe
845– Craniobuccal (Rathke's) pouch

For detailed list of structures of pituitary gland, see page 41

—0 DISEASES DUE TO GENETIC AND PRENATAL INFLUENCES

844–064	Cyst, vestigial, pituitary stalk	*8401*

—I DISEASES DUE TO INFECTION WITH LOWER ORGANISM

840–100.2	Abscess of pituitary gland. *Specify organism (page 57) when known*	*8410*
840–100.9	Degeneration of pituitary gland due to infection. *Specify organism (page 57) when known. Specify lobe if localized*	*8410*

—4 DISEASES DUE TO TRAUMA OR PHYSICAL AGENT

840–400.9	Degeneration of pituitary gland due to trauma. *Specify lobe if localized*	*8440*
840–436	Due to pressure of fractured bone. *Specify lobe if localized*	*8440*
840–4▲▲	Injury of pituitary gland. *Specify (page 83)*	*8440*

—50 DISEASES DUE TO CIRCULATORY DISTURBANCE
Record primary diagnosis when possible

840–512.9	Degeneration of pituitary gland due to embolism. *Specify lobe if localized*	*8450*
841–530	Hypopituitarism due to postpartum hemorrhage. *Record primary diagnosis*	*8450*
840–512	Infarction of pituitary gland due to embolism	*8450*

—6 DISEASES DUE TO OR CONSISTING OF STATIC MECHANICAL ABNORMALITY

845–600.8	Cyst of craniobuccal (Rathke's) pouch, nonneoplastic	*8460*
840–615	Pituitary calculus	*8460*

—7 DISEASES DUE TO DISORDER OF METABOLISM, GROWTH, OR NUTRITION

841–776	Anterior pituitary hyperfunction	*8470*
841–7761	Hypophysial gigantism	*8470*

841–7762	Acromegaly	*8470*
841–7763	Pituitary basophilism. *See also* Basophilic adenoma *following*	*8470*
841–7764	Premature puberty	*8470*
841–7765	Acromegalic gigantism	*8470*
841–777	Anterior pituitary hypofunction	*8470*
841–7771	Pituitary dwarfism	*8470*
841–7772	Juvenile hypopituitarism	*8470*
841–7773	Hypopituitary cachexia	*8470*
841–7774	Sex infantilism	*8470*
841–7775	Sex infantilism with obesity (adiposo-genital dystrophy)	*8470*
841–7776	Dwarfism and infantilism	*8470*
842–779	Diabetes insipidus due to unknown cause	*8470*

—8 NEW GROWTHS

841–8091	Adenocarcinoma of pituitary gland. *Specify behavior (page 99)*	*8480*
841–8091A	Adenoma of pituitary gland	*8480*
841–8055A	Basophilic adenoma of pituitary gland	*8480*
841–8067A	Chromophobe adenoma of pituitary gland	*8480*
841–8067	Chromophobe carcinoma of pituitary gland. *Specify behavior*	*8480*
841–8887	Craniopharyngioma of pituitary gland. *Specify behavior (page 99)*	*8480*
841–8045A	Eosinophilic adenoma of pituitary gland	*8480*
841–8▲▲▲	Unlisted tumor of pituitary gland. *Specify neoplasm and behavior (page 99)*	

—9 DISEASES DUE TO UNKNOWN OR UNCERTAIN CAUSE WITH THE STRUCTURAL REACTION MANIFEST

| 840–900.9 | Degeneration of pituitary gland due to unknown cause. *Specify lobe if localized* | *8490* |

—X DISEASES DUE TO UNKNOWN OR UNCERTAIN CAUSE WITH THE FUNCTIONAL REACTION ALONE MANIFEST

| 840–x10 | Obesity with pituitary disturbance | *8490* |

DISEASES OF THE PINEAL GLAND

850– Pineal gland

—4 DISEASES DUE TO TRAUMA OR PHYSICAL AGENT

850–4▲▲   Injury of pineal gland. *Specify (page
                   83)*   *8540*

—7 DISEASES DUE TO DISORDER OF METABOLISM, GROWTH, OR NUTRITION

850–780   Premature puberty due to pineal tumor.
                   Record primary diagnosis   *8570*

—8 NEW GROWTHS

850–8475   Glioma of pineal gland. *Specify behavior*   *8580*
850–8982   Pinealoma of pineal gland. *Specify
                   behavior*   *8580*
850–882   Teratoma of pineal gland. *Specify be-
                   havior (page 99)*   *8580*
850–8▲▲▲   Unlisted tumor of pineal gland. *Specify
                   neoplasm and behavior*   *8580*

**—9 DISEASES DUE TO UNKNOWN OR UNCERTAIN CAUSE WITH THE
STRUCTURAL REACTION MANIFEST**

850–923   Calcification of pineal gland due to un-
                   known cause   *8590*

DISEASES OF THE ADRENAL GLANDS

860– Adrenal glands
861– Cortex
862– Medulla
86x– Intrinsic vessels

—0 DISEASES DUE TO GENETIC AND PRENATAL INFLUENCES

860–012	Absence of adrenal gland	8601
860–031	Accessory adrenal gland	8601
860–050	Birth injury of adrenal gland	8601
860–064	Cyst of adrenal gland, congenital	8601
860–021	Displacement of adrenal gland	8601
860–014	Hyperplasia of adrenal gland, congenital	8601
860–013	Hypertrophy of adrenal gland, congenital	8601
860–016	Hypoplasia of adrenal gland, congenital	8601
860–0161	Virilizing with female pseudohermaphroditism	8601
860–0162	Virilizing with male macrogenitosomia precox	8601

—I DISEASES DUE TO INFECTION WITH LOWER ORGANISM

860–100	Acute adrenalitis. *Specify organism (page 57) when known*	8610
860–100.0	Chronic adrenalitis	8610
860–100.9	Degeneration of adrenal gland due to infection. *Specify organism (page 57) when known*	8610
860–100.7	Hemorrhage into adrenal gland due to infection. *Specify organism (page 57) when known*	8610
860–147.x	Syphilis of adrenal gland with cortical hypofunction	8610
860–123	Tuberculosis of adrenal gland	8610
860–123.x	Tuberculosis of adrenal gland with cortical hypofunction	8610

—4 DISEASES DUE TO TRAUMA OR PHYSICAL AGENT

860–4x7	Hemorrhage into adrenal gland due to trauma	8640
860–4▲▲	Injury of adrenal gland. *Specify (page 83)*	8640

—50 DISEASES DUE TO CIRCULATORY DISTURBANCE
Record primary diagnosis when possible

860–505.7	Hemorrhage into adrenal gland due to asphyxia	*8650*
860–540.7	Hemorrhage into adrenal gland due to blood dyscrasia	*8650*
860–500.1	Necrosis of adrenal gland	*8650*

—7 DISEASES DUE TO DISORDER OF METABOLISM, GROWTH, OR NUTRITION
Record primary diagnosis when possible

861–781	Adrenal cortical hyperfunction	*8678*
861–7814	With aldosteronism	*8678*
861–7813	With Cushing's syndrome	*8678*
861–7822	With hypoalderstonism	*8678*
861–7811	With premature puberty	*8678*
861–7812	With virilism	*8678*
861–782	Adrenal cortical hypofunction	*8679*
861–788	Secondary to excessive administration of hormones	*8679*
861–7821	Secondary to hypopituitarism	*8679*

—8 NEW GROWTHS

860–8091	Adenocarcinoma of adrenal gland. *Specify behavior (page 99)*	*8680*
860–8091.x	With Cushing's syndrome	*8680*
860–8091A	Adenoma of adrenal gland	*8680*
860–8091A.x	With Cushing's syndrome	*8680*
860–8051F	Feminizing adenocarcinoma of adrenal gland	*8680*
860–8051A	Feminizing adenoma of adrenal gland	*8680*
862–840A	Ganglioneuroma of medulla. *Specify behavior (page 99)*	*8680*
862–8431	Pheochromocytoma of medulla. *Specify behavior (page 99)*	*8680*
862–841F	Sympathicoblastoma of medulla	*8680*
860–8041F	Virilizing adenocarcinoma of adrenal gland	*8680*
860–8041A	Virilizing adenoma of adrenal gland	*8680*
860–8▲▲▲	Unlisted tumor of adrenal gland. *Specify neoplasm and behavior (page 99)*	*8680*

—9 DISEASES DUE TO UNKNOWN OR UNCERTAIN CAUSE WITH THE STRUCTURAL REACTION MANIFEST

861–911	Atrophy of adrenal cortex due to unknown cause	*8690*

DISEASES OF THE INSULAR TISSUE

See also Diseases of the pancreas, *page 295*

870– Insular tissue

—7 DISEASES DUE TO DISORDER OF METABOLISM, GROWTH, OR NUTRITION
Record primary diagnosis when possible

870–771	Diabetes mellitus with hyperthyroidism	*8778*
870–772	Diabetes mellitus with hypothyroidism	*8778*
870–776	Diabetes mellitus with hyperpituitarism	*8778*
870–777	Diabetes mellitus with hypopituitarism	*8778*
870–781	Diabetes mellitus with hyperadrenocorticism	*8778*
870–782	Diabetes mellitus with hypoadrenocorticism	*8778*
870–770	Diabetes mellitus with hyperfunction of chromaffin tissue	*8778*
870–785	Diabetes mellitus	*8778*
870–784	Hyperinsulinism, without tumor	*8770*

—8 NEW GROWTHS

870–8091	Adenocarcinoma of insular tissue. *Specify behavior (page 99)*	*8780*
870–8091A	Adenoma of insular tissue	*8780*
870–8044F	Functioning islet cell adenocarcinoma of insular tissue	*8780*
870–8044A	Functioning islet cell adenoma of insular tissue	*8780*
870–8074F	Nonfunctioning islet cell adenocarcinoma of insular tissue	*8780*
870–8074A	Nonfunctioning islet cell adenoma of insular tissue	*8780*
870–8▲▲▲	Unlisted tumor of insular tissue. *Specify neoplasm and behavior (page 99)*	*8780*

—9 DISEASES DUE TO UNKNOWN OR UNCERTAIN CAUSE WITH THE STRUCTURAL REACTION MANIFEST

870–953	Sclerosis of insular tissue due to unknown cause	*8790*
870–953.6	With diabetes mellitus	*8778*

—X DISEASES DUE TO UNKNOWN OR UNCERTAIN CAUSE WITH THE FUNCTIONAL REACTION ALONE MANIFEST

870–x10	Diabetes mellitus without known cause or structural change	*8778*

DISEASES OF GONADS

880– Gonads generally

DISEASES OF THE CAROTID GLAND

890– Carotid gland

—8 NEW GROWTHS

890–8981A	Carotid body tumor benign	*8980*
890–8981	Carotid body tumor malignant. *Specify behavior (page 99)*	*8980*
890–8▲▲▲	Unlisted tumor of carotid gland. *Specify neoplasm and behavior (page 99)*	*8980*

9– DISEASES OF THE NERVOUS SYSTEM

INTRODUCTION

The method of classifying diseases described in the general Introduction is applicable to diseases of the nervous system. Under System 9 of the Topographic Classification (page 41) will be found the arrangement of the structures which may be regarded as sites of specific diseases of the nervous system. The method of representing the etiologic factor and combining it with the site is explained in the general Introduction.

The sequelae of diseases of the nervous system are dealt with in one of two ways:

1. In a case of hemorrhage, for example, the site is the vessel, the cause being stated in each case. If the case later becomes one not of hemorrhage but of disease (in the broad sense) of the brain due to the hemorrhage, BRAIN (or some specified region of the brain) becomes the site, the cause now being HEMORRHAGE (Category 50, page 86).

The disease in question is to be diagnosed in terms of blood vessels when it is an acute condition and in terms of damage to the brain (encephalopathy, encephalomalacia) after the lapse of sufficient time to allow for the development of permanent changes in the brain.

2. In a case of acute anterior poliomyelitis, VENTRAL HORN CELLS are the site, the cause being the specific virus. If muscular paralyses or trophic diseases, etc., are present, they are to be recorded as secondary diagnoses (in Category 55 under the organ concerned). If, however, the disease or lesion of the nervous system has healed (e.g., anterior poliomyelitis, wound of nerve), the secondary diagnosis becomes the primary one.

Certain diseases of the nervous system, especially of the vegetative nervous system, are dealt with in this indirect way whenever it is impossible to define the underlying disease explicitly. All that can be said of these diseases is that distinct organs or tissues may manifest disease because of disturbance of sympathetic or other innervation.

As elsewhere, the diagnostic title expresses none of the symptomatic or other details of the particular case. The Supplementary Terms (page 501) is a list of symptoms and syndromes, with code numbers attached. In conformity with the requirements of the American Neurological Association, the syndromes present must be recorded as well as the basic diagnosis. The purpose of the numerical code is to permit these to be recorded in compact form. The complete diagnosis is therefore represented by the code for the basic diagnosis and codes for the syndromes, e.g.

4777–619 Thrombosis of lenticulostriate artery
969 Hemiplegia
901 Hemianesthesia

It may frequently occur that the primary neurologic diagnosis cannot be made, although there may be one or more important symptoms (page 501) which because of clinical or research interest should be recorded. Under these circumstances, the existence of these symptoms should be recognized and the diagnosis may read:

900–y00 Diagnosis deferred
631 Dysphagia

In this section the suffix -opathy is used to designate a tissue reaction of any nature due to causative factors of a noninfectious character; -itis is used to designate a condition which has an infectious or inflammatory basis.

401

DISEASES OF THE NERVOUS SYSTEM
GENERALLY

For Mental deficiency, *see page 110*
For Psychoses, *see page 110*
For Psychoneuroses, *see page 111*
For Diseases of endocrine glands and hormonal disturbances, *see page 387*

900–   Nervous system generally

Diseases affecting the nervous system generally or more than one of the chief divisions of the nervous system, named and numbered according to structures involved.

For detailed list of anatomic structures of nervous system, see page 41

—0 DISEASES DUE TO GENETIC AND PRENATAL INFLUENCES

903–092	Aplasia axialis extracorticalis congenita	*9001*
906–021	Caudal displacement of brain stem, cerebellum, and spinal cord	*9001*
906–1471	Cerebrospinal syphilis, congenital	*9001*
9▲▲–039	Constriction of . . . by anomalous meningeal bands or folds. *Specify region*	*9101*
9▲▲–077	Dysplasia, aplasia, hypoplasia, atrophy of . . . . *Specify site*	*9▲01*
901–027.8	Hydrencephalomeningocele	*9001*
9▲▲▲–093	Hyperplasia of . . . congenital. *Specify region*	*9▲01*

—I DISEASES DUE TO INFECTION WITH LOWER ORGANISM

The suffix—*radiculitis* may be added to the title of any of these combined diseases when applicable.

906–175	Encephalomyelitis. *The type or variety may be indicated by an additional digit (page 61)*	*9010*
906–100	Encephalomyelitis, acute. *Specify organism (page 57) when known*	*9010*
906–100.0	Encephalomyelitis, chronic. *Specify organism (page 57) when known*	*9010*
90x–147	Endarteritis, cerebrospinal syphilitic	*9010*
901–100	Meningoencephalomyelitis, acute. *Specify organism (page 57) when known*	*9010*
9011–1577	Meningoencephalomyelitis due to toxoplasma	*9010*

9011–100.0	Meningoencephalomyelitis, chronic, due to .... *Specify organism (page 57) when known*	*9010*
906–171	Poliomyelitis, acute bulbo-spinal	*9711*
900–147	Syphilis, cerebrospinal	*9010*
91x–147	Syphilis, meningovascular	*9010*
906–147	Tabes dorsalis	*9010*
900–153	Trypanosomiasis of nervous system	*9010*

—2 DISEASES DUE TO HIGHER PLANT OR ANIMAL PARASITE

9▲▲–2▲▲	Fungal or parasitic infection of .... *Specify site and organism, e.g.*	*9020*
901–218	Cryptococcosis of brain and meninges	*9020*

—3 DISEASES DUE TO INTOXICATION

906–3▲▲	Encephalomyelopathy due to . . . poison. *Specify (page 67)*	*9030*
946–399	Encephalomyelopathy due to Rh sensitization (kernicterus)	*9030*
900–3▲▲	Meningoencephalomyelopathy due to poison. *Specify (page 67)*	*9030*
901–3▲▲	Meningoencephalopathy due to . . . poison. *Specify (page 67)*	*9030*

—4 DISEASES DUE TO TRAUMA OR PHYSICAL AGENT

9▲▲–4▲▲	Injury of nervous system. *Specify injury (page 83), e.g.*	*9040*
900–485	Reaction to loss of cerebrospinal fluid	*9040*
901–400.4	Meningoencephalopathy due to trauma. *Indicate symptoms by use of term in list of supplementary terms (page 501)*	*9040*

—7 DISEASES DUE TO DISORDER OF METABOLISM, GROWTH, OR NUTRITION

902–755	Amaurotic familial idiocy (cerebromacular degeneration)	*9070*
902–7554	Infantile	*9070*
902–7552	Juvenile	*9070*
902–7551	Late infantile	*9070*
902–7553	Late juvenile	*9070*
906–785	Encephalomyelopathy due to diabetes	*9070*
906–7623	Encephalomyelopathy due to pellagra	*9070*

9▲▲–8▲▲▲   Neoplasm of nervous system, generally.
                  *Specify general region of nervous
                  system, neoplasm, and behavior (page
                  99)*   *9080*
9▲▲–8453A   Neurofibromatosis (plexiform neuroma)
                  of . . . . *Specify region*   *9080*

904–953   Amyotrophic lateral sclerosis (motor
                  neuron system disease)   *9092*
904–9531   Progressive muscular atrophy, spinal
                  type, familial   *9092*
904–9532   Progressive muscular atrophy, spinal
                  type, nonfamilial   *9092*
904–9533   Progressive muscular atrophy, bulbar
                  type, familial   *9092*
904–9534   Progressive muscular atrophy, bulbar
                  type, nonfamilial   *9092*
9041–953   Lateral sclerosis   *9092*
                  Pseudobulbar palsy
906–953   Multiple sclerosis (disseminated sclerosis) *9091*
9062–953   Optic pneuroencephalomyelopathy (neuro-
                  myelitis optica)   *9090*

90x– Vessels of nervous system

When disease of the vessels of the nervous system produces several
important neurologic symptoms, the latter should be coded and named after
the primary diagnosis. See Supplementary Classification, page 501.

90x–851   Hemangiomatosis of vessels of nervous
                  system. *Specify behavior (page 99)*   *9080*

90x–942   Cerebrospinal arteriosclerosis   *9594*
90x–952   Cerebrospinal endarteritis   *9090*
90x–930   Cerebrospinal thromboangiitis obliterans   *9090*
90x–931   Periarteritis nodosa of cerebrospinal
                  vessels   *9091*

DISEASES OF THE MENINGES

910–   Meninges
911–   Pachymeninges
912–   Leptomeninges
914–   Arachnoid
91x–   Intrinsic vessels

For detailed list of anatomic structures, see page 42

—0 DISEASES DUE TO GENETIC AND PRENATAL INFLUENCES

910x–025	Adhesions of . . . meninges, congenital. *Specify*	9101
91x▲–0▲▲	Anomaly of dural sinuses. *Specify anomaly*	9101
91▲▲–050	Birth injury: laceration of . . . meninges. *Specify*	9101
91▲▲–029	Congenital dermal sinus	9101
914▲–064	Cyst of arachnoid, congenital	9101
91▲▲–027	Meningocele of . . . . *Specify region*	9101

—I DISEASES DUE TO INFECTION WITH LOWER ORGANISM

915▲–100.2	Abscess, epidural of . . . . *Specify region and organism (page 57) when known, e.g.*	9110
9153–102.2	Epidural streptococcic abscess, temporal (right or left)	9110
913▲–100.2	Abscess, subdural, of . . . . *Specify region and organism (page 57) when known*	9110
913▲–1x8	Hygroma, subdural due to infection	9110
91▲–100	Meningitis, acute. *Specify organism (page 57) when known, e.g.*	9111
914–100	Arachnoiditis, acute	9111
912–100	Leptomeningitis, acute	9111
911–100	Pachymeningitis, acute	9111
91▲–100.0	Meningitis, chronic. *Specify organism and site when known, e.g.*	9111
914–100.0	Arachnoiditis, chronic	9111
912–100.0	Leptomeningitis, chronic	9111
911–100.0	Pachymeningitis, chronic	9111
910–189	Meningitis due to hepatic virus	9111
91▲–190	Meningitis, nonsuppurative. *Specify site, e.g.*	9111
914–190	Arachnoiditis, nonsuppurative	9111
912–190	Leptomeningitis, nonsuppurative	9111

911–190	Pachymeningitis, nonsuppurative	*9111*
91▲–1x0.4	Meningitis, adhesive, chronic. *Specify site, e.g.*	*9111*
914–1x0.4	Arachnoiditis, adhesive, chronic	*9111*
912–1x0.4	Leptomeningitis, adhesive, chronic	*9111*
911–1x0.4	Pachymeningitis, adhesive, chronic	*9111*
91▲–100.8	Meningitis, acute, serous. *Specify organism and site when known, e.g.*	*9111*
912–100.8	Leptomeningitis, acute, serous	*9111*
91▲–1x0.8	Meningitis, chronic, serous. *Specify site, e.g.*	*9111*
912–1x0.8	Leptomeningitis, chronic, serous	*9111*
91▲–100.6	Meningitis, hypertrophic. *Specify organism and site when known*	*9111*
91▲–160	Meningitis, lymphocytic, acute	*9111*
91▲–170	Meningitis due to mumps. *Specify site*	*9111*

—2 DISEASES DUE TO HIGHER PLANT OR ANIMAL PARASITE

| 9▲▲–2▲▲ | Fungal and parasitic infection of . . . . *Specify site and organism, e.g.* | *9120* |
| 910–209 | Moniliasis of meninges | *9120* |

—3 DISEASES DUE TO INTOXICATION

| 912–3931 | Meningismus, or aspetic meningitis, due to serum. *Specify* | *9130* |
| 912–3932 | Meningismus, or aseptic meningitis, due to vaccine. *Specify* | *9130* |

—4 DISEASES DUE TO TRAUMA OR PHYSICAL AGENT

913▲–4x7	Acute subdural hematoma of . . . . *Specify region*	*9140*
915▲–4x7	Epidural hematoma of . . . . *Specify region*	*9140*
915▲–427	Epidural aerocele of . . . . *Specify region*	*9140*
910▲–496	Foreign body in meninges. *Specify region*	*9140*
914–415.8	Hydrocephalus due to inadequate absorption following operation	*9261*
910▲–4▲▲	Injury of meninges. *Specify region and injury (page 83)*	*9140*
91041–412	Laceration of upper lumbar meninges	*9140*
912–438	Leptomeningopathy, aspetic, due to foreign body	*9140*
910▲–400.4	Meningeal adhesions due to trauma. *Specify region and injury (page 83), e.g.*	*9140*
91061–404.4	Meningeal adhesions, upper sacral, due to crushing	*9140*

918–415.8 Subarachnoid accumulation of cerebrospinal fluid, following operation *9140*
913–4x7.0 Subdural hematoma, chronic (internal hemorrhagic pachymeningopathy), of . . .
due to trauma. *Specify region* *9140*
913–4x7.9 Subdural hematoma, calcified, of . . . due
to trauma. *Specify region* *9140*
913▲–4x8 Subdural hygroma of . . . due to trauma.
Specify region *9140*

—8 NEW GROWTHS

91▲▲▲–872A Lipoma *9180*
9▲▲▲–8173 Melanoma of meninges. *Specify site and
behavior (page 99)* *9180*
91▲▲–846A Meningioma, benign. *Specify site* *9180*
91▲▲–846 Meningioma, malignant. *Specify site and
behavior (page 99)* *9180*
91▲▲–8▲▲▲ Unlisted tumor of meninges. *Specify site,
neoplasm, and behavior (page 99)* *9180*

**—9 DISEASES DUE TO UNKNOWN OR UNCERTAIN CAUSE WITH THE
STRUCTURAL REACTION MANIFEST**

91▲▲–923 Calcification of . . . due to unknown
cause. *Specify region* *9190*
913▲–9x7 Subdural hematoma of . . . due to unknown cause. *Specify region* *9190*

**—X DISEASES DUE TO UNKNOWN OR UNCERTAIN CAUSE WITH THE
FUNCTIONAL REACTION ALONE MANIFEST**

910–x20 Hypertensive meningeal hydrops *9190*

DISEASES OF MENINGEAL VESSELS

91x–   Meningeal vessels
  91x1–   Middle meningeal artery
  91x2–   Superior longitudinal sinus
  91x3–   Lateral sinus, right or left
  91x4–   Sigmoid sinus, right or left
  91x5–   Cavernous sinus, right or left
  91x6–   Straight sinus
  91x7–   Other sinuses

For list of anatomic structures, see page 43. If particular vessel cannot be identified, use generic code 91x–

—0 DISEASES DUE TO GENETIC AND PRENATAL INFLUENCES

91x–016.5	Arterial hypoplasia congenital of . . . with hemorrhage. *Special vessel when known*	*9101*
91x▲–050	Birth injury of . . . . *Specify vessel. To be diagnosed in cases of recent injury only. For delayed results see under Encephalomalacia, page 414*	*9101*
91x▲–015	Dilatation of . . . congenital. *Specify site*	*9101*
91x▲–077	Sinus pericranii. *Specify sinus if possible*	*9101*

—I DISEASES DUE TO INFECTION WITH LOWER ORGANISM

91x▲–100	Acute septic phlebitis of cranial sinus. *Specify sinus and organism*	*9110*
91x▲–100.4	Embolism of . . . by infected thrombus. *Specify vessel*	*9110*
91x▲–190	Phlebitis of . . . cranial sinus. *Specify sinus, e.g.*	*9110*
91x5–190	Of cavernous sinus	*9110*
91x▲–1x6.5	Subarachnoid hemorrhage of . . . due to rupture of embolic aneurysm. *Specify vessel and organism when known*	*9110*
91x▲–100.7	Thrombosis of . . . due to infection. *Specify vessel or sinus, e.g.*	*9110*
91x7–100.7	Of jugular bulb	*9110*
91x▲–1x0.7	Thrombosis of . . . due to remote infection. *Specify vessel and organism (page 57) when known, e.g.*	*9110*
91x4–101.7	Thrombosis of sigmoid sinus due to remote pneumococcic infection	*9110*

—4 DISEASES DUE TO TRAUMA OR PHYSICAL AGENT

91x▲–400.6	Aneurysm of . . . due to trauma. *Specify vessel, e.g.*	*9140*
91x1–400.6	Aneurysm of middle meningeal artery due to trauma	*9140*
91x▲–4x6	Arteriovenous aneurysm of . . . . *Specify vessel, e.g.*	*9140*
91x▲–4x6.5	Hemorrhage from arteriovenous aneurysm of . . . . *Specify*	*9140*
91x▲–4▲▲	Injury of meningeal vessel. *Specify injury (page 83) and vessel, e.g.*	*9140*
91x2–416	Hemorrhage from superior longitudinal sinus due to rupture	*9140*
91x1–412	Laceration of middle meningeal artery	*9140*

—50 DISEASES DUE TO CIRCULATORY DISTURBANCE
Record primary diagnosis when possible

91x▲–534.7	Marantic thrombosis of . . . . *Specify vessel, e.g.*	*9150*
91x5–534.7	Thrombosis of cavernous sinus	*9150*
91x–533.5	Subarachnoid hemorrhage due to vascular disease with hypertension	*9150*

—6 DISEASES DUE TO OR CONSISTING OF STATIC MECHANICAL ABNORMALITY

91x▲–619	Thrombosis of . . . . *Specify vessel*	*9160*

—8 NEW GROWTHS

91x▲–850A	Hemangioma of meningeal vessels. *Specify region*	*9180*
91x▲–8▲▲▲	Unlisted tumor of meningeal vessels. *Specify region, neoplasm, and behavior (page 99)*	*9180*

—9 DISEASES DUE TO UNKNOWN OR UNCERTAIN CAUSE WITH THE STRUCTURAL REACTION MANIFEST

91x▲–9x6	Aneurysm of . . . due to unknown cause. *Specify vessel*	*9190*
91x▲–900.7	Progressive thrombosis of . . . due to unknown cause. *Specify vessel or sinus*	*9190*

DISEASES OF THE BRAIN

930– Brain
920– Ventricles [1]

For detailed list of anatomic structures, see page 44

—0 DISEASES DUE TO GENETIC AND PRENATAL INFLUENCES

92▲▲▲–018	Atresia of ventricular system, congenital. *Specify region*	9201
946–092	Bilateral athetosis	9301
9▲▲▲–050	Birth injury of brain. *Specify region*	9301

The injury and its functional result are to be expressed by a combination of this code and that from the Supplementary Classification (page 501), as: 9334–050 (969) Birth palsy, hemiplegia (right or left). The actual significance of the first seven digits, as will be found on reference to the topographic and etiologic list: Birth injury of the precentral convolution.

93y–050	Birth injury of brain, unlocalized	9301
958–011	Cerebellar aplasia (right or left)	9301
930–076.6	Cerebral hemihypoplasia with compensatory cranial hemihyperplasia	9301
9334–076	Cerebral spastic infantile paralysis. *Indicate character by supplementary term (page 501), e.g.,* Monoplegia, Diplegia, Hemiplegia, Paraplegia, or Tetraplegia	
924–031	Congenital glial membrane of fourth ventricle	9201
932–045	Cortical disorders of association, developmental. *Specify type*	9301
926–064	Cyst of cavum septi pellucidi, congenital	9201
926–015	Dilatation of cavum septi pellucidi	9201
930–051	Encephalopathy, congenital due to maternal infection	9301
930–053	Encephalopathy, congenital due to maternal intoxication	9301
930–048	Encephalopathy due to anoxemia at birth	9301
930–050.x	Encephalopathy due to birth injury	9301
930–012	Hemianencephaly	9301
93▲▲–027	Herniation of brain. *Specify region*	**9301**
930–021	Heterotopia cerebralis	9301
920–063	Hydrocephalus, congenital, communicating	9202
920–064	Hydrocephalus, congenital, obstructive type	9202
932–013	Macrogyria, congenital	9301

[1] There are no diseases proper of the ventricles, but merely changes in size or contour, dependent on other disease.

901–019	Microcephaly, congenital	*9301*
901–019.8	Hydromicrocephaly, congenital	*9301*
932–076	Microgyria	*9301*
930–010	Multiple congenital anomalies of brain	*9301*
946–011	Nuclear aplasia of . . . . *Specify nuclei*	*9301*
930–090	Porencephaly, congenital	*9301*

—I DISEASES DUE TO INFECTION WITH LOWER ORGANISM

9▲▲–100.2	Abscess of . . . . *Specify region and organism (page 57) when known*	*9312*
958–100.2	Abscess of cerebellum	*9312*
933–100.2	Abscess of frontal lobe of brain	*9312*
935–100.2	Abscess of temporal lobe of brain	*9312*
930–196	Chorea	*9310*
9301–147.9	Dementia paralytica juvenilis	*9310*
930–147.9	Dementia paralytica without psychosis (general paresis)	*9310*
930–100	Encephalitis, acute. *Specify organism (page 57), e.g.*	*9311*
930–115	Acute encephalitis due to Bacterium typhosum	*9311*
930–100.0	Encephalitis, chronic. *Specify supplementary terms (page 501). Specify organism (page 57) when known as preceding*	*9311*
930–166	Encephalitis due to herpetic virus	*9311*
930–175	Encephalitis, epidemic, acute	*9311*
955–175	Midbrain type	*9311*
930–1▲▲.x	Encephalitis, postexanthema. *Specify*	*9311*
930–169.x	Following measles	*9311*
930–1761.x	Following smallpox	*9311*
930–1▲▲.x	Encephalitis, postinfectious. *Specify infection*	*9311*
930–115.x	Following typhoid	*9311*

ARTHROPOD-BORNE

955–1752	Eastern equine	*9311*
930–1755	Japanese B and other arthropod-borne types	*9311*
930–1753	St. Louis	*9311*
955–1751	Western equine	*9311*

OTHER TYPES

930–1756	Australian X	*9311*
930–175.0	Encephalitis, epidemic, chronic	*9311*

930–100.6	Encephalopathy due to remote infection. *Specify organism (page 57) when known, e.g.*	9310
930–115.6	Encephalopathy due to Bacterium typhosum	9310
927▲–100	Ependymitis, acute, of . . . . *Specify region and organism (page 57) when known, e.g.*	9210
9272–105	Staphylococcic ependymitis of third ventricle	9210
927–100.0	Ependymitis, chronic. *Specify organism (page 57) when known*	9210
927–100.8	Hydrocephalus due to inflammation of ependyma	9212
928▲–1x4.8	Hydrocephalus due to sclerosis of foramen. *Specify foramen*	9212
930–147.6	Syphilis, cerebral gumma	9310

—2 DISEASES DUE TO HIGHER PLANT OR ANIMAL PARASITE

| 9▲▲–2▲▲ | Parasitic infection of . . . . *Specify site* | 9320 |

—3 DISEASES DUE TO INTOXICATION

908–388	Chorea gravidarum	9330
930–3932	Encephalitis, post vaccination	9330
930–39321	Encephalitis, post smallpox vaccination	9330
930–39322	Encephalitis, post rabies vaccination	9330
930–3▲▲	Encephalopathy, toxic, due to poison. *Specify (page 67). See also under* Brain disorders *(page 107), e.g.*	
930–321	Due to arsenic	9330
930–3821	Due to extract of thyroid gland	9330
930–300.7	Encephalorrhagia, pericapillary, due to poison. *Specify (page 67)*	9330
927–3▲▲	Ependymopathy due to poison. *Specify (page 67), e.g.*	9230
927–3931	Ependymopathy due to serum	9230

—4 DISEASES DUE TO TRAUMA OR PHYSICAL AGENT

9▲▲–435	Compression of . . . by aneurysm of varix. *Specify region*	9340
9▲▲–438	Compression of . . . by foreign body. *Specify region*	9340
9▲▲–436	Compression of . . . by fractured bone. *Specify region*	9340

9▲▲–4362.x	Compression of . . . by scar tissue. *Specify region*	*9340*
930–428	Concussion (commotion) of brain	*9340*
9▲▲–402	Contusion of . . . (direct blow or contrecoup). *Specify region, e.g.*	*9340*
935–402	Contusion of temporal lobe	*9340*
9▲▲–4▲▲.8	Cyst, posttraumatic, of . . . due to . . . . *Specify region and injury (page 83), e.g.*	*9340*
958–414.8	Cyst of cerebellum due to bullet wound	*9340*
930–460	Electric shock of brain	*9340*
9▲▲–4x9	Encephalomalacia of . . . due to trauma. *Specify region*	*9340*
930–481	Encephalopathy due to cerebral anoxia, the result of high altitude	*9340*
930–436	Encephalopathy due to depressed fracture	*9340*
930–438	Encephalopathy due to foreign body	*9340*
930–445	Encephalopathy due to heat	*9340*
930–480	Encephalopathy due to hypobaropathy	*9340*
930–420.x	Encephalopathy due to remote trauma. *Indicate supplementary terms (page 501)*	*9340*
930–453	Encephalopathy due to sunstroke	*9340*
927–4742	Ependymopathy due to thorotrast	*9240*
9▲▲–4x4	Fibroastrial scar due to trauma. *Specify region*	*9340*
9▲▲–496	Foreign body in . . . . *Specify region*	*9340*
9▲▲–4x6	Gliosis of . . . due to trauma. *Specify region*	*9340*
93▲–400.9	Hernia of . . . . *Specify region*	*9340*
93▲▲–4x7	Intracerebral hematoma of . . . . *Specify region*	*9340*
9▲▲–4362	Irritation of . . . by scar tissue. *Specify region*	*9340*
9▲▲–412	Laceration of . . . . *Specify region*	*9340*
930–427	Pneumocephalus	*9340*
9▲▲–4x8.3	Porencephaly of . . . due to trauma. *Specify region*	*9340*
9▲▲–414	Wound, gunshot (missile) of . . . . *Specify region*	*9340*
9▲▲–410	Wound, penetrating, of . . . . *Specify region*	*9340*
9▲▲–411	Wound, stab of . . . . *Specify region*	*9340*

—50 DISEASES DUE TO CIRCULATORY DISTURBANCE
Record primary diagnosis when possible

9▲▲–5x0	Encephalomalacia due to circulatory disturbance	9351
	Specify site and nature of circulatory disturbance, e.g.	
946–512	Encephalomalacia of basal ganglia due to embolism	9351
945–532	Encephalomalacia of internal capsule due to hemorrhage	9351
955–511	Encephalomalacia of midbrain due to thrombosis	9351
9▲▲▲▲–516	Encephalomalacia of . . . due to arteriosclerosis. *Specify region*	9351
930–519	Encephalopathy due to cardiac standstill	9350
930–533	Encephalopathy due to arterial hypertension	9350
930–516	Encephalopathy due to arteriosclerosis	9350
9▲▲–549.7	Hemorrhage into . . . due to disturbance of clotting mechanism (*Diagnose disease*)	9350
932–500	Microgyria, acquired	9350

—6 DISEASES DUE TO OR CONSISTING OF STATIC MECHANICAL ABNORMALITY

93▲▲–639.7	Hemorrhage due to herniation of brain. *Specify region*	9360

—7 DISEASES DUE TO DISORDER OF METABOLISM, GROWTH, OR NUTRITION
Record primary diagnosis when possible

935–791	Deaf-mutism, acquired. *To be used when previous disease has interfered with normal development of central speech mechanism*	9370
930–705	Encephalopathy due to anoxia	9370
930–784	Encephalopathy due to hyperinsulinism	9370
930–701	Encephalopathy due to starvation	9370
930–760	Encephalopathy due to vitamin deficiency	9370
9462–740	Hepatolenticular degeneration	9370
953–762▲	Polioencephalopathy, superior, hemorrhagic, due to lack of vitamin. *Specify vitamin*	9370

—8 NEW GROWTHS

When a neoplasm involving the brain arises from the meninges or other neighboring structures, it should be diagnosed according to its anatomic site of origin, and its nature, if known, indicated (*e.g., 910–8451 Neurofibroma of brain*).

Complete topographic number by inserting digits representing region of brain involved (page 44)

9▲▲–8091	Adenocarcinoma. *Specify behavior (page 99)*	9380
9▲▲–8473	Astrocytoma. *Specify behavior (page 99)*	9380
9▲▲–812	Basal cell carcinoma. *Specify behavior (page 99)*	9380
9▲▲–873B	Chondroma	9380
9▲▲–8886	Chordoma. *Specify behavior (page 99)*	9380
9▲▲–8887	Craniopharyngioma. *Specify behavior (page 99)*	9380
9▲▲–848	Ependymoma. *Specify behavior (page 99)*	9380
9▲▲–814	Epidermoid carcinoma. *Specify behavior (page 99)*	9380
9▲▲–870A	Fibroma	9380
9▲▲–870F	Fibrosarcoma	9380
9▲▲–8471	Ganglioglioma. *Specify behavior*	9380
9▲▲–8474	Glioblastoma multiforme. *Specify behavior*	9380
9▲▲–8475	Glioma. *Specify behavior (page 99)*	9380
9▲▲–850B	Hemangioendothelioma	9380
95x–850A	Hemangioma of intrinsic vessels of brain	9380
9▲▲–872A	Lipoma	9380
9▲▲–830	Lymphosarcoma [1]	9380
9▲▲–842G	Medulloblastoma	9380
9▲▲–8173	Melanoma. *Specify behavior (page 99)*	9380
9▲▲–846	Meningioma. *Specify behavior (page 99)*	9380
9▲▲–842F	Neuroepithelioma	9380
9▲▲–8451	Neurofibroma (cerebellar pontine angle tumor). *Specify behavior (page 99)*	9380
9▲▲–8472	Oligodendroma. *Specify behavior*	9380
9▲▲–879	Sarcoma. *Specify behavior (page 99)*	9380
9▲▲–841F	Sympathicoblastoma	9380
9▲▲–841G	Sympathicogonioma	9380
9▲▲–882	Teratoma. *Specify behavior (page 99)*	9380
9▲▲–8▲▲▲	Unlisted tumor of brain. *Specify neoplasm and behavior (page 99)*	9380

[1] Use lymphoma behavior code (page 99).

958–953	Cerebellar atrophy	*9390*
930–910	Cerebral cortical atrophy, generalized	*9390*
939▲▲–910	Cerebral cortical atrophy, localized.	
	Specify site	*9390*
9461–953	Chronic progressive chorea (nonhereditary)	*9390*
908–953	Chronic progressive chorea with mental deterioration (nonhereditary)	*9390*
930–995	Diffuse, familial cerebral sclerosis	*9390*
958–9531	Dyssynergia cerebellaris progressiva	*9390*
950–9532	Dystonia musculorum deformans	*9390*
9273–956	Gliosis of cerebral aqueduct, with or without stenosis	*9390*
906–992	Hereditary cerebellar atrophy	*9390*
908–992	Hereditary chronic progressive chorea with mental deterioration	*9390*
950–9535	Intermittent spastic torticollis	*9390*
942–992	Leukodystrophia, cerebri progressiva hereditaria	*9390*
9591–953	Olivopontocerebellar atrophy	*9390*
9464–953	Paralysis agitans	*9395*
9586–911	Parenchymatous cortical cerebellar atrophy	*9390*
931–9x1	Poliodystrophia cerebri progressiva (infantilis)	*9390*
954–953	Progressive labioglossopharyngeal paralysis; bulbar palsy	*9390*
9462–9531	Progressive lenticular degeneration	*9390*
9385–953	Progressive subcortical encephalopathy	*9390*
950–9533	Pseudosclerosis	*9390*
959–992	Spinocerebellar atrophy, hereditary	*9390*
957–9x8	Syringobulbia	*9390*
930–997	Tuberous sclerosis	*9390*

93▲▲▲–x02	Focal, motor or sensory, cortical seizures. *Insert digits in the topographic portion of the code number to indicate the focal site of dysfunction*	*9391*
9334–x02	Focal motor cortical seizure (Jacksonian)	*9391*
930–x0x	Focal psychical (psychomotor)	*9391*
9341–x02	Focal sensory cortical seizure	*9391*
933–x021	Focal visceral seizure	*9391*
935–x02	Temporal lobe seizure	*9391*

930–x08	Grand and petit mal	*9391*
930–x01	Grand mal	*9391*
930–x07	Petit mal	*9391*
930–x06	Status epilepticus	*9391*
930–x05	Other types of seizure	*9391*

Other paroxysmal psychic disorders, see Supplementary Terms, *page 501*

930–x12	Akinetic seizure	*9391*
930–x52	Cataplexy	*9391*
930–x40	Migraine, cause unknown	*9393*
930–x46	Abdominal migraine	*9393*
930–x45	Cerebral migraine	*9393*
930–x48	Migrainous equivalents	*9393*
930–x42	Ophthalmic migraine	*9393*
930–x43	Ophthalmoplegic migraine	*9393*
930–x49	Other types of migraine (migraine variants)	*9393*
930–x41	Simple migraine (hemicrania)	*9393*
990–x53	Mixed paroxysmal disorders	*9390*
930–x50	Narcolepsy	*9390*
930–x51	Narcolepsy with cataplexy	*9390*
954–x30	Paroxysmal vasovagal attacks	*9390*
930–x30	Pyknolepsy	*9390*
990–x41	Sympatheticotonia	*9390*
990–x20	Vagotonia	*9390*

CEREBRAL VESSELS

477▲– Arteries of brain
92x–   Choroid plexus
94x–   Intrinsic arteries of brain
95x–   Intrinsic vessels of brain

For list of anatomic structures, see page 27. If particular vessel cannot be identified, use generic code 95x

When disease of the vessels of the brain produces one or more important neurologic symptoms, the latter should be coded and named after the primary diagnosis. See *Supplementary Terms, page 501.*

—0 DISEASES DUE TO GENETIC AND PRENATAL INFLUENCES

477▲–015	Aneurysm, congenital, of . . . *Specify vessel*	9501
477▲–015.5	Rupture of congenital aneurysm of . . . . *Specify vessel*	9501
95x▲–010	Anomaly of . . . . *Specify vessel*	9501
92x▲–01x	Anomaly of choroid plexus. *Specify region*	9501
95x▲–019	Atypical distribution of . . . . *Specify vessel*	9501
95x–029	Arteriovenous fistula, congenital	9501
477▲–050	Birth injury of . . . . *Specify vessel. To be diagnosed in cases of recent injury only. For late sequelae, see under* Encephalomalacia, *page 414*	9501

—1 DISEASES DUE TO INFECTION WITH LOWER ORGANISM

95x▲–100.6	Aneurysm, arteriovenous, of . . . due to infection. *Specify vessel*	9510
477–190	Cerebral essential angiitis	9510
477▲–190.5	Hemorrhage from . . . due to cerebral essential angiitis. *Specify vessel*	9510
477–100.6	Embolic aneurysm, multiple	9510
477▲–100.6	Embolic aneurysm of . . . . *Specify vessel*	9510
477▲–100.4	Embolism of . . . by infected thrombus. *Specify vessel and source*	9510
477▲–1x6.5	Hemorrhage from . . . due to rupture of embolic aneurysm. *Specify vessel*	9510
95x▲–157	Vascular occlusion by malarial parasites. *Specify vessel*	9510

—2 DISEASES DUE TO HIGHER PLANT OR ANIMAL PARASITES

477▲–2x6   Mycotic aneurysm of . . . . *Specify*
             vessel   *9520*

—4 DISEASES DUE TO TRAUMA OR PHYSICAL AGENT

477▲–427   Air embolism of . . . . *Specify vessel*   *9542*
477▲–400.6   Aneurysm of . . . due to trauma.
             Specify vessel   *9540*
95x▲–400.6   Arteriovenous aneurysm of . . . due to
             trauma. *Specify vessel*   *9540*
95x▲–4x6.5   Hemorrhage from arteriovenous an-
             eurysm of . . . . *Specify vessel*   *9542*
477▲–425   Embolism of . . . following operation.
             Specify vessel   *9542*
477▲–426   Fat embolism of . . . . *Specify vessel*   *9542*
95x▲–416   Hemorrhage from . . . due to trauma.
             Specify vessel   *9541*

—50 DISEASES DUE TO CIRCULATORY DISTURBANCE
Record primary diagnosis when possible

For Thrombosis and Hemorrhage *due to causes other than
blood disease, see under Categories 1, 4, 6, and 9, pages
418 to 420*

477▲–533.5   Cerebral hemorrhage due to hypertension *9551*
477▲–541.7   Thrombosis of . . . due to polycythemia.
             Specify vessel   *9553*
477▲–547.7   Thrombosis of . . . due to thrombotic
             thrombocytopenia. *Specify vessel*   *9553*

—55 DISEASES DUE TO DISTURBANCE OF INNERVATION

477▲–582   Angiospasm of . . . . *Specify vessel*   *9556*

**—6 DISEASES DUE TO OR CONSISTING OF STATIC MECHANICAL ABNOR-
MALITY**

477▲–618   Embolism of . . . due to unspecified
             cause. *Specify source as second diag-
             nosis*   *9562*
477▲–611   Foreign body embolism of . . . causing
             obstruction. *Specify vessel*   *9562*
477▲–619   Thrombosis of . . . due to unspecified
             cause. *Specify vessel*   *9563*

—8 NEW GROWTHS

477▲–850A	Hemangioma of intrinsic arteries of brain	*9580*
477▲–850F	Hemangiosarcoma of intrinsic arteries of brain	*9580*
94x–8▲▲▲	Unlisted tumor of . . . . *Specify neo-plasm and behavior (page 99)*	*9580*

—9 DISEASES DUE TO UNKNOWN OR UNCERTAIN CAUSE WITH THE STRUCTURAL REACTION MANIFEST

477▲–9x6	Aneurysm of . . . due to unknown cause. *Specify vessel*	*9590*
477▲–942	Arteriosclerosis of . . . . *Specify vessel*	*9590*
477▲–942.6	Arteriosclerotic aneurysm of . . . . *Specify*	*9594*
477▲–942.5	Hemorrhage from . . . due to arterio-sclerosis.[1] *Specify*	*9594*
95x▲–9x6	Arteriovenous aneurysm of . . . due to unknown cause. *Specify vessels*	*9590*
92x–923	Calcification of choroid plexus due to unknown cause	*9290*
477–942	Cerebral arteriosclerosis. *Diagnose.* Encephalopathy due to arteriosclerosis, *page 414 if present*	*9594*
477–930	Cerebral thromboangiitis obliterans	*9590*
477▲▲–930	Cerebral thromboangiitis obliterans of . . . . *Specify vessel*	*9590*
477▲–942.7	Cerebral thrombosis due to arterio-sclerosis.[1] *Specify vessel*	*9594*
477▲–997	Familial cerebral arterial calcification	*9594*
477▲–900.7	Progressive thrombosis, cerebral, due to unknown cause	*9590*

—Y DISEASES DUE TO CAUSE NOT DETERMINABLE IN THE PARTICULAR CASE

Y signifies an incomplete diagnosis. It is to be replaced whenever possible by a code digit signifying the specific diagnosis

477▲–yx7	Hemorrhage from . . . due to undetermined cause. *Specify vessel*	*0069*

[1] See Introduction, page 401.

DISEASES OF THE SPINAL CORD AND NERVE ROOTS

970– Spinal cord
978– Combined ventral and dorsal roots
9781– Ventral roots
9782– Dorsal roots
9783– Dorsal root ganglia

Conditions affecting the nerve roots may be diagnosed according to the terms used in the classification under SPINAL CORD, the digits for the topographic code and the written diagnosis being changed.

—0 DISEASES DUE TO GENETIC AND PRENATAL INFLUENCES

970–011	Amyelia	*9701*
972–090	Amyotonia congenita (flabby infant)	*9701*
97▲–011	Aplasia of . . . . *Specify site*	*9701*
972▲–011	Aplasia of ventral cell horn. *Specify region*	*9701*
970–012	Atelomyelia	*9701*
909▲▲–050	Birth injury; laceration of spinal cord and meninges at . . . . *Specify region*	*9701*
970–034	Diastematomyelia	**9701**
970–021	Heterotopia spinalis	*9701*
929–015	Hydromyelia	*9701*
97▲▲▲–093	Hyperplasia, congenital, of . . . . *Specify region*	*9701*
970–076	Micromyelia	*9701*
97▲▲–077	Myelodysplasia of . . . . *Specify region*	*9701*
909–027	Myelomeningocele	*9701*
970–037	Rachischisis of spinal cord	*9701*
978▲▲▲–0681	Radiculopathy of . . . by pressure from other forms of congenital malformation. *Specify roots*	*9701*
978▲▲▲–068	Radiculopathy of . . . by pressure of meningocele. *Specify roots*	*9701*

—I DISEASES DUE TO INFECTION WITH LOWER ORGANISM

970▲▲–100.2	Abscess of spinal cord. *Specify region and organism (page 57) when known, e.g.*	*9710*
97031–105.2	Staphylococcic abscess of spinal cord, upper thoracic region	**9710**
970–102	Disseminated streptococcic myelitis	*9710*
9783▲▲–1764.x	Ganglionitis, chronic; neuralgia following zoster	*9710*
9783▲▲–1764	Ganglionitis (zoster). *Specify ganglion as under 970, page 47*	*9710*

909–100	Meningomyelitis, acute. *Specify organism (page 57) when known*	9710
909–101	Acute pneumococcic meningomyelitis	9710
909–100.0	Meningomyelitis, chronic. *Specify organism (page 57) when known*	9710
909–147	Meningomyelitis, syphilitic	9710
970–100	Myelitis, acute; myelitis disseminated. *Specify organism (page 57) when known*	9710
97034–102	Streptococcic transverse myelitis, thoracolumbar	9710
970▲▲–100	Transverse myelitis at . . . . *Specify region and organism*	9710
971–100	Myelitis, ascending, acute	9710
970–100.0	Myelitis, chronic	9710
972▲▲–171	Poliomyelitis, anterior, acute, of . . . . *Specify region. If old poliomyelitis, diagnose under* Bone, Joint, *or* Muscle *affected, pages 152, 160, 169*	9711
972–171	Poliomyelitis, abortive, nonparalytic	9711
972▲▲–171.0	Poliomyelitis, anterior, chronic of . . . . *Specify region*	9711
972▲▲–147.0	Poliomyelitis, anterior, chronic, of . . . due to syphilis. *Specify region*	9710
974▲▲–100	Poliomyelitis, lateral, acute, of . . . . *Specify region*	9710
907–160	Polyradiculoneuropathy, acute infectious (Guillain-Barre syndrome)	9710
978▲▲–100	Radiculitis of . . . . *Specify region and organism when known*	9710
979–160	Virus myeloradiculitis	9710

—2 DISEASES DUE TO HIGHER PLANT OR ANIMAL PARASITE

909▲▲–2▲▲	Meningiomyelitis mycotic. *Specify fungus (page 63)*	9720
909▲▲–2▲▲	Parasitic infection of spinal cord and meninges. *Specify parasite (page 63)*	9720

—3 DISEASES DUE TO INTOXICATION

970–3▲▲	Myelopathy due to poison. *Specify (page 67)*	9730
970–321	Due to arsenic	9730
970–33212	Due to ethyl alcohol	9730
970–3238	Due to lead	9730
97▲▲–3▲▲	Myelopathy, transverse, at . . . due to poison. *Specify region and poison (page 67)*	9730

907▲▲–300   Myeloradiculopathy due to poison. *Spec-*
                 ify region (page 67)   9730
978▲▲–3▲▲   Radiculopathy of . . . due to poison.
                 Specify region and poison (page 67)   9730

—4 DISEASES DUE TO TRAUMA OR PHYSICAL AGENT

97844–4x4   Adhesions of cauda equina due to trauma   9740
978▲▲–409   Avulsion of . . . nerve roots. *Specify re-*
                 gion   9740
970▲▲–403   Compression, acute, of spinal cord at . . . .
                 Specify region and agent (page 83)   9740
970▲▲–43▲   Compression, chronic, of spinal cord at
                 . . . . *Specify region and agent (page*
                 83)   9740
970▲▲–437   Compression of spinal cord at . . . by
                 abscess or granuloma or by epidural
                 cellulitis. *Specify region. Record*
                 primary diagnosis   9740
970▲▲–435   Compression of spinal cord at . . . by
                 aneurysm. *Specify region*   9740
970▲▲–4361   Compression of spinal cord at . . . by
                 callus. *Specify region*   9740
970▲▲–43x   Compression of spinal cord at . . . by
                 contiguous hematoma. *Specify re-*
                 gion   9740
970▲▲–439   Compression of spinal cord at . . . by
                 contiguous neoplasm. *Specify re-*
                 gion   9740
970▲▲–4341   Compression of spinal cord at . . . by
                 extrusion of nucleus pulposus.
                 Specify region   9740
970–438   Compression of spinal cord at . . . by
                 foreign body. *Specify region*   9740
970▲▲–4353   Compression of spinal cord at . . . by
                 meningeal adhesions. *Specify level*   9740
970▲▲–4352   Compression of spinal cord at . . . by
                 osteoarthritic overgrowth. *Specify*
                 region   9740
970▲▲–4362   Compression of spinal cord at . . . by
                 scar tissue. *Specify region*   9740
970▲▲–4351   Compression of spinal cord at . . . by
                 varix. *Specify region*   9740
970▲▲–434   Compression of spinal cord at . . . by
                 vertebral dislocation. *Specify re-*
                 gion   9740
970▲▲–436   Compression of spinal cord at . . . by
                 vertebral fracture. *Specify region*   9740

978▲▲–4354	Compression of . . . nerve roots by hyper-trophied ligamentum flavum. *Specify region*	9740
970–428	Concussion, or commotion, general, of spinal cord	9740
970▲▲–428	Concussion, or commotion, of spinal cord at . . . . *Specify region*	9740
970▲▲–402	Contusion of spinal cord at . . . . *Specify region*	9740
970–460	Electrical shock of spinal cord	9740
970▲▲–4x6	Gliosis due to trauma at . . . . *Specify region*	9740
970▲▲–4x7	Hematomyelia at . . . . *Specify region*	9740
970▲▲–4051	Hemisection of spinal cord at . . . . *Specify region*	9740
970▲▲–4▲▲	Injury of spinal cord. *Specify region and injury (page 83)*	9740
970▲▲–412	Laceration of spinal cord at . . . . *Specify region*	9740
970–480	Myelopathy due to decompression disease	9740
970–481	Myelopathy due to hyperbaropathy	9740
970▲▲–410	Wound, penetrating, of spinal cord at . . . . *Specify region*	9740

—50 DISEASES DUE TO CIRCULATORY DISTURBANCE

970▲▲–516	Myelopathy at . . . due to arteriosclerosis. *Specify region*	9750
970–51▲	Myelopathy at . . . due to circulatory disturbance. *Specify region when known,* e.g.	9750
970▲▲–515	Myelopathy at . . . due to arteritis or phlebitis. *Specify region*	9750
970▲▲–512	Myelopathy at . . . due to embolism. *Specify region*	9750
970▲▲–532	Myelopathy at . . . due to hemorrhage. *Specify region*	9750
970▲▲–511	Myelopathy at . . . due to thrombosis. *Specify region*	9750

—7 DISEASES DUE TO DISORDER OF METABOLISM, GROWTH, OR NUTRITION
Record primary diagnosis when possible

975–785	Diabetic dorsal sclerosis	9770
970–704	Myelopathy due to anoxemia	9770
970–711	Myelopathy due to cachexia	9770
970–701	Myelopathy due to starvation	9770
970–760	Myelopathy due to vitamin deficiency, *e.g.*	9770
970–7621	Due to beriberi	9770

970–7623	Due to pellagra	*9770*
970–7625	Due to vitamin B$_{12}$	*9770*
907▲▲–785	Myeloradiculopathy due to diabetes. *Specify roots*	*9770*
977–7625	Posteriolateral spinal cord degeneration due to vitamin B$_{12}$	*9770*

—8 NEW GROWTHS

When a neoplasm involving the spinal cord arises from the meninges or other neighboring structures, it should be diagnosed according to its anatomic site of origin, and its nature, if known, indicated. Its code will begin with 910, to which are added two digits to define its particular site (see page 42). For example, 91021–8541 is the code for *Neurofibroma of the upper cervical meninges.*

Complete topographic number by inserting digits representing regions of spinal cord and nerve roots involved

970▲▲–848	Ependymoma. *Specify behavior (page 99)*	*9780*
970▲▲–8475	Glioma. *Specify behavior (page 99)*	*9780*
970▲▲–8451	Neurofibroma. *Specify behavior (page 99)*	*9780*
970▲▲–8▲▲▲	Unlisted tumor of spinal cord and nerve roots. *Specify neoplasm and behavior (page 99)*	*9780*

—9 DISEASES DUE TO UNKNOWN OR UNCERTAIN CAUSE WITH THE STRUCTURAL REACTION MANIFEST; AND HEREDITARY AND FAMILIAL DISEASES OF THIS NATURE

975–953	Dorsal sclerosis due to unknown cause	*9790*
972–992	Familial spinal muscular atrophy, infantile	*9790*
971–953	Myelopathic muscular atrophy [1]	*9790*
971–9531	Nonprogressive myelopathic muscular atrophy	*9790*
971–9530	Progressive myelopathic muscular atrophy	*9790*
970–915	Necrosis of spinal cord	*9790*
907▲▲–953	Progressive neuropathic (peroneal) muscular atrophy [1] of . . . . *Specify region*	*9790*
970▲▲–9x8	Syringomyelia of . . . . *Specify region*	*9790*
97x–	Vessels of spinal cord	

For list of anatomic structures, see page 47. If particular vessel cannot be identified, use generic code 97x–

When disease of the vessels of the spinal cord produces one or more important neurologic symptoms, the latter should be coded and named after the primary diagnosis. See *Supplementary Terms,* page 501.

1 Other disorders of the muscular system which cannot be referred definitely to structural or functional disturbance of the nervous system are listed on pages 167, 170.

—0 DISEASES DUE TO GENETIC AND PRENATAL INFLUENCES

97x▲▲–015	Aneurysm of . . . . *Specify vessel*	*9701*
97x▲▲–019	Atypical distribution of . . . . *Specify vessel*	*9701*
97x▲▲–010	Developmental defect of . . . . *Specify vessel*	*9701*
97x▲▲–076	Hypoplasia of . . . . *Specify vessel*	*9701*

—I DISEASES DUE TO INFECTION WITH LOWER ORGANISM

97x▲▲–100.6	Aneurysm, embolic, of . . . due to infection. *Specify vessel*	*9710*
97x▲▲–1x6.5	Hemorrhage from . . . due to rupture of aneurysm due to infection. *Specify vessel*	*9710*
97x–100	Arteritis and phlebitis of spinal cord due to infection	*9710*
97x▲▲–100.4	Embolism of . . . by infected thrombi. *Specify vessel*	*9710*
97x▲▲–100.7	Thrombosis of . . . due to infection. *Specify vessel and organism when known (page 57)*	*9710*
97x▲▲–1x0.7	Thrombosis of . . . due to remote infection. *Specify vessel*	*9710*

—4 DISEASES DUE TO TRAUMA OR PHYSICAL AGENT

97x▲▲–427	Air embolism of . . . . *Specify vessel*	*9740*
97x▲▲–400.6	Aneurysm of . . . due to trauma. *Specify vessel*	*9740*
97x–4x6	Arteriovenous aneurysm of intrinsic vessel of spinal cord	*9740*
97x▲▲–425	Embolism of . . . following operation. *Specify vessel*	*9740*
97x▲▲–426	Fat embolism of . . . . *Specify vessel*	*9740*
97x▲▲–4▲▲	Injury of spinal vessel. *Specify injury and region (page 83)*	*9740*

—55 DISEASES DUE TO DISTURBANCE OF INNERVATION

97x▲▲–582	Angiospasm of . . . . *Specify artery*	*9755*

—6 DISEASES DUE TO OR CONSISTING OF STATIC MECHANICAL ABNORMALITY

97x▲▲–618	Embolism of . . . due to unspecified cause. *Specify vessel*	*9760*
97x▲▲–619	Thrombosis of . . . due to unspecified cause. *Specify vessel*	*9760*

97x4▲▲–641   Varix of . . . spinal vein. *Specify region*
                     according to subdivision of spinal cord   9760

—8 NEW GROWTHS

97x▲▲–850A   Hemangioma of spinal vessels   *9780*
97x▲▲–850G   Hemangiosarcoma of spinal vessels   *9780*
97x▲▲–8▲▲▲   Unlisted tumor of spinal vessels   *9780*

—9 DISEASES DUE TO UNKNOWN OR UNCERTAIN CAUSE WITH THE STRUCTURAL REACTION MANIFEST

97x▲▲–942.6   Arteriosclerosis aneurysm of . . . . *Spec-*
                  ify vessel   *9790*
97x–942   Arteriosclerosis of vessels of spinal cord,
                  generalized   *9790*
   97x▲▲–942   Arteriosclerosis of . . . . *Specify vessel*   *9790*
97x▲▲–942.5   Hemorrhage from . . . due to arterio-
                  sclerosis. *Specify vessel*   *9790*
97x–930   Spinal thromboangiitis obliterans, general   *9790*
   97x▲▲–930   Spinal thromboangiitis obliterans of
                  . . . . *Specify region*   *9790*
97x–900.7   Thrombosis, progressive, spinal   *9790*

DISEASES OF THE PERIPHERAL NERVES
INCLUDING CRANIAL NERVES AND GANGLIA

960– Cranial nerves and ganglia
980– Peripheral nerves (cranial and spinal)
981– Spinal nerves

For list of anatomic structures, see page 47

—0 DISEASES DUE TO GENETIC AND PRENATAL INFLUENCES

When the condition involves the cranial nerves, use 96▲▲▲

98▲▲–011	Agenesis of . . . . *Specify nerve*	*9801*
98▲▲–019	Atypical distribution of . . . . *Specify nerve*	*9801*
98▲▲–050	Birth injury: laceration of . . . . *Specify nerve*	*9801*
983–021	Displacement of brachial plexus	*9801*
983–0212	Postfixed brachial plexus	*9801*
983–0211	Prefixed brachial plexus	*9801*

—I DISEASES DUE TO INFECTION WITH LOWER ORGANISM

980–100	Acute multiple neuritis. *Specify organism (page 57) when known*	*9810*
98▲▲–100	Acute neuritis of . . . due to . . . . *Specify nerve and organism (page 57) when known*	*9810*
98▲▲–100.0	Chronic neuritis of . . . . due to infection. *Specify nerve and organism (page 57) when known*	*9810*
96▲▲–100.9	Faulty regeneration, postinfectious (synkinesis). *Specify nerve*	*9610*
96▲▲–1764	Ganglionitis of . . . . *Specify ganglion, e.g.*	*9610*
9655–1764	Ganglionitis of geniculate ganglion	*9610*

—3 DISEASES DUE TO INTOXICATION

98▲▲–300.x	Neuralgia of . . . due to poison. *Specify nerve and poison (page 67)*	*9380*
98▲▲–3▲▲	Neuropathy of . . . due to poison. *Specify nerve if localized and poison (page 67)*	*9380*
98▲▲–321	Toxic neuropathy of . . . due to arsenic. *Specify nerve*	*9830*
98▲▲–33212	Toxic neuropathy of . . . due to ethyl alcohol. *Specify nerve*	*9380*

98▲▲–3238	Toxic neuropathy of . . . due to lead. *Specify nerve*	*9380*

—4 DISEASES DUE TO TRAUMA OR PHYSICAL AGENT

98▲▲–409	Avulsion of . . . . *Specify nerve*	*9840*
98▲▲–403	Compression, acute, of . . . . *Specify site*	*9840*
98▲▲–435	Compression of . . . by aneurysm. *Specify site*	*9840*
98▲▲–4x7	Compression of . . . by arteriosclerotic vessel. *Specify site*	*9840*
98▲▲–434	Compression of . . . by dislocation of contiguous joint. *Specify site*	*9840*
98▲▲–4341	Compression of . . . due to displacement or distortion. *Specify site*	*9840*
9833–4341	Compression of brachial plexus (medial cord) due to displacement	*9840*
98▲▲–438	Compression of . . . by foreign body. *Specify site*	*9840*
98▲▲–436	Compression of . . . by fracture of contiguous bone. *Specify site*	*9840*
98▲▲–43x	Compression of . . . by hemorrhage or clot. *Specify site*	*9840*
98▲▲–4362	Compression of . . . by scar tissue. *Specify site*	*9840*
96▲▲–4353	Compression of . . . cranial nerve by meningeal adhesions. *Specify nerve*	*9640*
98▲▲–402	Contusion of . . . . *Specify site*	*9840*
98▲▲–460	Electrical shock of . . . . *Specify site*	*9840*
98▲▲–4▲▲	Injury of . . . . *Specify nerve and trauma*	*9840*
98▲▲–4363	Irritation of . . . by scar tissue. *Specify site*	*9840*
98▲▲–412	Laceration of . . . . *Specify site*	*9840*
9874–430	Meralgia paresthetica	*9840*
98▲▲–400.x	Neuralgia of . . . due to trauma. *Specify site*	*9840*
98▲▲–4x6	Neuroma of . . . due to trauma. *Specify site*	*9840*
96▲▲–4351	Neuropathy of . . . cranial nerve following premature closure of cranial sutures. *Specify nerve*	*9640*
965–430	Neuropathy of facial nerve (Bell's palsy) due to pressure. *Distinguish from neuritis due to infection or acute compression of nerve. When palsy is not due to pressure, diagnose disease or other injury of nerve*	*9640*

96▲▲–415.x	Paralysis of . . . cranial nerve following operation. *Specify nerve*	*9640*
98▲▲–4091	Stretching of . . . . *Specify site*	*9840*

—50 DISEASES DUE TO CIRCULATORY DISTURBANCE
Record primary diagnosis when possible

98▲▲–514	Neuropathy, ischemic, of . . . due to circulatory obstruction. *Specify nerve*	*9850*
98▲▲–532	Neuropathy of . . . due to hemorrhage. *Specify nerve*	*9850*
98▲▲–563.x	Toxic neuralgia of . . . due to remote infection. *Specify nerve and organism when known as preceding*	*9855*
98▲▲–563	Toxic neuropathy of . . . due to remote infection. *Specify nerve and organism (page 88) when known, e.g.*	*9855*
9636–5631	Neuropathy of abducens nerve due to diphtheria toxin	*9655*

—7 DISEASES DUE TO DISORDER OF METABOLISM, GROWTH, OR NUTRITION

If multiple, use 980–. If not multiple, indicate specific nerve affected by means of digits and in the written diagnosis.

98▲▲–785	Diabetic neuropathy of . . . . *Specify nerve*	*9870*
98▲▲–711	Neuropathy due to cachexia	*9870*
98▲▲–781	Neuropathy of . . . due to hypercortisonism. *Specify nerve*	*9870*
98▲▲–784	Neuropathy of . . . due to hyperinsulinism. *Specify nerve*	*9870*
98▲▲–76▲▲	Neuropathy due to vitamin deficiency. *Specify (page 67)*	*9870*
98▲▲–749	Neuropathy of . . . due to porphyria. *Specify nerve*	*9870*
98▲▲–702	Peripheral neuropathy of . . . due to pernicious anemia. *Specify nerve*	*9870*

—8 NEW GROWTHS

When a neoplasm involving the peripheral nerves arises from the neighboring structures, it should be diagnosed according to its anatomic site of origin, and its nature, if known, indicated.

Diagnosis of neoplasm if not verified by operation or autopsy should have y at the end of the code.

98▲–8451	Neurofibroma. *Specify site and behavior*	*9880*
98▲–8453A	Neurofibromatosis. *Specify site*	*9880*
98▲–8453B	Plexiform neuroma. *Specify site*	*9880*

| 98▲–8452 | Schwannoma, malignant. *Specify behavior* | *9880* |
| 98▲–8▲▲▲ | Unlisted tumor of peripheral nerves. *Specify neoplasm and behavior* | *9880* |

—9 DISEASES DUE TO UNKNOWN OR UNCERTAIN CAUSE WITH THE STRUCTURAL REACTION MANIFEST; AND HEREDITARY AND FAMILIAL DISEASES OF THIS NATURE

98▲▲–922	Amyloidosis of . . . . *Specify nerve*	*9890*
9624–911	Primary optic atrophy, nonfamilial	*9690*
980–997	Progressive hypertrophic interstitial neuropathy	*9890*

—X DISEASES DUE TO UNKNOWN OR UNCERTAIN CAUSE WITH THE FUNCTIONAL REACTION ALONE MANIFEST

980–x10	Erythredema polyneuropathy	*9890*
965–x40	Facial nerve pain	*9690*
965–x20	Facial nerve pain, atypical	*9690*
9651–x30	Geniculate neuralgia	*9690*
967–x30	Glossopharyngeal neuralgia	*9690*
967–x301	Glossopharyngeal neuralgia with carotid sinus syndrome	*9690*
9▲▲–x30	Other types of neuralgia. *Specify nerve*	*9090*
99x2–x30	Sphenopalatine neuralgia	*9690*
964–x30	Trigeminal neuralgia	*9690*
9641–x30	Of first division	*9690*
9642–x30	Of second division	*9690*
9643–x30	Of third division	*9690*
9644–x30	Of mixed division	*9690*

DISEASES OF THE VEGETATIVE NERVOUS SYSTEM

The majority of disturbances of the vegetative nervous system are inserted either in the supplementary terms list or in the sections devoted to organs, regions, or the skin, owing to the fact that the relation of these diseases to the vegetative nervous system is uncertain or obscure. If in any case the disease can be clearly allocated to structures in the vegetative nervous system, it is to be inserted here under its proper etiologic category.

990– Vegetative nervous system

For detailed list of topographic classification, see page 49

—4 DISEASES DUE TO TRAUMA OR PHYSICAL AGENT

994–4▲▲▲x	Cervical sympathetic paralysis. *See also Supplementary Terms, page 501, for secondary paralysis*	*9940*
994–430.x	Cervical sympathetic paralysis due to pressure	*9940*
994–415.x	Cervical sympathetic paralysis following operation	*9940*
99▲–4▲▲	Injury of ganglion. *Specify ganglion (page 49) and injury (page 83)*	*9940*

—8 NEW GROWTHS

990–840A	Ganglioneuroma	*9980*
990–842F	Neuroepithelioma. *Specify behavior*	*9980*
990–8432	Paraganglioma. *Specify behavior*	*9980*
990–8431	Pheochromocytoma. *Specify behavior*	*9980*
990–841F	Sympathicoblastoma	*9980*
990–8▲▲▲	Unlisted tumor of vegetative nervous system. *Specify neoplasm and behavior*	*9980*

—X DISEASES DUE TO UNKNOWN OR UNCERTAIN CAUSE WITH THE FUNCTIONAL REACTION ALONE MANIFEST

994–x30	Autonomic faciocephalalgia	*9990*
994–x20	Facial neuralgia, atypical	*9990*
994–x40	Facial neuralgia, sympathetic	*9990*

X1– DISEASES OF THE EYE
DISEASES OF THE EYEBALL

See also under Orbit, *page 458*

x11– Eyeball
x19– Anterior chamber

—0 DISEASES DUE TO GENETIC AND PRENATAL INFLUENCES

x11–011	Anophthalmos	*5901*
x11–024	Cyclopia	*5901*
x11–050	Luxation of eyeball due to birth injury	*5901*
x11–076	Microphthalmos	*5901*
x11–012	Rudimentary eye	*5901*

—I DISEASES DUE TO INFECTION WITH LOWER ORGANISM

x11–100.1	Atrophy of eyeball due to infection	*5910*
x11–100	Panophthalmitis	*5910*

—3 DISEASES DUE TO INTOXICATION

x11–3▲▲	Chemical burn of eyeball. *Specify poison* (*page 67*)	*5930*
x11–3237	Siderosis of eyeball	*5930*

—4 DISEASES DUE TO TRAUMA OR PHYSICAL AGENT

x11–415.x	Absence of eyeball following operation	*5940*
x11–400.9	Atrophy of eyeball due to trauma	*5940*
x11–409	Avulsion of eyeball	*5940*
x19–496	Foreign body in anterior chamber	*5940*
x11–4▲▲	Injury of eyeball. *Specify (page 83), e.g.*	*5940*
x11–4111	Penetrating wound of eyeball	*5940*
x11–415	Surgical wound of eyeball	*5940*

—50 DISEASES DUE TO CIRCULATORY DISTURBANCE

x19–5x7	Hyphemia	*5950*

—7 DISEASES DUE TO DISORDER OF METABOLISM, GROWTH, OR NUTRITION

x11–771	Exophthalmos due to hyperthyroidism (*Record primary diagnosis*)	*5970*

—9 DISEASES DUE TO UNKNOWN OR UNCERTAIN CAUSE WITH THE STRUCTURAL REACTION MANIFEST

x11–9x9	Atrophy of eyeball due to unknown cause	*5990*

DISEASES OF THE CORNEA

x12–   Cornea
x121–   Superficial layer
x122–   Stroma
x123–   Deep layer
x124–   Descemet's membrane
x125–   Endothelium
x126–   Limbus

For detailed structures concerned in vision, see page 49

—0 DISEASES DUE TO GENETIC AND PRENATAL INFLUENCES

x12–092	Arcus juvenilis (embryotoxon), congenital	5901
x12–012	Changes, corneal, due to congenital defects in Descemet's membrane	5901
x12–0223	Cornea plana	5901
x12–0224	Keratoconus	5901
x12–019	Corneal opacity, congenital (leukoma)	5901
x12–027	Keratectasia	5901
x12–050	Keratitis due to injury at birth	5901
x12–1471	Keratitis, syphilitic, congenital	5901
x12–013	Megalocornea (without hypertension)	5901
x12–074	Melanosis of cornea, congenital	5901
x12–016	Microcornea	5901

—I DISEASES DUE TO INFECTION WITH LOWER ORGANISM

x12–100.2	Abscess of cornea. *Specify organism (page 57) when known*	5910
x124–100.9	Descemetocele	5910
x12–100.6	Ectasia cornea	5910
x12–100.3	Fistula of cornea due to infection	5910
x12–166	Herpes, keratitis disciformis	5913
x12–190	Infiltrate, corneal	5910
x12–147	Interstitial keratitis due to syphilis	5913
x123–147	Keratitis punctata profunda; keratitis pustuliformis profunda	5913
x123–130	Keratitis, deep. *Specify organism*	5913
x122–1762	Keratitis disciformis postvaccinulosa	5913
x122–130	Keratitis, parenchymatous	5913
x121–1235	Keratitis, phlyctenular	5913
x12–1x6	Keratocele	5910
x127–18x2	Keratoconjunctivitis, epidemic	5913
x12–124	Leprosy of cornea; keratitis punctata leprosa	5913

x12–1x0.9	Melanosis of cornea due to uveitis	*5910*
x12–100.4	Opacity of cornea due to infection. *Specify organism when known*	*5910*
x12–1x41	Nebula	*5910*
x12–1x42	Macula	*5910*
x12–1x43	Leukoma	*5910*
x12–194.6	Pannus due to trachoma	*5910*
x12–1x9.3	Perforation of cornea due to infection (ulcerative)	*5910*
x12–100.8	Staphyloma of cornea	*5910*
x12–123	Tuberculous keratitis	*5913*
x12–100.9	Ulcer, cornea, due to infection. *Specify organism (page 57) when known*	*5910*
x12▲–1x91	Ulcer, ring, of cornea	*5910*
x121–1x93	Ulcer, superficial marginal	*5910*
x12–101.9	Ulcus serpens, pneumococcic. *Specify when another organism is responsible*	*5910*
x12–1764	Zoster of cornea	*5910*

—2 DISEASES DUE TO HIGHER PLANT OR ANIMAL PARASITE

x12–2▲▲	Keratomycosis. *Specify fungus (page 63)*	*5920*

—3 DISEASES DUE TO INTOXICATION

x121–390.6	Allergic (eczematous) pannus	*5930*
x12–3253	Argyrosis of cornea	*5930*
x12–3231	Chalcosis of cornea	*5930*
x12–3▲▲	Chemical burn of cornea. *Specify poison (page 67)*	*5930*
x12–300	Metallic incrustation of cornea. *Specify metal*	*5930*
x12–3238	Lead incrustation of cornea	*5930*
x12–3▲▲.4	Opacity of cornea. *Specify poison*	*5930*
x12–33613	Opacity of cornea due to aniline	*5930*
x12–3237	Siderosis of cornea	*5930*
x12–300.8	Staphyloma of cornea due to poison. *Specify poison (page 67)*	*5930*
x12–3263	Zinc incrustation of cornea	*5930*

—4 DISEASES DUE TO TRAUMA OR PHYSICAL AGENT

x12–401	Abrasion of cornea	*5940*
x12–441	Burn of cornea	*5940*
x12–472.0	Burn of cornea from radium	*5940*
x12–471.0	Burn of cornea from roentgen rays (x-rays)	*5940*

x126–400.4	Cicatrix of limbus due to trauma. *Specify injury*	5940
x12–402	Contusion of cornea	5940
x12–400.4	Corneal opacity, due to trauma. *Specify injury*	5940
x126–400.8	Cystoid cicatrix of limbus due to trauma. *Specify injury*	5940
x124–416	Descemet's membrane, defect of	5940
x12–4x9	Erosion of cornea, recurrent	5940
x12–400.3	Fistula of cornea due to trauma. *Specify injury*	5940
x12–496	Foreign body in cornea	5940
x12–4▲▲	Injury of cornea. *Specify injury (page 83)*	5940
x12–430	Keratitis due to lagophthalmos. *When the lagophthalmos is the result of remote disease, show the latter in the primary diagnosis*	5940
x12–430.5	Rupture of cornea due to increased intraocular pressure	5940
x12–444	Scald of cornea	5940
x12–400.8	Staphyloma of cornea due to trauma. *Specify injury*	5940
x12–451	Sunburn (ultraviolet) of cornea	5940
x12–400.9	Ulcer of cornea due to trauma	5940
x12–41▲	Wound of cornea. *Specify type, e.g.*	5940
x12–412	Wound of cornea, lacerated	5940
x12–415	Wound of cornea, surgical	5940
x12–4111	Wound of cornea, penetrating	5940
x12–4101	Wound of cornea, perforating	5940

—50 DISEASES DUE TO CIRCULATORY DISTURBANCE
Record primary diagnosis when possible

x12–532	Blood staining of cornea	5950

—55 DISEASES DUE TO DISTURBANCE OF INNERVATION OR OF PSYCHIC CONTROL
Record primary diagnosis when possible

x12–565	Keratitis neuroparalytica	5955

—7 DISEASES DUE TO DISORDER OF METABOLISM, GROWTH, OR NUTRITION

x127–7x1	Keratoconjunctivitis, sicca	5970
x12–761	Keratomalacia	5970
x12–798	Linea corneae senilis	5970
x12–745	Melanosis of cornea	5970

—8 NEW GROWTHS

x12–814	Epidermoid carcinoma of cornea. *Specify behavior* (*page 99*)	*5980*
x12–8701A	Keloid of cornea	*5980*
x12–8451	Neurofibroma of cornea. *Specify behavior* (*page 99*)	*5980*
x12–8▲▲▲	Unlisted tumor of cornea. *Specify neoplasm and behavior* (*page 99*)	*5980*

—9 DISEASES DUE TO UNKNOWN OR UNCERTAIN CAUSE WITH THE STRUCTURAL REACTION MANIFEST

x126–950	Arcus senilis	*5990*
x12–995	Degeneration, corneal, familial	*5990*
x12–9951	Degeneration, corneal, familial, nodular	*5990*
x12–9952	Degeneration, corneal, familial, granular or macular	*5990*
x12–9953	Degeneration, corneal, familial, lattice or reticular	*5990*
x12–910	Dystrophy of cornea. *Specify type*	*5990*
x12–9101	Epithelial	*5990*
x12–9102	Endothelial (cornea guttata)	*5990*
x12–9103	Marginal	*5990*
x12–9x8	Keratitis bullosa due to unknown cause	*5990*
x12–912	Keratoconus	*5990*
x121–923	Keratopathy, band	*5990*
x12–921	Lipid degeneration of cornea following keratitis	*5990*
x12–952	Pannus degenerativus	*5990*
x12–924	Siderosis of cornea due to unknown cause	*5990*

DISEASES OF THE SCLERA

x13– Sclera

—0 DISEASES DUE TO GENETIC AND PRENATAL INFLUENCES

x13–074	Melanosis of sclera, congenital	*5901*

—I DISEASES DUE TO INFECTION WITH LOWER ORGANISM

x13–190	Annular scleritis	*5910*
x13–100.6	Ectasia of sclera	*5910*
x13–100	Scleritis, anterior, due to infection. *Specify organism when known*	*5910*
x13–100.8	Staphyloma of sclera due to infection. *Specify organism when known*	*5910*

—3 DISEASES DUE TO INTOXICATION

x13–390	Episcleritis periodica fugax (angioneurotic)	*5930*

—4 DISEASES DUE TO TRAUMA

x13–496	Foreign body in sclera	*5940*
x13–4..	Injury of sclera. *Specify (page 83)*	*5940*
x13–410	Wound of sclera	*5940*
x13–416	Rupture of sclera due to trauma	*5940*
x13–430.5	Rupture of sclera due to increased intraocular pressure (glaucoma)	*5940*

—8 NEW GROWTHS

x13–8...	Unlisted tumor of sclera. *Specify neoplasm and behavior (page 99)*	*5980*

—9 DISEASES DUE TO UNKNOWN OR UNCERTAIN CAUSE WITH THE STRUCTURAL REACTION MANIFEST

x13–996	Blue sclera (with fragility of bone and deafness)	*5990*
x13–952	Rheumatoid scleritis	*5990*

DISEASES OF THE IRIS

x15– Iris
x16– Ciliary body
x14– Uveal tract
x38– Mechanism for pupil

—0 DISEASES DUE TO GENETIC AND PRENATAL INFLUENCES

x15–079	Albinism	*5901*
x15–012	Aniridia	*5901*
x16–01x	Coloboma of ciliary body	*5901*
x15–016	Coloboma of iris, partial	*5901*
x15–01x	Coloboma of iris, complete	*5901*
x15–026	Corectopia	*5901*
x15–064	Cyst of iris, congenital	*5901*
x15–027	Ectropion uveae	*5901*
x15–074	Heterochromia iridis	*5901*
x15–0161	Notch of iris	*5901*
x15–019	Persistent pupillary membrane	*5901*
x15–034	Polycoria	*5901*

—1 DISEASES DUE TO INFECTION WITH LOWER ORGANISM

x15–100.9	Atrophy of iris. *Specify organism*	*5910*
x14–100	Endophthalmitis. *Specify organism* (*page 57*) *when known*	*5910*
x15–100.7	Hemorrhage of iris due to infection	*5910*
x15–100	Iritis; iridocyclitis. *Specify organism* (*page 57*) *when known*	*5910*
x15–100.6	Occlusion of pupil due to infection	*5910*
x15–1x4	Iris bombé	*5910*
x151–1x4	Synechia, anterior, due to infection	*5910*
x152–100.4	Synechia, posterior. *Specify organism when known*	*5910*
x14–130	Uveitis, sympathetic	*5910*
x15–1764	Zoster of iris	*5910*

—3 DISEASES DUE TO INTOXICATION

x15–390	Iritis (iridocyclitis) due to allergy. *Specify allergen* (*page 67*) *when known*	*5930*
x38–3483	Miosis due to opium or a derivative	*5930*
x38–34649	Miosis due to pilocarpine	*5930*
x38–34648	Miosis due to physostigmine	*5930*
x38–38▲	Mydriasis due to another plant or animal poison. *Specify* (*page 67*) *if known*	*5930*
x38–34652	Due to homatropine	*5930*

x38–34611	Due to epinephrine	*5930*
x14–390	Phaco-anaphylactic uveitis. *Record primary diagnosis*	*5930*
x14–393	Phaco-toxic uveitis. *Record primary diagnosis*	*5930*
x15–3237	Siderosis of iris	*5930*

—4 DISEASES DUE TO TRAUMA OR PHYSICAL AGENT

x15–400.4	Anterior synechia due to trauma. *Specify injury*	*5940*
x15–415.1	Coloboma of iris following operation	*5940*
x15–496	Foreign body in iris	*5940*
x15–400.8	Implantation cyst of iris	*5940*
x15–4▲▲	Injury of iris. *Specify (page 83) as*	*5940*
x15–4101	Perforation of iris	*5940*
x15–405	Iridodialysis due to trauma	*5940*
x15–4xx	Iridodonesis	*5940*
x15–4x9	Prolapse of iris	*5940*
x15–4x91	Incarceration of iris	*5940*
x15–4x93	Iridencleisis	*5940*
x15–4x94	Iridotasis	*5940*
x15–416	Rupture of iris	*5940*

—55 DISEASES DUE TO DISTURBANCE OF INNERVATION OR OF PSYCHIC CONTROL
Record primary diagnosis when possible

x38–580	Changes in pupil due to disturbance of sympathetic innervation	*5955*
x38–587	Miosis due to lesion of central nervous system	*5955*
x38–586	Mydriasis due to lesion of central nervous system	*5955*

—7 DISEASES DUE TO DISORDER OF METABOLISM, GROWTH, OR NUTRITION
Record primary diagnosis when possible

x15–798.5	Iridoschisis due to senile atrophy	*5970*

—8 NEW GROWTHS

x15–850A	Hemangioma of iris	*5980*
x15–866A	Leiomyoma of iris	*5980*
x14–8173	Melanoma, malignant, of uveal tract. *Specify behavior*	*5980*
x16–8170	Pigmented nevus of ciliary body. *Specify behavior*	*5980*
x15–8170	Pigmented nevus of iris. *Specify behavior*	*5980*
x15–8▲▲▲	Unlisted tumor of iris. *Specify neoplasm and behavior (page 99)*	

DISEASES OF THE CHOROID

x17–   Choroid
x24–   Choroid and retina

—0 DISEASES DUE TO GENETIC AND PRENATAL INFLUENCES

x17–01x	Coloboma of choroid	*5901*
x24–016	Crescent or conus, congenital	*5901*

—I DISEASES DUE TO INFECTION WITH LOWER ORGANISM

x17–100	Choroiditis. *Specify organism when known*	*5910*
x17–100.5	Detachment of choroid due to infection	*5910*

—4 DISEASES DUE TO TRAUMA OR PHYSICAL AGENT

x17–400.5	Detachment of choroid due to trauma	*5940*
x17–415.5	Detachment of choroid following operation	*5940*
x17–4..	Injury of choroid. *Specify (page 83)*	*5940*
x17–416	Rupture of choroid	*5940*

—50 DISEASES DUE TO CIRCULATORY DISTURBANCE
Record primary diagnosis when possible

x24–5x9	Atrophia gyrata of choroid and retina	*5950*
x17–532	Detachment of choroid due to hemorrhage	*5950*

—8 NEW GROWTHS

x17–850A	Hemangioma of choroid	*5980*
x17–8173	Melanoma, malignant, of choroid. *Specify behavior*	*5980*
x17–8451	Neurofibroma of choroid. *Specify behavior (page 99)*	*5980*
x17–8170	Pigmented nevus of choroid. *Specify behavior*	*5980*
x17–8▲▲▲	Unlisted tumor of choroid. *Specify neoplasm and behavior (page 99)*	*5980*

—9 DISEASES DUE TO UNKNOWN OR UNCERTAIN CAUSE WITH THE STRUCTURAL REACTION MANIFEST

x17–942	Arteriosclerosis of choroidal vessels	*5990*
x17–911	Atrophy of choroid	*5990*
x17–929	Colloid degeneration of choroid, familial	*5990*
x17–928	Drusen of choroid	*5990*

DISEASES OF THE CRYSTALLINE LENS

x20–   Crystalline lens
x21–   Capsule of lens

—0 DISEASES DUE TO GENETIC AND PRENATAL INFLUENCES

x20–011	Aphakia, congenital (absence of lens)	*5901*
x20–077	Cataract, congenital	*5901*
x20–01x	Coloboma of lens	*5901*
x20–026	Ectopia of lens, congenital	*5901*
x20–016	Microphakia	*5901*

—I DISEASES DUE TO INFECTION WITH LOWER ORGANISM

x20–100.9	Cataract due to uveitis	*5972*

—2 DISEASES DUE TO HIGHER PLANT OR ANIMAL PARASITE

x20–2▲▲	Parasites in lens. *Specify* (*page 63*)	*5920*

—3 DISEASES DUE TO INTOXICATION

x20–390	Cataract with atopic dermatitis	*5972*
x20–3▲▲	Cataract due to toxic agent. *Specify agent*	*5972*
x20–3231	Metallic deposit in lens. *Specify metal,* *e.g.*	*5930*
x20–3237	Siderosis in lens	*5930*

—4 DISEASES DUE TO TRAUMA OR PHYSICAL AGENT

x20–415.6	After cataract following operation	*5972*
x20–400.x	Aphakia due to trauma	*5940*
x20–415.x	Aphakia following operation	*5940*
x20–400.0	Cateract due to injury. *Specify injury*	*5972*
x20–4▲▲.x	Cataract due to physical agent	*5972*
x20–47▲	Cataract due to radiant injury	*5972*
x20–496	Foreign body in lens	*5940*
x20–4▲▲	Injury of lens. *Specify injury*	*5940*
x21–402	Lens, contusion lesion of (Vossius ring)	*5940*

—6 DISEASES DUE TO OR CONSISTING OF STATIC MECHANICAL ABNOR-MALITY
Record primary diagnosis when possible

x20–630	Luxation of lens	*5960*
x20–6301	Complete	*5960*
x20–6302	Partial	*5960*

—7 DISEASES DUE TO DISORDER OF METABOLISM, GROWTH, OR NUTRITION
Record primary diagnosis when possible

x20–772	Cataract in myxedema	*5972*
x20–785	Diabetic cataract	*5972*
x20–797	Senile cataract	*5972*
x20–774	Tetany cataract	*5972*

—9 DISEASES DUE TO UNKNOWN OR UNCERTAIN CAUSE WITH THE STRUCTURAL REACTION MANIFEST
Record primary diagnosis when known

x20–9x6	Cataract cause unknown	*5972*
x20–992	Cataract in myotonic dystrophy	*5972*

—X DISEASES DUE TO UNKNOWN OR UNCERTAIN CAUSE WITH THE FUNCTIONAL REACTION ALONE MANIFEST

x21–x21	Exfoliation of lens capsule	*5990*

DISEASES OF THE VITREOUS

x22–   Vitreous

—0 DISEASES DUE TO GENETIC AND PRENATAL INFLUENCES

x4x–019	Persistent hyaloid artery (generally incomplete)	5901
x22–01x	Persistent primary vitreous	5901
x22–019	Vestigial structures. *See also under* Diseases of the crystalline lens, *page 442*	5901
	Membrana capsularis lentis posterior	
	Remains of canal of Cloquet	
	Muscae volitantes ; myiodesopsia	
	Congenital fine vitreous opacities	

—I DISEASES DUE TO INFECTION WITH LOWER ORGANISM

x22–100.2	Abscess in vitreous. *Specify organism (page 57) when known*	5910
x22–1x6	Connective tissue formation in vitreous	5910
x22–100.5	Detachment of vitreous	5910
x22–1x0	New tissue formation in vitreous due to infection	5910
x221–1x9	Calcification of vitreous	5910
x222–1x9	Ossification of vitreous	5910
x22–100.4	Opacity in vitreous due to remote infection. *Specify organism (page 57) when known*	5910

—2 DISEASES DUE TO HIGHER PLANT OR ANIMAL PARASITE

x22–2▲▲	Parasites and fungi in vitreous. *Specify (page 63), e.g.*	5920
x22–240	Nematodes in vitreous	5920

—3 DISEASES DUE TO INTOXICATION

x20–3237	Siderosis of vitreous	5930

—4 DISEASES DUE TO TRAUMA OR PHYSICAL AGENT

x22–400.2	Abscess of vitreous due to trauma	5940
x22–496	Foreign body in vitreous	5940
x22–400.7	Hemorrhage in vitreous. *Specify injury*	5940
x22–400.9	Hernia of vitreous into anterior chamber. *Specify injury*	5940
x22–4▲▲	Injury of vitreous. *Specify (page 83)*	5940
x22–4111	Penetrating wound of vitreous	**5940**

| x22–406 | Prolapse of vitreous | *5940* |
| x22–4061 | Loss of vitreous | *5940* |

—50 DISEASES DUE TO CIRCULATORY DISTURBANCE
Record primary diagnosis when possible

| x22–500.7 | Hemorrhage in vitreous | *5950* |
| x22–5x7.9 | Opacities in vitreous due to hemorrhage | *5950* |

—7 DISEASES DUE TO DISORDER OF METABOLISM, GROWTH, OR NUTRITION
Record primary diagnosis when possible

| x22–797 | Senile synchysis of vitreous | *5970* |

—9 DISEASES DUE TO UNKNOWN OR UNCERTAIN CAUSE WITH THE STRUCTURAL REACTION MANIFEST

| x22–920 | Opacity in vitreous due to unknown cause | *5990* |

DISEASES OF THE RETINA

x23–   Retina
x24–   Retina and choroid
x25–   Central area
x26–   Peripheral area
x27–   Inner layer
x28–   Outer layer
x1x–   Intrinsic veins
x3x–   Intrinsic arteries
x2x–   Intrinsic vessels
932–   Cortex, generally

—0 DISEASES DUE TO GENETIC AND PRENATAL INFLUENCES

x23–041	Amaurosis, congenital	5901
x23–042	Amblyopia, congenital	5901
x2x–024	Anastomosis of retinal and choroidal vessels	5901
x25–016	Aplasia of fovea centralis	5901
x2x–029	Arteriovenous aneurysm of retina, congenital	5901
x3x–019	Cilioretinal artery, persistent	5901
x1x–019	Cilioretinal vein, persistent	5901
x23–019	Coloboma of retina	5901
x24–019	Coloboma of retina and choroid	5901
x23–0x4	Color blindness, congenital	5901

HERING CLASSIFICATION

x23–0x0	Achromatopsia, total color blindness	5901
x23–0x1	Anomalous trichromatopsia	5901
x23–0x2	Dichromatopsia (see blue and yellow, not red and green)	5901
x23–0x3	Trichromatopsia, normal	5901
x23–064	Cysts in retina	5901
x25–092	Degeneration, macular, congenital; infantile type of retinal atrophy	5901
x23–074	Grouped pigmentation of retina (nevoid pigmentation)	5901
x23–045	Night blindness, congenital	5901
x1x–013	Tortuous veins of retina	5901

—I DISEASES DUE TO INFECTION WITH LOWER ORGANISM

x23–100.9	Atrophy of retina due to infection	5910
x23–1x9.5	Detachment of retina due to atrophy	5910
x24–100	Chorioretinitis. *Specify organism when known*	5910

x23–100.5	Detachment of retina due to infection of uveal tract	5910
x1x–100	Endophlebitis of retinal veins due to infection. *Specify organism (page 57) when known*	5910
x3x–100.5	Hemorrhage in retina due to infection	5910
x1x–190	Periphlebitis. *Specify organism (page 57) when known*	5910
x23–100	Retinitis. *Specify organism (page 57) when known*	5912
x24–1x0	Retinochoroiditis juxtapapillaris	5912
x24–1471	Syphilis of retina, congenital and delayed (syphilis congenita et tarda)	5912
x23–1472	Neurorecidive syphilis of retina	5912
x23–123	Tuberculosis of retina	5912

—2 DISEASES DUE TO HIGHER PLANT OR ANIMAL PARASITE

| x23–266.5 | Detachment of retina due to subretinal cysticercosis | 5920 |

—3 DISEASES DUE TO INTOXICATION

x23–340	Cyanosis of retina due to intoxication by organic poison. *Specify (page 67)*	5930
x3x–3151	Hemorrhage of retina due to carbon monoxide poisoning	5930
x23–388	Retinitis gravidarum	5630
x23–351.6	Retrolental fibroplasia	5930
x3x–388	Spasm of retinal artery due to pregnancy	5630
932–389	Uremic amaurosis	5930
932–3891	Uremic amblyopia	5930

—4 DISEASES DUE TO TRAUMA OR PHYSICAL AGENT

x23–428	Commotio retinae	5940
x24–4x0	Chorioretinitis due to trauma	5940
x23–400.9	Degeneration of retina due to trauma	5940
x23–415.5	Detachment of retina following operation	5945
x23–400.5	Detachment of retina due to trauma	5945
x23–4▲▲	Injury of retina. *Specify (page 83)*	5940
x23–414	Gunshot wound of retina	5940
x23–4x3	Hole in retina due to trauma	5940

—50 DISEASES DUE TO CIRCULATORY DISTURBANCE

| x23–516 | Arteriosclerotic disease of retina | 5950 |
| x23–500.9 | Atrophy of retina due to circulatory disturbance | 5950 |

x23–511.9	Due to thrombosis	*5950*
x23–512.9	Due to embolism	*5950*
x23–532	Detachment of retina due to hemorrhage	*5950*
x2x–540.5	Hemorrhage of retina due to blood dyscrasia	*5950*
x2x–549.5	Hemorrhage of retina due to hemorrhagic purpura	*5950*
x2x–533	Hypertensive vascular disease of intrinsic vessels of retina	*5950*
x23–5x7	Infarction of retina	*5950*
x23–511	Due to thrombosis	*5950*
x23–512	Due to embolism	*5950*
x23–516.7	Ischemia of retina due to arteriosclerosis	*5950*
x28–532	Retinitis exudativa	*5950*
x23–532.5	Detachment of retina due to retinitis exudativa	*5950*
x27–532	Retinitis proliferans	*5950*
x23–510	Visual disturbances (blindness) from loss of blood	*5950*

—55 DISEASES DUE TO DISTURBANCE OF INNERVATION OR OF PSYCHIC CONTROL

x3x–582	Spasm of retinal artery	*5955*
x3x–590	Spasm of retinal artery due to arterio-sclerosis	*5955*

—6 DISEASES DUE TO OR CONSISTING OF STATIC MECHANICAL ABNOR-MALITY

x25–652	Chorioretinitis of progressive myopia	*5960*
x3x–618	Embolism of retinal artery	*5960*
x2x–619	Thrombosis of retinal vessel	*5960*
x2x–619.5	Retinal hemorrhage due to thrombosis	*5960*

—7 DISEASES DUE TO DISORDER OF METABOLISM, GROWTH, OR NUTRITION
Record primary diagnosis when possible

x23–757	Cholesterol deposit in retina	*5970*
x2x–763	Hemorrhage of retina due to scurvy	*5970*
x2x–785.5	Hemorrhage of retina due to diabetes	*5970*
x23–755	Lipemia, retinal	*5970*
x25–798	Macula, senile (including presenile) degeneration of	*5970*
x28–794	Medullated nerve fibers on retina	*5970*
x23–761	Night blindness due to xerophthalmia	*5970*
x25–797	Retinopathy, circinata	*5970*
x23–785	Retinopathy, diabetic	*5970*

—8 NEW GROWTHS

x23–850A	Hemangioma of retina	*5980*
x23–851	Hemangiomatosis of retina. *Specify behavior (page 99)*	*5980*
x23–842F	Neuroepithelioma (retinoblastoma)	*5980*
x23–8▲▲▲	Unlisted tumor of retina. *Specify neoplasm and behavior (page 99)*	*5980*

—9 DISEASES DUE TO UNKNOWN OR UNCERTAIN CAUSE WITH THE STRUCTURAL REACTION MANIFEST; HEREDITARY AND FAMILIAL DISEASES OF THIS NATURE

x3x–942	Arteriosclerosis of retinal vessels	*5990*
x3x–942.5	Retinal hemorrhage due to arteriosclerosis	*5990*
x23–992	Atrophy, progressive retinal	*5990*
x23–992.5	Detachment of retina due to progressive atrophy	*5990*
x27–996	Atrophy, retinal, in infantile amaurotic familial idiocy	*5990*
x28–996	Atrophy, retinal, in juvenile amaurotic familial idiocy	*5990*
x23–9x5	Detachment of retina due to unknown cause	*5990*
x23–9x5.5	Detachment of retina due to unknown cause, recurrent	*5990*
x1x–942	Endophlebitis of retinal vein due to unknown cause	*5990*
x1x–942.5	Hemorrhage of retina due to endophlebitis	*5990*
x25–911	Macula, degeneration of	*5990*
x25–9x8	Cystoid degeneration of macula	*5990*
x25–992	Hereditary degeneration of macula	*5990*
x25–9111	Infantile degeneration of macula	*5990*
x25–996	Macular heredodegeneration	*5990*
x26–996	Primary pigmentary degeneration at the retina	*5990*
x25–956	Retinitis disciformis	*5990*

DISEASES OF THE OPTIC NERVE

962–   Optic pathway
x29–   Optic papilla
9621–   Papillomacular bundle of optic nerve'
9622–   Peripheral fibers of optic nerve
9623–   Retrobulbar (orbital portion)
9624–   Intracranial portion
9625–   Canalicular portion
9626–   Optic chiasm
9627–   Optic tract
9362–   Cortical visual center
946–   Basal ganglia

For detailed list of structures, see page 46

—0 DISEASES DUE TO GENETIC AND PRENATAL INFLUENCES

x2x–010	Anomaly of vessels of papilla	*5901*
x2x–019	Anomaly of optico-ciliary vessels	*5901*
x2x–032	Vascular loop on papilla	*5901*
x29–016	Cavity of optic papilla	*5901*
962–01x	Coloboma of optic nerve	*9601*
x29–02x	Inversion of optic papilla	*5901*
x29–015	Large physiologic cup	*5901*
	Medullated nerve fibers on papilla. *See page 448*	
x29–039	Membrana epipapillaris	*5901*
x29–074	Pigmentation of optic papilla	*5901*
x29–013	Pseudoneuritis of optic papilla	*5901*

—1 DISEASES DUE TO INFECTION WITH LOWER ORGANISM

962–100.9	Atrophy of optic nerve due to infection	*9610*
962–147.9	Due to syphilis (including tabes dorsalis)	*9610*
962–100	Optic neuritis. *Specify organism (page 57) when known, e.g.*	*9610*
962–104	Meningococcic optic neuritis	*9610*
9623–1x0	Retrobulbar neuritis due to remote (focal) infection	*9610*
9641–1764	Zoster opthalmicus	*9610*

—3 DISEASES DUE TO INTOXICATION

9623–3▲▲.9	Atrophy of optic nerve due to poison. *Specify poison (page 67), e.g.*	*9630*
9623–3238.9	Due to lead	*9630*
9623–3238	Optic neuritis due to lead	*9630*

9623–3▲▲.x	Toxic amblyopia. *Specify poison* (*page 67*), *e.g.*	*9630*
9623–33131.x	Due to benzene, toluene, etc.	*9630*
9623–33212.x	Due to ethyl alcohol	*9630*
9623–3845.x	Due to Filix mas	*9630*
9623–33211.x	Due to methyl alcohol	*9630*
9623–36171.x	Due to nicotine; tobacco	*9630*
9623–34382.x	Due to quinine or optochin	*9630*
9623–3257.x	Due to thallium	*9630*

—4 DISEASES DUE TO TRAUMA OR PHYSICAL AGENT

962–430	Atrophy of optic nerve due to pressure of arteriosclerotic arteries (senile atrophy)	*9640*
962–400.9	Atrophy of optic nerve due to trauma	*9640*
962–409	Avulsion of optic nerve	*9640*
962–404	Crushing of optic nerve from fracture of bone	*9640*
962–4▲▲	Injury of optic nerve. *Specify injury*	*9640*
962–496	Foreign body in optic nerve	*9640*
x29–43x	Papilledema due to abnormally low intraocular tension	*5940*
x29–43x.9	Atrophy of optic nerve due to low intraocular tension	*5940*
x29–4x8	Papilledema due to trauma	*5940*
x29–435	Papilledema due to pressure	*5940*
x29–435.9	Atrophy of optic nerve due to pressure	*5940*
x29–434	Papilledema due to tower skull	*5940*
9623–435	Retrobulbar neuritis due to pressure	*9640*
962–414	Wound, gunshot, of optic nerve	*9640*

—50 DISEASES DUE TO CIRCULATORY DISTURBANCE

x29–500.9	Atrophy of optic nerve due to circulatory disturbance	*5950*
x29–540	Papilledema due to blood dyscrasia	*5950*
x29–532	Papilledema due to hematoma of orbit	*5950*
x29–501	Papilledema due to increased intracranial pressure	*5950*

—7 DISEASES DUE TO DISORDER OF METABOLISM, GROWTH, OR NUTRITION

962–713	Postretinal atrophy of optic nerve	*9670*

—8 NEW GROWTHS

962–8475	Glioma of optic nerve. *Specify behavior* (*page 99*)	*9680*

962–8451	Neurofibroma of optic nerve. *Specify behavior*	*9680*
962–8▲▲▲	Unlisted tumor of optic nerve. *Specify neoplasm and behavior (page 99)*	*9680*

—9 DISEASES DUE TO UNKNOWN OR UNCERTAIN CAUSE WITH THE STRUCTURAL REACTION MANIFEST

962–900.9	Atrophy of optic nerve due to unknown cause	*9690*
x29–928	Drusen of optic papilla	*5990*
9624–995	Hereditary atrophy of optic nerve	*9690*
962–940	Optic neuritis due to unknown cause	*9690*
9623–953	Optic neuritis (retrobulbar neuritis) in multiple sclerosis	*9690*

GLAUCOMA

x18–   Aqueous

—0 DISEASES DUE TO GENETIC AND PRENATAL INFLUENCES

x11–017   Hydrophthalmos infantile glaucoma   *5901*

—6 DISEASES DUE TO OR CONSISTING OF STATIC MECHANICAL ABNOR-MALITY

x18–600.8   Buphthalmos (hydrophthalmos) due to
                   lesions of early life   *5961*
x18–616   Glaucoma, narrow angle, obstructive type *5961*
x18–6xx   Glaucoma, secondary. *Diagnose primary*
                   disease   *5961*
x18–610.x   Glaucoma, simple (open angle; non-
                   obstructive, noncongestive)   *5961*
x18–610   Glaucoma, type not specified   *5961*
x18–6x0   Glaucoma, without increased intraocular
                   pressure   *5961*

ERRORS OF REFRACTION

x11– Eyeball
x12– Cornea
x20– Lens

—0 DISEASES DUE TO GENETIC AND PRENATAL INFLUENCES

x11–010	Anisometropia	*5901*
x11–016	Hypermetropia, congenital	*5901*
x11–0131	Myopia, congenital	*5901*

—I DISEASES DUE TO INFECTION WITH LOWER ORGANISM

x12–1xx	Irregular astigmatism due to infection.	
	Include astigmatism due to opacity	*5910*

—6 DISEASES DUE TO OR CONSISTING OF STATIC MECHANICAL ABNOR-MALITY

x12–657	Astigmatism, corneal, irregular	*5960*
x11–655	Astigmatism, hypermetropic	*5960*
x11–6551	Astigmatism, hypermetropic, compound	*5960*
x11–654	Astigmatism, mixed	*5960*
x11–656	Astigmatism, myopic	*5960*
x11–6561	Astigmatism, myopic, compound	*5960*
x20–637	Astigmatism due to tilting of lens (includes subluxation)	*5960*
x11–65x	Emmetropia	*5960*
x11–651	Hypermetropia	*5960*
x20–636.x	Hypermetropia due to displacement of lens	*5960*
x11–652	Myopia, axial	*5960*
x11–653	Myopia, curvature	*5960*
x20–635.x	Myopia due to displacement of lens	*5960*
x20–6xx	Myopia due to increased refraction of nucleus of lens	*5960*
x11–6521	Myopia, progressive	*5960*

—7 DISEASES DUE TO DISORDER OF METABOLISM, GROWTH, OR NUTRITION

x20–785.x	Change of refraction due to diabetes. *Record primary diagnosis*	*5970*
x20–79x	Presbyopia	*5970*

ANISEIKONIA

x10–400	Aniseikonia, due to unilateral aphakia	*5940*
x10–650	Aniseikonia, undifferentiated	*5960*

DISEASES OF THE OCULAR NEUROMUSCULAR
MECHANISM FOR BINOCULAR VISION

x30– Neuromuscular mechanism for binocular vision
x31– Mechanism for conjugate lateral movement
x32– Mechanism for convergence
x33– Mechanism for divergence
x34– Mechanism for conjugate movement upward
x35– Mechanism for conjugate movement downward
x36– Mechanism for disjunctive vertical movement
x37– Mechanism for cyclovergence
x38– Mechanism for pupil
x39– Mechanism for accommodation
x40– Extrinsic muscles of eye
2717– Superior rectus
27112– Inferior oblique
27110– Medial (internal) rectus
2718– Inferior rectus
27111– Superior oblique
2719– Lateral (external) rectus

—0 DISEASES DUE TO GENETIC AND PRENATAL INFLUENCES

27▲–012   Absence, partial, of extrinsic muscle,
                congenital   2701
2719–012   Absence, partial, of external rectus, con-
                genital (congenital enophthalmos)   2701
27▲–011   Agenesis of extrinsic muscle. *Specify site.*
                See also Agenesis of extrinsic muscle,
                preceding, and Agenesis of (cranial)
                nerve (*page 428*)   2701
x30–045   Nystagmus, congenital   5901
27▲–04▲   Paralysis of extrinsic muscle, congenital.
                Specify (*page 56*). *See also* Agenesis
                of extrinsic muscle, *preceding, and*
                Agenesis of (cranial) nerve (*page
                428*)   2701
27▲▲–050   Paralysis of extrinsic muscle due to birth
                injury. *Specify site*   2701
x32–043   Strabismus, congenital   5901

—1 DISEASES DUE TO INFECTION WITH LOWER ORGANISM

x3▲–100   Disturbed mechanism. *Specify mechanism
                and organism when known*   5910

—2 DISEASES DUE TO HIGHER PLANT OR ANIMAL PARASITE

x40–200.x   Strabismus due to parasite. *Specify*
                (*page 63*)   5920

—4 DISEASES DUE TO TRAUMA OR PHYSICAL AGENT

x32–4▲▲.x	Esotropia following trauma. *Specify trauma*	*5940*
x33–4▲▲.x	Exotropia following trauma. *Specify trauma*	*5940*
27▲▲–415.9	Strabismus, postoperative. *Specify muscle, e.g.*	*2740*
27110–415.9	Strabismus, postoperative (medial rectus)	*2740*
27▲▲–400.9	Strabismus due to trauma. *Specify muscle, e.g.*	*2740*
2719–400.9	Strabismus due to trauma (lateral rectus)	*2740*

—55 DISEASES DUE TO DISTURBANCE OF INNERVATION OR OF PSYCHIC CONTROL

Record primary diagnosis when possible

x32–595	Esophoria due to error of refraction (hypermetropia)	*5955*
x32–596	Exophoria due to error of refraction (myopia)	*5955*
x37–597	Cyclotropia	*5955*
x32–597	Esotropia	*5955*
x32–5973	Alternating	*5955*
x33–597	Exotropia	*5955*
x33–5973	Alternating	*5955*
x36–597	Hypertropia	*5955*
x30–577.x	Nystagmus of amblyopia	*5955*
x40–567	Paralysis of extrinsic muscles	*5955*
x40–5672	Paralysis of extrinsic muscles (nuclear)	*5955*
x40–5691	Paralysis of extrinsic muscles (nerve root)	*5955*
x40–5692	Paralysis of extrinsic muscles (nerve trunk, intracranial)	*5955*
x40–5693	Paralysis of extrinsic muscles (nerve trunk, intraorbital)	*5955*
27▲▲–56▲	Secondary contracture of extrinsic muscle following paralysis of antagonist. *Specify (page 88)*	*5955*
x39–561	Spasm of accommodation	*5955*
x30–560	Strabismus due to paralysis of ocular muscles	*5955*
x31–567	Paralysis of conjugate lateral movement (cortical)	*5955*
x31–5671	Paralysis of conjugate lateral movement (supranuclear)	*5955*

x32–5672	Paralysis of convergence (nuclear)	*5955*
x33–5672	Paralysis of divergence (nuclear)	*5955*
x34–567	Paralysis of conjugate movement upward (cortical)	*5955*
x34–5671	Paralysis of conjugate movement upward (supranuclear)	*5955*
x35–567	Paralysis of conjugate movement downward (cortical)	*5955*
x35–5671	Paralysis of conjugate movement downward (supranuclear)	*5955*

—7 DISEASES DUE TO DISORDER OF METABOLISM, GROWTH, OR NUTRITION

x30–712	Nystagmus due to fatigue of oculomotor nucleus	*5970*

—X DISEASES DUE TO UNKNOWN CAUSE WITH THE FUNCTIONAL REACTION ALONE MANIFEST

x37–x30	Cyclophoria	*5990*
x32–x21	Esophoria	*5990*
x33–x21	Exophoria	*5990*
x32–x15	Esotropia	*5990*
x33–x15	Exotropia	*5990*
x36–x15	Hypertrophia	*5990*
27112–x201	Overaction of inferior oblique, right eye	*2790*
27112–x202	Overaction of inferior oblique, left eye	*2790*

DISEASES OF THE ORBIT

x50– Orbit
x51– Contents of orbit, generally
x11– Eyeball
x46– Vessels of orbit
x44– Veins of orbit
473– Internal carotid artery
90x– Intrinsic vessels of brain and cranium
210– Bones of orbit

—0 DISEASES DUE TO GENETIC AND PRENATAL INFLUENCES

x11–022	Exophthalmos due to premature closure of sutures due to tower skull	5901
210–012	Partial absence of bony wall of orbit	2101
x46–015	Varix of orbit, congenital	5901

—I DISEASES DUE TO INFECTION WITH LOWER ORGANISM

x51–100.2	Abscess of orbit. *Specify organism (page 57) when known*	5910
x50–190	Chronic inflammation of orbit	5910
x51–100.6	Deformity of orbit due to infection	5910
x51–100.4	Enophthalmos following infection of orbital tissue	5910
x50–100.3	Fistula of orbit due to infection	5910
x50–100.6	Granuloma of orbit	5910
x51–100	Orbital cellulitis. *Specify organism (page 57) when known*	2110
210.4–100	Orbital periostitis. *Specify organism (page 57) when known*	2110
x111–100	Tenonitis	5910

—4 DISEASES DUE TO TRAUMA OR PHYSICAL AGENT

x45–400.6	Aneurysm in orbit due to trauma	5940
x51–415.4	Deformity of orbit following operation	5940
x11–436	Displacement of eyeball due to fracture	5940
x50–4x8	Edema of orbit due to trauma	5940
x51–427	Emphysema of orbit	5940
x11–4x1	Enophthalmos due to loss of orbital tissue	5940
x11–415.1	Enophthalmos following operation	5940
x50–496	Foreign body in orbit	5940
210–416	Fracture of bone of orbit	5940
x50–4x7	Hematoma of orbit due to trauma	5940
x50–4▲▲	Injury of orbit. *Specify (page 83)*	5940

—50 DISEASES DUE TO CIRCULATORY DISTURBANCE

x50–5x8	Edema of orbit, circulatory	*5950*
x11–522	Exophthalmos due to orbital edema	*5950*
x46–5x7	Hemorrhage in orbit due to disturbance of circulation	*5950*
x50–522	Passive congestion of oribt	*5950*

—6 DISEASES DUE TO OR CONSISTING OF STATIC MECHANICAL ABNOR-MALITY

x51–600.8	Cyst of orbit	*5960*
x11–630	Displacement of eyeball due to unspecified cause	*5960*
x44–641	Varix of orbit	*5960*

—7 DISEASES DUE TO DISORDER OF METABOLISM, GROWTH, OR NUTRITION

x11–711	Enophthalmos due to emaciation	*5970*
x11–708	Enophthalmos due to loss of water	*5970*
x11–798	Enophthalmos due to senile atrophy	*5970*
x51–798	Protrusion of orbital fat due to senile atrophy	*5970*

—8 NEW GROWTHS

x51–870A	Fibroma of orbit	*5980*
x51–870F	Fibrosarcoma of orbit	*5980*
x51–850A	Hemangioma of orbit	*5980*
x51–866A	Leiomyoma of orbit	*5980*
x51–866F	Leiomyosarcoma of orbit	*5980*
x51–872A	Lipoma of orbit	*5980*
x51–839	Lymphoma of orbit.[1] *Specify behavior*	*5980*
x51–830	Lymphosarcoma of orbit. *Specify behavior*	*5980*
x51–8173	Melanoma, malignant, of orbit. *Specify behavior*	*5980*
x51–8451	Neurofibroma of orbit. *Specify behavior*	*5980*
210–876A	Osteoma of orbital bone	*5980*
x51–8170	Pigmented nevus of orbit. *Specify behavior*	*5980*
x51–867A	Rhabdomyoma of orbit	*5980*
x51–8▲▲▲	Unlisted tumor of orbit. *Specify neoplasm and behavior (page 99)*	*5980*

[1] Use lymphoma behavior code (page 99).

460 EYE

—9 DISEASES DUE TO UNKNOWN OR UNCERTAIN CAUSE WITH THE STRUCTURAL REACTION MANIFEST

x45–942.6   Aneurysm in orbit due to arteriosclerosis   *5990*
x46–9x6   Arteriovenous aneurysm, retro-orbital, due
                to unknown cause   *5990*
210–943   Exostosis of orbit   *2190*

DISEASES OF THE EYELIDS

x52– Eyelids
x53– Upper eyelid
x54– Lower eyelid
x55– Tarsus
x57– Tarsal conjunctiva
2716– Levator palpebrae muscle
965– Seventh nerve
132– Skin of eyelid and adjacent skin
163– Eyebrows
164– Cilia including glands of hair follicle
x61– Meibomian gland
x60– Other glands of eyelid
27117– Orbicularis muscle of eyelid

—0 DISEASES DUE TO GENETIC AND PRENATAL INFLUENCES

x52–022	Absence of eyelid fold	*5901*
x52–011	Absence of eyelid	*5901*
x52–012	Absence of eyelid, partial	*5901*
x52–024	Anklyoblepharon filiforme, congenital	*5901*
x52–027	Atrophy or insufficiency, congenital, of tarso-orbital fascia causing fat hernia of eyelid	*5901*
x52–017	Blepharophimosis	*5901*
x52–01x	Coloboma of eyelid, congenital	*5901*
x52–018	Cryptophthalmos; ankyloblepharon totale	*5901*
164–022	Distichia	*1600*
x54–013	Epiblepharon	*5901*
210–016	Epicanthus (deficient bone)	*2101*
132–013	Epicanthus (excessive skin)	*1301*
x52–013	Excess of eyelid fold, ptosis adiposa	*5901*
164–014	Hypertrichosis, congenital	*1600*
164–012	Hypotrichosis, congenital	*1600*
132–014	Ichthyosis of eyelid	*1301*
x54–016	Narrowness of eyelid, abnormal	*5901*
163–074	Poliosis of eyebrow	*1600*
164–079	Poliosis of lashes	*1600*
2716–042	Ptosis of eyelid, congenital	*2701*
x52–019	Symblepharon, congenital	*5901*
132–079	Vitiligo of eyelid	*1301*

—I DISEASES DUE TO INFECTION WITH LOWER ORGANISM

x52–100.2	Abscess of eyelid. *Specify organism (page 57) when known*	*5910*

x68–100.2	Abscess of canthus. *Specify organism (page 57) when known*	*5910*
x52–119	Anthrax of eyelid	*5910*
x52–105	Blepharitis	*5910*
x52–105.9	Blepharitis ulcerative	*5910*
x52–100.4	Deformity of eyelid due to infection	*5910*
132–100.4	Ectropion, cicatricial	*1310*
x55–100.4	Entropion, cicatricial	*5910*
x52–146	Frambesia, lesions of eyelid in	*5910*
132–166	Herpes of eyelid	*1310*
164–105	Hordeolum externum	*1610*
x61–105	Hordeolum internum	*5910*
164–100.1	Hypotrichosis due to infection. *Specify organism when known*	*1610*
132–100	Infection of skin of eyelid. *Specify organism when known*	*1310*
x52–152	Leishmaniasis of lid	*5910*
x52–124	Leprosy of lid	*5910*
132–185	Molluscum contagiosum of eyelid	*1310*
2716–1xx	Ptosis of eyelid due to infection	*2710*
132–130	Rhinoscleroma of eyelid	*1310*
132–1236	Scrofuloderma of eyelid	*1310*
x55–100	Tarsitis. *Specify organism when known*	*5910*
164–1x4	Trichiasis, cicatricial	*1610*
132–1762	Vaccinia, lesions of eyelid in	*1310*
132–1761	Variola, lesions of eyelid in	*1310*
132–1764	Zoster of eyelid	*1310*

—2 DISEASES DUE TO HIGHER PLANT OR ANIMAL PARASITE

| 132–213 | Favus of eyelid | *1320* |

—3 DISEASES DUE TO INTOXICATION

132–390	Allergic eczema of eyelid	*1330*
132–3253	Argyrosis of eyelid	*1330*
132–321▲	Arsenic pigmentation of eyelid	*1330*
132–3▲▲	Dermatitis of eyelid due to poison. *Specify (page 67)*	*1330*
x52–3▲▲	Injury of eyelid by poison. *Specify poison (page 67)*	*5930*
x52–32131	By arsine	*5930*
x52–34651	By atropine	*5930*
x52–3243	By mercury salts	*5930*

—4 DISEASES DUE TO TRAUMA OR PHYSICAL AGENT

x52–415.x	Absence of eyelid following operation	*5940*
x52–415.4	Ankyloblepharon following operation	*5940*
132–454	Chloasma of eyelid due to trauma	*1340*

132–415.4	Ectropion, cicatricial, following operation	*1340*
132–400.4	Ectropion, cicatricial, due to trauma	*1340*
x52–427	Emphysema of eyelid due to trauma	*5940*
x55–415.4	Entropion, cicatricial, following operation	*5940*
x55–400.4	Entropion, cicatricial, due to trauma	*5940*
x52–4x7	Hematoma of eyelid due to trauma	*5940*
x52–4▲▲	Injury of eyelid due to trauma. *Specify trauma*	*5940*
x521–4▲▲	Injury of medial palpebral ligament due to trauma. *Specify trauma*	*5940*
x522–4▲▲	Injury of lateral palpebral ligament due to trauma. *Specify trauma*	*5940*
2716–410	Ptosis of eyelid due to trauma	*2740*
164–400.4	Trichiasis due to trauma	*1600*

—50 DISEASES DUE TO CIRCULATORY DISTURBANCE

x52–501	Elephantiasis of eyelid (nonfilarial)	*5950*
132–521	Rosacea of eyelid	*1350*

—55 DISEASES DUE TO DISTURBANCE OF INNERVATION OR OF PSYCHIC CONTROL

Record primary diagnosis when possible

132–580	Angioneurotic edema of eyelids	*1355*
132–581	Anhidrosis of eyelid, neurogenic	*1355*
x69–590	Blepharospasm	*5955*
x52–560	Ectropion, paralytic	*5955*
x52–561	Ectropion, spastic	*5955*
x69–561	Entropion, spastic	*5955*
132–582	Hyperhidrosis of eyelid	*1355*
x69–560	Lagophthalmos	*5955*
2716–561	Pseudoptosis of eyelid	*2755*
2716–560	Ptosis of eyelid, paralytic	*2755*

—6 DISEASES DUE TO OR CONSISTING OF STATIC MECHANICAL ABNORMALITY

x60–600.8	Cyst of gland of Moll	*5960*
x61–615	Meibomian infarct	*5960*
132–6x8	Milium of eyelid	*1161*

—7 DISEASES DUE TO DISORDER OF METABOLISM, GROWTH, OR NUTRITION

x52–711	Atrophy of eyelid, marantic	*5970*
x52–798	Atrophy of eyelid, senile	*5970*
x52–7x1	Blepharitis squamosa	*5970*
x61–7x8	Chalazion	*5971*
132–711	Chloasma cachecticorum	*1370*
132–789	Chloasma gravidarum	*1370*
132–771	Chloasma of eyelid, hyperthyroid	*1370*

132–748	Chloasma in hemochromatosis	*1370*
132–742	Chloasma in ochronosis	*1370*
132–7xx	Chromhidrosis of eyelid	*1370*
x52–797	Ectropion, senile	*5970*
164–794	Hypertrichosis of eyelid, acquired	*1600*
163–747	Poliosis of eyebrow	*1600*
164–747	Poliosis of lashes	*1600*
132–770	Scleroderma of eyelid	*1370*
132–747	Vitiligo of eyelid	*1370*
132–757	Xanthelasma of eyelid	*1370*

—8 NEW GROWTHS

x60–8091A	Adenoma of glands of Krause, glands of Moll or glands of Zeis	*5980*
x52–8091A	Adenoma of eyelid glands	*5980*
x61–8091A	Adenoma of Meibomian gland	*5980*
x68▲–812	Basal cell carcinoma of canthus of eyelid. *Specify site and behavior*	*5980*
132–812	Basal cell carcinoma of eyelid. *Specify behavior*	*1382*
x52–873B	Chondroma of eyelid	*5980*
x68▲–814	Epidermoid carcinoma of canthus. *Specify site and behavior (page 99)*	*5980*
x52–870A	Fibroma of eyelid	*5980*
x52–850A	Hemangioma of eyelid	*5980*
x52–872A	Lipoma of eyelid	*5980*
x52–854A	Lymphangioma of eyelid	*5980*
x52–830	Lymphosarcoma of eyelid. *Specify behavior*	*5980*
x52–8173	Melanoma, malignant, of eyelid. *Specify behavior*	*5980*
132–8451	Neurofibroma of eyelid; molluscum fibrosum. *Specify behavior (page 99)*	*1384*
132–8170	Pigmented nevus of eyelid. *Specify behavior*	*1385*
x52–867A	Rhabdomyoma of lid	*5980*
x52–879	Sarcoma of eyelid. *Specify behavior (page 99)*	*5980*
x52–8▲▲▲	Unlisted tumor of eyelid. *Specify neoplasm and behavior (page 99)*	*5980*

—9 DISEASES DUE TO UNKNOWN OR UNCERTAIN CAUSE WITH THE STRUCTURAL REACTION MANIFEST

132–911	Blepharochalasis	*1390*
132–929	Colloid degeneration of skin of eyelid	*1390*

—X DISEASES DUE TO UNKNOWN OR UNCERTAIN CAUSE WITH THE FUNCTIONAL REACTION ALONE MANIFEST

| x61–x20 | Hypersecretion of Meibomian glands | *5990* |

DISEASES OF THE LACRIMAL TRACT

x62– Lacrimal glands
x63– Lacrimal passages
x64– Lacrimal papillae
x65– Canaliculus
x66– Lacrimal sac
x67– Lacrimonasal duct

—0 DISEASES DUE TO GENETIC AND PRENATAL INFLUENCES

x64–011	Absence of canaliculus and punctum, congenital	*5901*
x63–018	Atresia or stenosis of lacrimal passage, congenital	*5901*
x67–018	Atresia or stenosis of lacrimonasal duct, congenital	*5901*
x67–031.8	Cyst due to supernumerary lacrimonasal duct	*5901*
x64–021	Displacement of canaliculus and punctum due to amniotic deformities	*5901*
x62–031	Supernumerary lacrimal gland	*5901*
x67–031	Supernumerary lacrimonasal duct	*5901*

—I DISEASES DUE TO INFECTION WITH LOWER ORGANISM

x62–100.6	Achroacytosis of lacrimal gland due to infection. *Specify organism (page 57) when known, e.g.*	*5910*
x62–123.6	Achroacytosis of lacrimal gland, tuberculous	*5910*
x62–100	Dacryoadenitis, acute. *Specify organism (page 57) when known*	*5910*
x62–100.0	Dacryoadenitis, chronic. *Specify organism when known*	*5910*
x66–100	Dacryocystitis, acute. *Specify organism (page 57) when known*	*5910*
x66–100.0	Dacryocystitis, chronic. *Specify organism when known*	*5910*
x64–100.6	Eversion of punctum due to infection	*5910*
x62–100.3	Fistula of lacrimal gland due to infection	*5910*
x66–100.3	Fistula of lacrimal sac due to infection	*5910*
x65–100.6	Granuloma (polyp) in canaliculus	*5910*
x66–100.6	Granuloma (polyp) in lacrimal sac	*5910*
x63–100	Infection of lacrimal passage. *Specify organism (page 57) when known*	*5910*
x62–100.5	Luxation of lacrimal gland due to infection	*5910*

x66–130	Rhinoscleroma of lacrimal sac	*5910*
x65–100.4	Stenosis of canaliculus, cicatricial, due to infection	*5910*
x67–100.4	Stenosis of lacrimonasal duct, cicatricial, due to infection	*5910*

—4 DISEASES DUE TO TRAUMA OR PHYSICAL AGENT

x62–400.3	Fistula of lacrimal gland due to trauma	*5940*
x66–400.3	Fistula of lacrimal sac due to trauma	*5940*
x67–400.3	Fistula of lacrimonasal duct due to trauma	*5940*
x62–435	Dislocation of lacrimal gland	*5940*
x62–4x6	Eversion of punctum due to trauma or following operation	*5940*
x65–496	Foreign body in canaliculus	*5940*
x66–496	Foreign body in lacrimal sac	*5940*
x62–406	Luxation of lacrimal gland due to trauma	*5940*
x65–400.4	Stenosis, cicatricial, of canaliculus, due to trauma	*5940*
x67–400.4	Stenosis, cicatricial, of lacrimonasal duct, due to trauma	*5940*
x63–415.4	Stenosis of lacrimal passage following operation	*5940*
x65–410	Wound of canaliculus	*5940*
x62–410	Wound of lacrimal gland	*5940*
x66–410	Wound of lacrimal sac	*5940*

—6 DISEASES DUE TO OR CONSISTING OF STATIC MECHANICAL ABNORMALITY

x62–615	Calculus of lacrimal gland	*5960*
x62–600.8	Retention cyst of lacrimal gland; dacryops	*5960*

—7 DISEASES DUE TO DISORDER OF METABOLISM, GROWTH, OR NUTRITION

x64–797	Senile eversion of punctum	*5970*

—8 NEW GROWTHS

x62–8091	Adenocarcinoma of lacrimal gland. *Specify behavior (page 99)*	*5980*
x62–814	Epidermoid carcinoma of lacrimal gland. *Specify behavior (page 99)*	*5980*
x62–830	Lymphosarcoma of lacrimal gland. *Specify behavior*	*5980*
x62–8852	Mixed tumor salivary type of lacrimal gland. *Specify behavior (page 99)*	*5980*

x62–8032A   Multiple benign cystic epithelioma   *5980*
x62–8▲▲▲   Unlisted tumor of lacrimal gland. *Spec-*
                   ify neoplasm and behavior (page 99)   *5980*

—9 DISEASES DUE TO UNKNOWN OR UNCERTAIN CAUSE WITH THE STRUCTURAL REACTION MANIFEST

x62–954   Achroacytosis of lacrimal gland due to
                       unknown cause   *5990*

—X DISEASES DUE TO UNKNOWN OR UNCERTAIN CAUSE WITH THE FUNCTIONAL REACTION ALONE MANIFEST

x62–x20   Epiphora due to hypersecretion by lacri-
                       mal glands   *5990*

DISEASES OF THE CONJUNCTIVA

x56– Conjunctiva
x57– Tarsal conjunctiva
x58– Bulbar conjunctiva
x59– Caruncle
x18– Aqueous
x56x– Vessels of conjunctiva

—0 DISEASES DUE TO GENETIC AND PRENATAL INFLUENCES

x56–025	Adhesions of conjunctiva, congenital	5901
x56–050	Birth injury of conjunctiva	5901

—I DISEASES DUE TO INFECTION WITH LOWER ORGANISM

x56–100.2	Abscess of conjunctiva. *Specify organism (page 57) when known*	5910
x59–100.2	Abscess of caruncle. *Specify organism (page 57) when known*	5910
x56–190	Blennorrhea, inclusion	5910
x56–100.0	Conjunctivitis, chronic	5911
x56–100.8	Follicular conjunctivitis	5911
x56–100	Conjunctivitis, infectious, acute. *Specify organism (page 57) when known, e.g.*	5911
x56–111	Conjunctivitis due to Morilla lacunta (Morax-Axenfeld bacillus, Hemophilos duplex)	5911
x56–107	Conjunctivitis tularensis	5911
x56–103	Gonococcic conjunctivitis	5911
x56–1101	Hemophilus aegypti (Koch-Weeks) conjunctivitis	5911
x56–101	Pneumococcic conjunctivitis	5911
x56–105	Staphylococcic conjunctivitis	5911
x56–102	Streptococcic conjunctivitis	5911
x56–125	Diphtheria of conjunctiva	5911
x56x–190	Herpes iris of conjunctiva (erythema multiforme)	5911
x56–166	Herpes of conjunctiva	5911
x56–124	Leprosy of conjunctiva	5911
x56–147	Syphilis of conjunctiva; syphilid of conjunctiva	5911
x56–194	Trachoma	5911
x56–194.0	Trachoma, chronic	5911
x56–194.4	Trachomatous contraction of conjunctiva	5911
x56–123	Tuberculosis of conjunctiva	5911
x56–100.9	Ulceration of conjunctiva due to infection	5911

x56–1762	Vaccinia of conjunctiva	*5911*
x56–1761	Variola of conjunctiva	*5911*
x56–1764	Zoster of conjunctiva	*5911*

—2 DISEASES DUE TO HIGHER PLANT OR ANIMAL PARASITE

x56–2542.8	Conjunctival edema due to Trichinella	*5920*
x56–299	Conjunctivitis, caterpillar	*5920*
x56–2952	Myiasis of conjunctiva	*5920*

—3 DISEASES DUE TO INTOXICATION

x56–390	Allergic conjunctivitis; eczematous conjunctivitis	*5930*
x56–3901	Allergic phlyctenulosis, nontuberculous	*5930*
x56–3903	Hay fever conjunctivitis	*5930*
x56–395	Urticaria of conjunctiva	*5930*
x56–3902	Vernal conjunctivitis (spring catarrh)	*5930*
x56–3▲▲	Conjunctivitis due to poison. *Specify poison (page 67), e.g.*	*5930*
x56–31▲	Due to alkali, acid or inorganic salt. *Specify agent*	*5930*
x56–3162	Due to ammonia	*5930*
x56–34651	Due to atropine	*5930*
x56–380	Due to caterpillar hairs (ophthalmia nodosa)	*5930*
x56–3123	Due to potassium hydroxide (caustic potash)	*5930*
x56–319▲	Due to a gas. *Specify agent*	*5930*
x56–3126	Due to lime	*5930*
x56–3253	Due to silver (argyrosis)	*5930*
x57–300.4	Symblepharon due to poison. *Specify poison (page 67) when known, e.g.*	*5930*
x57–3126.4	Symblepharon due to lime	*5930*

—4 DISEASES DUE TO TRAUMA OR PHYSICAL AGENT

x56–441	Burn of conjunctiva	*5940*
x56–4x0	Conjunctivitis, chronic, from physical agent. *Specify agent*	*5940*
x56–494	Conjunctivitis, chronic, due to smoke	*5940*
x56–430	Conjunctivitis due to lagophthalmos. *When the lagophthalmos is due to remote disease, include latter in primary diagnosis*	*5940*
x56–400.8	Cyst, conjunctival	*5940*
x59–415.9	Deformity of caruncle following operation	*5940*
x56–427	Emphysema of conjunctiva	*5940*

x56–496	Foreign body in conjunctiva	*5940*
x56–415.0	Granulation of conjunctiva following operation	*5940*
x56–420.7	Hemorrhage, subconjunctival, due to remote injury	*5940*
x56–43x	Hyperemia, conjunctival, due to eyestrain	*5940*
x56–4▲▲	Injury of conjunctiva. *Specify (page 83)*	*5940*
x56–401	Abrasion of conjunctiva	*5940*
x56–412	Lacerated wound of conjunctiva	*5940*
x57–438.1	Necrosis of orbital conjunctiva due to foreign body	*5940*
x56–467	Ophthalmia electrica	*5940*
x56–451	Photophthalmia due to ultraviolet rays	*5940*
x56–439	Pressure of prosthesis, lesion due to	*5940*
x58–415.6	Pterygium following operation	*5940*
x56–472.1	Radium necrosis of conjunctiva	*5940*
x56–471.0	Roentgen ray (x-ray) burn of conjunctiva	*5940*
x57–400.4	Symblepharon due to trauma	*5940*
x57–415.4	Symblepharon following operation	*5940*

—50 DISEASES DUE TO CIRCULATORY DISTURBANCE

x56–521	Acne rosacea conjunctivitis	*5950*
x56–5x2	Cyanosis of conjunctiva	*5950*
x56–500.7	Hemorrhage of conjunctiva due to unknown cause	*5950*
x56–501	Lymphangiectasis of conjunctiva	*5950*

—55 DISEASES DUE TO DISTURBANCE OF INNERVATION
Record primary diagnosis when possible

| x56–565 | Conjunctivitis due to paralysis of fifth nerve | *5955* |
| x56x–581 | Hyperemia of conjunctiva due to paralysis of sympathetic nervous system | *5955* |

—7 DISEASES DUE TO DISORDER OF METABOLISM, GROWTH, OR NUTRITION

| x56–798 | Senile atrophy of conjunctiva | *5970* |
| x56–761 | Xerosis of conjunctiva | *5970* |

—8 NEW GROWTHS

| x56–812 | Basal cell carcinoma of conjunctiva. *Specify behavior* | *5980* |
| x56–814 | Epidermoid carcinoma of conjunctiva. *Specify behavior (page 99)* | *5980* |

x56–870A	Fibroma of conjunctiva	*5980*
x56–850A	Hemangioma of conjunctiva	*5980*
x56–872A	Lipoma of conjunctiva	*5980*
x56–854A	Lymphangioma of conjunctiva	*5980*
x56–839	Lymphoma[1] of conjunctiva. *Specify be-havior*	*5980*
x56–830	Lymphosarcoma of conjunctiva. *Specify behavior*	*5980*
x56–8173F	Malignant melanoma of conjunctiva	*5980*
x56–8451	Neurofibroma of conjunctiva. *Specify behavior (page 99)*	*5980*
x56–8170	Pigmented nevus of conjunctiva. *Specify behavior*	*5980*
x56–879	Sarcoma of conjunctiva. *Specify be-havior (page 99)*	*5980*
x56–8▲▲▲	Unlisted tumor of conjunctiva. *Specify neoplasm and behavior (page 99)*	*5980*

—9 DISEASES DUE TO UNKNOWN OR UNCERTAIN CAUSE WITH THE STRUCTURAL REACTION MANIFEST

x56–922	Amyloidosis of conjunctiva	*5990*
x56–923	Concretions in conjunctiva	*5990*
x56–928	Hyaline degeneration of conjunctiva	*5990*
x56–980	Pemphigus of conjunctiva	*5990*
x58–929	Pinguecula	*5990*
x56–944	Polyp, simple of conjunctiva	*5990*
x58–9x4	Pseudopterygium	*5990*
x58–956	Pterygium	*5990*
x57–9x4	Symblepharon	*5990*

[1] Use lymphoma behavior code (page 99).

X7– DISEASES OF THE EAR

x70–   Acoustic sense
x71–   Ear

For detailed list of structures of ear, see page 52

—0 DISEASES DUE TO GENETIC AND PRENATAL INFLUENCES

—1 DISEASES DUE TO INFECTION WITH LOWER ORGANISM

x71–100	Panotitis. *Specify organism (page 57) when known*	5811
x71–123	Tuberculosis of ear, diffuse	5811

—4 DISEASES DUE TO TRAUMA OR PHYSICAL AGENT

x70–400	Acoustic trauma, acute or chronic, resulting in deafness. *Specify trauma (page 83) when known*	5840

—55 DISEASES DUE TO DISTURBANCE OF INNERVATION OR OF PSYCHIC CONTROL

x71–593	Reflex otalgia	5855

—6 DISEASES DUE TO OR CONSISTING OF STATIC MECHANICAL ABNORMALITY

x71–646	Otalgia due to malocclusion of temporomandibular joint	5860

—8 NEW GROWTHS

x71–8091	Adenocarcinoma of ear. *Specify behavior (page 99)*	5880
x71–8091A	Adenoma of ear	5880
x71–812	Basal cell carcinoma of ear. *Specify behavior*	5880
x71–873B	Chondroma of ear	5880
x71–814	Epidermoid carcinoma of ear. *Specify behavior (page 99)*	5880
x71–870A	Fibroma of ear	5880
x71–870F	Fibrosarcoma of ear	5880
x71–8532	Glomangioma of ear. *Specify behavior*	5880
x72–850A	Hemangioma of auricle	5880
x71–872A	Lipoma of ear	5880
x72–854A	Lymphangioma of auricle	5880
x72–8451	Neurofibroma of auricle. *Specify behavior (page 99)*	5880
x71–8170	Pigmented nevus of ear. *Specify behavior*	5880

| x71–879 | Sarcoma of ear. *Specify behavior (page 99)* | 5880 |
| x71–8▲▲▲ | Unlisted tumor of ear. *Specify neoplasm and behavior (page 99)* | 5880 |

DISEASES OF THE EXTERNAL EAR

x72–   Auricle
x79–   Cartilagenous meatus
x78–   Lobule
x75–   External auditory canal
x76–   Osseous meatus
x77–   Tympanic membrane

—0 DISEASES DUE TO GENETIC AND PRENATAL INFLUENCES

x72–011	Absence of auricle, congenital	5801
x72–010	Deformity of auricle, congenital (pointed ear, macacus ear, dog ear, lop ear, cat's ear, ridged ear, Darwin's tubercle)	5801
x72–021	Displacement of auricle (melotus)	5801
x75–011	External auditory canal, absence of, congenital	5801
x75–018	External auditory canal, atresia of, congenital	5801
x75–017	External auditory canal, narrowing of, congenital	5801
x72–029	Fistula of auricle, congenital	5801
x78–011	Lobule, absence of, congenital	5801
x78–032	Lobule, duplication of	5801
x78–013	Lobule, enlargement of	5801
x78–034	Lobule, fissure of, congenital	5801
x78–016	Lobule, rudimentary	5801
x78–031	Lobule, supernumerary	5801
x72–013	Macrotia	5801
x72–016	Microtia	5801
x76–018	Osseous meatus, atresia of, congenital	5801
x76–093	Osseous meatus, exostosis of, congenital	5801
x72–031	Polyotia	5801
x72–019	Preauricular sinus, congenital	5801
x72–064	Preauricular cyst, congenital	5801
x72–022	Prominence of auricle, congenital	5801
x72–01x	Sinus of auricle	5801

—I DISEASES DUE TO INFECTION WITH LOWER ORGANISM

x72–100.2	Abscess of auricle. *Specify organism (page 57) when known as*	5801
x72–105.2	Staphylococcic abscess of auricle	5810
x75–100.2	Abscess of external auditory canal. *Specify organism (page 57) when known*	5810
x72–118	Anthrax of auricle	5810

x72–100.4	Deformity of auricle due to infection	*5810*
x72–125	Diphtheria of external ear	*5810*
x75–100.0	Furunculosis of external auditory canal, circumscribed or diffuse	*5810*
x72–100.1	Gangrene of auricle due to infection (noma)	*5810*
x72–100	Infection of auricle. *Specify organism (page 57) when known*	*5810*
x75–100	Infection of external auditory meatus, diffuse. *Specify organism (page 57) when known*	*5810*
x77–100	Myringitis, acute. *Specify organism (page 57) when known*	*5810*
x77–100.8	Myringitis, bullous	*5810*
x77–100.0	Myringitis, chronic. *Specify organism (page 57) when known*	*5810*
x74–100	Perichondritis of auricle. *Specify organism (page 57) when known*	*5810*

—2 DISEASES DUE TO HIGHER PLANT OR ANIMAL PARASITE

x75–297	Myiasis of ear	*5820*
x75–2▲▲	Otomycosis. *Specify fungus*	*5820*

—3 DISEASES DUE TO INTOXICATION

x72–32▲	Chemical burn of auricle. *Specify poison (page 67)*	*5830*
x77–32▲	Chemical burn of tympanic membrane. *Specify poison (page 67)*	*5830*
x75–300.0	Inflammation of external auditory meatus due to chemical irritant. *Specify irritant (page 67)*	*5830*
x75–3122.4	Stricture of external auditory canal due to sodium hydroxide (caustic soda; lye)	*5830*

—4 DISEASES DUE TO TRAUMA OR PHYSICAL AGENT

x77–482	Blast injury of tympanic membrane	*5840*
x77–482.5	Blast injury with rupture of tympanic membrane	*5840*
x72–441	Burn of auricle, from heat	*5840*
x72–400.4	Deformity of external ear due to trauma	*5840*
x75–44x.6	Exostosis of external auditory canal due to cold (cold water immersion)	*5840*
x75–496	Foreign body in external auditory canal	*5840*
x76–416	Fracture of osseous meatus	*5840*
x72–448	Frostbite of auricle	*5840*

x72–4x7	Hematoma of auricle	*5840*
x72–4▲▲	Injury of auricle. *Specify (page 83)*	*5840*
x75–4▲▲	Injury of external auditory canal. *Specify (page 83)*	*5840*
x77–4x0	Myringitis, acute, due to trauma	*5840*
x77–416	Rupture of tympanic membrane due to trauma	*5480*
x75–400.4	Stricture of external auditory canal due to trauma	*5840*
x75–415.4	Stricture of external auditory canal following operation	*5840*

—50 DISEASES DUE TO CIRCULATORY DISTURBANCE

x72–501	Lymphangiectatic elephantiasis of external ear	*5840*

—55 DISEASES DUE TO DISTURBANCE OF INNERVATION

x72–573	Pruritus of auricle	*5855*

—6 DISEASES DUE TO OR CONSISTING OF STATIC MECHANICAL ABNOR-MALITY

x75–616	Impacted cerumen	*5860*

—8 NEW GROWTHS

See under Ear, *page 472. Change 3d digit to indicate site.*

—9 DISEASES DUE TO UNKNOWN OR UNCERTAIN CAUSE WITH THE STRUCTURAL REACTION MANIFEST

x74–923	Calcification of auricle	*5890*
x74–940	Chondrodermatitis nodular of ear	*5890*
x76–944	Exostosis of osseous meatus	*5890*
x77–941	Tympanosclerosis	*5890*

DISEASES OF THE MIDDLE EAR

x80– Middle ear
x81– Auditory ossicles
x83– Eustachian tube
x84– Mastoid antrum and mastoid air cells

—0 DISEASES DUE TO GENETIC AND PRENATAL INFLUENCES

x83–021	Abnormal course of Eustachian tube	5801
x80–011	Absence of middle ear	5801
x81–011	Absence of ossicles, congenital	5801
x81–077	Deformity of ossicles, congenital	5801
x83–036	Diverticulum of Eustachian tube, congenital	5801
x81–024	Fusion of ossicles, congenital	5801
x83–017	Narrowing of Eustachian tube, congenital	5801
x80–017	Narrowing of middle ear, congenital	5801
x8x–019	Persistence of arteria stapedia	5801
x81–031	Supernumerary ossicles	5801

—I DISEASES DUE TO INFECTION WITH LOWER ORGANISM

x81–100.4	Ankylosis of incudostapedial joint due to infection	5810
x80–100.6	Granuloma (polyp) of middle ear	5810
x84–100	Mastoiditis, acute. *Specify organism (page 57) when known, e.g.*	5812
x84–101	Due to Pneumococcus	5812
x84–102	Due to Streptococcus	5812
x84–1x6	Mastoiditis, acute coalescent. *Specify organism (page 57) when known*	5812
x84–1x7	Mastoiditis, acute hemorrhagic. *Specify organism (page 57) when known*	5812
x84–1x1	Mastoiditis, acute necrotic. *Specify organism (page 57) when known*	5812
x84–100.0	Mastoiditis, chronic	5812
x84–1x0	Mastoiditis, recurrent	5812
x81–100.1	Necrosis of ossicles	5811
x80–190	Otitis media, serous (otitis media with effusion, secretory otitis, hydrotympanum)	5811
x80–190.0	Otitis media, mucopurulent (mucoid, glue ear, catarrhal otitis, exudative catarrah)	5811
x80–100	Otitis media, suppurative, acute. *Specify organism (page 57) when known*	5811
x80–101	Due to Pneumococcus	5811

x80–105	Due to Staphylococcus	*5811*
x80–102	Due to Streptococcus	*5811*
x80–100.0	Otitis media, suppurative, chronic. *Specify organism (page 57) when known*	*5811*
x8x–100	Petrositis. *Specify organism (page 57) when known*	*5810*
x83–100	Salpingitis, Eustachian, acute. *Specify organism (page 57) when known*	*5810*
x83–100.0	Salpingitis, Eustachian, chronic	*5810*
x83–100.4	Stricture of Eustachian tube due to infection	*5810*
x84–123	Tuberculosis of mastoid	*5812*
x80–123	Tuberculosis of middle ear	*5811*

—3 DISEASES DUE TO INTOXICATION

x80–390	Allergy of middle ear. *Specify allergen (page 67) when known*	*5830*

—4 DISEASES DUE TO TRAUMA OR PHYSICAL AGENT

x91–482	Blast injury of ossicular chain	*5840*
x81–400.5	Disruption of ossicular chain due to trauma	*5840*
x84–415.3	Fistula of mastoid following operation	*5840*
x84–496	Foreign body in mastoid	*5840*
x84–416	Fracture of petrous pyramid and mastoid	*5840*
x80–415.0	Granulations in middle ear following operation	*5840*
x80–481	Otitis media, nonsuppurative, acute, due to rapid change in air pressure (aerotitis media)	*5840*

—8 NEW GROWTHS

See under Ear, *page 472. Change 3d digit to indicate site.*

—9 DISEASES DUE TO UNKNOWN OR UNCERTAIN CAUSE WITH THE STRUCTURAL REACTION MANIFEST

x80–956	Otitis media, suppurative, chronic, due to cholesteatoma (genuine or primary acquired, primary pseudocholesteatoma)	*5890*
x80–956.5	Otitis media, suppurative, chronic, due to cholesteatoma (secondary cholesteatoma)	*5890*

DISEASES OF THE INTERNAL EAR

x85– Internal ear
x86– Osseous labyrinth
x88– Organ of Corti
x89– Perilabyrinthine tissues
x93– Semicircular canals
x94– Utricle and saccule
966– Acoustic nerve

—0 DISEASES DUE TO GENETIC AND PRENATAL INFLUENCES

x88–011	Absence of organ of Corti, congenital	*5801*
x85–011	Aplasia of labyrinth, congenital	*5801*
x85–018	Collapse of membranous labyrinth, congenital	*5801*
x88–022	Defect of organ of Corti, congenital	*5801*
x88–0421	Sensory, neural deafness (high frequency)	*5801*
x88–0422	Sensory, neural deafness (low frequency)	*5801*
x88–0423	Sensory, neural deafness	*5801*
x85–092	Degeneration (epithelial metaplasia) of membranous labyrinth, congenital	*5801*
x94–092	Degeneration of saccule, congenital	*5801*
x94–015	Dilatation of saccule, congenital	*5801*

—1 DISEASES DUE TO INFECTION WITH LOWER ORGANISM

x85–100	Acute labyrinthitis, diffuse (suppurative or destructive). *Specify organism (page 57) when known, e.g.*	*5810*
x85–104	Due to Meningococcus	*5810*
x85–1x0.0	Chronic labyrinthitis, diffuse (dead labyrinth due to previous infection). *Specify organism (page 57) when known*	*5810*
x85–1x8	Diffuse serous labyrinthitis	*5810*
x93–100.3	Fistula of semicircular canal due to infection	*5810*
x89–100	Perilabyrinthitis. *Specify organism (page 57) when known*	*5810*

—3 DISEASES DUE TO INTOXICATION

x85–390	Allergy of internal ear. *Specify allergen (page 67) when known*	*5830*
x85–3▲▲	Labyrinthitis due to poison. *Specify*	*5830*
x88–3▲▲.x	Sensory, neural deafness due to drug. *Specify agent*	*5830*

—4 DISEASES DUE TO TRAUMA OR PHYSICAL AGENT

x85–482	Blast injury of labyrinth	*5840*
x93–415.3	Fistula of semicircular canal following operation	*5840*
x86–416	Fracture of osseous labyrinth and internal ear	*5840*
x85–4x0	Labyrinthitis due to trauma	*5840*
x88–400.x	Sensory, neural deafness, due to trauma	*5840*

—50 DISEASES DUE TO CIRCULATORY DISTURBANCE
Record primary diagnosis when known

x85–520	Congestion of labyrinth	*5850*
x85–532	Hemorrhage of labyrinth	*5850*
x85–510	Ischemia of labyrinth	*5850*

—7 DISEASES DUE TO DISORDER OF METABOLISM, GROWTH, OR NUTRITION

x86–7x9.4	Otosclerosis, conduction deafness, with fixation of stapes	*5870*
x86–7x9	Otosclerosis, primary nerve deafness, without stapes fixation	*5870*
x86–7x9.6	Otosclerosis with round window closure	*5870*
x86–7x1	Otosclerosis without impaired hearing	*5870*
966–79x	Presbycusis	*5870*
x88–79x	Senile degeneration of organ of Corti	*5870*
x88–7x9.x	Sensory neural deafness, due to otosclerosis	*5870*

—8 NEW GROWTHS

See under Ear, *page 472. Change 3d digit to indicate site.*

—9 DISEASES DUE TO UNKNOWN OR UNCERTAIN CAUSE WITH THE STRUCTURAL REACTION MANIFEST

966–9x9	Deafness due to degeneration of acoustic nerve due to unknown cause	*5890*
x93–9x3	Fistula of semicircular canals	*5890*
x85–9x8	Hydrops of the labyrinth (Ménière's syndrome)	*5890*
x85–910	Labyrinthitis due to unknown cause	*5890*

NONDIAGNOSTIC TERMS FOR
HOSPITAL RECORD

011–33212	Alcoholic intoxication (simple drunkenness)
y00–y01	Boarder only
y00–00x	Convulsive disorder, non-epileptic
y00–0031	Cytology test
y00–00312	Atypical
y00–00314	Malignancy indicated
y00–00311	Negative
y00–00313	Suspected
y00–yyy	Dead on arrival
y02–000	Diet, for adjustment of
y00–000	Disease none. *Change first three digits to indicate suspected system or organ*
y00–009	Donor of blood
y00–0091	Donor of blood marrow
y01–009	Donor of bone
y00–00y	Donor of skin
y00–y02	Examination, none
y00–002	Examination only. *Change first three digits as needed*
y00–004	Experiment only. *Change first three digits as needed*
410–yx0	Heart disease, possible
0193–100	Inoculation before pregnancy
0192–100	Inoculation before traveling
0194–100	Inoculation, mass
0191–100	Inoculation triple typhoid
y00–005	Malingerer
000–000	Mental disorder, none
000–y00	Mental disorder, undiagnosed
y00–800	Neoplasm of unknown primary site. *Change last two digits to indicate specific neoplasm when known*
785–003	No disease of the endometrium (premenstrual stage)
785–0001	No disease of the endometrium (proliferative stage)
785–0002	No disease of the endometrium (secretory stage)
y00–001	Observation. *Change first three digits as needed*
y00–003	Tests only. *Change first three digits as needed*
y01–001	Serological reaction, false positive
y01–000	Serological reaction negative
y00–147	Serological reaction positive

OBSTETRICAL TERMS

7x2–y60	Abnormal labor
7x2–y604	Due to abnormal muscular contractions
7x2–y603	Due to abnormality of cervix
7x2–y606	Due to drugs
7x2–y601	Due to malpresentation
7x2–y602	Due to pelvic distortion
7x2–y605	Due to premature rupture of membranes
7x2–y607	Due to unknown cause
y00–008	Child, nursing
7x2–y01	Died, undelivered
7x2–y02	Discharged before delivery
y00–300	Medical induction
y00–007	Postpartum admission
y00–006	Pregnant, not
790–y03	Immature birth, neonatal death
790–y09	Multiple birth, neonatal death
790–y02	Premature birth, neonatal death
790–y04	Postmature birth, neonatal death
790–y01	Term birth, neonatal death
790–y08	Triplets, neonatal death
790–y05	Twins, neonatal death
790–y06	Twins, single ovum, neonatal death
790–y07	Twins, double ovum, neonatal death

SUPPLEMENTARY TERMS

TOPOGRAPHIC SYSTEMS

0 to X

Note.—These terms may be used as supplements to any of the diagnoses in the NOMENCLATURE OF DISEASES section.

484

0– SUPPLEMENTARY TERMS

0 *Supplementary terms of the body as a whole (including supplementary terms of the psyche and of the body generally) and those not affecting a particular system exclusively*

088	Acarophobia
089	Acrophobia
08x	Agoraphobia
044	Antisocialism
084	Anxiety
0x1	Asthenia
030	Breath holding
098	Bruxism
00x	Cachexia
090	Cancerophobia
016	Causalgia
091	Claustrophobia
020	Cheiromegaly (enlargement of hands and fingers)
0x3	Chills
0x4	Chilly sensations
0x9	Collapse
01x	Compulsions
079	Counting (steps, etc.)
063	Criminality
052	Cruelty
046	Deficiency, moral
010	Dehydration
078	Délire de toucher
080	Depersonalization
021	Deposition of iron Compound
085	Depression
053	Destructiveness
02x	Diabetes insipidus
076	Dipsomania
051	Disobedience
077	Echolalia or praxis
001	Edema of cardiovascular origin
002	Edema due to lymphatic obstruction
018	Edema, hysterical
005	Edema of renal origin
0x7	Edema, other types
043	Emotional instability
065	Encopresis
05x	Enuresis
057	Erotomania
019	Facetiousness

0x0	Fatigue, abnormal
087	Fears, mixed
035	Feeding problem in children
059	Folie du doute
055	Forgery
028	Fugue
006	Gain in weight
036	Homosexuality
064	Hypochondriasis
	Hyperthemia. *See* Pyrexia
000	Hypothermia
004	Jaundice
069	Kleptomania
008	Loss in weight
	Malingering. *See* Simulation
037	Mania
034	Masturbation
047	Mendacity pathologic: untruthfulness
03x	Misanthropy
039	Misogyny
014	Moria (Witzelsucht)
086	Mysophobia
031	Nail biting
029	Negativism
09x	Nephrotic glycosuric hypophosphatemic dwarfism associated with rickets: hereditary cystinuria (de Toni-Fanconi Syndrome)
022	Neurovisceral central syndrome; pilous adiposity
068	Nymphomania
007	Obesity
045	Overactivity
0x2	Pain, general
083	Panic
082	Panic, acute homosexual
023	Paralysis agitans
081	Paranoid trends
072	Paroxysmal automatism
074	Paroxysmal clouded states
073	Paroxysmal furor
071	Paroxysmal psychic equivalents
027	Personality, dual
026	Personality, dissociated
040	Personality, hysterical
041	Personality, hypochondriacal
042	Personality, syntonic
093	Phthisiophobia

017	Positive Castaneda's stain for rickettsia
015	Positive Weil-Felix reaction
003	Pyrexia; hyperthermia
056	Pyromania; setting fires
050	Quarrelsomeness
061	Sexual immaturity
060	Sex offenses
062	Sexual perversion
0x8	Shock
011	Simulation; malingering
024	Somnambulism
025	Somniloquism
054	Stealing
06x	Swindling
0xx	Syncope
092	Syphilophobia
033	Tantrums
0x5	Tetany
0x6	Tetany due to hyperventilation
032	Thumb sucking
038	Tongue swallowing
012	Trance
066	Trichokryptomania
067	Trichotillomania
04x	Truancy
013	Urge to say words
075	Use of alcohol
058	Use of drugs
048	Vagabondage
049	Vagrancy
009	Xanthomatosis (symptomatic)

1– SUPPLEMENTARY TERMS

1 *Supplementary terms of the integumentary system (including subcutaneous areolar tissue, mucous membranes of orifices, and the breast)*

110	Abnormality of heat elimination
121	Acroasphyxia
122	Acrocyanosis
155	Anhidrosis
103	Blushing
141	Cutaneous nodules
104	Cyanosis
132	Dermatographia (excessive local circulatory reaction due to scratching the skin)
105	Erythema, general
106	Erythema, local
161	Hirsutism
153	Hyperhidrosis, general
154	Hyperhidrosis, local
156	Hyperhidrosis, nocturnal
157	Increased pigmentation of skin, not abnormal
199	Intermediate reaction to smallpox vaccination (vaccinoid)
162	Loss of hair
158	Melanosis
186	Negative reaction to blastomycin
184	Negative reaction to coccidioidin
190	Negative reaction to Dick test
193	Negative reaction to histoplasmin test
195	Negative reaction to Schick test
198	Negative reaction to smallpox vaccination
188	Negative reaction to toxocara canis
177	Negative reaction to toxoplasma
192	Negative reaction to tuberculin test
125	Night sweats
196	No-take reaction to smallpox vaccination
101	Pallor
134	Petechiae
182	Pilomotor disturbances
102	Polydactyly
185	Positive reaction to blastomycin
183	Positive reaction to coccidioidin
18x	Positive reaction to Dick test
179	Positive reaction to Echinococcus (Casoni test)
180	Positive reaction to Frei test
189	Positive reaction to histoplasmin test
194	Positive reaction to Schick test

19x	Positive reaction to smallpox vaccination (vaccinia)
181	Positive reaction to test for trichinosis
187	Positive reaction to toxocara canis
178	Positive reaction to toxoplasma
191	Positive reaction to tuberculin test
143	Pruritus
133	Purpura
197	Successful vaccination
151	Trophedema
152	Trophoneuroses
159	Ulceration
140	Zoster

2– SUPPLEMENTARY TERMS

2 Supplementary terms of the musculoskeletal system

270	Amyotrophy
206	Arthralgia (general joint pain)
246	Arthropathy
271	Ataxia; incoordination
272	Atonia (loss of muscle tone)
208	Coccygodynia .
241	Contracture
202	Hydrarthrosis
242	Kyphosis
243	Lordosis
207	Lumbago (lumbosacral pain)
231	Muscular cramp
251	Myalgia (muscle pain)
230	Myoidema (local increased muscular irritability)
232	Myotonia (increased muscular irritability)
203	Osteoporosis
20x	Postures, hysterical
212	Retardation of ossification of epiphysis
244	Scoliosis
201	Swelling of joint or joints

3– SUPPLEMENTARY TERMS

3 *Supplementary terms of the respiratory system*

393	Acid fast bacilli in sputum
396	Animal parasites in sputum
322	Aphonia (nonneurogenic)
326	Asthma
392	Bronchial casts in sputum
31x	Bronchial spasm
320	Change in voice
394	Charcot-Leyden crystals in sputum
314	Cough
390	Dittrich plugs in sputum
311	Dyspnea
395	Elastic fibers in sputum
301	Epistaxis
309	Hemoptysis
305	Hemorrhage from lung (terminal)
300	Hemorrhage from respiratory tract
321	Hoarseness
365	Hydropneumothorax
340	Hydrothorax
310	Incoordination of vocal cords
397	Lung stones in sputum
317	Malignant tumor cells in bronchial secretions
316	Malignant tumor cells in pleural fluid
398	Molds and yeasts in sputum
312	Orthopnea
330	Pain in thorax (noncardiac)
323	Paralysis of larynx
313	Paroxysmal dyspnea
324	Pulmonary edema
325	Rales in lung
383	Radiopaque body in lung
327	Respiratory insufficiency
381	Roentgenogram characteristic of tuberculosis
373	Roentgenogram characteristic of tuberculosis, combined types
371	Roentgenogram characteristic of tuberculosis, proliferative
385	Sinus, clouded on transillumination or x-ray
318	Sneezing, intractable
315	Sputum
319	Stridor
391	Tubercle bacillus in sputum
331	Weakness in chest wall (flail chest)

4— SUPPLEMENTARY TERMS

4 *Supplementary terms of the cardiovascular system*

SYMPTOMS AND CLINICAL SYNDROMES

455	Adams-Stokes syndrome
401	Anginal syndrome
43x	Atrioventricular nodal tachycardia, paroxysmal
429	Atrioventricular nodal premature contractions
404	Cardiac insufficiency
462	Carotid sinus syndrome
403	Coronary insufficiency (myocardial ischemia)
40x	Neurocirculatory asthenia (cardiopsychoneurosis)
402	Palpitation
42x	Postpericardiotomy syndrome
400	Precordial pain of cardiac origin
409	Raynaud's phenomenon

PHYSIOLOGIC FEATURES

408	Aortic valve incompetency
499	Aortic valve stenosis, not congenital
451	Arrhythmia generally and unspecified
420	Atrial arrhythmia, unspecified
426	Atrial fibrillation, chronic
425	Atrial fibrillation, paroxysmal
424	Atrial flutter, chronic
423	Atrial flutter, paroxysmal
421	Atrial premature contraction
422	Atrial tachycardia, paroxysmal
460	Atrial tachycardia, unspecified
436	Atrioventricular block, complete
4361	First degree
4362	Second degree
4363	Third degree
434	Atrioventricular block, prolonged conduction only
446	Atrioventricular dissociation, not due to bundle block
433	Atrioventricular nodal rhythm
4x3	Blood pressure diastolic depressed
4x2	Blood pressure diastolic elevated
4x4	Blood pressure systolic depressed
4x5	Blood pressure systolic elevated
418	Bradycardia (sinus)

438	Bundle branch block, left
437	Bundle branch block, right
480	Cardiac thrombosis within chamber
426	Chronic atrial fibrillation
424	Chronic atrial flutter
453	Coupled rhythm (bigeminal)
452	Gallop rhythm
427	Infundibular stenosis, aortic
428	Infundibular stenosis, pulmonary
430	Junctional arrhythmia, unspecified
432	Junctional paroxysmal tachycardia
431	Junctional premature contractions
407	Mitral incompetency
498	Mitral valve stenosis, not congenital
461	Murmur of unknown origin
456	Premature beats, unspecified
406	Pulmonic valve incompetency
497	Pulmonic valve stenosis, not congenital
454	Pulsus alternans
417	Pulsus deletus
470	Recanalization of vein
416	Sinoatrial block
411	Sinus arrest
412	Sinus arrhythmia
413	Sinus bradycardia
450	Sinus rhythm normal
414	Sinus tachycardia
460	Tachycardia, paroxysmal, unspecified
405	Tricuspid valve incompetency
496	Tricuspid valve stenosis
440	Ventricular arrhythmia, unspecified
443	Ventricular escape
445	Ventricular fibrillation
441	Ventricular premature contractions
444	Ventricular standstill
442	Ventricular tachycardia paroxysmal
415	Wandering pacemaker

CARDIAC FUNCTION CAPACITY

457	Class I Cardiac disease exists without resulting limitation of physical activity
458	Class II Cardiac disease resulting in slight limitation of physical activity
459	Class III Cardiac disease resulting in marked limitation of physical activity
45x	Class IV Cardiac disease resulting in discomfort after any physical activity

5– SUPPLEMENTARY TERMS

5 Supplementary terms of the hemic and lymphatic systems

509	Abnormal sedimentation rate of erythrocytes
500	Abnormal viscosity of blood
51x	Abnormality in bleeding time
527	Abnormality of spleen
542	Acidosis
541	Alkalosis
503	Anhydremia
533	Anisocytosis
540	Anoxemia
551	Azotemia; uremia
583	Blood group A
584	Blood group B
585	Blood group AB
586	Blood group M
587	Blood group N
588	Blood group O
589	Blood group Rh negative
590	Blood group Rh positive
564	Carotenemia
501	Change in blood volume
502	Change in proportion of blood plasma to cells
580	Cholemia
5x2	Cryoglobulinemia
555	Decrease in amino acids in blood
526	Decrease in cevitamic acid in blood
559	Decrease in cholesterol esters
520	Decrease in coagulation time
572	Decrease in phenols in blood
573	Decreased carbon dioxide combining power of blood plasma
506	Decreased fragility of erythrocytes
554	Disturbance of creatine and creatinine metabolism
529	Enlargement of lymph nodes
513	Eosinophilia
5x0	Fibrinogenopenia
57x	Galactemia
565	Galactosemia
512	Granulocytopenia
530	Hemolysis
534	High icterus index
582	Hypercalcemia
562	Hyperchloremia

557	Hypercholesteremia
536	Hyperchromasia
546	Hypercupremia
5x4	Hypergammaglobulinemia
568	Hyperglobulinemia
571	Hyperglycemia. For Increased dextrose tolerance (test). *See Section 8, page 500*
59x	Hypenatremia
538	Hypernitremia
544	Hyperphosphatemia
592	Hyperpotassemia
545	Hyperproteinemia
567	Hypocalcemia
563	Hypochloremia
558	Hypocholesteremia
537	Hypochromasia
58x	Hypocupremia
5x1	Hypogammaglobulinemia
56x	Hypoglobulinemia
574	Hypoglycemia. For Decreased dextrose tolerance (test). *See Section 8, page 500*
599	Hyponatremia
539	Hyponitremia
549	Hypophosphatemia
593	Hypopotassemia
576	Hypoproteinemia
547	Hypoproteinemia with reversed albumin-globulin ratio
52x	Hypoprothrombinemia
553	Increase in amino acids in blood
575	Increase in bleeding time
579	Increase in cevitamic acid in blood
577	Increase in coagulation time
516	Increase in other leukocytes
552	Increase in phenols in blood
578	Increased carbon dioxide combining power of blood plasma
505	Increased fragility of erythrocytes
543	Ketosis
531	Leukemoid blood picture
510	Leukocytosis, simple
50x	Leukopenia, simple
556	Lipemia
514	Lymphocytosis
55x	Macrocytosis
5x3	Macroglobulinemia
581	Methemoglobinemia
532	Microcytosis

515	Monocytosis
535	Multiple capillary hemorrhages
511	Neutrophilia
54x	Oligocythemia
550	Poikilocytosis
594	Polychromatophilia
595	Polycythemia
596	Positive heterophil antibody test
597	Presence of immature cells in blood
598	Reticulocytosis
548	Sensitization Rh-Hr
528	Splenomegaly
507	Stippling of erythrocytes
519	Thrombocytopenia
518	Thrombocytosis
517	Toxic neutrophils
591	Tubercle bacilli in blood
561	Uricacidemia

6– SUPPLEMENTARY TERMS

6 *Supplementary terms of the digestive system*

620	Abdominal mass
645	Abnormality of duodenal filling
655	Abnormality of gallbladder after administration of dye
647	Abnormality of intestinal filling
650	Abnormality of opaque enema
680	Abnormal function of liver
659	Abnormal opacity in peritoneal cavity
661	Achlorhydria
662	Achylia
693	Acid bacilli, nonpathogenic, in gastric contents
617	Aerophagia
612	Anorexia (loss of appetite)
621	Ascites (hydroperitoneum)
668	Blood in gastric contents
669	Blood in feces, occult
694	Boas-Oppler bacilli in gastric contents
616	Bulimia (excessive appetite)
630	Constipation
635	Diarrhea
631	Dysphagia (difficulty in swallowing)
615	Eructation
641	Filling defect of stomach
695	Flexner agglutination, positive
601	Gastric crisis
643	Gastric hypermotility
644	Gastric hypomotility
642	Gastric stasis
619	Halitosis
600	Hemorrhage from gastrointestinal tract or peritoneum
622	Hepatomegaly
671	Hiccup (singultus)
663	Hyperchlorhydria
664	Hypersecretion, gastric
666	Hypochlorhydria
639	Incontinence of feces
649	Intestinal hypermotility
64x	Intestinal hypomotility
633	Intestinal obstruction
632	Intestinal stasis
665	Lactic acid in gastric contents
670	Melanosis of colon

611	Nausea
648	Obstipation
613	Odor in gastric contents in the newborn
625	Pain in abdomen
624	Pain in epigastrium; heartburn; purosis; cardialgia
628	Paralysis of uvula
6x1	Pathogenic bacteria in feces
672	Petechiae of jejunum
608	Pica
638	Proctalgia
60x	Ptyalism (salivation)
618	Pyloric obstruction
626	Rigidity of abdomen, general or local
623	Rumination or merycism
61x	Thirst, excessive; polydipsia
627	Tympanites
692	Tubercle bacilli in ascitic fluid
691	Tubercle bacilli in gastric or intestinal contents
6x8	Tumor cells in ascitic or peritoneal fluid
6x6	Tumor cells in gastric secretions
6x7	Tumor cells in sputum
627	Tympanites
6x5	Undigested fat in feces
6x4	Undigested protein in feces
6x3	Undigested starch in feces
614	Vomiting
609	Xerostomia
6x2	Yeast and molds in feces

7– SUPPLEMENTARY TERMS

7 *Supplementary terms of the urogenital system*

730	Abnormal acidity of urine
731	Abnormal alkalinity of urine
745	Abnormal content of electrolyte in urine
720	Abnormal phenosulphonphthalein excretion
755	Abnormal secretion of dye by kidney
723	Abnormal urea excretion
740	Acetonuria
793	**Acid fast bacilli, nonpathogenic, in urine**
733	Albuminuria
761	Amenorrhea
748	Aminoaciduria
708	Ammoniacal urine
703	Anuria
772	Aspermia
777	Asthenospermia
771	Azoospermia
790	Bacteriuria
734	Bence-Jones protein in urine
709	Bile pigments in urine
714	Calcification
715	Calculi
732	Casts in urine
751	**Decreased concentrating power of kidney**
766	Delayed menstruation
765	Dysmenorrhea
768	Dyspareunia
704	Dysuria
70x	Epithelial cells in urine
706	Frequency of micturition
707	Frequency of micturition, nocturnal
76x	Frigidity
743	Fructosuria
744	Galactosuria
718	Galacturia
741	Glycosuria
700	Hematuria
735	Hemoglobinuria
75x	Hemospermia
71x	Hyperoxaluria
719	Hyperuricemia
778	Impotence
721	Incontinence of urine
750	Increased concentrating power of kidney
742	Lactosuria

767	Leukorrhea
716	Lone kidney
763	Menorrhagia
764	Metrorrhagia
774	Necrospermia
737	Negative reaction to Aschheim-Zondek or similar test
724	Nocturnal emissions
762	Oligomenorrhea
773	Oligospermia
702	Oliguria
749	Other abnormal chemical substances in urine
781	Ovulation bleeding
780	Ovulation pain (Mittelschmerz)
747	Oxaluria
770	Pain referable to female genital organs
775	Pain referable to male genital organs
710	Pain referable to urinary system
746	Phosphaturia
701	Polyuria
736	Porphyrinuria
738	Positive reaction to Aschheim-Zondek or similar test
725	Premature ejaculation of semen
776	Priapism
795	Pyuria
711	Renal colic
705	Retention of urine
779	Spermatozoa count below normal
77x	Spermaturia
769	Sterility, circumstantial sterility
783	Superfecundation
782	Superfetation
791	Tubercle bacillus in urine
796	Tumor cells in cervical or vaginal secretions
797	Tumor cells in kidney secretions
798	Tumor cells in urinary secretions
760	Vaginal bleeding
717	Vaginismus
712	Vesical pain
713	Vesical tenesmus
792	Yeast cells in urine

8– SUPPLEMENTARY TERMS

8 *Supplementary terms of the endocrine system*

804	Aldosteronism
821	Decreased dextrose tolerance (test)
802	Depressed basal metabolism
801	Elevated basal metabolism
800	Hemorrhage from endocrine gland
811	Hibernation; somnolence
822	Increased dextrose tolerance (test)
806	Male climacteric
805	Menopausal syndrome
803	Thyroid crisis

9– SUPPLEMENTARY TERMS

9 *Supplementary terms of the nervous system*

9525	Absence of sensation of cold
9521	Absence of sensation of heat
9531	Absence of vibratory sensibility
992	Acalculia (inability to do simple arithmetic)
90x1	Adie syndrome (tonic pupil, reduction or loss in lower extremity tendon reflex activity)
984	Agnosia, acoustic; (loss of ability to recognize significance of sounds)
981	Agnosia, anosognosia: (loss of ability to recognize disease)
985	Agnosia, localization: (loss or diminution of localization sense, topagnosis)
986	Agnosia, position: (loss or diminution of position sense, acragnosis)
983	Agnosia, tactile: (loss or diminution of form sense, astereognosis)
988	Agnosia, texture: (loss or diminution of texture sense)
982	Agnosia, visual: (loss of ability visually to recognize objects)
987	Agnosia, weight: (loss or diminution of weight sense, baragnosis)
980	Agnosia: others
9551	Agrammatism aphasia (jargon aphasia)
955	Agraphia, developmental
951	Agraphia (inability to write or produce written or drawn symbols)
952	Alexia (inability to read)
967	Alexia developmental (strephosymbolia symbol reversal)
927	Allochiria (symmetrical contralateral identification of body areas stimulated)
921	Amentia
920	Amimia (loss of ability to mimic)
911	Amnesia
989	Amusia (inability to recognize musical sounds)
903	Analgesia (loss of pain sensitivity)
957	Anarthria (inability to express words or symbols properly)
902	Anesthesia, hysterical
900	Anesthesia (loss of feeling)
9550	Aphasia (difficulty in formulating, expressing or understanding speech symbols)
9552	Aphasia, amnestic (loss of memory for words)

976	Aphasia, developmental
95x	Aphasia, dysarthric
9553	Aphasia, expressive (motor)
9554	Aphasia, global
9557	Aphasia, nominal (anomia)
955x	Aphasia, receptive (sensory)
9561	Aphasia, semantic
9562	Aphasia, syntactic (mistakes in syntax)
9563	Aphasia, verbal
9564	Aphasia, visual
954	Aphemia
990	Aphonia, developmental
956	Aphonia (inability to vocalize speech)
9630	Apraxia (difficulty in performance of skilled acts)
991	Apraxia, developmental
9632	Apraxia, ideational
9633	Apraxia, ideomotor
9634	Apraxia, motor
942	Astasia abasia (hysterical inability to stand)
950	Asymbolia (inability to understand or make symbols and signs)
9xx	Asymmetry of ventricles demonstrable by roentgen ray
944	Asynergia (ataxia) (disturbance in coordination)
9211	Athetosis (successive pattern movements, vermicular in character)
921x	Athetosis, bilateral (acquired)
9011	Auriculotemporal nerve syndrome
972	Autotopagnosia (illusion of absence of paralyzed extremity)
970	Autotopagnosia (inability to recognize defects in one's body scheme)
975	Autotopagnosia (phantom limb)
9012	Brown-Sequard syndrome (hemi-involvement of spinal cord)
936	Cataplexy (falling caused by emotional influences)
939	Catatonia (maintenance of fixed postures)
9x5	Cerebral dysrhythmia (electroencephalographic)
996	Cerebrospinal fluid, abnormal cell count
997	Cerebrospinal fluid, decrease in sugar
998	Cerebrospinal fluid, increase in globulins
999	Cerebrospinal fluid, increased pressure of
99x	Cerebrospinal fluid, increase in proteins
9x0	Cerebrospinal fluid, increase in sugar

949	Cerebrospinal otorrhea (loss of cerebrospinal fluid from the external auditory meatus)
94x	Cerebrospinal rhinorrhea (loss of cerebrospinal fluid from the nose)
9026	Cestan syndrome (disseminated pontine)
9213	Chorea (isolated twitching movements of muscles)
9215	Choreoathetosis (combination of chorea and athetosis)
9014	Claude syndrome (rubrospinal cerebellar peduncle)
9x1	Colloidal benzoin test, positive
9x2	Colloidal gold test, positive
932	Coma
922x	Combined forms of abnormal involuntary movements
9x3	Confabulation
908	Compulsive talking
9631	Constructional apraxia
934	Convulsions, generalized
918	Crying, forced
993	Deafness, word, developmental
9015	Dejerine-Roussy syndrome (thalamic hyperesthetic anesthesia)
9301	Delayed speech with mental deficiency
9303	Delayed speech without mental deficiency
931	Delirium
925	Delusions
922	Dementia
947	Diataxia, cerebral, infantile
9522	Diminution of sensation of heat
9526	Diminution of sensation of cold
9532	Diminution of vibratory sensibility
960	Diplegia
9016	Dorsolateral medullary syndrome (posterior inferior cerebellar artery)
9038	Dorsal sclerosis (dorsal column degeneration)
9039	Dorsolateral sclerosis (dorsal and lateral column degeneration)
904	Dream states
977	Dysautonomia
943	Dysbasia (difficulty in standing)
906	Dysesthesia (perverted objective sensitivity)
958	Dyslexia (difficulty in reading)
945	Dysmetria (incorrect measuring of movements)
953	Dysphasia (difficulty in speech)

959	Dyspraxia (difficulty in performance of skilled acts)
9216	Dystonic movements (intermittent hyper-and hypotonia)
928	Echolalia (echoing speech of examiner)
962	Edema, cerebral
963	Encephalomalacia (softening of the brain)
938	**Erythromelalgia** (pain and redness of extremities due to nervous influence)
90x	Extinction (suppression of one stimulation by another)
937	Flexibilitas cerea (cataleptic retention of postures)
9217	Forced grasping and groping
9x17	Foville syndrome (lateral gaze paralysis, unilateral or bilateral)
974	Gerstmann syndrome (finger agnosia, right-left disorientation, acalculia, agraphia)
9018	Gradenigo syndrome (petrous osteomyelitis or meningitis with abducens nerve palsy)
901x	Guillain-Barré syndrome (virus encephalomyelitis)
9226	Habit spasm
910	Hallucinosis, general
9101	Hallucinosis, hypnagogic (on going to sleep)
9102	Hallucinosis, hypnopompic (on awakening)
961	Headache; cephalalgia
9513	Hemianalgesia
901	Hemianesthesia
9212	Hemiathetosis
9210	Hemiballismus (gross throwing movements of upper and/or lower extremities)
9214	Hemichorea
9514	Hemihypalgesia
917	Hemihypesthesia
968	Hemiparesis
969	Hemiplegia
9013	Horner syndrome (irritative cervical sympathetic paralysis, miosis, enophthalmos, ptosis)
964	Hydrocephalus
965	Hydrocephalus, external
9512	Hypalgesia (reduction of pain sensitivity)
9515	Hyperalgesia (increased pain sensitivity)
905	Hyperesthesia (increased sensitivity)
9516	Hyperpathia (increased effect from painful stimuli)
914	Hypersomnia

913	Hypesthesia (reduction of feeling)
97x	Hypsarhythmia
926	Illusions
9527	Increase of sensation of cold
9523	Increase of sensation of heat
916	Insomnia; hyposomnia
9555	Interjectional speech
946	Irreminiscence (difficulty in recall of auditory, visual or directional engrams)
935	Jacksonian seizures (motor or sensory)
903x	Lateral sclerosis (lateral column degeneration)
909	Lateropulsion (deviation of gait or station to one side)
919	Laughter, forced
9304	Letter sound substitution
9541	Loss or diminution of sense of position and movement
9543	Loss or diminution of tactile discrimination (circles of Weber)
9542	Loss or diminution of tactile localization
9063	Manometric block (interference with transmission of spinal fluid pressures)
9218	Mass movements
9x6	Mastic test, cerebrospinal syphilitic reaction
9x7	Mastic test, paretic reaction
9x8	Mastic test, tabetic reaction
979	Meningismus
91x	Mental deficiency
923	Mental deterioration
92x	Migraine
948	Monoplegia
9219	Myoclonus (muscle contractions of a rhythmical character)
9220	Myokymia (fasciculation without atrophy)
930	Narcolepsy (excessive inclination to sleep)
9519	Neuralgia, facial, atypical
915	Neurotic excoriations
9227	Occupation spasm or tic
9501	Pain asymbolia (loss of pain symbolism)
973	Palilalia (repetition of words)
9558	Paragrammatism (ungrammatical speech)
9571	Paralysis abducens, facial, hemiplegic, alternating (Millard-Gubler syndrome)
9570	Paralysis of accommodation
9572	Paralysis, alternating abducens, hemiplegic
9573	Paralysis, alternating (facial) lateral gaze, hemiplegic
9574	Paralysis, alternating, hypoglossal, hemiplegic

9575	Paralysis, alternating, oculomotor, hemiplegic (Weber paralysis)
9576	Paralysis, ambiguoaccessorius
9577	Paralysis, ambiguoaccessorius-hypoglossal
9578	Paralysis, ambiguo-hypoglossal
9579	Paralysis, ambiguospinothalamic (Avellis)
957x	Paralysis, brachial plexus, upper or lower
9580	Paralysis, bulbar
9581	Paralysis, cerebral diplegic, infantile
9582	Paralysis, cerebral hemiplegic, infantile
9583	Paralysis, cerebral, hereditary, spastic
9585	Paralysis, cerebral, infantile
9947	Paralysis, cerebral, infantile, ataxia
9584	Paralysis, cerebral, infantile, choreoathetoid
9586	Paralysis, cerebrocerebellar, diplegic, infantile
9587	Paralysis, cerebrospinal, hereditary; hemiplegia, diplegia, paraplegia or tetraplegia
9588	Paralysis, cruciate, hemiplegic (one upper opposite lower extremity)
9589	Paralysis, medullary, tegmental (Babinski-Nageotte) mixed gray and white involvement of medulla
958x	Paralysis, mesencephalic, tegmental (Benedikt)
9x29	Paralysis, oculomotor, external, bilateral
9590	Paralysis, oculomotor, tetraplegic
9591	Paralysis, pseudobulbar (upper motor neurone bulbar palsy)
9592	Paralysis, spinal, hereditary, spastic
9559	Paraphasia (central aphasia)
971	Paraphasia (misuse of words)
941	Paraplegia
907	Paresthesia (tingling, numbness, burning, bursting, crawling, tickling, etc.)
9024	Parinaud syndrome (lateral rectus paralysis with spasm of contralateral medial rectus)
9221	Paramyoclonus (spontaneous involuntary contractions of muscles or fasciculi without atrophy)
929	Perseveration (repetition of patient's own words, phrases or movements)
93x	Petit mal
9025	Posterior lacerated (jugular) foramen syndrome, Villaret IX, X, XI cerebral nerves
940	Pyknolepsy (short lapses of consciousness)
9027	Retroparotid space (Villaret) IX, X, XI, XII cerebral nerves, plus cervical sympathetic
912	Retropulsion (deviation of gait or posture backward)

98x	Simultanagnosia (inability to synthesize elements into a whole)
9222	Spasm; torticollis; hemispasm facialis
9330	Spasm of glottis
9224	Spasmus nutans (nodding of head)
994	Special spelling disability
9305	Speech disorder due to habit (after repair of cleft palate)
9028	Striocerebellar syndrome
933	Stupor
966	Subarachnoid hemorrhage
9029	Supranuclear bulbar, bulbar palsy (upper motor neurone bulbar involvement)
9302	Stuttering (including stammering)
924	Synesthesia (simultaneous feeling of stimulation in unstimulated areas)
96x	Tetraplegia; quadriplegia
9225	Tic (muscle contraction, irregular)
9223	Torsion spasm (torsion of shoulder or pelvic girdle)
9228	Tremor
978	Triplegia (three extremities)
9x9	Tumor cells in cerebrospinal fluid
995	Vasomotor disturbances

X– SUPPLEMENTARY TERMS

X *Supplementary terms of the organs of special sense*

x11	Achromatopsia (color blindness)
x12	Amaurosis (blindness)
x13	Amblyopia (dimness of vision)
x41	Anosmia
x44	Asthenopia
x09	Conduction deafness
x122	Day blindness; hemeralopia
x08	Deaf mutism, symptomatic
x59	Deafness, neural, cause unknown
x47	Deafness, neural, due to vascular lesion of higher centers
x56	Deafness sensory, cause unknown
x58	Deafness, sensory-neural, cause unknown
x06	Deafness unspecified
x071	Diplacusis (hearing of one sound as two sounds)
x22	Diplopia
x70	Disturbances of facial nerve
x80	Disturbances of glossopharyngeal and vagal nerves
x83	Disturbances of glossopharyngeal and vagal nerves, laryngoplegia
x81	Disturbances of glossopharyngeal and vagal nerves, palatoplegia
x82	Disturbances of glossopharyngeal and vagal nerves, pharyngoplegia
x07	Disturbances of hearing
xx0	Disturbances of hypoglossal nerve
x40	Disturbances of olfactory nerve
x50	Disturbances of optic nerve
x78	Disturbances of secretory and vasomotor nerves
x90	Disturbances of spinal accessory nerves
x60	Disturbances of trigeminal nerve
x20	Enophthalmos
x21	Exophthalmos
x32	Extrinsic muscles (eye), paralysis (including ptosis)
x33	Extrinsic muscles (eye), skew deviation
x31	Extrinsic muscles (eye), spasm (including blepharospasm)
x71	Facial nerve paralysis, central
x72	Facial nerve paralysis, peripheral

x43	Hallucinations
x432	Hallucinations of hearing
x435	Hallucinations of smell
x431	Hallucinations of taste: ageusia, parageusia
x433	Hallucinations of vision
x15	Hemianopsia, binasal
x16	Hemianopsia, bitemporal
x17	Hemianopsia, homonymous
x14	Hemianopsia, macular involving
x19	Hemianopsia, macular sparing
x18	Hemianopsia, quadrantic
x45	Hyperosmia
xx1	Hypoglossal nerve, atrophy
xx2	Hypoglossal nerve, paralysis
x35	Intrinsic muscles (eye), paralysis (reflex rigidity of pupil)
x34	Intrinsic muscles (eye), spasm
x00	Ménière syndrome (labyrinthine syndrome)
x01	Middle ear deafness
x02	Nerve deafness
x121	Night blindness; nyctalopia
x2x	Nystagmus
x28	Oculogyric paralysis, convergence
x29	Oculogyric paralysis, divergence
x27	Oculogyric paralysis, lateral gaze
x26	Oculogyric paralysis, vertical gaze
x25	Oculogyric spasm, convergent
x24	Oculogyric spasm, lateral
x23	Oculogyric spasm, vertical
x52	Optic atrophy
x51	Optic neuritis or neuropathy
x48	Otalgia
xy1	Other disturbances of intrinsic muscles
x10	Other disturbances of vision
x54	Other intraocular changes
x2y	Other oculogyric disturbances
x49	Otorrhagia
x4x	Otorrhea
x53	Papilledema
x42	Parosmia
x55	Photophobia
x46	Proptosis
x123	Psychic blindness
x1x	Scotoma
x91	Spinal accessory nerve, atrophy
x92	Spinal accessory nerve, paralysis (cephalogyric disturbances)
x04	Tinnitus

x68	Trigeminal nerve, atrophy facial
x69	Trigeminal nerve, hemiatrophy facial
x62	Trigeminal nerve, motor paralysis
x61	Trigeminal nerve, motor spasm (trismus)
x6x	Trigeminal nerve, secretory disturbances
x64	Trigeminal nerve, sensory disturbance, glossodynia (pain in tongue)
x66	Trigeminal nerve, sensory disturbance of pain
x67	Trigeminal nerve, sensory disturbance of temperature
x65	Trigeminal nerve, sensory disturbance of touch
x0x	Vertigo
x124	Word blindness
x03	Word deafness

STANDARD NOMENCLATURE
OF OPERATIONS

STANDARD NOMENCLATURE OF OPERATIONS

INTRODUCTION

Topographic numbers, i.e., those digits appearing before the dash, correspond exactly with those used in the Standard Nomenclature of Diseases, the listing of which begins on page 3. The operative procedure completes the code and is expressed by the digits following the dash. The key, or meaning of the digits, is given on page 517. The main operative procedures are:

-0 Incision
-1 Excision
-2 Amputation
-3 Introduction
-4 Endoscopy
-5 Repair
-6 Destruction
-7 Suture
-8 Manipulation

The classification has been made as complete and as detailed as was believed necessary for the use of the average general hospital. For the use of certain types of institutions and in various surgical specialties it may be desirable to carry out further subdivisions of the listed procedures. This can be done readily within the present framework. The procedure codes may be used arbitrarily where applicable.

It will be noted that in some cases special operative methods may be specified in relation to the fundamental surgical procedures. The manner by which these may be indicated generally is noted on page 517; and at appropriate points in the text. In a few instances there are alternative methods of approach, which may also be indicated as shown in the key on page 517.

The term "excision of lesion" of an organ or structure is used to differentiate an essentially local excision, such as that of a tumor, cyst, or ulcer, from a wide excision, which is generally referred to as a resection. In some cases this is of necessity an arbitrary distinction.

Hospitals are encouraged to carry out the maximum degree of refinement in classification of operative procedures which their facilities will permit. A number of terms which have appeared in previous publications have been omitted because of ambiguous interpretation or lack of sufficient specificity or because in the light of present day standards of surgery they do not represent generally accepted operative procedures. Synonymous terms are separated by a colon. Closely allied but not synonymous terms are separated by a semicolon. Names of persons as applied to operative procedures have been placed in the index whenever possible.

513

Lists of anesthetic agents and methods appear on page 607.   Hospital record libraries may, if desired, record these code numbers for purposes of additional information or for clinical research in anesthesia.

The Committee on Operations under the chairmanship of Hilger Perry Jenkins, M.D., has contributed substantial assistance in the preparation of the classification.   The committee members are

BURRILL B. CROHN, M.D.
MONTAGUE L. BOYD, M.D.
H. HOUSTON MERRITT, M.D.
JOHN D. STEELE, M.D.
HAROLD E. B. PARDEE, M.D.
J. P. GREENHILL, M.D.
M. EDWARD DAVIS, M.D.
HAROLD HAYES, D.D.S.
M. M. HIPSKIND, M.D.
ARTHUR GROLLMAN, M.D.
JOHN H. DUNNINGTON, M.D.
LOUIS R. LIMARZI, M.D.
H. EARLE CONWELL, M.D.
HERBERT RATTNER, M.D.

Questions relative to the section on operations may be sent directly to the editors.

EDWARD T. THOMPSON, M.D., *Editor*

CLASSIFICATION OF OPERATIVE
PROCEDURES

CLASSIFICATION OF OPERATIVE PROCEDURES

—0 INCISION
—1 EXCISION
—2 AMPUTATION
—3 INTRODUCTION
—4 ENDOSCOPY
—5 REPAIR
—6 DESTRUCTION
—7 SUTURE
—8 MANIPULATION

CLASSIFICATION OF OPERATIVE PROCEDURES [1,2]

—0 INCISION

–00	Incision, generally or unspecified (suffix -tomy) [1]
–01	Incision, exploratory
–02	Incision and drainage [1]
–020	"Closed tube" drainage
–021	Radical drainage
–023	Puncture for aspiration (suffix -centesis)
–03	Incision and removal (*foreign body, calculus, plates, nails, screws*) [1]
–030	Incision and removal of foreign body, partial
–031	Magnet removal
–04	Cesarean section
–05	Reopening of recent operative *wound*
–06	Transection, cutting or division [1]
–060	Partial transection
–07	Preliminary or preparatory incision
–070	Incision and packing of *wound* (prior to drainage, etc.)
–071	Incision and exteriorization of organ or *lesion* thereof (prior to excision)
–072	Incision and resuture of *wound* (plastic operation)
–073	Incision and tubing (pedicle graft)
–08	Decompression

—1 EXCISION

–10	Excision, generally or unspecified (suffix -ectomy) [3]
–101	Wedge excision
–11	Local excision of *lesion* of organ [3]
–111	Partial excision of *lesion*
–12	Complete or total excision of organ [3]
–121	Fistulectomy

1 Special operative method may be indicated where applicable by appropriate 3d digit as follows:

▲▲2	Electrocoagulation
▲▲3	Aspiration
▲▲4	Curettage
▲▲5	Cauterization
▲▲6	Fulguration
▲▲7	Endothermy
▲▲8	Punch
▲▲9	Other special methods: avulsion, snare, constriction

2 Approach may be indicated where two or more standard methods are in use, as:

▲▲x	Alternate method of approach, *to be specified*
▲▲y	Combined approach or second alternate method of approach, *to be specified*

3 Special operative method may be indicated by appropriate 3d digit. See above.

--13	Partial or subtotal excision of organ: resection of organ [1]
–14	Radical excision of organ [1] or structure or *lesion* thereof
–15	Excision or resection of exteriorized organ [1]
–16	Biopsy [1]
–163	Needle biopsy
–168	Punch biopsy
–17	Excision of tissue for grafting (to designate donor site) [1]

—2 AMPUTATION

–20	Amputation
–21	Disarticulation

—3 INTRODUCTION

–30	Injections
–300	Serum, immunizing
–301	Air or other gases (oxygen, helium, ethylene)
–302	Radiopaque substance
–303	Dye, nonopaque
–304	Alcohol
–305	Oil
–306	Sclerosing solution
–307	Antibiotic (sulfanilamide, penicillin, streptomycin, aureomycin, bacitracin)
–308	Irritant
–31	Transfusion
–310	Refusion of blood
–311	Plasma
–312	Serum
–313	Replacement of blood
–314	Removal, processing and replacement of blood
–32	Introduction or implantation of radioactive substances
–320	Radium
–321	Radon
–322	Other radioactive substances
–323	Roentgen radiation delivered through open wound
–33	Insertion of metal device (without open reduction)
–330	Wire
–331	Metal pin or nail
–332	Caliper
–333	Threaded wire
–334	Beaded wire or pin

1 Special operative method may be indicated by appropriate 3d digit. See page 517.

–335	Metal periosteal implant
–336	Orthodontic appliance
–3361	Space maintainer
–3362	Stabilizing appliance
–338	Denture
–34	Insertion of collapsible bag
–35	Insertion of pack, tampon, plug, or prosthetic device
–351	Paraffin
–352	Plastic
–353	Glass
–37	Irrigation
–38	Insertion of catheter or tube: catheterization or intubation
–381	Rubber tube; T tube
–382	Plastic tube
–383	Metal tube (Vitallium)
–384	Glass tube
–39	Introduction of or implantation of endocrine products
–391	Artificial insemination

—4 ENDOSCOPY

–40	Endoscopy, generally or for exploration (suffix-scopy)
–41	Endoscopic biopsy [1]
–42	Endoscopic excision [1]
–43	Endoscopic drainage [1]
–44	Endoscopic removal (*calculus, foreign body*)
–45	Endoscopic dilation
–46	Endoscopic division of adhesions [1]
–47	Endoscopic injection of fluid
–470	For irrigation
–471	Diagnostic
–472	Therapeutic
–48	Endoscopic insertion of radioactive substance
–49	Endoscopic insertion of catheter or tube
–4x	Endoscopic control of *hemorrhage* [1]

—5 REPAIR

–50	Plastic repair, generally or unspecified (suffix -plasty)
–500	Lengthening
–5001	By oblique transection and resuture
–5002	By flap

[1] Special operative method may be indicated by appropriate 3d digit. See page 517.

−5003	By Z – plastic
−5004	By fragmentation and mechanical or synthetic device
−501	Shortening
−5011	By plication or overlapping
−502	Plastic repair with aid of metal, mechanical or synthetic device
−5021	Restoration of tooth structure
−503	Plastic closure of wound
−5031	By pedicle of tube flaps
−50311	Open
−50312	Closed by skin graft
−50313	Closed by tubing
−5032	By advanced flap (sliding flap)
−5033	By double pedicle flap
−504	Plastic reconstruction with excision of
−5041	Bone
−5042	Cartilage
−5043	Skin
−5044	Restoration gingival tissue
−505	Plastic repair with bone shifting
−506	Revision of pedicle
−5061	Defatting of skin
−5062	Defatting of skin and fat transplant
−51	Graft
−510	Pinch graft, skin
−512	Split thickness or partial thickness graft, skin
−514	Full thickness graft, skin
−516	Bone graft
−5161	Tooth germ graft
−5162	Autogenous
−5163	Heterogenous
−5164	Homogenous
−517	Cartilage graft
−5172	Autogenous
−5173	Heterogenous
−5174	Homogenous
−518	Fascial graft
−519	Fat graft
−51x	Blood vessel graft
−52	Anastomosis (suffix -stomy)
−53	Fistulization (suffix -stomy). *When performed primarily for drainage classify as* Incision and drainage −02
−54	Open reduction
−540	And fixation with suture
−541	**And fixation with metal nail, pin, or screw**
−542	And fixation with plate or band

–543	And fixation with metal rod, intramedullary
–544	And fixation with insertion of prosthesis
–56	Fixation; suspension (suffix -pexy)
–560	Attachment; reattachment
–561	Advancement
–562	Recession
–563	By aid of metal, mechanical or synthetic device
–564	Attachment
–57	Fusion; stabilization (suffix -desis)
–571	With aid of metallic device
–58	Transplantation

—6 DESTRUCTION

–60	Destructive procedure, generally or unspecified [1]
–609	Surgical abrasion
–61	Debridement
–63	Fracturing; refracturing (suffix -clasis)
–631	Fracture with rodding
–64	Crushing (suffixes -tripsy, -trity)
–65	Freeing or division of *adhesions* (suffix -lysis) [1]
–66	Stripping

—7 SUTURE

–70	Suture or closure, generally or unspecified (suffix -rrhaphy)
–71	Suture or closure of *wound* (suffix -rrhaphy)
–710	Suture of *wound* following debridement
–72	Closure of *fistula*
–73	Secondary suture or closure of *wound;* resuture of *wound*
–730	Delayed suture of *wound;* closure of *granulating wound*
–74	Ligation
–75	Occlusion; exclusion

—8 MANIPULATION

–80	Manipulation: manual procedures, generally
–81	Manipulation and application of plaster, splint or traction apparatus (correction of angulation or other procedure where ends are in apposition)
–82	Closed reduction and application of plaster, splint or traction apparatus
–83	Removal of drains, dressings, packing, bag, sutures, wire, caliper, traction, etc.

[1] Special operative method may be indicated by appropriate 3d digit. See page 517.

–84	Dilation or stretching, manual (suffixes -tasia, -tasis)
–840	Dilation or stretching, instrumental
–85	Application of or delivery by forceps
–850	Low
–851	Mid
–852	High
–86	Version
–860	External
–861	Internal
–862	Combined
–87	Conversion of position, manual
–870	Conversion of position, instrumental
–88	Extraction, obstetric
–89	Delivery, obstetric

NOMENCLATURE OF OPERATIONS

O– OPERATIONS ON REGIONS
OF THE BODY

(Not Associated with a Single Anatomic System)

Specify region by inserting digits when indicated. See page 3.

—0 INCISION

0▲▲–01	Exploratory incision
0▲▲–02	Incision and drainage (*abscess,* subcutaneous or not involving an organ) [1]
0▲▲–03	Incision and removal (*foreign body*)
0▲▲–05	Reopening of recent operative incision (for exploration or for control of *hemorrhage*)
0▲▲–06	Cutting of pedicle or tube graft
0▲▲–060	Partial cutting of pedicle or tube graft
0▲▲–07	Preparation of pedicle or tube graft
0▲▲–070	Incision and packing of *wound* (with elevation of pedicle from its bed)
0▲▲–072	Incision and resuture of *wound* (to establish cicatricial barriers)
0▲▲–073	Incision and tubing of pedicle

—1 EXCISION

0▲▲–11	Local or simple excision of *lesion* [1]
0▲▲–111	Partial excision of *lesion*
0▲▲–13	Wide excision of *lesion* (especially *malignant neoplasm*) [1]
0▲▲–16	Biopsy [1]
0▲▲–163	Aspiration or needle biopsy
0▲▲–164	Biopsy by curettage
0▲▲–168	Punch biopsy

—5 REPAIR

0582–53	Marsupialization of pilonidal sinus
0▲▲–50	Plastic operation on region of body
022–50	Forehead
027–50	Face
028–50	Cheek
029–50	Chin
0▲▲–503	Plastic closure of *wound*
0▲▲–5031	By pedicle of tube flaps

[1] Special operative method may be indicated by appropriate 3d digit. See page 517.

525

0▲▲–5032	By advanced flap (sliding flap)
0▲▲–5033	By double-pedicled flap
0▲▲–504	Plastic reconstruction with excision of
0▲▲–5041	Bone
0▲▲–5042	Cartilage
0▲▲–5043	Skin
0▲▲–505	Plastic repair with bone shifting
0▲▲–506	Revision of pedicle
0▲▲–5061	Defatting of skin
0▲▲–5062	Defatting of skin and fat transplant
0▲▲–51	Plastic operation on region of body involving graft
0▲▲–516▲	Bone graft (autogenous, homologous, or heterologous)
0▲▲–517▲	Cartilage graft (autogenous, homologous, or heterologous)
0▲▲–518	Fascial graft
0▲▲–519	Fat graft
0▲▲–514	Full thickness graft, skin
0▲▲–512	Split thickness or partial thickness graft, skin
0▲▲–510	Pinch graft, skin

To indicate donor site:

2▲▲–17	Bone
2290–17	Rib cartilage
297–17	Thigh fascia
13▲–17	Skin
18▲–17	Subcutaneous tissue

—6 DESTRUCTION

0▲▲–60	Destruction of *lesion* [1]
0▲▲–604	By curettage
0▲▲–605	By cauterization
0▲▲–606	By fulguration
0▲▲–61	Debridement [1]

—7 SUTURE

▲▲▲–72	Fistulectomy and closure
0▲▲–71	Suture of *wound*
0▲▲–710	Suture of *wound* following debridement
0▲▲–73	Secondary suture of *wound;* resuture of *wound*
0▲▲–730	Delayed suture of *wound;* closure of *granulating wound*

—8 MANIPULATION

0▲▲–83	Removal of drains, packs, dressings, etc.

[1] Special operative method may be indicated by appropriate 3d digit. See page 517.

OPERATIONS ON THE MEDIASTINUM

—0 INCISION

039–00   Mediastinotomy [1]
  039–01   With exploration
  039–02   With drainage (*abscess*)
  039–03   With removal (*foreign body*)

—I EXCISION

039–11   With excision of *lesion* (*cyst, tumor*)
039–16   With biopsy

For operations on other structures in this region see Heart and pericardium, *page 547, and* Lung and pleura, *page 645.*

[1] Posterior approach may be indicated by x added at end of code to differentiate from anterior approach.

1– OPERATIONS ON THE INTEGU-MENTARY SYSTEM

OPERATIONS ON THE SKIN AND SUBCUTANEOUS AREOLAR TISSUE

Specify region by inserting digits when indicated. See page 3.

—0 INCISION

1▲▲–02	Incision and drainage of *infection* of skin. *For drainage of subcutaneous abscess, classify under* Regions, *page 525*
15▲–02	Of glands of skin (*infected steatoma*)
16▲–02	Of hair follicles (*furuncle*)
17▲–02	Of nail bed or fold (*onychia, paronychia, infected ingrowing toenail*)
18▲–02	Of subcutaneous areolar tissue (*cellulitis*)

—1 EXCISION

1▲▲–11	Local excision of *lesion* of skin (*cicatricial, inflammatory, congenital,* or *benign neoplastic lesion*) [1]
15▲–11	Of glands of skin (*steatoma*)
16▲–11	Of hair follicles
18▲–11	Of subcutaneous tissue (*lipoma*)
1▲▲–13	Wide excision of *lesion* of skin (especially malignant *neoplasm*) [1]
1▲▲▲–14	Radical excision of lesion of skin (*For* excision involving underlying or adjacent structures)
1▲▲–16	Biopsy of skin or subcutaneous tissue [1]
1▲▲–17	Excision of skin for graft (to designate donor site)
17▲–10	Excision of nail, nail bed, or nail fold
17▲–12	Complete excision of nail, nail bed, or nail fold
17▲–13	Partial excision of nail, nail bed, or nail fold

—3 INTRODUCTION

18▲–39	Implantation of desoxycorticosterone in subcutaneous tissue

[1] Special operative method may be indicated by appropriate 3d digit. See page 517.

528

—5 REPAIR

For all superficial plastic operations see Plastic operations on region of body.

1▲▲–5003   Z Plastic relaxing operation

OPERATIONS ON THE BREAST

For male breast substitute 199 for 190

—0 INCISION

190–00	Mastotomy: mammotomy
190–01	With exploration
190–02	With drainage (*abscess*)
190–03	With removal (*foreign body*)

—I EXCISION

190–10	Mastectomy: mammectomy: amputation of breast
190–11	Local excision of *lesion* of breast (*cyst, fibro-adenoma, or aberrant breast tissue*). *Ordinarily classify as* Partial mastectomy
190–12	Complete (simple) mastectomy
190–13	Partial mastectomy
190–14	Radical mastectomy (breast, pectoral muscles, and axillary lymph nodes)
190–16	Biopsy of breast
193–11	Excision of *lesion* of ducts
194–12	Excision of nipple

—3 INTRODUCTION

190–352	Plastic operation on breast with insertion of plastic implant

—5 REPAIR

190–50	Mastoplasty: plastic operation on breast
194–50	Mammilliplasty: plastic operation on nipple
194–514	With free graft of nipple
194–515	With transposition of nipple
190–56	Mastopexy: fixation of pendulous breast

—7 SUTURE

190–71	Suture of breast (*wound, injury*)

2– OPERATIONS ON THE MUSCULO-SKELETAL SYSTEM

OPERATIONS ON BONES

Specify bone by inserting digits where indicated. See page 8.

—0 INCISION

2▲▲–01	Exploration of bone
2▲▲–02	Drainage of bone (*osteomyelitis, abscess*)
2▲▲.4–02	By incision of periosteum; periosteotomy
2▲▲.5–02	By drilling or "windowing" of cortex
2▲▲–03	Removal (sequestrum, foreign body, metal plate, band, screw, nail, etc.)
2▲▲–06	Osteotomy: cutting, division or transection of bone
227–06	Clavicotomy
22x3–06	Pubiotomy
22x–06	Ischiopubiotomy
2203–06	Laminotomy
228–06	Sternotomy

—1 EXCISION

22▲6–10	Facetectomy
2▲▲–10	Ostectomy: excision or resection of bone or lesion of bone. *Specify complete or partial*
229–10	Costectomy
233▲–10	Carpectomy
23x–10	Metatarsectomy
2▲▲–11	Local excision of *lesion* of bone (*bone cyst, chondroma*).[1] *Ordinarily classify* Partial ostectomy
2▲▲–12	Complete ostectomy: complete excision of bone
2392–12	Astragalectomy
225–12	Coccygectomy
2▲▲–13	Partial ostectomy: resection of bone: partial excision of bone: craterization, guttering or saucerization of bone: diaphysectomy
2▲▲▲▲–13	Condylectomy
2464–13	Costotransversectomy
2▲▲–101	Wedge ostectomy of bone . . . . *Specify bone*
2▲▲–16	Biopsy of bone
2▲▲.x–16	Biopsy of marrow (bone), *e.g.*

1 Special operative method may be indicated by appropriate 3d digit. See page 517.

530

228.x–163	Sternal puncture-by aspiration
228.x–164	Sternal puncture by curettage
2▲▲–17	Excision of bone for graft (to designate donor site)

—3 INTRODUCTION

2▲▲–33	Insertion or application of traction device (without incision)
2▲▲–330	Insertion of wire (Kirschner wire)
2▲▲–331	Insertion of metal pin (Steinmann pin)
2▲▲–332	Insertion or application of caliper traction apparatus (ice tongs)
2▲▲–333	Insertion of threaded wire
229.x–332	Venography, costal intra-osseus

—5 REPAIR

2▲▲–50	Osteoplasty
2▲▲–500	Lengthening of bone
2▲▲–5004	Lengthening of bone by fragmentation and metal, mechanical or synthetic device
2▲▲–501	Shortening of bone
2▲▲–516▲	Bone graft. *Specify autogenous, homologenous or heterologenous if desired*
2x53–516	Metacarpal bone graft (Thompson procedure)
2▲▲.4–516	Periosteal graft; osteoperiosteal graft
2▲▲–54	Open reduction of *fracture:* osteosynthesis
2▲▲–540	With suture (surgical gut, kangaroo tendon, or wire) : osteorrhaphy
2▲▲–541	With metal screw, nail or pin
2▲▲–542	With metal band or plate (Parham band, Lane or Sherman plate)
2▲▲–543	With metal rod, intramedullary
2▲▲–544	With insertion of prosthesis
226–56	Scapulopexy
2▲▲–57	Fusion of bone
2▲▲.2–57	Epiphysial-diaphysial fusion : epiphysial arrest : arrest of longitudinal growth of bone
220–57	Spinal fusion : spondylosyndesis
220–570	Correction of angulation (Harrington strut)
2414–57	Lumbosacral fusion

—6 DESTRUCTION

2▲▲–61	Debridement (*compound fracture*)
2▲▲–63	Fracture or refracture of bone: osteoclasis
2▲▲–65	Freeing of bone (*adhesions, callus, synostosis*)

—8 MANIPULATION

2▲▲–81   Manipulation of *fracture* and application of cast,
                 splint, or traction apparatus (correction of
                 angulation or other procedure where ends
                 are in opposition)
2▲▲–82   Closed reduction of *fracture* and application of
                 cast, splint, or traction apparatus. *See also*
                 Insertion or application of traction device
                 (without incision) preceding.
2▲▲–83   Removal of wire, pins or other metal device used
                 in maintaining apposition of fractured frag-
                 ments which does not require incision. If
                 incision is required *see* Removal (by incision)
                 page 530

OPERATIONS ON THE JOINTS (CAPSULE, SYNOVIAL MEMBRANE, CARTILAGES, AND LIGAMENTS)

Specify site by inserting digits where indicated. See page 13.

—0 INCISION

24▲–00   Arthrotomy
24▲–01   With exploration
24▲–02   With drainage, arthrostomy
24▲–03   With removal (*foreign body, osteocartilaginous
                   loose body*)
2493–06   Section, midtarsal joint region; medial joint
                 section
246▲–06   Synchondrotomy: division of synchondrosis
25▲–06   Chondrotomy: division of cartilage
26▲–06   Cutting or division of ligaments: desmotomy
24▲.4–06   Capsulotomy (joint): cutting or division of joint
                 capsule
24▲–023   Puncture for aspiration of joint: arthrocentesis

—I EXCISION

24▲–12   Arthrectomy: excision of joint
25▲–10   Chondrectomy: excision of cartilage
251–13   Excision of intervertebral cartilage, partial
                   (*prolapsed disk*)
253–10   Excision of semilunar cartilage of knee joint:
                   meniscectomy
2291–10   Excision of costal cartilage
26▲–10   Excision or resection of ligament

2▲▲.7–10	Synovectomy: excision or resection of synovial membrane of joint
24▲–11	Local excision of lesion of joint (osteochondritis dissecans)
2▲▲–16	Biopsy

—3 INTRODUCTION

24▲–301	Arthrography: injection of air into joint and roentgen examination

—5 REPAIR

24▲–50	Arthroplasty: plastic or reconstruction operation on joint; shelf operation
24▲–502	Arthroplasty with mechanical device (metal cup, etc.)
24▲–51	Arthroplasty with graft
24▲–516	Bone graft
24▲–518	Fascial graft
24x▲–50	Bunionectomy
2▲▲▲–517	Cartilage graft
24▲–57	Arthrodesis: fusion of joint to produce ankylosis. *For* Spinal fusion, *see* Operations on Bones, *page 531*
24▲–570	Stabilization of joint by bone block (to limit motion of joint)
24921–570	Stabilization of calcaneoastragaloid joint (Grice procedure)
24▲–54	Open reduction of *dislocation* or *fracture-dislocation* and fixation or repair
24▲–540	With suture (surgical gut, kangaroo tendon or wire)
24▲–541	With metal nail, pin or screw
24▲–542	With metal band or plate
24▲–543	With metal rod, intramedullary

—7 SUTURE

24▲.4–71	Suture or repair of joint capsule: capsulorrhaphy
26▲–71	Suture of ligament (*torn, ruptured, or severed*)

—8 MANIPULATION

24▲–80	Manipulation of joint
24▲–81	Manipulation of joint and application of cast, splint or traction apparatus

24▲–82   Closed reduction of *dislocation* or *fracture-dislocation* and application of cast, splint, or traction apparatus. *For special skeletal traction devices, see* Operations on Bones, *page 530*

OPERATIONS ON BURSAS

Specify bursa by inserting 3d digit. See page 14.

—0 INCISION

25▲–02   Incision and drainage of bursa
25▲–03   Incision and removal of *calcareous deposit* in bursa

—1 EXCISION

25▲–12   Excision of bursa: bursectomy
25▲–16   Biopsy of bursa

OPERATIONS ON MUSCLES

Specify muscle by inserting 3d digit. See page 15.

—0 INCISION

27▲–01   Exploration of muscle
27▲–02   Drainage of muscle (*abscess, hematoma, infection*)
27▲–03   Removal (*foreign body*)
27▲–06   Myotomy: cutting, division, or transection of muscle
2x71–06   Myotomy of gluteus minimus and gluteus medius (Durham procedure)

—1 EXCISION

27▲–10   Myectomy
27▲–11   Local excision of *lesion* of muscle (*myositis ossificans, neoplasm*)
27▲–13   Resection of muscle
27▲–16   Biopsy of muscle

—5 REPAIR

27▲–50   Myoplasty: plastic operation on muscle
27▲–51   Graft of muscle, free

27▲–515	Pedicle flap of muscle
27▲–58	Transplantation of muscle. *Specify muscle*
27▲–560	Transplantation of muscle origin: transference of origin with reattachment

—7 SUTURE

| 27▲–71 | Myorrhaphy: myosuture: suture of muscle (divided or severed) |

—8 MANIPULATION

| 27▲–81 | Manipulation of muscle and application of cast (for spasm) |
| 27▲–84 | Stretching of muscle: myotasis |

OPERATIONS ON TENDONS, TENDON SHEATHS, AND FASCIA

Specify site by inserting 3d digit.   See page 19.

—0 INCISION

28▲–01	Exploration of tendon
28▲.9–01	Exploration of tendon sheath
29▲–01	Exploration of fascia
28▲.9–02	Drainage of tendon sheath (*infection, tenosynovitis*)
28▲.9–03	Removal of *foreign body* or *rice bodies* in tendon sheath
29▲–03	Removal of *foreign body* in fascia
28▲–06	Tenotomy: cutting, division or transection of tendon: myotenotomy
2x82–06	Tenotomy of gastrocenemius and soleus
278–06	Myotenotomy of hip (Soutter procedure)
29▲–06	Fasciotomy: aponeurotomy: cutting or division of fascia
297–06	Fasciotomy of thigh (Yount procedure)

—1 EXCISION

28▲–11	Excision of *lesion* of tendon (*ganglion, xanthoma*)
28▲.9–11	Excision of *lesion* of tendon sheath (*ganglion, xanthoma*)
28▲.9–13	Excision or resection of tendon sheath: tenosynovectomy
29▲–13	Excision of fascia: fasciectomy

28▲–16   Biopsy of tendon or tendon sheath
29▲–16   Biopsy of fascia

—5 REPAIR

28▲–50   Tenoplasty: plastic operation on tendon
   28▲–500   With lengthening of tendon
   28▲–501   With shortening of tendon
   28▲–51   With graft of tendon
29▲–50   Fascioplasty
   2▲▲▲–518   Graft of fascia
28▲–56   .   Transposition of tendon (for transplantation of body of tendon into a new position)
28▲–560   Reattachment of tendon (for transplantation of tendon insertion)
   28819–561   Advancement of patellar tendon
   28▲–561   Advancement of tendon
   28▲–564   Attachment of tendon. *Specify tendon*
   28▲–562   Recession of tendon
28▲–57   Tenodesis: suture of tendon to skeletal attachment (when tendon is torn at point of insertion)
2896–560   Reattachment tendon, extensor hallucis longus
2896–5601   Reattachment tendon, extensor hallucis longus with fusion (Jones procedure)
2x64–560   Reattachment tendons of hamstring muscles (Eggers procedure)
2x61–560   Reattachment iliacus and psoas major tendons (Mustard procedure)
2875–560   Reattachment flexor digitorum sublimis tendon (Royal procedure)
2x63–5601   Reattachment of tendons of flexor muscles of elbow to humerus (Steindler procedure)
2x63–5602   Reattachment of tendons of flexor muscles of elbow to radius (Tubby-Steindler procedure)
2x84–560   Reattachment anterior tibial and peroneal tendons (Farill procedure)
29▲–57   Fasciodesis: suture of fascia to skeletal attachment

—7 SUTURE

28▲–71   Tenorrhaphy: tenosuture: suture of tendon (*divided or ruptured*)
29▲–71   Fasciorrhaphy: aponeurorrhaphy: suture of fascia or aponeurosis (*torn or divided*)

OPERATIONS ON THE EXTREMITIES

See also Operations on Regions of the Body, *page 525.*

—0 INCISION

Incision and drainage (*infection*)

2961–02	Of dorsal subaponeurotic space
2962–02	Of hypothenar space
2963–02	Of thenar space
2964–02	Of middle palmar space
2966–02	Of distal anterior closed space of finger
1871–02	Of web space

—2 AMPUTATION

Amputation at upper, middle, or lower portion of bone may be specified by appropriate additional topographic digits. See page 8.

Upper extremity

226–20	Interthoracoscapular amputation
242–21	Disarticulation of shoulder
230–20	Amputation of arm through humerus
243–21	Disarticulation of elbow
2x1–20	Amputation of forearm through radius and ulna
244–21	Disarticulation of wrist
2442–21	Radiocarpal
2443–21	Midcarpal
2444–21	Carpometacarpal
234–20	Amputation of hand through metacarpal bones
245▲–21	Amputation of finger by disarticulation
2451–21	Of metacarpophalangeal joint of thumb
2452–21	Of metacarpophalangeal joint of index finger
2453–21	Of metacarpophalangeal joint of middle finger
2454–21	Of metacarpophalangeal joint of ring finger
2455–21	Of metacarpophalangeal joint of little finger
234▲–20	Amputation of finger by dismemberment
2341–20	Through first metacarpal
2342–20	Through second metacarpal
2343–20	Through third metacarpal
2344–20	Through fourth metacarpal
2345–20	Through fifth metacarpal
2346–20	Through phalanges of thumb
2347–20	Through phalanges of index finger
2348–20	Through phalanges of middle finger
2349–20	Through phalanges of ring finger
234x–20	Through phalanges of little finger

Lower extremity

22x–20	Interpelviabdominal amputation
247–21	Disarticulation of hip joint
235–20	Amputation at thigh through femur
2353–20	Amputation at knee through condyles of femur: Gritti-Stokes amputation
248–21	Disarticulation of knee
2x2–20	Amputation of leg through tibia and fibula
2x23–20	Amputation at ankle through malleoli of tibia and fibula: Syme's amputation: Pirogoff's amputation
2493–21	Amputation of foot by midtarsal disarticulation; Chopart's amputation
2494–21	Amputation of foot between tarsus and metatarsus: Hey's amputation
24x▲–21	Amputation of toe by disarticulation
24x1–21	Of metatarsophalangeal joint of great toe
24x2–21	Of metatarsophalangeal joint of second toe
24x3–21	Of metatarsophalangeal joint of third toe
24x4–21	Of metatarsophalangeal joint of fourth toe
24x5–21	Of metatarsophalangeal joint of fifth toe
23x▲–20	Amputation of toe by dismemberment
23x1–20	Through first metatarsal
23x2–20	Through second metatarsal
23x3–20	Through third metatarsal
23x4–20	Through fourth metatarsal
23x5–20	Through fifth metatarsal
23x6–20	Through phalanges of great toe
23x7–20	Through phalanges of second toe
23x8–20	Through phalanges of third toe
23x9–20	Through phalanges of fourth toe
23xx–20	Through phalanges of fifth toe

3– OPERATIONS ON THE RESPIRATORY SYSTEM

OPERATIONS ON THE NOSE

—0 INCISION

310–02	Drainage of nose (*abscess*)
313–02	Drainage of septum (*abscess*)
216–06	Osteotomy of nasal bones (*deformity*)
310–00	Rhinotomy

—1 EXCISION

310–11	Excision of *lesion* of nose (*polyp, tumor, etc.*)
313–11	Of septum
315–11	Of turbinates
318–11	Of nasopharynx
133–11	Of skin of nose (*rhinophyma, tumor*)
216–11	Of nasal bones (*excess callus, hump, etc.*)
310–13	Resection of nose
313–13	Septectomy : submucous resection
315–10	Turbinectomy
315–12	Complete
315–13	Partial
310–16	Biopsy of nose

—3 INTRODUCTION

310–302	Radiopaque substance
310–303	Dye injected into nose
315–306	Sclerosis solution injected into turbinates
310–320	Introduction of radium
310–321	Introduction of radon

—4 ENDOSCOPY

310–44	Rhinoscopy with removal of *foreign body* in nose

—5 REPAIR

310–50	Rhinoplasty : plastic reconstruction of nose
310–5041	With excision of bone
310–5042	With excision of cartilage
310–5043	With excision of skin
310–51▲	With free skin graft. *Specify type (page 520)*
310–515	With pedicle skin graft
310–516	With bone graft

| 310–517 | With cartilage graft |
| 313–502 | With metal or plastic implant |

—6 DESTRUCTION

315–63	Infraction of turbinate
216–63	Fracture or refracture of nasal bones
31x–605	Cauterization of nose

—7 SUTURE

| 310–71 | Suture of nose (*wound, injury*) |

—8 MANIPULATION

| 216–82 | Closed reduction of nasal bones (*fracture*) |

OPERATIONS ON THE ACCESSORY SINUSES

Specify sinus by inserting 3d digit. See page 22.

—0 INCISION

32▲–02	Sinusotomy
321–02	Maxillary sinusotomy, simple: antrum window operation
321–021	Maxillary sinusotomy, radical: maxillary antrotomy, radical
322–02	Frontal sinusotomy, intranasal, simple
322–02x	Frontal sinusotomy, external, simple
322–021	Frontal sinusotomy, external, radical
323–02	Ethmoidotomy
324–02	Sphenoid sinusotomy, intranasal; sphenoidotomy
324–02x1	Transanthral-ethmoidal sphenoid sinusotomy
320–021	Combined external frontal, ethmoid, and sphenoid sinusotomy
324–02x	Sphenoid sinusotomy, external
32▲–023	Puncture of sinus, for aspiration or irrigation

—I EXCISION

32▲–11	Excision of *lesion* of accessory sinus (*polyp*)
32▲–16	Biopsy of accessory sinus
323–10	Ethmoidectomy
323–12	Complete ethmoidectomy, intranasal
323–13	Partial ethmoidectomy, intranasal
323–10x	Ethmoidectomy, external
322–12x	Transanthral ethmoidectomy

—3 INTRODUCTION

32▲–38   Insertion of canula into accessory sinus (for as-
              piration or irrigation)
32▲–302   Introduction of radiopaque substance

—7 SUTURE

3021–72   Closure of oral *fistula* of maxillary sinus

OPERATIONS ON THE LARYNX

Specify site by inserting 3d digit.   See page 22.

—0 INCISION

330–00   Laryngotomy
              Median—laryngofissure: thyrotomy: thyro-
                  chondrotomy
              Inferior—thyrocricotomy: intercricothyrotomy
330–01   With exploration
330–03   With removal (*foreign body*)
              With biopsy or excision of *lesion. See* Excision,
                  following
33▲–02   Incision and drainage of larynx (*abscess, peri-
                  chondritis*)
330–023   Laryngocentesis: puncture of larynx

—1 EXCISION

33▲–11   Local excision of *lesion* of larynx (by laryngot-
                  omy)
330–10   Laryngectomy
330–12   Complete or total laryngectomy
330–13   Partial laryngectomy: hemilaryngectomy
330–14   Laryngopharyngectomy
331–12   Epiglottidectomy
332–12   Arytenoidectomy
336–138   Ventriculocordectomy: punch resection of vocal
                  cords
33▲–16   Biopsy of larynx

—3 INTRODUCTION

330–302   Injection of radiopaque substance (oil) into larynx
                  (for bronchography)
330–38   Insertion of tube into larynx: intubation. *If with
                  laryngoscope, classify under* Laryngoscopy,
                  following

—4 ENDOSCOPY

330–40	Laryngoscopy
33▲–41	With biopsy [1]
33▲–42	With excision of *lesions* [1]
33▲–43	With drainage
330–44	With removal (*foreign body*)
330–45	With dilation (*stenosis*)
330–46	With division of laryngeal *adhesions* (*congenital web, synechia*) [1]
330–471	With instillation of diagnostic fluid (radiopaque oil or solution)
330–472	With instillation or application of therapeutic agent
330–48	With insertion of radioactive substance (radium, radon)
330–49	With insertion of tube: intubation; mold

—5 REPAIR

330–50	Laryngoplasty: plastic operation on larynx
330–53	Laryngostomy: fistulization of larynx
336–56	Cordopexy
332–56	Arytenoidopexy

—7 SUTURE

330–71	Laryngorrhaphy: suture of larynx (*wound or injury*)
330–72	Closure of laryngostomy or laryngeal *fistula*

OPERATIONS ON THE TRACHEA AND BRONCHI

—0 INCISION

340–00	Tracheotomy; tracheofissure; cricotracheotomy: laryngotracheotomy
340–01	With exploration
340–03	With removal (*foreign body*)
	With biopsy or excision of *lesion*. *See* Excision, (*following*)
350–00	Bronchotomy
350–01	With exploration
350–03	With removal (*foreign body*)
	With biopsy or excision of *lesion*. *See* Excision, (*following*)

[1] Special operative method may be indicated by appropriate 3d digit. See page 517.

—1 EXCISION

340–11	Local excision of *lesion* of trachea (by tracheotomy) [1]
350–11	Local excision of *lesion* of bronchus (by bronchotomy) [1]
3▲▲–16	Biopsy of trachea or bronchus. *Specify* (*page 23*)

—4 ENDOSCOPY

340–40	Tracheoscopy
340–41	With biopsy [1]
340–42	With excision of *lesion* [1]
340–44	With removal (*foreign body*)
340–45	With dilation (*stenosis*)
340–470	With irrigation, lavage
340–471	With instillation of diagnostic fluid (radiopaque)
340–48	Insertion of radioactive substance (radium, radon)
350–40	Bronchoscopy
350–41	With biopsy [1]
350–42	With excision of *lesion* [1]
350–43	With drainage or aspiration of bronchus or cavity
360–43	With drainage or aspiration of lung (*abscess*)
350–44	With removal (*foreign body*)
350–45	With dilation (*stenosis*)
350–470	With irrigation of bronchus or *bronchiectatic cavities*
360–470	With irrigation of pulmonary *abscess*
350–471	With instillation of diagnostic fluid (radiopaque oil, etc.)
350–472	With application of therapeutic agent
350–48	With insertion of radioactive substance (radium, radon)
350–49	With insertion of catheter or tube

—5 REPAIR

340–50	Tracheoplasty
340–52	Tracheostomy, anastomosis
340–53	Tracheostomy: fistulization of trachea: fenestration
340–51	Tracheostomy, graft
350–50	Bronchoplasty
350–52	Anastomosis of bronchus

1 Special operative method may be indicated by appropriate 3d digit. See page 517.

350–53   Bronchostomy: fistulization of bronchus through
                          chest wall

—7 SUTURE

340–71   Tracheorrhaphy: suture of trachea (*wound, in-
                          jury*)
340–72   Closure of tracheostomy or tracheal *fistula*
350–72   Bronchorrhaphy: suture of bronchus (*wound, in-
                          jury, incision*)
3051–72   Closure of bronchopleural *fistula*
305–72   Closure of bronchocutaneous *fistula*

OPERATIONS ON THE LUNG AND PLEURA

—0 INCISION

3074–00   Thoracotomy
3074–01   With exploration: exploratory thoracotomy
3074–02   With open drainage
3074–020   With closed drainage (for tube drainage with
                                  negative pressure)
3074–03   With removal (*foreign body, blood residue*)
                              With division of intrapleural *adhesions*. *See*
                                  Pneumonolysis, intrapleural, open, *page 546*
360–00   Pneumonotomy (approach by thoracotomy im-
                          plied)
360–01   With exploration: exploratory pneumonotomy
360–02   With open drainage (pulmonary *abscess or
                                  cyst*); *cavernostomy* (tuberculous cavity)
360–020   With closed drainage
360–03   With excision of *lesion*. *See* Excision, *follow-
                                  ing*
360–023   Pneumonocentesis: puncture of lung for aspira-
                          tion (*abscess, cyst*)
3074–020   Thoracentesis with closed tube drainage
3074–023   Thoracentesis: paracentesis thoracis: pleurocen-
                          tesis: puncture of pleural cavity for aspiration
3074–070   Incision and packing of *wound,* in preparation for
                          subsequent drainage of pulmonary *abscess:*
                          first stage drainage of lung: abscess or cav-
                          ernostomy

—I EXCISION

360–10   Pneumonectomy (approach by thoracotomy im-
                          plied)

360–12	Complete or total pneumonectomy
	Partial pneumonectomy. *Classify as* Lobectomy, complete or partial
	Code lobectomy of two lobes as for two operations using code number for each lobe
36▲–12	Complete lobectomy. *Specify lobe (page 23)*
36▲–13	Segmental pulmonary resection. *Specify segment (page 23)*
36▲–11	Subsegmental pulmonary resection for local excision of lesion. *Specify lobe (page 23)*
360–11	Local excision of *lesion* of lung (by pneumonotomy) [1]
360–16	Biopsy of lung [1]
370–10	Pleurectomy
370–11	Excision of *lesion* of pleura
372–11	Decortication of lung: excision of *thickened scar* deposited on visceral pleura
3074–14	Resection of parietal pleura, ribs and intercostal muscle bundles; Schede's operation
370–16	Biopsy of pleura [1]

—3 INTRODUCTION

307–308	Pleuropexy

—4 ENDOSCOPY

3074–40	Thoracoscopy, for exploration
3074–41	With biopsy [1]
3074–42	With excision [1]
3074–44	With removal (*foreign body*)
3074–46	With division (intrapleural *adhesions*): closed intrapleural pneumonolysis [1]
3074–4x	With control of intrapleural *hemorrhage* [1]

SURGICAL COLLAPSE THERAPY

229–102	Thoracoplasty: extrapleural resection of ribs [2]
229–122	Complete thoracoplasty
229–132	Partial thoracoplasty
229–504	Thoracoplasty with reduction of bony cage
	Pneumonolysis
3074–65	Extrapleural pneumonolysis. *Record following associated procedures as secondary operation:*

---

[1] Special operative method may be indicated by appropriate 3d digit. See page 517.
[2] Third digit in operative procedure code is used arbitrarily to indicate multiple excision or resection of ribs.
Note: Y indicates cervical approach.

	Filling of extrapleural space with
376–301	Air: extrapleural pneumothorax
376–351	Paraffin: plombage
376–352	Plastic: plombage
	Extraperiosteal pneumonolysis
034–351	Paraffin
034–352	Plastic
	Intrapleural pneumonalysis
370–65	Open intrapleural pneumonolysis: thoracotomy with division of intrapleural *adhesions*
	Closed intrapleural pneumonolysis. *See* Thoracoscopy with division of intrapleural *adhesions, page 645*
	Apicolysis
3761–65	Extrafascial apicolysis: Semb's operation (done as part of apical thoracoplasty)
3074–301	Pneumothorax: intrapleural injection of air
3074–305	Oleothorax: intrapleural injection of oil
9824–06	Phrenicotomy: division or transection of phrenic nerve
9824–64	Phrenicotripsy: phrenemphraxis: crushing of phrenic nerve

4– OPERATIONS ON THE CARDIO-VASCULAR SYSTEM

OPERATIONS ON THE HEART AND PERICARDIUM

—0 INCISION

410–00	Cardiotomy
410–01	With exploration
410–03	With removal (*foreign body*)
410–023	Cardiocentesis
457–06	Division of chordae tendinae
437–06	Division of papillary muscle
420–00	Pericardiotomy
420–01	With exploration: exploratory pericardiotomy
420–02	With drainage: pericardiostomy
420–03	With removal (*foreign body*)
420–08	With decompression (by evacuation of *hematoma*)
420–023	Pericardiocentesis
45▲–06	Valvulotomy (cardiac)
453–06	Pulmonary valvulotomy
454–06	Mitral valvulotomy
455–06	Aortic valvulotomy
45▲1–06	Commissurotomy. *Specify valve*

—1 EXCISION

4171–12	Auricular ligation
420–13	Pericardiectomy
412–13	Production of interatrial septal defect
420–16	Biopsy of pericardium
45▲–12	Valvulectomy. *Specify valve*

—3 INTRODUCTION

420–308	Cardiopericardiopexy (introduction of irritant)
410–38	Catheterization of heart
418–38	Left
416–38	Right
410–302	Cardiography (angiocardiography)

—5 REPAIR

412–56	Atrioseptopexy
412–50	Atrioseptoplasty
412–502	Atrioseptoplasty with prosthetic device
454–560	Neostrophingic mobilization of mitral valve hingeing

41▲–50	Repair of septal defect. *Specify septum*
45▲–50	Valvuloplasty. *Specify valve*
413–56	Ventriculoseptopexy
413–50	Ventriculoseptoplasty
413–502	Ventriculoseptoplasty with prosthetic device

—6 DESTRUCTION

410–65	Cardiolysis
420–65	Pericardiolysis

—7 SUTURE

410–71	Cardiorrhaphy: suture of heart (*wound, injury*)
420–71	Pericardiorrhaphy: suture of pericardium (*wound, injury*)

—8 MANIPULATION

410–80	Cardiac massage

OPERATIONS ON ARTERIES AND VEINS

Specify site by inserting digits where indicated. See page 26.

—0 INCISION

4▲▲–00	Arteriotomy
4▲▲–01	With exploration
4▲▲–03	With removal of *embolus:* embolectomy
46▲–00	Aortotomy
46▲–01	With exploration
46▲–03	With removal of *embolus:* embolectomy
48▲–00	Phlebotomy: venotomy
48▲–01	With exploration
4▲▲–023	Arterial puncture
4▲▲–03	With removal of thrombus: thrombectomy
48▲–023	Venipuncture
4▲▲–06	Transection (or division) of artery (ligation or suture implied, when only ligation is done, file 4▲▲–74)
40x–06	Transection of ductus arteriosus
48▲–06	Transection of vein (ligation implied, when only ligation is done, file 48▲–74)

—1 EXCISION

46▲.1–13	Decortication of adventitial coat of artery. *Specify artery:* periarterial sympathectomy

46▲.3–13	Endarterectomy: intimectomy
4▲▲–11	Excision of *lesion* of artery
411–12	Excision of arterial *aneurysm;* aneurysmectomy
461–11	Excision of *coarctation* of aorta (with anastomosis)
402▲–11	Excision of *lesion* of artery and vein
402▲–12	Excision of arteriovenous *aneurysm* or fistula
46▲–13	Arteriectomy
46▲–16	Biopsy of artery
48▲–16	Biopsy of vein
4612–12	Infundibulectomy, aortic
4712–12	Infundibulectomy, pulmonary
48▲–13	Phlebectomy: venectomy: excision or resection of vein

—3 INTRODUCTION

46▲–302	Arteriography
461–302	Aortography
477–302	Cerebral arteriography (angiography)
48▲–302	Venography
480–31	Blood transfusion
480–310	Refusion of blood
480–311	Plasma transfusion
480–312	Serum transfusion
480–313	Replacement transfusion
480–314	Removal, processing, and replacement of blood
47▲–31	Arterial transfusion of blood

—5 REPAIR

46▲–50	Arterioplasty: plastic or reconstruction operation on artery
40236–51	Pericardial transventricular graft
402▲–50	Plastic operation for repair of arteriovenous *fistula* or *aneurysm*
45▲–502	Reconstruction of valve by prosthesis
46▲–502	Reconstruction of artery by prosthesis
40235–52	Transplantation of internal mammary artery to myocardium
4▲▲–51x	Reconstruction of artery by blood vessel graft
46▲–52	Arterial anastomosis
461–52	Aortic anastomosis
4035–52	Subclavian aortic anastomosis
4051–52	Pulmonary aortic anastomosis (Pott's)
4052–52	Pulmonary subclavian anastomosis (Blalock)
4053–52	Pulmonary innominate anastomosis (Blalock)
48▲–52	Venous anastomosis: venovenostomy
4061–52	Porta-caval anastomosis (portal vein and *in*ferior vena cava) end to side

4061–521	Porta-caval anastomosis (portal vein and inferior vena cava) side to side
4062–52	Superior mesenteric-caval anastomosis
4063–52	Splenorenal anastomosis (splenic vein and renal vein)
402▲–52	Arteriovenous anastomosis

—7 SUTURE

46▲–71	Arteriorrhaphy: suture of artery
46▲–74	Ligation of artery
40x–74	Ligation of ductus arteriosus
48▲–71	Phleborrhaphy: suture of vein
48▲–74	Ligation of vein
4▲▲–71	Aneurysmorrhaphy: suture of aneurysm
402▲–74	Ligation of artery and concomitant vein

5– OPERATIONS ON THE HEMIC AND LYMPHATIC SYSTEMS

OPERATIONS ON THE SPLEEN AND MARROW

—0 INCISION

520–00	Splenotomy
520–01	With exploration
520–02	With drainage (*abscess*)
520–023	Splenic puncture

—I EXCISION

520–12	Splenectomy
520–16	Biopsy of spleen

—3 INTRODUCTION

54▲–302	Lymphangiography

—5 REPAIR

520–56	Splenopexy: fixation of spleen

—7 SUTURE

520–71	Splenorrhaphy: suture of spleen (*wound, injury*)

OPERATIONS ON THE LYMPHATIC CHANNELS

Specify channel by inserting 3d digit. See page 29.

—0 INCISION

54▲–00	Lymphangiotomy

—I EXCISION

54▲–11	Excision of *lesion* of lymphatic channel (*lymphangioma, hygroma*)
54▲–16	Biopsy of lymphatic channel

—5 REPAIR

54▲–50	Lymphangioplasty: plastic operation on lymphatic channel
541–53	Lymphaticostomy: fistulization of thoracic duct

552

HEMIC AND LYMPHATIC SYSTEMS

OPERATIONS ON THE LYMPH NODES

Specify node by inserting 3d digit. See page 29.

—0 INCISION

55▲–02   Incision and drainage of lymph nodes: lymph-
                adenotomy (*abscess, lymphadenitis*)

—I EXCISION

55▲–12   Local or simple excision of lymph nodes:
                lymphadenectomy
55▲–14   Radical excision or resection of lymph nodes:
                radical lymphadenectomy
55▲–16   Biopsy of lymph node

6– OPERATIONS ON THE DIGESTIVE SYSTEM

OPERATIONS ON THE MOUTH

—0 INCISION

610–02 | Incision and drainage of mouth (*abscess*)
6102–02 | Incision and drainage of floor of mouth

—1 EXCISION

610–11 | Excision of *lesion* of mouth [1]

—5 REPAIR

610–50 | Stomatoplasty: plastic or reconstruction operation on mouth
610–51 | Plastic repair with skin graft. *Specify type of graft, page 520*

—7 SUTURE

610–71 | Suture of mouth (*wound, injury*)
610–72 | Closure of external *fistula* of mouth

OPERATIONS ON THE LIPS

—0 INCISION

611–02 | Incision and drainage of lip (*abscess*)

—1 EXCISION

611–11 | Local excision of *lesion* of lip [1]
123–11 | Of mucous membrane of lip
134–11 | Of skin of lip
156–11 | Of mucous glands of lip
611–13 | Resection of lip (for wide excision of *malignant growth*) [1]
611–16 | Biopsy of lip [1]

—5 REPAIR

611–50 | Cheiloplasty: plastic or reconstruction on lip: plastic repair of *cleft lip*

[1] Special operative method may be indicated by appropriate 3d digit. See page 517.

—7 SUTURE

611–71 Suture of lip (*wound, injury*)

OPERATIONS ON THE TONGUE

—0 INCISION

612–00 Glossotomy
612–02 With drainage (*abscess*)
612–03 With removal (*foreign body*)
6121–00 Clipping of frenulum linguae

—I EXCISION

612–10 Glossectomy
612–11 Local excision of *lesion* of tongue.[1] *Ordinarily classify as* Partial glossectomy
612–12 Complete or total glossectomy [1]
612–13 Partial glossectomy: resection of tongue; hemiglossectomy [1]
612–16 Biopsy of tongue [1]

—5 REPAIR

612–50 Glossoplasty: plastic operation on tongue
61431–50 Plastic repair of alveolus

—7 SUTURE

612–71 Glossorrhaphy: suture of tongue (*wound, injury*)
612–72 Suture of tongue to lower lip for micrognathia

OPERATIONS ON THE TEETH AND GINGIVA

—0 INCISION

614▲–02 Incision and drainage (dentigerous lesion, cyst)
Specify structure, e.g.
6143–02 Incision and drainage of alveolus (alveolar abscess), approach unspecified
6143–02x Through pulp canal
6143–02y Through alveolar plate
613–00 Odontomy

1 Special operative method may be indicated by appropriate 3d digit. See page 517.

—I EXCISION

6136–13	Apicoectomy
6143–13	Alveolectomy
6142–16	Biopsy of gingiva
6142–11	Enucleation of cyst
6142–111	Removal of cyst, partial (Partsch operation)
613–129	Forceps extraction of tooth
6142–13	Gingivectomy
6132–12	Pulpectomy, complete
6132–13	Pulpectomy, partial
613▲–11	Removal of odontogenic tumor. *Specify structure, e.g.*
6133–11	Removal of ameloblastoma
6131–11	Removal of cementoma
6134–11	Removal of odontoma (dentinoma)
613–12	Surgical removal of tooth
613–121	Surgical removal of tooth with resection (odontomy)

—3 INTRODUCTION

6135▲–338	Denture, fixed. *Specify site*
6135▲–3381	Denture, removable. *Specify site*
6135–336	Orthodontic appliance
6135–3361	Space maintainer
6135–3362	Stabilizing appliance for loose tooth
6145–335	Subperiosteal implant

—5 REPAIR

6145–5041	Alveoloplasty
6135–502	Equilibration
6132–5021	Filling of pulp canal
6142–5044	Gingivoplasty
613–5161	Plantation of tooth or tooth germ
61431–50	Plastic repair of alveolus
613–5021	Restoration of tooth structure (crown or filling)
6103–500	Vestibuloplasty

—6 DESTRUCTION

613–614	Dental debridement (subgingival curettage)
6137–61	Crown debridement (prophylaxis)

—7 SUTURE

6142–71	Suture of gingiva

OPERATIONS ON THE PALATE AND UVULA

—0 INCISION

616–02   Incision and drainage of palate (*abscess*)

—I EXCISION

616–11   Local excision of *lesion* of palate
616–13   Resection of palate (for wide excision of *lesion*)
617–12   Uvulectomy: excision of uvula
616–16   Biopsy of palate

—5 REPAIR

616–50   Palatoplasty: plastic operation on palate (*cleft palate*)
   616–500   Palate lengthening

—7 SUTURE

616–71   Suture of palate (*wound, injury*)

OPERATIONS ON THE SALIVARY GLANDS AND DUCTS

Specify gland by inserting digits where indicated. See page 33.

—0 INCISION

62▲–01   Exploration of salivary gland or duct
62▲–02   Incision and drainage of salivary gland
62▲–03   Incision and removal of salivary *calculus:* sialolithotomy

—I EXCISION

62▲–11   Excision of *lesion* of salivary gland (*ranula, mixed tumor*)
62▲–12   Excision of salivary gland: sialoadenectomy
62▲–14   Radical excision of salivary glands
   621–12   Parotidectomy
62▲–16   Biopsy of salivary gland

—5 REPAIR

62▲–50   Plastic repair of salivary duct: sialodochoplasty

—7 SUTURE

—7 SUTURE

62▲–72   Closure of salivary *fistula*

—8 MANIPULATION

62▲–80   Removal of salivary *calculus* (without incision)
62▲–84   Dilation of salivary duct: ptyalectasis

OPERATIONS ON THE PHARYNX, ADENOIDS, AND TONSILS

—0 INCISION

631–00   Pharyngotomy
  631–01   With exploration
  631–02   With drainage (retropharyngeal *abscess*)
              Incision and drainage (*abscess*)
634–02   Of tonsil
636–02   Of peritonsillar tissues
639–02   Of retropharyngeal tissues (for external incision)
630–070   Incision and packing of wound, in preparation for subsequent excision of pharyngoesophageal *diverticulum*

—I EXCISION

630–11   Excision of pharyngoesophageal *diverticulum*
631–11   Local excision of *lesion* of pharynx (branchial *cyst* or *vestige*)
631–13   Pharyngectomy: resection of pharynx
              Laryngopharyngectomy. *See under* Larynx, *page 541*
632–12   Tonsillectomy and adenoidectomy
633–12   Adenoidectomy
  633–11   Excision of adenoid tag
634–12   Tonsillectomy
  634–11   Excision of tonsil tag
635–12   Excision of lingual tonsil
63▲–16   Biopsy of pharynx. *Specify* (*page 33*)

—5 REPAIR

631–50   Pharyngoplasty: plastic or reconstruction operation on pharynx
  631–5031   Pharyngeal flap of palate

—7 SUTURE

631–71   Suture of pharynx (*wound or injury*)
631–72   Closure of *fistula* into pharynx (branchial cleft)

OPERATIONS ON THE ESOPHAGUS

—0 INCISION

637–00   Esophagotomy
  637–01   With exploration: exploratory esophagotomy
  637–03   With removal (*foreign body*)

—I EXCISION

637–11   Local excision of *lesion* of esophagus (esophageal *diverticulum:* diverticulectomy, esophageal; intrathoracic portion of esophagus)
(*For excision of diverticulum in neck, see* Excision of pharyngoesophageal *diverticulum*), *page 557*
637–13   Esophagectomy: resection of esophagus
6001–13   Esophagogastrectomy
637–16   Biopsy of esophagus

—4 ENDOSCOPY

637–40   Esophagoscopy
  637–41   With biopsy [1]
  637–42   With excision [1]
  637–43   With drainage (intramural *abscess*)
  637–44   With removal (*foreign body*)
  637–45   With dilation (*stenosis, stricture*)
  637–470   With irrigation
  637–471   With instillation of diagnostic agent, radiopaque
  637–48   With insertion of radioactive substance
63x–472   Injection of esophageal varices endoscopically

—5 REPAIR

637–50   Esophagoplasty: plastic repair or reconstruction of esophagus
6003–50   Esophagojejunoplasty (interposition operation)
6001–50   Esophagogastroplasty; cardioplasty
6001–52   Esophagogastrostomy
6002–52   Esophagoduodenostomy
6003–52   Esophagojejunostomy

[1] Special operative method may be indicated by appropriate 3d digit. See page 517.

637–52	Esophagoesophagostomy: anastomosis of esophagus (after local excision of *lesion* of esophagus or in atresia of esophagus)
637–53	Esophagostomy: fistulization of esophagus, external

—7 SUTURE

637–71	Suture of esophagus (*wound, injury, rupture*)
637–72	Closure of esophagostomy or other external esophageal *fistula*
3041–72	Closure of tracheoesophageal *fistula*
63x–74	Ligation of esophageal varices

—8 MANIPULATION

637–840	Dilation of esophagus (by sound, bougie, or bag)
6373–840	Dilation of cardiac sphincter

OPERATIONS ON THE STOMACH

—0 INCISION

640–00	Gastrotomy
640–01	With exploration: exploratory gastrotomy
640–03	With removal (*foreign body, hair ball*)
640–079	With injection of gastric varices
648–06	Pyloromyotomy: cutting, division, or transection of pyloric muscle: Fredet-Ramstedt operation
6001–06	Esophagastromyotomy (Heller procedure)

—I EXCISION

640–10	Gastrectomy
640–100	With vagisection
640–11	Local excision of *lesion* of stomach (*ulcer or benign neoplasm*). *Ordinarily classify as* Partial gastrectomy
640–12	Complete or total gastrectomy with esophago-duodenostomy
640–13	Partial or subtotal gastrectomy: resection of stomach
642–13	Fundectomy of stomach
6012–12	Complete gastroduodectomy
640–14	Radical gastrectomy (when portion of adjacent organ such as liver, pancreas, or colon are removed)
640–16	Biopsy of stomach

6012–11	Excision of gastroduodenal *lesion* (gastroduo-denal, marginal, or stoma *ulcer* secondary to gastroduodenostomy)
6013–11	Excision of gastrojejunal *lesion* (gastrojejunal, jejunal, marginal, or stoma *ulcer* secondary to gastrojejunostomy)
647–13	Excision of prolapsed mucosa of stomach

—4 ENDOSCOPY

640–40	Gastroscopy
640–41	Gastroscopy for biopsy
640–411	Gastroscopy for cytology

—5 REPAIR

640–50	Gastroplasty
645–50	Pyloroplasty
640–52	Gastrogastrostomy
6012–52	Gastroduodenostomy
6013–52	Gastrojejunostomy
6011–53	Gastrostomy

—7 SUTURE

640–71	Gastrorrhaphy: suture of stomach (*perforated gastric ulcer, wound, injury*)
6012–72	Closure or taking down of gastroduodenal anasto-mosis (gastroduodenostomy)
6013–72	Closure or taking down of gastrojejunal anasto-mosis (gastrojejunostomy)
6016–72	Closure of gastroileal anastomosis
6014–72	Closure of gastrocolic *fistula*
6015–72	Closure of gastrojejunocolic *fistula*
6011–72	Closure of gastrostomy, pylorostomy, or other ex-ternal *fistula* of stomach
645–75	Pyloric occlusion or exclusion operation

OPERATIONS ON THE INTESTINE
(EXCEPT THE RECTUM)

Specify site by inserting digits where indicated. See page 34.

—0 INCISION

| 6▲▲–00 | Enterotomy [1] |
| | Small intestine |

1 When done for exploration, substitute 01 for 00: when done for removal of foreign body, substitute 03 for 00.

651–00	Duodenotomy [1]
653–00	Jejunotomy [1]
654–00	Ileotomy [1]
	Large intestine
660–00	Colotomy [1]
662–00	Cecotomy [1]
666–00	Sigmoidotomy [1]
60▲▲–071	Exteriorization of intestine, preliminary to resection: first stage Mikulicz resection of intestine

—1 EXCISION

6▲▲–11	Local excision of *lesion* of intestine (not requiring anastomosis, exteriorization, or fistulization)
660–12	Complete or total colectomy (cecum, colon, sigmoid colon, and sometimes rectum)
6038–11	Excision of redundant mucosa of colostomy
6▲▲–13	Resection of intestine: enterectomy
	Small intestine
651–13	Of duodenum: duodenectomy
	Pancreatoduodenectomy. *See* Operations on pancreas
653–13	Of jejunum: jejunectomy
654–13	Of ileum: ileectomy
	Small and large intestine
6045–13	Of ileum (terminal) and cecum
6046–13	Of ileum (terminal), cecum, and ascending colon
	Large intestine
662–12	Of cecum: cecectomy
6031–13	Of cecum and ascending colon
660–13	Of colon: colectomy, partial
666–13	Of sigmoid colon: sigmoidectomy
60▲▲–15	Resection of exteriorized intestine: second stage Mikulicz resection of intestine; obstruction resection of intestine
6▲▲–16	Biopsy of intestine

—3 INTRODUCTION

650–38	Intubation of small intestine (Miller-Abbott, Johnson, Harris, Cantor, Honore-Smathers tubes)

—4 ENDOSCOPY

660–40x	Colonoscopy transabdominal

[1] When done for exploration, substitute 01 for 00: when done for removal of foreign body, substitute 03 for 00.

—5 REPAIR

6027–50	Plastic operation on ileostomy
6038–50	Plastic operation on colostomy
6023–5011	Plication of small intestine
653–5011	Plication of jejunum
6▲▲–52	Anastomosis of intestines: enteroenterostomy: enteroanastomosis

Small intestine to small intestine

651–52	Duodenoduodenostomy
6021–52	Duodenojejunostomy
6022–52	Duodenoileostomy
653–52	Jejunojejunostomy
6023–52	Jejunoileostomy
654–52	Ileoileostomy

Small intestine to large intestine

6041–52	Jejunocecostomy
6042–52	Jejunocolostomy
6045–52	Ileocecostomy
6046–52	Ileocolostomy
6046–521	With transection of ileum
6047–52	Ileosigmoidostomy

Large intestine to large intestine

6031–52	Cecocolostomy
6032–52	Cecosigmoidostomy
660–52	Colocolostomy
6034–52	Colosigmoidostomy
6035–52	Coloproctostomy: colorectostomy
666–52	Sigmoidosigmoidostomy
6048–52	Ileoproctostomy
6036–52	Sigmoidoproctostomy: sigmoidorectostomy
60▲▲–53	Enterostomy: fistulization of intestine. *Specify*
6025–53	Duodenostomy
6026–53	Jejunostomy
6027–53	Ileostomy
6027–531	With plication of ileum
6037–53	Cecostomy
6038–53	Colostomy
6039–53	Sigmoidostomy
6▲▲–54	Reduction (*volvulus, intussusception, or hernia*)
6037–56	Cecopexy: fixation of cecum to abdominal wall
6039–56	Sigmoidopexy: fixation of sigmoid colon to abdominal wall

—6 DESTRUCTION

6▲▲–65	Division or freeing of *adhesions* of intestine; enterolysis

—7 SUTURE

6▲▲–71	Suture of intestine: enterorrhaphy: duodenorraphy; jejunorraphy, etc. (*perforated ulcer, wound, injury, rupture*)
651–71	Suture or closure of perforated duodenal *ulcer*
6049–72	Closure of enterostomy or *fecal fistula*
6025–72	Closure of duodenostomy or duodenal *fistula*
6026–72	Closure of jejunostomy or jejunal *fistula*
6027–72	Closure of ileostomy or *fecal fistula* of ileum
6037–72	Closure of cecostomy or *fecal fistula* of cecum
6038–72	Closure of colostomy or *fecal fistula* of colon

—8 MANIPULATION

6049–80	Reduction of *prolapse* of enterostomy
6038–80	Reduction of *prolapse* of colostomy
6027–80	Reduction of *prolapse* of ileostomy
6049–84	Dilation of enterostomy (for stenosis)
6038–84	Dilation of colostomy (for stenosis)
6027–84	Dilation of ileostomy (for stenosis)

OPERATIONS ON MECKEL'S DIVERTICULUM AND THE MESENTERY

—1 EXCISION

658–12	Excision of *Meckel's diverticulum:* diverticulectomy, Meckel's
659–11	Local excision of *lesion* of mesentery
659–13	Resection of mesentery
659–16	Biopsy of mesentery

—5 REPAIR

659–56	Mesopexy

—7 SUTURE

659–71	Suture of mesentery

OPERATIONS ON THE APPENDIX

—0 INCISION

661–02	Incision and drainage of appendical *abscess*

—I EXCISION

661–12   Appendectomy

—5 REPAIR

661–53   Appendicostomy: fistulization of appendix, external

—7 SUTURE

661–72   Closure of appendicostomy or other *fistula* of appendix

OPERATIONS ON THE RECTUM

—0 INCISION

668–00   Proctotomy
668–01   With exploration
668–02   With drainage (perirectal *abscess*)
668–08   With decompression (*imperforate anus*)
603x–071   Exteriorization of rectum (preliminary to resection)
669–02   Incision and drainage, external, of perirectal tissues (*abscess*)

—I EXCISION

668–10   Proctectomy
668–12   Complete proctectomy[1]
668–13   Partial proctectomy: resection of rectum[1]
668–121   Proctectomy, pull through
6036–13   Proctosigmoidectomy[1]
6036–131   Proctosigmoidectomy, pull through
668–15   Resection of exteriorized rectum
6036–13y   Proctosigmoidectomy, abdominal
668–11   Local excision of *lesion* of rectum (*fistula* opening into rectum)
669–11   Excision of lesion of perirectal tissue (*fistula* not opening into rectum)

—4 ENDOSCOPY

668–40   Proctoscopy
668–41   With biopsy[2]

[1] Perineal approach may be indicated by adding x at end of code: combined abdominal-perineal approach may be indicated by adding y.
[2] Special operative method may be indicated by appropriate 3d digit. See page 517.

668–42	With excision (*papilloma, polyps*) [1]
668–44	With removal (*foreign body*)
668–45	With dilation
668–46	With division of *adhesions, scar, stricture:* proctotomy, internal
668–48	With insertion of radioactive substance
666–40	Sigmoidoscopy. *Use subdivisions as for Proctoscopy*

—5 REPAIR

668–50	Proctoplasty: rectoplasty
668–52	Anastomosis of rectum
668–53	Proctostomy: rectostomy
668–56	Proctopexy: rectopexy
6036–56	Proctosigmoidopexy

—7 SUTURE

668–71	Proctorrhaphy: suture of rectum
7085–72	Closure of rectovesical *fistula*
709–72	Closure of rectourethral *fistula*
70x2–72	Closure of rectovaginal *fistula*

—8 MANIPULATION

668–80	Reduction of *prolapse* of rectum
668–84	Dilation of rectum, manual
668–840	Instrumental dilation of rectum (sound, bougie)

OPERATIONS ON THE ANUS

—0 INCISION

670–02	Incision of anal *fistula:* fistulotomy, anal
677–02	Incision and drainage of perianal *abscess*
672–06	Sphincterotomy, anal: division of anal sphincter

—I EXCISION

670–11	Local excision of *lesion* of anus (*fissure fistula*)
67x–11	Hemorrhoidectomy, internal and/or external
670–12	Excision of anus, complete
670–16	Biopsy of anus [1]
143–11	Excision of *lesion* of perianal skin (skin tabs)
670–13	Excision of *lesion* of anus: fistulectomy

[1] Special operative method may be indicated by appropriate 3d digit. See page 517.

—3 INTRODUCTION

67x–306   Injection of hemorrhoids, internal and/or external

—4 ENDOSCOPY

670–40   Anoscopy
   670–41   With biopsy of anus [1]
   670–42   With excision [1]
   670–44   With removal (*foreign body*)
   670–46   With cutting or division (*stricture*) [1]
   670–48   With insertion of radioactive substance

—5 REPAIR

670–50   Anoplasty: plastic or reparative operation on anus
672–50   Sphincteroplasty, anal: plastic operation for repair of anal sphincter
   671–50   Repair of internal anal sphincter only

—6 DESTRUCTION

670–604   Curettage of *lesion* of anus (*fissure, fistula*)
670–605   Cauterization of *lesion* of anus (*fissure*)
670–606   Fulguration of *lesion* of anus

—8 MANIPULATION

672–84   Dilation of anal sphincter

OPERATIONS ON THE LIVER

—0 INCISION

680–00   Hepatotomy [2]
   680–01   With exploration
   680–02   With drainage (*abscess, cyst*)
   680–03   With removal (*foreign body*)
680–070   Incision and packing of *wound* in preparation for subsequent drainage of liver: "first stage drainage" of liver (*abscess* or *cyst*)

—I EXCISION

680–10   Hepatectomy
   680–11   Local excision of *lesion* of liver
   680–13   Resection of liver: partial hepatectomy
680–16   Biopsy of liver

---

1 Special operative method may be indicated by appropriate 3d digit. See page 517.
2 Transpleural approach may be indicated by adding x at end of code to differentiate from abdominal approach; extrapleural approach may be indicated by adding y.

680–42   Biopsy of liver, endoscopically

680–53   Marsupialization of *cyst* or *abscess* of liver

680–71   Hepatorrhaphy: suture of liver (*wound, injury*)

OPERATIONS ON THE BILIARY TRACT

Specify site by inserting digits where indicated. See page 36.

68▲–00	Incision of bile ducts
684–00	Hepaticotomy
684–01	With exploration
684–02	With drainage: hepaticostomy
684–03	With removal of *calculus:* hepaticolithotomy
685–00	Choledochotomy
685–01	With exploration
685–02	With drainage: choledochostomy
685–03	With removal of *calculus:* choledocho-lithotomy
6092–00	Duodenocholedochotomy
6092–01	With exploration
6092–03	With removal of *calculus:* transduodenal choledocholithotomy
6511–00	Incision of sphincter of Oddi: sphincterotomy, Oddi
682–01	Exploration of bile ducts (when identity of bile ducts cannot be established)
687–00	Cholecystotomy
687–01	With exploration
687–02	With drainage: cholecystostomy
687–03	With removal of *calculus*
6871–03	Removal of gall stone (outside of gallbladder or bile ducts)

68▲–11	Excision of lesion of bile ducts
685–12	Choledochectomy
688–12	Excision of ampulla of Vater, transduodenal (with reimplantation of bile and main pancreatic ducts into duodenum)

687–12	Cholecystectomy
686–13	Excision remnant of cystic duct
68▲–16	Biopsy of biliary tract. *Specify site*

—3 INTRODUCTION

682–302	Cholangiography; introduction of radiopaque medium into bile ducts (through tube in ducts or gall bladder) and roentgen examination
682–381	Insertion of T tube into bile ducts
682–382	Insertion of metal tube (Vitallium) into bile ducts

—5 REPAIR

68▲–50	Plastic repair or reconstruction of bile ducts
685–50	Choledochoplasty
	Anastomosis of bile duct
682–52	To bile duct
6091–52	To stomach
6092–52	To duodenum
6093–52	To jejunum
6051–52	Cholecystogastrostomy
6053–52	Cholecystoduodenostomy
6054–52	Cholecystojejunostomy
	Implantation of biliary fistulous tract
6091–521	Into stomach
609▲–521	Into intestine

—7 SUTURE

68▲–71	Suture of bile ducts
685–71	Choledochorrhaphy
687–71	Cholecystorrhaphy
68▲–72	Closure of biliary *fistula*
605–72	Closure of cholecystogastrostomy or cholecystogastric *fistula*
6053–72	Closure of cholecystoduodenostomy or cholecystoduodenal *fistula*
6054–72	Closure of cholecystojejunostomy or cholecystojejunal *fistula*

OPERATIONS ON THE PANCREAS

—0 INCISION

| 690–00 | Pancreatotomy |
| 690–01 | With exploration |

690–02   With drainage
690–03   With removal of *calculus:* Pancreolithotomy

—I EXCISION

690–10   Pancreatectomy
 690–11   Local excision of *lesion* of pancreas (adenoma)
 6062–12   Complete pancreatectomy and duodenectomy: pancreatoduodenectomy
 690–13   Partial pancreatectomy: resection of pancreas
  6062–13 With duodenectomy: pancreatoduodenectomy

—5 REPAIR

6061–52   Pancreaticogastrostomy
6062–52   Pancreaticoduodenostomy
6063–52   Pancreaticojejunostomy, side to side
 6063–521   Retrograde
692–53   Marsupialization of *cyst* of pancreas
6061–53   Anastomosis pancreas due to stomach
6062–53   Anastomosis pancreas due to duodenum
6063–53   Anastomosis pancreas due to jejunum

—7 SUTURE

690–71   Suture of pancreas (*wound, injury*)

OPERATIONS ON THE ABDOMEN, PERITONEUM, AND OMENTUM

—0 INCISION

060–01   Laparotomy, exploratory: celiotomy, exploratory
060–02   Drainage (peritoneal *abscess,* localized *peritonitis*)
 063–02   Subdiaphragmatic [1]
 064–02   Subhepatic
 065–02   Retroperitoneal [2]
 066–02   Pelvic-peritoneal [3]
 067–02   Omental
 528–02   Perisplenic
 649–02   Perigastric
        Appendical (*See operations on appendix, page 563*)

[1] Transpleural approach may be indicated by adding x at end of code to differentiate from abdominal approach; extrapleural approach may be indicated by adding y.
[2] Extraperitoneal approach may be indicated by adding x at end of code to differentiate from abdominal approach.
[3] Vaginal approach (by colpotomy) may be indicated by adding x at the end of code to differentiate from abdominal approach; rectal approach (by proctotomy) may be indicated by adding y.

060–03	Removal, peritoneal (*foreign body*)
	Incision and drainage
042–02	Of abdominal wall (*abscess, infection*)
044–02	Of umbilicus (*abscess, omphalitis*)
042–03	Incision and removal of *foreign body* in abdominal wall
042–05	Reopening of recent laparotomy incision (for exploration, removal of *hematoma,* control of *bleeding,* etc.)
060–023	Peritoneocentesis: abdominal paracentesis
06▲–070	Incision and packing of wound in preparation for subsequent drainage: "first stage drainage." *Specify site* (*page 4*)

—I EXCISION

042–11	Excision of *lesion* of abdominal wall
044–12	Umbilectomy: omphalectomy: excision of umbilicus
067–13	Omentectomy: epiploectomy: resection of omentum
0▲▲–16	Biopsy. *Specify site* (*page 4*)

—3 INTRODUCTION

049–384	Insertion of glass tube with flange between peritoneal cavity and subcutaneous tissue (Crosby-Cooney operation for ascites)
060–301	Intraperitoneal injection of air: pneumoperitoneum
065–301	Retroperitoneal injection of air

—4 ENDOSCOPY

060–40	Peritoneoscopy

—5 REPAIR

	Hernioplasty: Herniorrhaphy: Herniotomy: repair of *hernia*
0601–50	Inguinal
0602–50	Femoral
042–50	Ventral (incisional)
043–50	Epigastric
044–50	Umbilical
056–50	Lumbar
057–50	Ischiatic
063–50	Diaphragmatic [1]

1 Abdominal approach (laparotomy) is implied; thoracic approach (thoracotomy) may be indicated by adding x at end of code.

066–50	Ischiorectal (cul de sac of Douglas)
091–50	Obturator
0▴▴–518	Hernioplasty with fascial graft. *Specify site as under* Hernioplasty, etc. *preceding*
0▴▴–502	Hernioplasty with plastic mesh. *Specify site*
067–54	Reduction of *torsion* of omentum (by laparotomy)
067–56	Omentopexy: epiplopexy: omentofixation (for establishing collateral circulation in portal *obstruction*)

—6 DESTRUCTION

042–61	Debridement of abdominal wall (*wound, injury*)
060–65	Division of peritoneal *adhesions*

—7 SUTURE

042–71	Suture of abdominal wall (*wound, injury*) laparorrhaphy
042–710	Suture of abdominal wall following debridement
042–73	Secondary suture of abdominal wall (*evisceration, disruption*): resuture of abdominal wall
042–730	Secondary, or delayed, closure of *granulating wound* of abdominal wall
067–71	Omentorrhaphy: epiplorrhaphy: suture of omentum (*wound, injury*). *For fixation to abdominal wall see* Omentopexy, *preceding.*

7– OPERATIONS ON THE UROGENITAL SYSTEM

OPERATIONS ON THE URINARY SYSTEM

OPERATIONS ON THE KIDNEY

—0 INCISION

710–02	Drainage of kidney (*abscess*)
716–01	Exploration of perirenal tissues
716–02	Drainage of perirenal tissues (*abscess*)
716–03	Removal of *calculus* or *foreign body* in perirenal tissues
719–00	Nephrotomy
719–01	With exploration
719–02	With drainage: nephrostomy
719–03	With removal of calculus: nephrolithotomy
71x–06	Division or transection of aberrant renal vessels
722–00	Pyelotomy
722–01	With exploration
722–02	With drainage: pyelostomy
722–03	With removal of *calculus:* pyelolithotomy

—I EXCISION

710–12	Nephrectomy, complete
710–13	Partial nephrectomy: heminephrectomy
721–13	Calycectomy
710–121	Subcapular nephrectomy
715–12	Decapsulation of kidney: renal capsulectomy
710–16	Biopsy of kidney
710–168	Needle biopsy

—5 REPAIR

722–50	Pyeloplasty: plastic operation on renal pelvis
710–56	Nephropexy: fixation, suspension of movable kidney
718–54	Reduction of *torsion* of pedicle of kidney

—6 DESTRUCTION

710–65	Nephrolysis

—7 SUTURE

710–71	Nephrorrhaphy: suture of kidney
710–72	Closure of nephrostomy, pyelostomy, or other renal *fistula*

OPERATIONS ON THE URETER

—0 INCISION

723–023	Ureterocentesis
723–00	Ureterotomy
723–01	With exploration
723–02	With drainage. *See also* Ureterostomy, external
723–03	With removal of *calculus:* ureterolithotomy; removal of foreign body
723–06	Division of ureter, transection

—I EXCISION

723–10	Ureterectomy
723–12	Complete ureterectomy
723–13	Partial ureterectomy
723–16	Biopsy of ureter

—5 REPAIR

723–52	Anastomosis of ureter
7076–52	Uretero-ileostomy
7076–53	Uretero-ileostomy, external
723–50	Ureteroplasty: plastic operation on ureter (*stricture*)
7012–52	Ureteropyelostomy: anastomosis of ureter and renal pelvis
7011–52	Ureterocystostomy: anastomosis of ureter to bladder: reimplantation of ureter into bladder
7073–52	Ureterocolostomy
7074–52	Ureterosigmoidostomy
723–52	Ureteroureterostomy
723–53	Ureterostomy, external or cutaneous: transplantation of ureter to skin

—6 DESTRUCTION

723–65	Ureterolysis: freeing of ureter (adhesions)

—7 SUTURE

723–71	Ureterorrhaphy: suture of ureter
723–72	Closure of *fistula* of ureter
7022–72	Closure of ureterovaginal *fistula*

OPERATIONS ON THE BLADDER

—0 INCISION

730–00	Cystotomy
730–01	With exploration
730–02	With drainage: cystostomy
730–03	With removal of *calculus:* cystolithotomy; removal of foreign body
739–01	Exploration of perivesical tissues or prevesical space
739–02	Drainage of perivesical tissues or prevesical space

—I EXCISION

730–10	Cystectomy
730–11	Local excision of *lesion* of bladder; diverticulectomy.[1] *Ordinarily classified as* Partial cystectomy
730–12	Complete cystectomy
730–13	Partial cystectomy: resection of bladder
732–138	Punch operation on neck of bladder
730–16	Biopsy of bladder

—4 ENDOSCOPY

730–40	Cystoscopy
730–41	With biopsy [1]
730–42	With excision
730–43	With drainage; evacuation of *blood clots*
730–44	With removal (*foreign body, calculus*)
	With dilation
723–45	Of ureter (*stricture*)
727–45	Of ureterovesical orifice
730–45	Of bladder
732–46	With division of neck of bladder (*contracture*) [1]
730–470	With irrigation of bladder
720–470	With irrigation of renal pelvis and ureter
720–471	With instillation of diagnostic fluid into renal pelvis and roentgen examination: pyelography
730–471	With instillation of diagnostic fluid into bladder and roentgen examination: cystography
730–48	With insertion of radioactive substance
730–4x	With control of *bleeding* [1]
727–46	Ureteralmeatotomy to enlarge orifice

[1] Special operative method may be indicated by appropriate 3d digit. See page 517.

—5 REPAIR

730–50   Cystoplasty: plastic or reconstruction operation on bladder
7081–50   Ileocystoplasty

—6 DESTRUCTION

730–64   Litholapaxy: crushing of *calculus* in bladder and removal of fragments; lithotripsy: crushing of *calculus*

—7 SUTURE

730–71   Cystorrhaphy: suture of bladder (*wound, injury, rupture*)
730–72   Of cystostomy or external *fistula* of bladder
7031–72   Of vesicovaginal *fistula*
7032–72   Of vesicouterine *fistula*
708▲–72   Of vesicoenteric *fistula*.   *Specify site*
7083–72   Of vesicocolic *fistula*
7085–72   Of vesicorectal *fistula*
7301–74   Ligation of urachus

OPERATIONS ON THE URETHRA

—0 INCISION

740–00   Urethrotomy, external
740–01   With exploration
740–02   With drainage, by fistulization: urethrostomy
740–03   With removal (*calculus, foreign body*)
746–06   Meatotomy: cutting of meatus
747–02   Drainage of bulbourethral gland (*abscess*)
748–02   Drainage of periurethral tissues (*abscess, extravasated urine*)

—I EXCISION

740–11   Excision of *lesion* of urethra (external approach) [1]
740–16   Biopsy of urethra (external approach) [1]
747–12   Excision of bulbourethral gland

—4 ENDOSCOPY

740–40   Urethroscopy
740–41   With biopsy [1]
740–42   With excision [1]

[1] Special operative method may be indicated by appropriate 3d digit. See page 517.

740–422	By electrocoagulation
740–43	With drainage
740–44	With removal (*calculus, foreign body*)
740–45	With dilation
740–46	With cutting or division (*adhesions, scar, stric-ture*) : internal urethrotomy
740–470	With irrigation of urethra
740–471	With instillation of diagnostic fluid
740–472	With instillation of therapeutic agent
740–48	With insertion of radioactive substance
740–49	With insertion of catheter, tube

—5 REPAIR

| 740–50 | Urethroplasty: plastic or reconstruction operation on urethra |

—7 SUTURE

740–71	Urethrorrhaphy: suture of urethra (*wound, injury*)
	Closure
740–72	Of urethrostomy or *fistula* of urethra
7042–72	Of urethrovaginal *fistula*
709–72	Of urethrorectal *fistula*

—8 MANIPULATION

| 740–840 | Dilation of urethra by passage of sound (*stricture*). *See also under* Endoscopy |

75– OPERATIONS ON THE GENITAL SYSTEM

OPERATIONS ON THE MALE GENITAL SYSTEM

OPERATIONS ON THE PENIS

—0 INCISION

753–06   Dorsal or lateral "slit" of prepuce

—1 EXCISION

751–10   Amputation of penis
  751–12   Complete excision of penis
  751–13   Partial excision or resection of penis
  751–14   Radical excision of penis
751–11   Local excision of *lesion* of penis [1]
751–16   Biopsy of penis [1]
753–13   Circumcision

—5 REPAIR

751–50   Plastic or reconstruction operation on penis
  752–50   Plastic operation on glans penis: balanoplasty

OPERATIONS ON THE TESTIS

—0 INCISION

755–02   Incision and drainage of testis (*abscess*)

—1 EXCISION

755–12   Orchiectomy
  755–122   Castration: bilateral complete orchiectomy
755–16   Biopsy of testis

—5 REPAIR

755–50   Orchioplasty: plastic operation on testis
755–54   Reduction of *torsion* of testis: detorsion of testis
755–56   Orchiopexy

---

[1] Special operative method may be indicated by appropriate 3d digit.   See page 517.

755–71   Suture of testis

OPERATIONS ON THE EPIDIDYMIS

—0 INCISION

756–02   Epididymotomy and drainage

—I EXCISION

756–11   Excision of *lesion* of epididymis (*spermatocele*)
756–12   Epididymectomy
756–13   Partial epididymectomy
756–16   Biopsy of epididymis

—5 REPAIR

7561–52   Epididymovasostomy: anastomosis of epididymis to vas deferens

OPERATIONS ON THE TUNICA VAGINALIS

—0 INCISION

757–02   Incision and drainage of tunica vaginalis

—I EXCISION

757–11   Excision of *lesion* of tunica vaginalis (*hydrocele*)

OPERATIONS ON THE SCROTUM

—0 INCISION

758–02   Incision and drainage of scrotum
758–03   Incision and removal (*foreign body*)

—I EXCISION

758–11   Local excision of *lesion* of scrotum
758–13   Resection of scrotum: scrotectomy

—5 REPAIR

758–50   Plastic operation on scrotum: scrotoplasty

—7 SUTURE

758–71   Suture of scrotum

OPERATIONS ON THE VAS DEFERENS

—0 INCISION

761–06   Vasotomy: division or transection of vas

—1 EXCISION

761–10   Vasectomy
761–12   Complete vasectomy
761–13   Partial vasectomy

—5 REPAIR

761–52   Anastomosis of vas deferens

—6 DESTRUCTION

761–64   Crushing of vas deferens

—7 SUTURE

761–74   Ligation of vas: vasoligation

OPERATIONS ON THE SPERMATIC CORD

—0 INCISION

762–02   Incision and drainage of spermatic cord
762–06   Transection of spermatic cord

—1 EXCISION

762–11   Excision of *hydrocele* of spermatic cord
76x–11   Excision of *varicocele* of spermatic cord

OPERATIONS ON THE SEMINAL VESICLES

—0 INCISION

763–02   Vesiculotomy

—1 EXCISION

763–12   Vesiculectomy

OPERATIONS ON THE PROSTATE

—0 INCISION

764–00   Prostatotomy [1]
  764–02   With drainage (*abscess*) [1]
  764–03   With removal of *calculus:* prostatolithotomy [1]

—I EXCISION

764–168   Needle biopsy of prostate
764–10   Prostatectomy [1] (suprapubic approach)
  764–12   Complete prostatectomy [1]
  764–138   Partial prostatectomy, by punch
  764–10x   Perineal approach
  764–14   Radical prostatectomy [1]
  764–10y   Retropubic approach

—4 ENDOSCOPY

764–4x2   Transurethral electrocoagulation of prostate to control hemorrhage
764–427   Transurethral electroresection of prostate
764–43   Transurethral drainage of prostate (*abscess*)

[1] Perineal approach may be indicated by adding x at the end of code, and retropubic approach may be indicated by adding y at the end of the code.

OPERATIONS ON THE FEMALE GENITAL SYSTEM
OPERATIONS ON THE VULVA

—0 INCISION

774–00	Episiotomy [1]
776–00	Hymenotomy
774–02	Incision and drainage of vulva (*abscess*)
777–02	Incision and drainage of Bartholin's gland (*abscess*)
7461–02	Incision and drainage of Skene's glands (*abscess*)

—I EXCISION

774–10	Vulvectomy
774–12	Complete vulvectomy
774–13	Partial vulvectomy
774–14	Radical vulvectomy (includes regional lymph nodes)
77▲–11	Local excision of *lesion* of external female organ (vulva, labia, canal of Nuck, etc. *See page 39*)
772–12	Excision of labia majora
773–12	Excision of labia minora
775–12	Clitoridectomy: excision or amputation of clitoris
775–13	Circumcision, female: clitoridotomy
777–12	Excision of Bartholin's gland
7461–12	Excision of Skene's glands

—5 REPAIR

774–50	Episioplasty: plastic repair of vulva
7740–50	Episioperineoplasty: plastic repair of vulva and perineum
749–50	Plastic operation on urethral sphincter, female

—7 SUTURE

774–71	Episiorrhaphy: suture of vulva (recent *injury*) [1]
7740–71	Episioperineorrhaphy: suture of vulva and perineum (recent *injury*)

[1] To distinguish obstetric procedures 7x4– may be substituted for 774–.

OPERATIONS ON THE VAGINA

—0 INCISION

781–00	Colpotomy: vaginotomy
781–01	With exploration: diagnostic or exploratory colpotomy
066–02x	With drainage (*pelvic abscess*)

—I EXCISION

781–10	Colpectomy: colpocleisis: obliteration of vagina
781–12	Complete colpectomy
781–13	Partial colpectomy
781–11	Local excision of *lesion* of vagina
781–16	Biopsy of vagina

—3 INTRODUCTION

781–34	Insertion of vaginal bag [1]
781–35	Insertion of vaginal pack or tampon [1]

—4 ENDOSCOPY

7813–40	Culdoscopy

—5 REPAIR

Colpoplasty or colpoperineoplasty

781–512	Plastic construction of vagina with skin graft for congenital absence
7812–50	Repair of anterior vaginal wall; repair of *cystocele*
7813–50	Repair of posterior vaginal wall; repair of *rectocele;* repair of *enterocele* (*see also* Perineoplasty)
781–50	Repair of anterior and posterior vaginal wall; repair of cystocele and rectocele
781–56	Colpopexy

—7 SUTURE

781–71 [1]	Colporrhaphy: suture of vagina (recent *injury*) [1]
7811–71	Colpoperineorrhaphy: suture of vagina and perineum (recent *injury*) [1]
7022–72	Closure of ureterovaginal *fistula*
70x2–72	Closure of rectovaginal *fistula*

[1] To distinguish procedures related to **pregnancy**, 7x1 may be substituted for 781 as the topographic code.

—8 MANIPULATION

781–84   Dilation of vagina, manual [1]
781–840   Dilation of vagina, instrumental [1]

OPERATIONS ON THE FALLOPIAN TUBE (OVIDUCT)

—0 INCISION

787–06   Transection of tube

—I EXCISION

780–10   Supravaginal hysterectomy, bilateral; salpingo-
                     oophorectomy
780–12   Total hysterectomy bilateral; salpingo-oophorec-
                     tomy
787–00   Salpingotomy
787–10   Salpingectomy
  787–12   Complete salpingectomy
  787–13   Partial salpingectomy
7803–10   Salpingo-oophorectomy
  7803–12   Bilateral
  7802–13   Unilateral

—3 INTRODUCTION

7801–302   Hysterosalpingography

—5 REPAIR

787–50   Salpingoplasty
787–53   Salpingostomy
7801–50   Tubal implantation into uterus

—7 SUTURE

787–74   Ligation of tube

OPERATIONS ON THE OVARY

—0 INCISION

788–02   Drainage of ovary (*cyst, abscess*)

---

[1] To distinguish procedures related to pregnancy, 7x1 may be substituted for 781 as the topographic code.

—I EXCISION

788–10	Oophorectomy (one ovary)
788▲–11	Local excision of *lesion* of ovary. *For lesion derived from epoophoron (Gartner's duct), paroophoron, etc., add appropriate topographic digit, see page 39*
788–12	Bilateral oophorectomy
788–13	Oophorocystectomy
788–122	Castration, female: bilateral complete oophorectomy
788–131	Wedge resection of ovary

OPERATIONS ON THE UTERUS AND CERVIX UTERI

—0 INCISION

782–00	Hysterotomy [1]
783–00	Trachelotomy: hysterotrachelotomy [1]
782–023	Uterocentesis

—I EXCISION

782–10	Hysterectomy [2]
782–12	Complete or total hysterectomy (corpus and cervix)
782–11	Hysteromyomectomy: fibroidectomy or myomectomy, uterine; local excision of *fibroid tumor* of uterus
7801–12	Hysterosalpingectomy
782–13	Supracervical hysterectomy; partial or subtotal hysterectomy
7820–12	Excision of fundus of uterus: fundectomy, uterine
782–14	Radical hysterectomy (Wertheim's operation)
7062–14	Pelvic organ exenteration [radical excision of uterus (corpus, cervix, and adnexa), vagina, urinary bladder, rectum, and portion of sigmoid]
783–11	Local excision of lesion of cervix [3]
783–12	Trachelectomy: cervicectomy: amputation of cervix [3]

[1] To distinguish procedures related to pregnancy, 7x3 may be substituted for 783, and 7x2 may be substituted for 782 as the topographic code.

[2] Vaginal approach may be indicated by adding x at the end of code to differentiate from abdominal approach.

[3] Special operative method may be indicated by appropriate 3d digit. See page 517.

783–13	Partial excision of cervix; conization of cervix [1]
783–16	Biopsy of cervix [1]
785–104	Dilation and curettage of uterus [2]
785–164	Diagnostic dilation and curettage
7x5–104	Dilation and curettage for termination of pregnancy
789▲–11	Excision of *lesion* of uterine supporting structures. *Specify, page 39*

—3 INTRODUCTION

782–302	Hysterography
782–35	Insertion of intrauterine pack [2]
783–34	Insertion of intracervical bag [2]
783–35	Insertion of intracervical pack
782–32▲	Insertion of radioactive substance into uterus. *Specify, page 518*
783–32▲	Insertion of radioactive substance into cervix. *Specify, page 518*
782–301	Insufflation of uterus with air (Rubin test)

—5 REPAIR

782–56	Hysteropexy
782–560	With ventrosuspension: ventrofixation
782–56x	With interposition operation
7891–501	With shortening of round ligaments
7893–501	With shortening of sacrouterine ligaments
7894–501	With shortening and suture of endopelvic fascia: parametrial fixation: Manchester type operation
7801–52	Hysterosalpingostomy
783–50	Tracheloplasty: plastic repair of uterine cervix

—6 DESTRUCTION

782–65	Hysterolysis: freeing of uterus (*adhesions, etc.*)

—7 SUTURE

782–71	Hysterorrhaphy: suture of uterus (*rupture*) [2]
783–71	Trachelorrhaphy: hysterotrachelorrhaphy: suture of uterine cervix (recent *injury, laceration*) [2]

—8 MANIPULATION

783–84	Dilation of cervix, manual [2]
783–840	Dilation of cervix, instrumental [2]

1 Special operative method may be indicated by appropriate 3d digit. See page 517.
2 To distinguish procedures related to pregnancy, 7x3 may be substituted for 783; and 7x2 may be substituted for 782 as the topographic code. 7x5 may be substituted for 785 as a topographic code.

OPERATIONS ON THE PERINEUM

—0 INCISION

074–00	Perineotomy
074–02	With drainage (*abscess*)
074–03	With removal (*foreign body*)

—5 REPAIR

074–50	Perineoplasty: plastic repair of perineum

—7 SUTURE

074–71	Perineorrhaphy: suture of perineum
074–72	Closure of perineal *fistula*

OPERATIONS ON THE FETUS AND FETAL STRUCTURES

—0 INCISION

7x2–04	Cesarean section
7x23–04	Classic cesarean section
7x24–04	Low cervical (lower uterine segment) cesarean section
7x2–041	Cesarean section and hysterectomy: Porro's cesarean section
7x2–04x	Extraperitoneal cesarean section
7x3–04	Vaginal cesarean section
795–023	Artificial rupture of membranes

—I EXCISION

79▲–12	Removal of fetal structures
790–12	Of *embryo* [1]
7942–12	Of *placenta fragment* [1]
794–12	Of *retained placenta* [1]
7941–12	Of *retained placenta and membranes* [1]
797–11	Removal of *lesion* of chorionic villi (*hydatidiform mole*) [1]
794–16	Biopsy of placenta [1]

—6 DESTRUCTION

790–60	Embryotomy
7902–601	Cranial puncture
7902–60	Craniotomy, fetal

[1] Special operative method may be indicated by appropriate 3d digit. See page 517.

7902–64	Cranioclasis: basiotripsy
7905–63	Cleidotomy
7902–609	Decapitation

—8 MANIPULATION

790–85	Application of, or delivery by, obstetric forceps
790–850	Low [1]
790–851	Mid [1]
790–852	High [1]
790–86	Version [2]
790–860	External [2]
790–861	Internal [2]
790–862	Combined (external and internal) [2] (Braxton-Hicks)
790–87	Conversion of position (*malposition of head, etc.*) [3]
790–88	Extraction [3]
790–89	Obstetric delivery
790–891	Spontaneous breech delivery
790–892	Partial breech extraction
790–893	Total breech extraction
799–80	Replacement of umbilical cord

[1] Low forceps is the application of forceps when the head is visible during pain, the skull is on the perineal floor, and the sagittal suture is in the anterior-posterior or oblique diameter of the pelvis.

Mid forceps is the application of forceps before the criteria of low forceps have been met as stated above, but after engagement has taken place, that is, after the plane of greatest cephalic diameter (bi-parietal) has passed the inlet. Rotation is usually incomplete.

High forceps is the application of forceps before engagement has taken place. A subdivision of high forceps is forceps on the floating head.

[2] Cephalic version may be indicated by use of topographic code 7902; podalic version by 790x1.

[3] 790 Fetus generally:

7901–	Scalp
7902–	Head
7903–	Neck
7904–	Thorax
7905–	Shoulder
7906–	Arm
7907–	Abdomen
7908–	Back
7909–	Buttocks
790x–	Leg
790x1–	Foot

8– OPERATIONS ON THE ENDOCRINE SYSTEM

OPERATIONS ON THE THYROID GLAND

—0 INCISION

810–00	Thyroidotomy
810–01	With exploration
810–02	With drainage (*abscess, cyst*)
813–06	With division or transection of thyroid isthmus
810–05	Reopening of thyroid *wound* (for removal of *hematoma* and control of *hemorrhage*)
815–02	Incision and drainage of thyroglossal cyst (infected)

—I EXCISION

810–10	Thyroidectomy
810–11	Local excision of *lesion* of thyroid (*small cyst* or *adenoma*). *Ordinarily classify as* Partial thyroidectomy
810–12	Complete, or total, thyroidectomy
810–13	Partial, or subtotal, thyroidectomy
81▲–13	Hemithyroidectomy: lobectomy, thyroid
813–12	Excision of thyroid isthmus: isthmectomy
814–10	Excision of aberrant thyroid or *lesion* thereof
815–10	Excision of thyroglossal duct, *cyst* or *sinus*
810–16	Biopsy of thyroid

—5 REPAIR

810–51	Graft of thyroid: transplantation of thyroid tissue or tissue culture

—7 SUTURE

81x–74	Ligation of thyroid arteries
81x1–74	Of superior thyroid artery
81x2–74	Of inferior thyroid artery

OPERATIONS ON THE PARATHYROID, THYMUS, PITUITARY, PINEAL, ADRENAL, AND CAROTID GLANDS

Specify site by inserting digits where indicated.   See page 40.

—0   INCISION

8▲▲–01   Exploration of endocrine gland

—1   EXCISION

820–1▲   Parathyroidectomy [1]
830–1▲   Thymectomy [1]
84▲–1▲   Hypophysectomy [1]
850–1▲   Pinealectomy [1]
860–1▲   Adrenalectomy [1]
8▲▲–11   Local excision of *lesion* of endocrine gland
8▲▲–16   Biopsy of endocrine gland

[1] Specify complete or partial excision.   See page 588.

9– OPERATIONS ON THE NERVOUS SYSTEM

OPERATIONS ON STRUCTURES OVERLYING THE MENINGES, BRAIN, AND SPINAL CORD

Specify site by inserting 3d digit. See page 9.

—0 INCISION

21▲–00	Craniotomy [1]
21▲–01	Exploration of skull
21▲–02	Drainage of skull (*osteomyelitis*)
21▲–08	Decompression
211–08	Orbital, intracranial approach. *For antral approach, see* Decompression of orbit, *page 601* . .
213–08	Subtemporal
214–08	Suboccipital
2203–01	Exploration of spinal canal (without laminectomy)

—1 EXCISION

21▲–13	Craniectomy [1]
21▲–16	Biopsy of skull
2203–12	Laminectomy [1]
2203–13	Hemilaminectomy [1]

—5 REPAIR

21▲–50	Cranioplasty: Plastic operation on skull for *defects* or *deformities*
21▲–502	With metal or plastic plate
21▲–516	With bone graft
2203–50	Repair of *defect* of vertebral arch and spine (*spina bifida* with *meningocele* or *meningomyelocele*)
21▲–54	Open reduction of *fracture* of skull, with elevation or removal of fragments

—6 DESTRUCTION

21▲–61	Debridement of *compound fracture* of skull

[1] These operations indicate method of approach to meninges, brain, or spinal cord.

OPERATIONS ON THE MENINGES AND MENINGEAL VESSELS

Specify site by inserting digits where indicated. See page 42.

—0 INCISION

910▲–01	Exploration of meninges [1]
910▲–02	Drainage of meninges [1]
913▲–02	Drainage of subdural space (*abscess, hematoma, hygroma*)
915▲–02	Drainage of cerebral epidural space (*abscess, hematoma, hygroma*)
916▲–02	Drainage of spinal epidural space (*abscess, hematoma, hygroma*)
917▲–02	Drainage of subarachnoid space (*abscess, hematoma, hygroma*)
910▲–03	Removal (*foreign body*) [1]
917▲–023	Puncture of subarachnoid space, for aspiration: rachicentesis
9171–023	Cranial puncture; cisternal puncture
9172–023	Spinal puncture; lumbar puncture
91x▲–02	Drainage of cranial sinus (*phlebitis, thrombosis*)
91x3–02	Drainage of lateral sinus (*phlebitis, thrombosis*)
91x4–02	Drainage of sigmoid sinus (*phlebitis, thrombosis*)

—I EXCISION

910▲–11	Excision of *lesion* of meninges (*meningioma, cyst, meningocele,*[1] *congenital dermal sinus* extending to or involving meninges)
9102▲–11	Cervical
9103▲–11	Thoracic
9104▲–11	Lumbar
9106▲–11	Sacral
910▲–16	Biopsy of meninges [1]

—3 INTRODUCTION

917–301	Encephalography: injection of air (or oxygen helium, ethylene) into subarachnoid space by lumbar spinal puncture and roentgen examination

[1] Approach to cerebral meninges is by craniotomy, craniectomy, or trephination; to spinal meninges, by laminectomy. **See preceding section, page 590.**

9172–302   Myelography; injection of radiopaque substance into spinal canal and roentgen examination

—5 REPAIR

917▲–53   Fistulization of subarachnoid space
910▲–50   Plastic repair of meninges; duraplasty [1]
   910–51   Graft of dura [1]
910▲–53   Marsupialization of *lesion* of meninges (*cyst, abscess*) [1]

—7 SUTURE

910▲–71   Suture of meninges; dura [1]
91x–74   Ligation of meningeal vessels [1]
   91x1–74   Ligation of middle meningeal artery
   91x2–74   Ligation of superior longitudinal sinus

OPERATIONS ON THE BRAIN

Specify site by inserting digits as indicated. See page 44.

—0 INCISION

9▲▲–01   Exploration of brain
   9▲▲–010   Exploratory puncture
9▲▲–02   Drainage (*abscess*)
9▲▲–03   Removal (*foreign body*)
9▲▲–060   Cutting or division of brain tissue
   93▲–060   Lobotomy; leukotomy
   957–060   Tractotomy of medulla oblongata
   955–060   Tractotomy of mesencephalon
920–020   Insertion of tube (metal, rubber, plastic) into lateral ventricle for continuous drainage
9464–00   Pallidotomy
9▲▲–023   Puncture of brain, for aspiration (*cyst, abscess*)
920–023   Puncture of ventricles, for aspiration

—I EXCISION

9▲▲–11   Local excision of *lesion* of brain (*cyst, neoplasm, scar, fungus cerebri*) [2]
9▲▲–13   Resection of brain tissue; topectomy [2]

---

[1] Approach to cerebral meninges is by craniotomy, craniectomy, or trephination; to spinal meninges, by laminectomy. See preceding section, page 590.
[2] Special operative method may be indicated by appropriate 3d digit.

93▲–12	Excision of lobe of brain [1]
933–12	Of frontal lobe [1]
934–12	Of parietal lobe [1]
935–12	Of temporal lobe [1]
936–12	Of occipital lobe [1]
92x▲–12	Excision of choroid plexus [1]
9▲▲–16	Biopsy of brain [1]

—3 INTRODUCTION

920–301	Ventriculography: injection of air into lateral ventricles and roentgen examination

—5 REPAIR

9011–52	Ventriculocisternostomy by tube: Torkildsen's operation (plastic tube, polyethylene)
92▲–53	Ventriculostomy
9▲▲–53	Marsupialization of *lesion* of brain (*cyst, abscess*)
9▲▲–61	Debridement of *contused* brain tissue
9▲▲–65	Division of cortical *adhesions*

OPERATIONS ON THE SPINAL CORD AND NERVE ROOTS

Specify site by inserting 4th digit. See page 47.
For operations on intervertebral disk, see page 532.

—0 INCISION

970▲–01	Exploration of spinal cord [2]
970▲–02	Drainage of spinal cord (*cyst*).[2] *For operations on epidural space, such as drainage of abscess, evacuation of hematoma, or removal of foreign body, see* Operations on Meninges, etc., *page 591*
970▲–060	Chordotomy: tractotomy or division or transection of nerve tracts in cord [2]
978▲–06	Rhizotomy: division or transection of nerve roots
9781–06	Ventral nerve roots
9782–06	Dorsal nerve roots
970▲–08	Decompression of spinal cord (by removal of *hematoma, bone fragments*) [2]

[1] Special operative method may be indicated by appropriate 3d digit.
[2] Approach by laminectomy is implied.

—I EXCISION

970▲–11   Excision of *lesion* of spinal cord (*neoplasm, cyst*) [1]
970▲–16   Biopsy of spinal cord [1]

OPERATIONS ON THE PERIPHERAL NERVES, CEREBRAL NERVES, AND GANGLIA

Specify region by inserting digits as indicated. See page 47.

—0 INCISION

9▲▲–01   Exploration of nerve
9▲▲–06   Neurotomy: cutting, division, or transection of nerve
  96▲–06   Of cranial nerves
    9647–06   Retrogasserian neurotomy: transection of sensory root of trigeminal nerve
    966–06   Acoustic neurotomy
    968–06   Vagotomy: transection of vagus nerve
  98▲–06   Of spinal nerves
    9824–06   Phrenicotomy: transection of phrenic nerve
9▲▲–060   Partial transection of nerve. *Specify as for Neurotomy, preceding*
  967–06   Glossopharyngeal neurotomy

—I EXCISION

9▲▲–11   Excision of *lesion* of nerve (*neuroma*)
9▲▲–13   Neurectomy
  96▲–13   Of cranial nerves
  98▲–13   Of spinal nerves
    9824–13   Phrenicectomy: resection of phrenic nerve
9▲▲–139   Neurexeresis: avulsion of nerve
  9824–139   Phrenicoexeresis: avulsion of phrenic nerve
9▲▲–12   Ganglionectomy. *See also* Sympathectomy, *page 595*
  96▲–12   Cerebral nerve ganglia
    9645–12   Gasserian ganglionectomy
9▲▲–16   Biopsy of nerve

—3 INTRODUCTION

9▲▲–30   Injection into nerve. *Specify substance injected*

[1] Approach by laminectomy is implied.

—5 REPAIR

9▲▲–50   Neuroplasty: plastic repair of nerve (old *injury* of nerve)

9▲▲–51   Graft of nerve

9▲▲–52   Anastomosis of nerves: neuroanastomosis

  9601–52   Spinal accessory-facial neuroanastomosis

  9602–52   Hypoglossal-facial neuroanastomosis

  9603–52   Spinal accessory-hypoglossal neuroanastomosis

—6 DESTRUCTION

9▲▲–64   Neurotripsy: crushing of nerve

  9824–64   Phrenicotripsy: phrenemphraxis

9▲▲–65   Neurolysis: freeing of nerve (*adhesions, callus*); transposition of nerve

—7 SUTURE

9▲▲–71   Neurorrhaphy: suture of nerve (recent *injury*)

—8 MANIPULATION

9▲▲–84   Stretching of nerve: neurectasia

OPERATIONS ON THE VEGETATIVE NERVOUS SYSTEM

Specify nerve by inserting 4th digit. See page 49.

        Sympathectomy

99▲▲–06   Transection, cutting or division

  994▲–06   Of preganglionic nerves

  995▲–06   Of ganglionated chains

  996▲–06   Of postganglionic nerves

    9961–06   Splanchnicotomy

  997▲–06   Of mixed plexus nerves

99▲▲–13   Resection

  994▲–13   Of preganglionic nerves

  996▲–13   Of postganglionic nerves

    9961–13   Splanchnicectomy

  997▲–13   Of mixed plexus nerves

    9977–13   Presacral neurectomy (hypogastric plexus)

99▲▲–12   Excision of ganglionated chains, mixed plexuses, ganglia: ganglionectomy

  995▲–12   Excision of ganglionated chains: sympathetic ganglionectomy

997▲–12   Excision of mixed plexuses
99x▲–12   Excision of mixed ganglia associated with cere-
                 bral nerves
   99x2–12   Sphenopalatine (Meckel's) ganglionectomy
          Sympathicotripsy
99▲▲–64   Crushing of nerve, ganglion or plexus of vegeta-
                 tive nervous system. *Specify as under* Sym-
                 pathectomy, *preceding*

X- OPERATIONS ON THE ORGANS OF SPECIAL SENSE

X1- OPERATIONS ON THE EYE

OPERATIONS ON THE EYEBALL

—0 INCISION

x13–024   Goniotomy

—1 EXCISION

x11–12   Enucleation of eyeball
x11–13   Evisceration of eyeball

—3 INTRODUCTION

x111–353   Orbital implant

—5 REPAIR

x11–50   Plastic operation on eyeball

—7 SUTURE

x11–71   Suture of eyeball (*wound, injury*)

OPERATIONS ON THE CORNEA

—0 INCISION

x12–00   Keratotomy
  x12–06   Delimiting keratotomy : Gifford's operation
x12–023   Keratocentesis
x12–03   Removal of *foreign body* in cornea
  x12–031   With magnet

—1 EXCISION

x12–10   Keratectomy
  x12–12   Complete
  x12–13   Partial

—3 INTRODUCTION

x12–30   Tattoo of cornea, mechanical (with needle) or
                 chemical

597

—5 REPAIR

x12–50　　　　　Keratoplasty
　x12–51　　　　　　Graft of cornea

—7 SUTURE

x12–71　　　　　Suture of cornea

OPERATIONS ON THE SCLERA

—0 INCISION

x13–00　　　　　Sclerotomy
　x13–01　　　　　　With exploration
　x13–02　　　　　　With drainage: scleral fistula operation: scler-
　　　　　　　　　　　ostomy
　x13–03　　　　　　With removal of *foreign body*

—1 EXCISION

x13–13　　　　　Sclerectomy
　x13–131　　　　　By scissors (Lagrange's operation)
　x13–138　　　　　By punch (Holth's operation)
　x13–139　　　　　By trephining (Elliot's operation)

—5 REPAIR

x13–50　　　　　Plastic operation on sclera: scleroplasty
　x13–501　　　　　Scleral shortening

—7 SUTURE

x13–71　　　　　Suture of sclera (*wound, injury*)

OPERATIONS ON THE IRIS AND CILIARY BODY

—0 INCISION

x15–00　　　　　Iridotomy: sphincterotomy
　x15–06　　　　　　With transfixion of iris (*iris bombé*): iriden-
　　　　　　　　　　cleisis

—1 EXCISION

x15–10　　　　　Iridectomy
　x15–11　　　　　　Excision of lesion of iris
　x15–13　　　　　　"Complete" iridectomy; optical iridectomy; pre-
　　　　　　　　　　liminary iridectomy
　x15–131　　　　　Peripheral iridectomy

—5 REPAIR

x15–50   Coreoplasty

—6 DESTRUCTION

x16–606   Diathermy of the ciliary body; cyclodiathermy
x16–609   Cycloelectrolysis
x15–65   Iridodialysis
x151–651   Iridodialysis, anterior
x152–651   Iridodialysis, posterior
x16–65   Cyclodialysis

—7 SUTURE

x15–71   Suture of iris

—8 MANIPULATION

x15–84   Iridotasis: stretching of iris; iridencleisis

OPERATIONS ON THE CHOROID

—1 EXCISION

x17–16   Biopsy of choroid

—5 REPAIR

x17–560   Repair of choroid; reattachment of choroid
x24–560   Repair of choroid and retina; reattachment of choroid and retina

OPERATIONS ON THE CRYSTALLINE LENS

—0 INCISION

x20–06   Discission: needling of lens
x21–00   Capsulotomy

—1 EXCISION

x20–121   Extraction of subluxated lens
x20–12   Extraction of lens, intracapsular
x20–14   Extraction of lens and capsulectomy: extracapsular extraction of lens
x21–12   Capsulectomy

OPERATIONS ON THE VITREOUS

—0 INCISION

x22–023   Aspiration of vitreous

—5 REPAIR

x22–51   Vitreous replacement

OPERATIONS ON THE RETINA

—5 REPAIR

x23–560   Repair of retina; reattachment of retina
x24–560   Repair of retina and choroid; reattachment of retina and choroid

OPERATIONS ON THE OCULAR MUSCLES

Specify muscle by inserting 3d digit. See page 15.

—0 INCISION

27▲–06   Myotomy of ocular muscle
28▲–06   Tenotomy of ocular tendon
27▲–060   Partial transection of ocular muscle or tendon

—1 EXCISION

28▲–10   Tenectomy of ocular muscle
27▲–10   Myectomy of ocular muscle
27▲–13   "Resection": excision of segment of ocular muscle and suture

—5 REPAIR

27▲–50   Transplantation of ocular muscle
27▲–501   Shortening of ocular muscle by tucking, plicating, folding, or "cinching"
27▲–561   Advancement of ocular muscle
27▲–562   Recession of ocular muscle

OPERATIONS ON THE ORBIT

—0 INCISION

x50–00	Orbitotomy. *Specify type*
x50–01	With exploration
x50–02	With drainage
x50–03	With removal (*foreign body*)
x50–08	Decompression of orbit, antral approach. *For intracranial approach, see* Decompression, orbital, *page 590*

—I EXCISION

x50–11	Excision of lesion of orbit
x51–12	Exenteration or evisceration of orbital contents
x50–16	Biopsy of orbit

—5 REPAIR

x50–50	Plastic repair of orbit

OPERATIONS ON THE EYELIDS

—0 INCISION

x52–00	Blepharotomy
x52–02	With drainage of eyelid (abscess)
x61–02	With drainage of Meibomian glands (*hordeolum*)
x68–06	Canthotomy: division of canthus
2716–06	Tenotomy of levator palpebrae muscle

—I EXCISION

x52–11	Excision of *lesion* of eyelids; blepharectomy
132–11	Of skin of eyelids
x61–11	Of Meibomian glands (*chalazion*)
x55–10	Tarsectomy: excision of tarsal cartilage
164–12	Excision of cilia base
164–10	Epilation
164–106	Electrolytic
164–109	Mechanical

—5 REPAIR

x52–50	Blepharoplasty: plastic repair of eyelid
x52–51	Graft to eyelid. *Specify type*

x52–514	Full thickness skin graft
x52–518	Fascial graft (fascia lata)
x68–50	Canthoplasty: plastic repair of canthus
x55–50	Tarsoplasty: plastic repair of tarsal cartilage
163–51	Plastic restoration of eyebrow (by graft)
164–50	Reposition of cilia base

—7 SUTURE

x52–71	Blepharorrhaphy: suture of eyelid
x55–71	Tarsorrhaphy: suture of tarsal cartilage
x68–71	Canthorrhaphy: suture of palpebral fissure of canthus

OPERATIONS ON THE CONJUNCTIVA

—0 INCISION

x56–03   Removal of *foreign body*

—I EXCISION

x56–11   Excision of lesion of conjunctiva (*cyst, epithelioma, nevus, pterygium*)

x56–114   Grattage: scraping of conjunctiva (*trachoma follicles*)

x56–13   Peritectomy: peritomy: excision of ring of conjunctiva around cornea (*pannus*)

x56–16   Biopsy of conjunctiva

—5 REPAIR

x56–50	Conjunctivoplasty
x56–51	Free graft of conjunctiva
x56–511	Free graft of mucous membrane of lip
x56–515	Flap operation: "flapping" of conjunctiva

—7 SUTURE

x56–71   Suture of conjunctiva

—8 MANIPULATION

x56–80   Rolling conjunctiva: expression (*trachoma follicles*)

OPERATIONS ON THE LACRIMAL TRACT

—0 INCISION

x62–02	Drainage of lacrimal gland (*abscess*)
x66–02	Drainage of lacrimal sac: dacryocystostomy: dacryocystotomy
x64–00	Splitting of lacrimal papilla

—I EXCISION

x62–12	Excision of lacrimal gland: dacryoadenectomy
x66–12	Excision of lacrimal sac: dacryocystectomy

—3 INTRODUCTION

x67–38	Catheterization of lacrimonasal duct

—5 REPAIR

x65–50	Plastic operation on canaliculi
x66–53	Dacryocystorhinostomy: fistulization of lacrimal sac into nasal cavity

—8 MANIPULATION

x64–840	Dilation of punctum
x67–840	Probing of lacrimonasal duct

X7- OPERATIONS ON THE EAR

OPERATIONS ON THE EXTERNAL EAR

—0 INCISION

x7▲–02	Incision and drainage of ear
x72–02	Of auricle (*abscess*)
x75–02	Of external auditory canal (*abscess*)
135–02	Of skin of ear (*furuncle*)

—1 EXCISION

x72–11	Local excision of *lesion* of ear
x72–12	Complete excision of ear: amputation of ear
x72–13	Partial excision of ear
x75–11	Excision of *lesion* of external auditory canal
x7▲–16	Biopsy of ear. *Specify site (page 52)*

—4 ENDOSCOPY

x75–44	Otoscopy and removal of *foreign body* in external auditory canal

—5 REPAIR

x75–50	Canaloplasty (surgical correction, stenosis of external auditory canal)
x7▲–50	Otoplasty: plastic operation on ear
x72–50	Of auricle
x74–50	Of cartilage (*"lop ear"*)
x78–50	Of lobule
x7▲–51	Reconstruction of ear with graft
x71–512	With split thickness or partial thickness skin graft
x71–514	With full thickness skin graft
x71–517	With cartilage graft

—7 SUTURE

x72–71	Suture of ear (*wound, injury*)

OPERATIONS ON THE MIDDLE EAR

—0 INCISION

x84–00	Atticotomy
x77–02	Myringotomy: tympanotomy: plicotomy
x8x–01	Exploration of petrous pyramid air cells

x84–01	Exploratory mastoidectomy by removal of mastoid cortex
x77–01	Exploratory tympanotomy by transtympanic route
x8x–02	Drainage of petrous pyramid air cells (*petrositis*) [1]

—1 EXCISION

x84–131	Atticoantrotomy, outer attic wall removed but bridge remains intact
x8x–13	Exenteration of air cells of petrous pyramid [1]
x84–10	Mastoidectomy
x84–13	Simple mastoidectomy: cortical not complete; mastoid antrotomy
x84–14	Radical mastoidectomy
x84–141	Modified radical bridge taken down and incus and heart of whole malleus sacrificed
x81–12	Ossiculectomy

—3 INTRODUCTION

x80–35	Insertion of pack or tampon into middle ear
x80–382	Insertion of plastic tube
x81–382	Insertion of plastic tube between incus and footplate of stapes
x81–330	Insertion of wire loop between incus and footplate of stapes
x83–38	Intubation or catheterization of eustachian tube

—5 REPAIR

x81–50	Mobilization of auditory ossicles (stapes) [1]
x81–53	Perforation of the footplate of the stapes
x81–505	Plastic repair with bone shifting
x81–51x	Repair with vein graft after removal of stapes
x81–502	Stapedectomy with tissue graft and introduction of prosthesis
x81–5021	Partial stapedectomy with introduction of prosthesis
x77–50	Tympanoplasty, total
x771–50	Epitympanic, type I
x772–50	Columnellar, type II
x773–50	Tympanoplasty, type III
x774–50	Other types

1 Intrapetrosal approach may be indicated by adding x at end of code to differentiate from extrapetrosal approach.

—6 DESTRUCTION

x80–65	Division of adhesions
x81–65	Division of otosclerotic processes which have fixed the stapes to the oval window
x81–63	Fracture of the curb and/or footplate of the stapes
x93–602	Electrocoagulation of semicircular canals
x93–609	Special methods of destruction, *e.g.,* ultrasound application to canals

—7 SUTURE

x84–72	Closure of *fistula* of mastoid

—8 MANIPULATION

x84–83	Removal of packing, mastoid spaces
x80–83	Removal of packing, middle ear spaces

OPERATIONS ON THE INTERNAL EAR

—0 INCISION

x85–02	Labyrinthotomy
x87–02	Of cochlea
x91–02	Of vestibule; vestibulotomy
x93–02	Of semicircular canals
x82–02y	Labyrinthotomy, transtympanic

—I EXCISION

x85–13	Labyrinthectomy

—5 REPAIR

x93–53	Fenestration of semicircular canals

ANESTHESIA

Agents

1 and 2   GASEOUS AND VOLATILE AGENTS

10   Carbon dioxide
11   Chloroform
12   Cyclopropane
13   Divinyl ether (Vinethene)
14   Ethyl chloride
15   Diethyl oxide (Ethyl ether)
16   Ethylene
17   Nitrous oxide
18   Trichloroethylene (Trilene; Trimar)
19   Halothane (Fluothane)
20   Oxygen
21   Vinyl-ethyl ether (Vinemar)
22   Helium
23   Nitrogen
24   Other halogenated agents
29   Other gaseous and volatile agents

3   BARBITURATES

30   Hexobarbital (Evipal)
31   Thiopental (Pentothal)
32   Thialbarbitone (Kemithal)
33   Thiamylal (Surital)
34   Pentobarbital (Nembutal)
35   Amobarbital (Amytal)
36   Secobarbital (Seconal)
39   Other barbiturates

4   LOCAL ANALGESIC AGENTS

40   Cocaine
41   Piperocaine (Metycaine)
42   Dibucaine (Nupercaine)
43   Tetracaine (Pontocaine)
44   Procaine (Novocaine)
45   Lidocaine (Xylocaine)
46   Hexylcaine (Cyclaine)
47   Butacaine (Butyn)
49   Other locally acting analgesic agents

5 and 6   BASAL HYPNOTIC AND NARCOTIC AGENTS

50   Alcohol
51   Ether in oil

52 Paraldehyde
53 Tribromethanol in amylene hydrate (Avertin liquid)
55 Phenothiazine derivations
56 Other tranquilizers
59 Other basal hypnotic agents
60 Morphine
61 Meperidine (Demerol)
62 Alphaprodine (Nisental)
63 Dilaudid
69 Other narcotic agents

7 PHYSICAL AND PSYCHIC AGENTS

70 Thermal
71 Electronarcosis
72 Hypnosis
73 Hypotensive
79 Other physical and psychic agents

8 MUSCLE RELAXANTS

80 d-Tubocurarine (Curare)
81 Gallamine (Flaxedil)
82 Benzoquinonium chloride (Mytolon)
84 Other synaptic blocking agents
85 Succinyl choline (Anectine; Quelicin; Sucostrin)
86 Decamethonium bromide (Syncurine)
89 Other depolarizing relaxants

9 ADJUNCTIVE AGENTS

90 N-allyl morphine (Nalline)
91 Nallorphan (Lorfan)
92 Other narcotic antagonists
93 Corticosteroids
95 Edrophonium (Tensilon)
96 Anticholinesterase (Neostigmine, etc.)
97 Barbiturate antagonists
98 Vasopressor agents
99 Other adjunctive agents

Methods of Administration of Inhalation Anesthetics

00 None
01 Open
02 Open, endotracheal
03 Nonrebreathing (semi-open)
04 Semi-open, endotracheal
05 Insufflation, pharyngeal
06 Insufflation, endotracheal

07   Semi-open, T-tube (Ayres) technique
08   Closed, no absorption
10   Partial rebreathing (semi-closed) respiration unassisted
11   Semi-closed (respiration assisted)
14   Semi-closed, endotracheal (unassisted respiration)
15   Semi-closed, endotracheal (assisted respiration)
17   Semi-closed, endobronchial (unassisted respiration)
18   Semi-closed, endobronchial (assisted respiration)
20   Absorption, to and fro (unassisted respiration)
21   Absorption, to and fro (assisted respiration)
22   Absorption, to and fro (controlled respiration)
24   Absorption, to and fro, endotracheal (unassisted respiration)
25   Absorption, to and fro, endotracheal (assisted respiration)
26   Absorption, to and fro, endotracheal (controlled respiration)
27   Absorption, to and fro, endobronchial (unassisted respiration)
28   Absorption, to and fro, endobronchial (assisted respiration)
29   Absorption, to and fro, endobronchial (controlled respiration)
30   Absorption in circuit (respiration unassisted)
31   Absorption in circuit (assisted respiration)
32   Absorption in circuit (controlled respiration)
34   Absorption in circuit, endotracheal (unassisted respiration)
35   Absorption in circuit, endotracheal (assisted respiration)
36   Absorption in circuit, endotracheal (controlled respiration)
37   Absorption in circuit, endobronchial (unassisted respiration)
38   Absorption in circuit, endobronchial (assisted respiration)
39   Absorption in circuit, endobronchial (controlled respiration)

Other Anesthetic Methods

40   Intravenous
50   Rectal
60   Topical
61   Infiltration
62   Field block
63   Nerve block, cervical plexus
64   Nerve block, brachial plexus
65   Nerve block, thoracic

66 Nerve block, lumbar
67 Nerve block, thoracolumbar combined
68 Splanchnic block
69 Miscellaneous nerve blocks
70 Sacral block
71 Caudal block
72 Continuous caudal analgesia
73 Combined sacral and caudal block (transsacral)
74 Peridural, epidural, single injection
75 Continuous peridural
79 Other block techniques
80 Spinal (no adrenergic drug)
81 Spinal (with adrenergic drug)
82 Spinal, hyperbaric saddle block
83 Spinal, hypobaric
84 Spinal, isobaric
90 Hypothermia—surface cooling
91 Hypothermia—body cavity cooling
92 Hypothermia—extracorporeal exchange
93 Hypothermia—drug-induced
94 Extracorporeal circulation

Time of administration and special procedures may be indicated when applicable by appropriate third digit added to the method code as follows:

▲▲0 Prior to anesthesia
▲▲1 Induction
▲▲2 Maintenance (during procedure)
▲▲3 Closing
▲▲4 Postoperative
▲▲5 Mechanical ventilation
▲▲9 Other methods

INDEX
TO
NOMENCLATURE OF DISEASE

The number in parentheses refers to etiologic category.

A

Abdomen. *See also* Gastrointestinal tract; Pelvis; Peritoneum
abnormal communication between uterus and anterior abdominal wall, 306 (0)
abscess of wall, 298 (1)
carcinomatosis, generalized, 129 (8)
diseases, 298 ff.
ectopia of viscera due to defect in wall, 240 (0)
fatty necrosis due to unknown cause, 302 (9)
fistula
due to infection, 298 (1)
due to trauma, 299 (4)
following operation, 299 (4)
vesicoabdominal, following operation, 319 (4)
foreign body in wall, due to trauma or following operation, 299 (4)
hernia. *See* Hernia, ventral
pain: *supplementary term,* 497. *Diagnose disease*
rigidity, general or local: *supplementary term,* 497. *Diagnose disease*
sarcoma, 301 (8)
transposition of viscera, 298 (0)
tumors, unlisted, 301 (8)
wound
penetrating, 127 (4)
of wall, 127 (4)
Abdominal mass: *supplementary term,* 496. *Diagnose disease*
Abdominal pregnancy, 380 (7)
Abnormalities. *See also under organ, region or structure affected*
list, 55
Abortion, 378
accidental, following operation, 378
complete, 378
habitual
due to syphilis, 380 (1)
due to undetermined cause, 380 (y)
incomplete, 378
inevitable, 378

Abortion—Continued
missed, 378
threatened, 378
Abrasion, 136 (4). *See also under organ, region or structure affected*
Abrikossoff's tumor. *Diagnose as* Granular cell myoblastoma, 96
Abruptio placentae. *See* Placenta, premature separation, 383 (4), 384 (9)
Abscess, 123 (1). *See also under organ, region or structure affected*
amebic. *See* Amebiasis, 114 (1)
Brodie's, 148 (1)
compression of spinal cord, 423 (4)
due to stitch, 136 (4)
due to trauma, 125 (4)
epidural, 405 (1)
following operation, 125 (4)
ischiorectal, 284 (1)
multiple, 114 (1)
of operative wound, 125 (4)
palmar, 123 (1)
retrocecal, 298 (1)
retroperitoneal, 298 (1)
of subcutaneous areolar tissue, 132 (1)
subdiaphragmatic, 298 (1)
subdural, 405 (1)
subgaleal, 123 (1)
subhepatic, 298 (1)
Absence. *See also under organ, region or structure affected*
congenital, 122 (0)
due to trauma, 125 (4)
following operation, 125 (4)
Acalculia: *supplementary term,* 501. *Diagnose disease*
Acanthoameloblastoma. *Diagnose as* Ameloblastoma, 98
Acanthoma
adenoides cysticum. *Diagnose as* Neoplastic cyst, not otherwise specified, 93
benign. *Diagnose as* Squamous cell papilloma, 94

Acanthoma—Continued
  malignant. *Diagnose* as Epidermoid
    carcinoma, 94
Acanthosis
  nigricans, 140 (9)
  of tongue, 246 (9)
Acardia, 201 (0)
Acarodermatitis, 134 (2)
Acarophobia: *supplementary term,*
    484. *Diagnose disease*
Accessory. *See under organ, region
    or structure affected*
Accessory sinuses. *See* Sinuses, ac-
    cessory
Accidents. *See* Injuries; Trauma
Accommodation
  paralysis of: *supplementary term,*
    505. *Diagnose disease*
  spasm of, 456 (5)
Acetabulum
  pelvic protrusion, 154 (9)
Acetanilid poisoning, 117 (3)
Acetonuria: *supplementary term,* 498.
    Diagnose disease
Achalasia, 261 (55)
  cardiospasm, congenital, 263 (0)
  cardiospasm reflex, 261 (55)
  dilatation of esophagus due to, 261
    (55)
Achlorhydria
  due to chronic atrophic gastritis,
    265 (9)
  due to poison, 264 (3)
  supplementary term, 496. *Diagnose
    disease*
Achondroplasia
  complete (dwarfism) or incomplete,
    146 (0)
Achroactyosis
  of lacrimal gland
    due to infection, 465 (1)
    due to unknown cause, 467 (9)
Achromatopsia, 446 (0)
  supplementary term, 508. *Diagnose
    disease*
Achylia
  gastrica, atrophy of mucous mem-
    brane of tongue in, 246 (9)
  supplementary term, 496. *Diagnose
    disease*
Acid. *See also under name of acid*
  conjunctivitis due to, 469 (3)

Acid-base equilibrium
  disorders, 152 (7)
  nephrosis due to disturbance of acid-
    base balance, 311 (7)
Acid-fast bacilli
  in gastric contents: *supplementary
    term,* 496. *Diagnose disease*
  nonpathogenic, in urine: *supplemen-
    tary term,* 498. *Diagnose disease*
  in sputum: *supplementary term,* 490.
    Diagnose disease
Acidosis
  not due to diabetes, 120 (7)
  supplementary term, 493. *Diagnose
    disease*
Aclasis
  metaphysial, 147 (0)
Acne, 138 (7)
  chéloidique. *See* Folliculitis keloid-
    alis, 132 (1)
  conglobate, 132 (1)
  conjunctivitis, 470 (5)
  rosacea with, 137 (5), 463 (5)
  varioliformis, 140 (9)
Aconitine
  poisoning of heart by, 209 (3)
Acosta's disease. *See* Hypobaropa-
    thy, 118 (4)
Acoustic nerve
  degeneration, deafness due to, 480
    (9)
  tumor. *Diagnose as* Schwannoma, 95
Acoustic trauma
  resulting in deafness, 472 (4)
Acragnosis: *supplementary term,* 501.
    Diagnose disease
Acroasphyxia: *supplementary term,*
    487. *Diagnose disease*
Acrocephalia, 122 (0)
Acrocyanosis, 127 (5), 137 (5)
  supplementary term, 487. *Diagnose
    disease*
Acrodermatitis
  atrophic chronic, 140 (9)
  entropathia, 121 (9)
  persistent, 132 (1)
Acromegaly, 394 (7)
  of skin, 138 (7)
  stricture of larynx due to, 185 (7)
Acromelalgia. *See* Erythromelalgia,
    217 (55)
Acroparesthesia, 138 (55)

Acrophobia: *supplementary term,* 484. *Diagnose disease*

Actinic elastosis, 136 (4)

Actinomycosis, 124 (2). *See under organ, region or structure affected. See also* Mycosis, generalized, 116 (2)

Activity. *See* Overactivity: *supplementary term,* 485

Adamantinoacanthoma. *Diagnose as* Squamous cell papilloma, 94

Adamantinocarcinoma, 98

Adamantinoma
except tibia. *Diagnose as* Ameloblastoma, 98
infiltrating. *Diagnose as* Adamantinocarcinoma, 98
metastasizing. *Diagnose as* Adamantinocarcinoma, 98
of tibia. *Diagnose as* Carcinoma, not otherwise specified, 94

Adamantoblastoma
not otherwise specified. *Diagnose as* Ameloblastoma, 98

Adamanto-odontoma. *Diagnose as* Odontogenic tumor, benign, 98

Adams-Stokes syndrome: *supplementary term,* 491. *Diagnose disease*

Addiction, 112 (x)
alcohol, 112 (x)
drug, 112 (x)

Addison's anemia. *See* Anemia, pernicious, 229 (7)

Addison's disease. *See* Adrenal cortical hypofunction, 397 (7); Tuberculosis of adrenal gland with cortical hypofunction, 396 (1)

Adenitis. *See also* Lymphadenitis
of Bartholin's gland, 352 (1)
of bulbourethral gland (Cowper's), 322 (1)
lacrimal. *See* Dacryoadenitis, 465 (1)
of Skene's glands, acute, 323 (1)
venereal. *See* Bubo, inguinal, 235 (1)

Adenoacanthoma. *Diagnose as* Adenocarcinoma, 94

Adenoameloblastoma. *Diagnose as* Ameloblastoma, 98

Adenoangiosarcoma. *Diagnose as* Mesenchymal mixed tumor, 98

Adenocancroid. *Diagnose as* Adenocarcinoma, 94

Adenocanthoma. *Diagnose as* Adenocarcinoma, 94

Adenocarcinoma, 94
chromophobe. *Diagnose as* Chromophobe tumor, 94
colloid. *Diagnose as* Mucinous carcinoma, 93
feminizing. *Diagnose as* Feminizing tumor, 93
Hürthle cell. *Diagnose as* Hürthle cell tumor, 94
islet cell. *Diagnose as* Non-functioning islet cell tumor, 94
islet cell, functioning. *Diagnose as* Functioning islet cell tumor, 93
mucoid. *Diagnose as* Mucinous carcinoma, 93
papillary
except of breast and sweat gland. *Diagnose as* Serous papillary cystic tumor, 93
sweat gland. *Diagnose as* Sweat gland tumor, 94
scirrhous. *Diagnose as* Adenocarcinoma, 94
sudoriferous or sudoriferum. *Diagnose as* Sweat gland tumor, 94
sweat gland. *Diagnose as* Sweat gland tumor, 94
of testis. *Diagnose as* Embryonal carcinoma of testis, 98
virilizing. *Diagnose as* Virilizing tumor, 93

Adenochondroma
salivary gland type. *Diagnose as* Mixed tumor, salivary gland type, 98

Adenocystoma
except of sweat gland. *Diagnose as* Neoplastic cyst, not otherwise specified, 93
of sweat gland. *Diagnose as* Sweat gland tumor, 94

Adenocystosarcoma (breast). *Diagnose as* Cystosarcoma phyllodes, 97

Adenofibroma, 97

Adenofibrosis
endometrioid. *Diagnose as* Adenomyosis, 98

Adenoid(s)
diseases, 258 ff.
hemorrhage after operation, 258 (4)
hypertrophy
due to infection, 258 (1)
due to unknown cause, 259 (9)
Adenoides peritonitis. *Diagnose as*
Adenomyosis, 98
Adenoiditis, 258 (1)
Adenoleiomyoma. *Diagnose as* Adenomyosis, 98
Adenolymphoma, 98
papillary. *Diagnose as* Adenolymphoma, 98
Adenoma, 94
acidophilic
except of pituitary, sweat gland.
Diagnose as Adenoma, 94
of pituitary. *Diagnose as* Eosinophilic tumor, not otherwise
specified, 93
sweat gland. *Diagnose as* Sweat
gland tumor, 94
apocrine. *Diagnose as* Sweat gland
tumor, 94
basophilic. *Diagnose as* Basophilic
tumor, 94
chromophobe. *Diagnose as* Chromophobe tumor, 94
cylindroid
of bronchus. *Diagnose as* Adenoma, 94
except of bronchus. *Diagnose as*
Sweat gland tumor, 94
cystic. *Diagnose as* Neoplastic cyst,
not otherwise specified, 93
destruens. *Diagnose as* Adenocarcinoma, 94
eccrine. *Diagnose as* Sweat gland
tumor, 94
endometrioid. *Diagnose as* Adenomyosis, 98
eosinophilic
except of pituitary, sweat gland.
Diagnose as Adenoma, 94
of pituitary. *Diagnose as* Eosinophilic tumor, not otherwise
specified, 93
sweat gland. *Diagnose as* Sweat
gland tumor, 94
feminizing. *Diagnose as* Feminizing
tumor, 93

Adenoma—Continued
functionally hyperactive. *Diagnose*
as Functionally hyperactive thyroid tumor, 93
functioning islet cell. *Diagnose as*
Functioning islet cell tumor, 93
Hürthle cell. *Diagnose as* Hürthle
cell tumor, 94
with hyperparathyroidism. *Diagnose*
as Neoplastic cyst, 93
hyperplastic (thyroid). *Diagnose as*
Functionally hyperactive thyroid
tumor, 93
intracanalicular papillary. *Diagnose*
as Adenofibroma, 97
islet cell. *Diagnose as* Non-functioning islet cell tumor, 94
malignum. *Diagnose as* Adenocarcinoma, 94
Menge's. *Diagnose as* Adenomyosis,
98
mesenchymale malignum. *Diagnose*
as Mesenchymal mixed tumor,
98
nephrogenic. *Diagnose as* Mesothelioma, 97
oxyphilic or oxyphylic granular cell
except of salivary gland. *Diagnose*
as Adenoma, 94
of salivary gland. *Diagnose as*
Adenolymphoma, 98
papillary
except of intestines, ovary, rectum
and stomach. *Diagnose as* Papillary tumor, not otherwise
specified, 93
of ovary, rectum, stomach and thyroid. *Diagnose as* Serous papillary cystic tumor, 93
pleomorphic, salivary gland type.
Diagnose as Mixed tumor, salivary gland type, 98
pseudomucinous solid. *Diagnose as*
Pseudomucinous cystic tumor,
93
malignant. *Diagnose as* Mucinous
carcinoma, 93
rete cell. *Diagnose as* Rete cell tumor, 94
rete ovarii. *Diagnose as* Virilizing
tumor, 93
sebaceous. *Diagnose as* Sebaceous
tumor, 94

Adenoma—Continued

sebaceum, congenital. *Diagnose as* Neoplastic cyst, not otherwise specified, 93

solitary

except of thyroid. *Diagnose as* Adenoma, 94

sudoriferous. *Diagnose as* Sweat gland tumor, 94

of sweat gland, not otherwise specified. *Diagnose as* Sweat gland tumor, 94

testicular or testicular tubular. *Diagnose as* Virilizing tumor, 93

thyroid. *See under* Thyroid gland

tubular (ovary). *Diagnose as* Virilizing tumor, 93

virilizing. *Diagnose as* Virilizing tumor, 93

Wolffian. *Diagnose as* Virilizing tumor, 93

Adenomatoid tumor

of bronchus. *Diagnose as* Adenoma, 94

except of bronchus and testis. *Diagnose as* Mesothelioma, 97

of testis. *Diagnose as* Embryonal carcinoma of testis, 98

Adenomatosis

of breast, 145 (9)

cancerous pulmonary. *Diagnose as* Bronchiolar carcinoma, 94

neoplastic pulmonary (lung). *Diagnose as* Bronchiolar carcinoma, 94

Adenomyoepithelioma. *Diagnose as* Myoepithelial tumor, 98

Adenomyohyperplasia. *Diagnose as* Adenomyosis, 98

Adenomyoleioma. *Diagnose as* Adenomyosis, 98

Adenomyoma. *Diagnose as* Adenomyosis, 98

Adenomyometritis. *Diagnose as* Adenomyosis, 98

Adenomyosarcoma, 98

embryonal

except of kidney. *Diagnose as* Mesenchymal mixed tumor, 98

of kidney. *Diagnose as* Nephroblastoma, 98

Adenomyosis, 98

of stomach, 265 (8)

of uterus, 364 (8)

Adenomyositis, seroepithelial. *Diagnose as* Adenomyosis, 98

Adenomyxochondrosarcoma

salivary gland type. *Diagnose as* Mixed tumor, salivary gland type, 98

Adenomyxoma. *Diagnose as* Cystosarcoma phyllodes, 97

Adenosarcoma. *Diagnose as* Cystosarcoma phyllodes, 97

embryonal. *Diagnose as* Nephroblastoma, 98

Adenosis benigna (uterus). *Diagnose as* Adenomyosis, 98

Adhesions. *See also under organ, region or structure affected*

congenital, 122 (0)

Adie syndrome: *supplementary term,* 501. *Diagnose disease*

Adiponecrosis neonatorum, 136 (4)

Adiposis dolorosa, 120 (7)

Adiposity. *See also* Obesity

pilous: *supplementary term. See* Neurovisceral central syndrome, 485

Adiposogenital dystrophy, 394 (7)

Adjustment reaction

of adolescence, 112 (x)

of childhood, 112 (x)

of infancy, 112 (x)

of late life, 112 (x)

Adolescence. *See also* Puberty

adjustment reaction, 112 (x)

mastitis of, 144 (7)

Adrenal clear cell tumor (ovary). *Diagnose as* Virilizing tumor, 93

Adrenal cortex

hyperfunction

bone changes associated with, 153 (7)

Adrenal cortical carcinoma (ovary). *Diagnose as* Virilizing tumor, 93

Adrenal cortical rest tumor, 94

Adrenal gland(s)

absence, 396 (0)

accessory, 396 (0)

adenoma, 397 (8)

feminizing, 397 (8)

virilizing, 397 (8)

adenocarcinoma, 397 (8)

feminizing, 397 (8)

virilizing, 397 (8)

Adrenal gland(s)—Continued
arterial hypertension due to disease of, 218 (7)
atrophy of cortex due to unknown cause, 397 (9)
birth injury, 396 (0)
cortical hyperfunction, 397 (7)
cortical hypofunction, 397 (7)
  secondary to excessive administration of hormones, 397 (7)
  secondary to hypopituitarism, 397 (7)
cyst, congenital, 396 (0)
degeneration due to infection, 396 (1)
diseases, 396 ff.
displacement, 396 (0)
ganglioneuroma of medulla, 397 (8)
hemorrhage into
  due to asphyxia, 397 (5)
  due to blood dyscrasia, 397 (5)
  due to infection, 396 (1)
  due to trauma, 396 (4)
hypertrophy, congenital, 396 (0)
hyperplasia, congenital, 396 (0)
hypoplasia, congenital, 396 (0)
hypotension due to disease of, 218 (7)
injury, 396 (4)
necrosis, 397 (5)
neoplasms, 397 (8)
pheochromocytoma of medulla, 397 (8)
sympathicoblastoma of medulla, 397 (8)
syphilis, 396 (1)
tuberculosis, 396 (1)
tumors, unlisted, 397 (8)
Adrenalitis, 396 (1)
Aerocele
epidural, 406 (4)
Aerophagia: *supplementary term,* 496. *Diagnose disease*
Aerotitis media, 478 (4)
Agalactia, 145 (x)
Agammaglobulinemia
acquired, 237 (x)
congenital, 237 (0)
Agenesis. *See under organ or structure affected*
Ageusia. *See* Hallucinations of taste: *supplementary term,* 509
Aggressive personality, 112 (x)
Aglossia, 245 (0)

Agnosia: *supplementary terms,* 501. *Diagnose disease*
acoustic, 501
anosognosia, 501
localization, 501
position, 501
tactile, 501
texture, 501
visual, 501
weight, 501
Agoraphobia: *supplementary term,* 484. *Diagnose disease*
Agrammatism aphasia: *supplementary term,* 501. *Diagnose disease*
Agranulocytosis. *See also* Granulocytopenia
due to intoxication or drug reaction, 228 (3)
due to splenic diseases, 228 (5)
generally and unspecified, 229 (7)
Agraphia: *supplementary term,* 501. *Diagnose disease*
Ainhum, 129 (9)
Air blast injury, 118 (4)
Air pressure
change in, otitis media due to, 478 (4)
increased, disease due to. *See* Caisson disease, 118 (4)
reduced, disease due to. *See* Hypobaropathy, 118 (4)
Air sickness, 119 (55)
Air swallowing. *See* Aerophagia: *supplementary term,* 496
Albers-Schönberg disease: *See* Osteopetrosis, 147 (0)
Albinism. *See also* Albinismus
of iris, 439 (0)
Albinismus, 131 (0). *See also* Albinism
Albright's syndrome. *See* Polyostotic fibrous dysplasia, 147 (0)
Albuminuria
orthostatic, 310 (6)
supplementary term, 498. *Diagnose disease*
Alcohol. *See also* Alcoholism, 112 (x)
amblyopia due to, 451 (3)
intoxication, 481
  acute brain syndrome, 106 (3)
  chronic brain syndrome, 107 (3)
methyl. *See* Methyl alcohol

Alcohol—Continued
myelopathy due to, 422 (3)
poisoning, 117 (3)
fatty liver due to, 288 (3)
toxic neuropathy due to, 428 (3)
use of: *supplementary term,* 486.
Diagnose disease
Alcoholism, 112 (x)
Aldosteronism: *supplementary term,*
500. *Diagnose disease.* See Adrenal
cortical hyperfunction, 397 (7)
Aleukemia. *Diagnose as* Leukemia,
type unspecified, 230 (8)
Alexia
developmental, 501
supplementary term, 501. *Diagnose*
disease
Alimentary tract
absence, 240 (0)
diseases, 240
Alkali
conjunctivitis due to, 469 (3)
Alkalosis, 120 (7)
nephrosis of, 311 (7)
supplementary term, 493. *Diagnose*
disease
tetany due to, 120 (7)
Allergy. *See also* Anaphylaxis
arthritis due to, 158 (3)
capillary purpura due to, 226 (3)
conjunctivitis due to, 469 (3)
cystitis due to, 318 (3)
eczema due to
of eyelid, 462 (3)
of scrotum, 339 (3)
endophthalmitis due to, 439 (1)
food, 117 (3)
gastrointestinal, 267 (3)
of internal ear, 475 (3)
iritis (iridocyclitis) due to, 439 (3)
of middle ear, 478 (3)
pannus due to, 435 (3)
physical, 136 (3)
rhinitis due to, 177 (3)
urethritis due to, 324 (3)
Allochiria: *supplementary term,* 501.
Diagnose disease
Alopecia
areata, 138 (55)
capitis total, 138 (55)
celsi. *See* Alopecia areata
cicatrisata (pseudopelade), 132 (1)
circumscripta. *See* Alopecia areata

Alopecia—Continued
congenital, 131 (0)
disseminated, 138 (55)
due to favus, 134 (2)
due to pregnancy, 135 (3)
due to undetermined cause, 142 (y)
furfuracea. *See* Alopecia hereditary
hereditary, premature and senile, 140
(9)
postfebrile, 132 (1)
due to influenza, 132 (1)
due to syphilis, 132 (1)
due to typhoid fever, 132 (1)
universal, 138 (55)
Altitude, high
encephalopathy due to cerebral anoxia from, 413 (4)
Alveolar. *See* Alveolus
Alveolitis, 248 (4)
Alveolus(i)
abnormal alveolar ridge, 247 (0)
cleft, 247 (0)
hemorrhage from
due to trauma, 248 (4)
following extraction, 248 (4)
osteitis, 248 (4)
resorbed ridge, 248 (4)
sequestrum formation of arches, due
to infection, 248 (1)
Amaurosis
amaurotic familial idiocy, 403 (7)
infantile, 403 (7)
juvenile, 403 (7)
congenital, 446 (0)
supplementary term, 508. *Diagnose*
disease
uremic, 447 (3)
Amblyopia
congenital, 446 (0)
nystagmus of, 456 (5)
supplementary term, 508. *Diagnose*
disease
toxic, 451 (3)
uremic, 447 (3)
Amebiasis, 114 (1). *See also un-*
der organ, region or structure
affected
of skin, 132 (1)
Amebic dysentery. *See* Colitis, amebic, 276 (1)
Ameloblastoma, 98, 249 (8)
follicular. *Diagnose as* Ameloblastoma, 98

Ameloblastoma—Continued
plexiform. *Diagnose as* Ameloblastoma, 98
primitive. *Diagnose as* Ameloblastoma, 98
stellate. *Diagnose as* Ameloblastoma, 98
Ameloblastosarcoma. *Diagnose as* Adamantinocarcinoma, 98
Amenorrhea
due to anemia, 362 (5)
due to debility, 363 (7)
due to obesity, 363 (7)
due to persistence of corpus luteum, 363 (7)
due to surgery, 361 (4)
hyperhormonal. *See* Endometrium, hyperplasia secondary to basophilic hyperpituitarism, 364 (7)
primary (functional), 365 (x)
supplementary term, 498. Diagnose disease
Amentia: *supplementary term, 501. Diagnose disease*
Ametropia. *See* Astigmatism; Hypermetropia; Myopia
Amimia: *supplementary term, 501. Diagnose disease*
Aminoaciduria: *supplementary term, 498. Diagnose disease*
Ammonia
conjunctivitis due to, 469 (3)
Amnesia: *supplementary term, 501. Diagnose disease*
Amnion
adhesions to fetus, 383 (7)
cyst, 384 (9)
oligohydramnios, 384 (x)
polyhydramnios, 384 (x)
Amniotic fluid
pneumonia due to aspiration of, 196 (4)
pulmonary embolism due to, 195 (4)
Ampulla of Vater
variations of common bile duct and pancreatic duct openings into, 292 (0)
Amputation
due to accident, 125 (4)
stump, abnormal, 125 (4)
Amusia: *supplementary term, 501. Diagnose disease*
Amyelia, 421 (0)

Amygdalolith. *See* Tonsil, calculus in, 259 (6)
Amylene hydrate
with tribromethanol poisoning, 118 (3)
Amyloid degeneration. *See* Amyloid disease
Amyloid disease (amyloidosis)
of bladder, 321 (9)
of bone marrow, 239 (9)
of conjunctiva, 471 (9)
due to unknown cause, 129 (9)
generalized
due to infection, 114 (1)
due to tuberculosis, 114 (1)
due to unknown cause, 121 (9)
of heart, due to unknown cause, 212 (9)
of intestine, due to infection, 272 (1)
of kidney
due to infection, 308 (1)
due to unknown cause, 312 (9)
of liver
due to infection, 287 (1)
due to unknown cause, 289 (9)
of nerve, 431 (9)
of skin, 140 (9)
of spleen, 233 (9)
Amyoplasia congenita, 167 (0)
Amyotonia congenita, 167 (0), 421 (0)
Amyotrophy: *supplementary term, 289. Diagnose disease*
Anal. *See* Anus
Analgesia: *supplementary term, 501. Diagnose disease*
Anaphylaxis. *See also* Allergy
generalized reaction, 117 (3)
local reaction, 125 (3)
shock, 117 (3)
Anarthria: *supplementary term, 501. Diagnose disease*
Ancylostomiasis, 124 (2)
Andreioblastoma. *Diagnose as* Virilizing tumor, 93
Androblastoma. *Diagnose as* Virilizing tumor, 93
Anemia
amenorrhea due to, 362 (5)
aplastic, 229 (7)
Cooley's, 231 (9)
due to malaria, 228 (1)

Anemia—Continued
fatty degeneration of heart due to, 210 (5)
of heart, due to blood disease, 209 (5)
hemolytic, acquired, 228 (3)
 due to cold agglutinins, 228 (3)
 due to sensitization to Rh-Hr or other erythrocytic agglutinogens, 228 (3)
 due to sulfonamide, 228 (3)
hemolytic, hereditary, 230 (9)
hemorrhage in vitreous due to, 445 (5)
hypochromic microcytic, 229 (7)
idiopathic hypoplastic, 229 (7)
macrocytic, not pernicious type, 229 (7)
megaloblastic, 229 (7)
menorrhagia due to, 362 (5)
nonspherocytosis, hereditary, 230 (9)
normocytic
 cause undetermined, 231 (y)
 cause unknown, 230 (9)
 due to acute blood loss, due to trauma, 228 (4)
 due to congestive splenomegaly, 228 (5)
 due to erythrocytic destruction, 228 (5)
 due to erythrocytic hypoplasia, 229 (7)
 due to erythrocytic hypoplasia, congenital, 227 (0)
 due to erythrocytic hypoplasia from infection, 227 (1)
normocytic hemolytic
 due to infection, 227 (1)
 due to parasite, 228 (2)
 normocytic hypoplastic (pancytopenia), 229 (7)
 congenital, 227 (0)
 due to infection, 227 (1)
 due to poison, 228 (3)
 due to radiation, 228 (4)
normocytic metabolic, 229 (7)
 due to hypothyroidism, 229 (7)
 due to protein deficiency, 229 (7)
 due to sprue, 229 (7)
normocytic myelophthisic, 230 (9)
pernicious, 229 (7)
 atrophy of mucous membrane of tongue in, 246 (9)

Anemia—Continued
pernicious—continued
 peripheral neuropathy due to, 430 (7)
sickle cell (sicklemia), 230 (9)
 atrophy of spleen secondary to, 232 (7)
 polyarthritis due to, 164 (9)
spherocytic. *See* Spherocytosis, 230 (9)
Anesthesia
hysterical: *supplementary term,* 501. *Diagnose disease*
supplementary term, 501. *Diagnose disease*
Anesthetic
atony of pregnant uterus due to, 374 (3)
gas, poisoning, 117 (3)
Aneurysm. *See also under* Artery *and name of vessel or organ affected*
arteriovenous. *See* Arteriovenous aneurysm
circoid. *Diagnose as* Hemangioma (angioma), 96
compression of nerve by, 429 (4)
compression of spinal cord, 423 (4)
malignant. *Diagnose as* Hemangiosarcoma, 96
malignant, of bone. *Diagnose as* Osteosarcoma (osteogenic sarcoma), 97
venous racemose or racemose. *Diagnose as* Hemangioma (angioma), 96
Aneurysmal tumor. *Diagnose as* Hemangioma (angioma), 96
Angiitis. *See also* Arteritis; Endothelioangiitis, diffuse; Thromboangiitis obliterans; *and under name of specific vessel*
cerebral essential, 418 (1)
gangrene due to, 128 (5)
Angina
pectoris. *See* Anginal syndrome: *supplementary term,* 491
Anginal syndrome: *supplementary term,* 491. *Diagnose disease*
Angioblastic meningioma, neoplasm *or* **sarcoma.** *Diagnose as* Hemangiosarcoma, 96
Angioblastoma. *Diagnose as* Hemangiosarcoma, 96

Angiochondroma. *Diagnose as* Mesenchymoma, 98
malignant. *Diagnose as* Mesenchymal mixed tumor, 98
Angioendothelioma. *Diagnose as* Hemangioendothelioma, 96
of bone (Ewing's). *Diagnose as* Ewing's sarcoma, 97
Angiofibrosarcoma. *Diagnose as* Hemangiosarcoma, 96
Angiokeratoma, 137 (5)
Angiolipoma. *Diagnose as* Lipoma, 97
Angioma. *See also* Hemangioma of conjunctiva, 471 (8)
Angiomatosis
generalized. *Diagnose as* Hemangiomatosis, 96
multiple hereditary. *Diagnose as* Hemangiomatosis, 96
multiple punctate. *Diagnose as* Hemangiomatosis, 96
not otherwise specified. *Diagnose as* Hemangiomatosis, 96
Angiomyolipoma (adrenal). *Diagnose as* Mesenchymoma, 98
Angiomyoneuroma. *Diagnose as* Glomangioma, 96
Angioneurofibroma. *Diagnose as* Neurofibroma, 95
Angioneuroma. *Diagnose as* Glomangioma, 96
Angioneuromyoma. *Diagnose as* Glomangioma, 96
Angioneurotic edema, 138 (55)
of eyelids, 463 (55)
of larynx, 184 (3)
Angiosarcoma
capillary. *Diagnose as* Hemangiosarcoma, 96
multiplex. *Diagnose as* Multiple hemorrhagic hemangioma of Kaposi, 96
not otherwise specified. *Diagnose as* Hemangiosarcoma, 96
Angiosis, progressive multiform. *Diagnose as* Hemangiomatosis, 96
Angiospasm
of arteries of leg and foot, 217 (5)
of cerebral vessels, 419 (55)
peripheral. *See* Raynaud's disease, 217 (55)
of spinal vessels, 426 (55)

Angiovenosum. *Diagnose as* Hemangioma (angioma), 96
Anhidrosis, 138 (55)
of eyelid, neurogenic, 463 (55)
supplementary term, 487. *Diagnose disease*
Anhydremia: *supplementary term,* 493. *Diagnose disease*
Aniline
corneal opacity due to, 435 (3)
poisoning, 117 (3)
Aniridia, 439 (0)
Aniseikonia, 454 (4) (6)
Anisocytosis: *supplementary term,* 493. *Diagnose disease*
Anisometropia, 454 (0)
Ankle
fracture, trimalleolar, 151 (4)
sprain, 159 (4)
Ankyloblepharon
filiforme, congenital, 461 (0)
following operation, 462 (4)
totale, 461 (0)
Ankyloglossia, 245 (0)
Ankylosis. *See also under name of joint*
bony or fibrous
due to trauma, 158 (4)
following operation, 158 (4)
Ankylostomiasis. *See* Ancylostomiasis, 124 (2)
Anoderm
moniliasis, 285 (2)
Anodontia, 247 (0)
Anomalies. *See also under organ, region or structure affected*
congenital, 122 (0)
undiagnosed, 122 (0)
list, 55
Anonychia, 131 (0)
Anophthalmos, congenital, 433 (0)
Anorchism, 332 (0)
Anorexia: *supplementary term,* 496. *Diagnose disease*
Anosmia
due to infection, 176 (1)
due to unknown cause, 179 (x)
supplementary term, 508. *Diagnose disease*
Anosognosia. *See* Agnosia, anosognosia, *supplementary term,* 501

Anoxemia
arterial, erythrocytoses due to, 229 (7)
at birth, encephalopathy due to, 410 (0)
myelopathy due to, 424 (7)
supplementary term, 493. *Diagnose disease*

Anoxia
cerebral, from high altitude, encephalopathy due to, 413 (4)
due to drowning, 119 (7)
encephalopathy due to, 413 (4)

Anterior chamber
foreign body in, 433 (4)
hemorrhage into. *See* Hyphemia, 433 (5)
hernia of vitreous into, due to trauma, 444 (4)

Anthracosis, 196 (4)
lymphadenitis due to, 235 (4)

Anthrax, 132 (1)
of auricle, 474 (1)
of eyelid, 462 (1)
infection, generalized, 114 (1)
of lung, 192 (1)

Antimony
liver degeneration due to, 288 (3)

Antisocial personality, 112 (x)

Antisocialism: *supplementary term,* 484. *Diagnose disease*

Anuria: *supplementary term,* 498. *Diagnose disease*

Anus. *See also* Rectum; Sphincter ani
aberrant sebaceous glands of mucocutaneous junction, 284 (0)
abscess
following operation, 285 (4)
ischiorectal, 284 (1)
marginal, 284 (1)
of perianal tissue, 284 (1)
posterior anal triangle tissue, 284 (1)
subcutaneous, 284 (1)
absence, congenital, 284 (0)
adenocarcinoma, 286 (8)
artificial (colostomy), 277 (4)
atresia
ani perinealis, 284 (0)
ani urethralia, 284 (0)
ani vaginalis, 284 (0)
ani vesicalis, 284 (0)

Anus—Continued
atresia—continued
congenital, 284 (0)
fibrous, 284 (0)
membranous, 284 (0)
chancroid, 284 (1)
chemical burn, 285 (3)
cicatrix due to infection, 284 (1)
condyloma acuminatum, 284 (1)
condyloma lata, syphilitic, 284 (1)
crypt
enlarged, 286 (9)
foreign body in, 285 (4)
diseases, 284 ff.
epidermoid carcinoma, 286 (8)
fibroma, 286 (8)
fibrous anal tags, 286 (6)
fissure, 285 (4)
fistula
anovaginal, following parturition, 356 (4)
congenital, 284 (0)
due to infection, 284 (1)
foreign body in, 285 (4)
hypertrophy of anal skin, 286 (9)
imperforate, rupture of cecum during birth with, 276 (0)
injury, 285 (4)
laceration, 285 (4)
malfunctioning colostomy, 277 (4)
neoplasms, 286 (8)
papillae
hypertrophy, 286 (9)
infected, 284 (1)
pigmented nevus, 286 (8)
prolapse of anal canal, 286 (6)
pruritus, 285 (55)
skin tabs, 286 (9)
stenosis, due to infection, 284 (1)
stricture
due to operation, 285 (4)
due to poison, 285 (3)
tumors, unlisted, 286 (8)
ulcer, due to unknown cause, 286 (9)
ulceration due to poison, 285 (3)

Anusitis, 284 (1)

Anxiety
reaction, 111 (x)
supplementary term, 484. *Diagnose disease*

Aorta. *See also* Aortitis
abdominal
  arteriosclerosis of, 221 (9)
aneurysm
  arteriosclerotic, rupture into pulmonary artery, 221 (9)
  dissecting, due to cystic medial necrosis, 221 (9)
  dissecting, due to unknown cause, 221 (9)
  dissecting, with coarctation, 204 (0)
  due to arteriosclerosis, 221 (9)
    abdominal, 221 (9)
    thoracic, 221 (9)
  due to infection, 220 (1)
  due to medial necrosis, 221 (9)
  due to syphilis, 220 (1)
  of right aortic sinus, 204 (0)
    congenital ruptured, 204 (0)
  syphilitic, rupture into pulmonary artery, 220 (1)
arteriosclerosis, 221 (9)
coarctation
  adult type, 204 (0)
  with bicuspid aortic valve, 204 (0)
  with dissecting aneurysm, 204 (0)
  with dissecting aneurysm and rupture of aorta, 204 (0)
  infantile type, 204 (0)
degeneration, medial (not due to syphilis), 221 (9)
dextroposition, 204 (0)
  in tetralogy of Fallot, 203 (0)
  with ventricular septal defect (Eisenmenger complex), 203 (0)
dilatation
  due to arteriosclerosis, 221 (9)
  due to infection, 220 (1)
  dynamic, 220 (5)
diseases, 204, 220 ff.
fatty infiltration, 220 (7)
hypoplasia, 204 (0)
injury, 220 (4)
obstruction due to arteriosclerosis, 221 (9)
pulmonary septal defect, 204 (0)
rupture
  due to arteriosclerosis, 221 (9)
  due to infection, 220 (1)
  due to medial degeneration, 221 (9)

Aorta—Continued
rupture—continued
  due to trauma, 220 (4)
  of syphilitic aneurysm of, into pulmonary artery, 220 (1)
  saddle embolus, 220 (6)
  thrombosis, due to arteriosclerosis, 221 (9)
  transposition, 205 (0)
Aortic arch, persistent
double, 204 (0)
right, 204 (0)
  with left descending aorta, 205 (0)
Aortic valve
atresia, 203 (0)
bicuspid, 203 (0)
  with coarctation of aorta, 204 (0)
calcification, 212 (9)
fenestration of aortic cusps, 204 (0)
fusion or defect of aortic cusps, 204 (0)
incompetency: *supplementary term,* 491. *Diagnose disease*
stenosis, not congenital: *supplementary term,* 491. *Diagnose disease*
supernumerary aortic cusps, 204 (0)
Aortitis
acute bacterial, 220 (1)
acute rheumatic, 221 (9)
subacute bacterial, 220 (1)
syphilitic, 220 (1)
Aphakia
aniseikonia due to, 454 (4)
congenital, 442 (0)
due to trauma, 442 (4)
following operation, 442 (4)
Aphasia
agrammatism: *supplementary term,* 501. *Diagnose disease*
amnestic: *supplementary term,* 501. *Diagnose disease*
central (paraphasia): *supplementary term,* 506. *Diagnose disease*
developmental, 502
dysarthric: *supplementary term,* 502. *Diagnose disease*
expressive (motor): *supplementary term,* 502. *Diagnose disease*
global: *supplementary term,* 502. *Diagnose disease*
nominal (anomia): *supplementary term,* 502. *Diagnose disease*

Aphasia—Continued
  receptive (sensory) : *supplementary term, 502. Diagnose disease*
  semantic : *supplementary term, 502. Diagnose disease*
  supplementary term, 501. Diagnose disease
  syntactic : *supplementary term, 502. Diagnose disease*
  verbal : *supplementary term, 502. Diagnose disease*
  visual : *supplementary term, 502. Diagnose disease*
Aphemia : *supplementary term, 502. Diagnose disease*
Aphonia
  developmental, 502
  non-neurogenic : *supplementary term, 490. Diagnose disease*
  supplementary term, 502. Diagnose disease
Aphthous stomatitis, 241 (1)
Aphthous ulcer of larynx, 186 (9)
Apical cyst, 247 (1)
Apical granuloma, 247 (1)
Apical infection, 247 (1)
Aplasia. *See under organ or structure affected*
Apocrine tumor. *Diagnose as* Sweat gland tumor, 94
Apophysitis of os calcis. *See* Osteochondrosis of calcaneus, 155 (9)
Appendage cell tumor (skin). *Diagnose as* Adenoma, 94
Appendices epiploicae
  gangrene, 277 (5)
  infarction, 277 (5)
Appendicitis. *See also* Appendix
  acute, 279 (1)
    with abscess, 279 (1)
    with gangrene, 279 (1)
    with perforation, 279 (1)
    chronic recurrent, 279 (1)
Appendix. *See also* Appendicitis
  absence, congenital, 279 (0)
  adenocarcinoma, 280 (8)
  argentaffinoma, 280 (8)
  diseases, 279 ff.
  displacement, retrocecal, 279 (0)
  diverticulum due to unknown cause, 280 (6)
  duplication, with duplication of cecum, 276 (0)

Appendix—Continued
  excessively long, 279 (0)
  excessively short, 279 (0)
  fecalith in, 280 (6)
  fibrosis, noninflammatory, 280 (7)
  fistula due to infection, 279 (1)
  foreign body in, 280 (6)
  injury, 279 (4)
  intussusception, 280 (6)
  kinking, 280 (6)
  lymphoid hyperplasia, 280 (9)
  mucocele due to obstruction, 280 (6)
  neoplasms, 280 (8)
  obstruction due to helminthiasis, 279 (2)
  strangulation, 279 (5)
  transposition (in situs transversus), 279 (0)
  tumors, unlisted, 280 (8)
Appetite
  excessive. *See* Bulimia : *supplementary term, 496*
  loss of. *See* Anorexia : *supplementary term, 496*
Apraxia
  developmental, 502
  ideational : *supplementary term, 502. Diagnose disease*
  ideomotor : *supplementary term, 502. Diagnose disease*
  motor : *supplementary term, 502. Diagnose disease*
  supplementary term, 502. Diagnose disease
Arachnodactyly, 114 (0)
Arachnoid
  congenital cyst, 405 (0)
Arachnoiditis
  acute, 405 (1)
  chronic, 405 (1)
  chronic adhesive, 406 (1)
  nonsuppurative, 405 (1)
Aran-Duchenne muscular atrophy. *See* Myelopathic muscular atrophy, 425 (9)
Arcus
  juvenilis, 434 (0)
  senilis, 437 (9)
Areola, hypoplasia, 143 (0)
Areolar subcutaneous tissue. *See* Subcutaneous areolar tissue
Argentaffinoma, 95

Argyll Robertson pupil. *See* Intrinsic muscles of eye, paralysis: *supplementary term,* 509
Argyria (argyrosis), 135 (3). *See also* Silver, poisoning, 118 (3)
  of conjunctiva, 469 (3)
  of cornea, 434 (3)
  of eyelid, 462 (3)
Arithmetic disability. *See* Acalculia: *supplementary term,* 501
Arm
  causalgia, 128 (55)
  elephantiasis, congenital, 122 (0)
  hypoplasia, congenital, 122 (0)
Arnold-Chiari syndrome. *See* Caudal displacement of brain stem, cerebellum and spinal cord, 402 (0)
Arrhenoblastoma, 93
  of ovary, 370 (8)
Arrhenoma *or* **arrhenonoma.** *Diagnose as* Arrhenoblastoma, 93
Arrhythmia
  atrial, unspecified: *supplementary term,* 491. *Diagnose disease*
  generally and unspecified: *supplementary term,* 491. *Diagnose disease*
  junctional, unspecified: *supplementary term,* 492. *Diagnose disease*
  neurogenic, 211 (55)
  reflex, 211 (55)
  sinus
    due to unknown cause, 214 (x)
    supplementary term, 491. *Diagnose disease*
    unspecified: *supplementary term,* 491. *Diagnose disease*
  vagal, 211 (55)
  ventricular, unspecified: *supplementary term,* 492. *Diagnose disease*
Arsenic
  encephalopathy due to, 412 (3)
  keratosis due to, 135 (3)
  liver degeneration due to, 288 (3)
  myelopathy due to, 422 (3)
  pigmentation of lid due to, 462 (3)
  poisoning, 117 (3)
    of heart by, 209 (3)
  toxic neuropathy due to, 428 (3)
Arsine
  injury of eyelid by, 462 (3)
Arteria stapedia, persistence, 477 (0)

Arterial hypertension. *See* Hypertension
Arterial hypotension. *See* Hypotension
Arteries. *See* Artery
Arteriolar sclerosis. *See also* Nephrosclerosis, arteriolar, 310 (5)
  generalized, 219 (9)
Arteriosclerosis. *See also* Arteriolar sclerosis; Atherosclerosis; *and under name of specific vessel*
  aneurysm
    of aorta due to, 221 (9)
    of artery due to, 218 (9)
    of cerebral vessel, 420 (9)
    of coronary artery due to, 212 (9)
    in orbit due to, 460 (9)
    of pulmonary artery due to, 223 (9)
  atrophy of bone due to, 152 (5)
  cerebral, 420 (9)
  cerebral thrombosis due to, 420 (9)
  cerebrospinal, 404 (9)
  of choroidal vessels, 441 (9)
  coronary thrombosis due to, 212 (9)
  dilatation of aorta due to, 221 (9)
  disease of retina, 447 (5)
  encephalomalacia due to, 414 (5)
  encephalopathy due to, 414 (5)
  gangrene due to, 128 (5)
  general, 218 (9)
  heart disease, 210 (5)
  ischemia of retina due to, 448 (5)
  lead, 217 (3)
  of lesser circulation, 223 (9)
  medial, 218 (9)
  myelopathy due to, 424 (5)
  with narrowing of coronary artery, 212 (9)
  obliterans, 218 (9)
  obstruction of aorta due to, 221 (9)
  retinal hemorrhage due to, 449 (9)
  of retinal vessels, 449 (9)
  rupture of aorta due to, 221 (9)
  rupture of artery due to, 218 (9)
  spasm of retinal artery due to, 448 (55)
  spinal, 427 (9)
  thrombosis of aorta due to, 221 (9)
  thrombosis of artery secondary to, 219 (9)
  ulcer due to, 128 (5)
  of uterine vessels, 364 (9)

Arthropathy—Continued
  supplementary term, 489. *Diagnose*
    disease
  tabetic, of knee, 162 (55)
Arthus' phenomenon. *See* Anaphy-
    lactic reaction, generalized, **117**
    (3) ; Anaphylactic reaction, local,
    125 (3)
Articulation. *See* Joints
  of larynx. *See* Larynx
Asbestosis, 195 (4)
Ascariasis, 124 (2)
  intestinal, 272 (2)
Aschheim-Zondek test
  reactions to: *supplementary terms,*
    499. *Diagnose disease*
Ascites
  chylous (nonfilarial), 300 (5)
  due to tuberculous peritonitis, 299
    (1)
  due to venous congestion (portal sta-
    sis), 300 (5)
  supplementary term, 496. *Diagnose*
    disease
  tubercle bacilli in ascitic fluid: *sup-
    plementary term,* 497. *Diagnose*
    disease
  tumor cells in ascitic fluid: *supple-
    mentary term,* 497. *Diagnose*
    disease
Aspergillosis, 124 (2)
Aspermia: *supplementary term,* 498.
    Diagnose disease
Asphyxia, fetal
  due to interference with fetal circu-
    lation, 381 (5)
  due to trauma, 381 (4)
Asphyxiation
  due to trauma, 118 (4)
  not due to trauma, 119 (7)
Astasia abasia: *supplementary term,*
    502. *Diagnose disease*
Asteatoses, 132 (0)
Astereognosis: *supplementary term,*
    501. *Diagnose disease*
Asthenia
  supplementary term, 484. *Diagnose*
    disease
Asthenopia: *supplementary term,* 508.
    Diagnose disease
Asthenospermia: *supplementary*
    term, 498. *Diagnose disease*

Asthma, 190 (3)
  supplementary term, 490. *Diagnose*
    disease
Astigmatism
  due to tilting of lens, 454 (6)
  hypermetropic, 454 (6)
    compound, 454 (6)
  irregular
    corneal, 454 (6)
    due to infection, 454 (1)
  mixed, 454 (6)
  myopic, 454 (6)
Astroblastoma
  except of nose. *Diagnose as* Astro-
    cytoma, 96
Astrocytoma, 96
  of brain, 415 (8)
  fibrillary. *Diagnose as* Astrocytoma,
    96
  gigantocellure. *Diagnose as* Astro-
    cytoma, 96
  piloid. *Diagnose as* Astrocytoma, 96
  protoplasmic. *Diagnose as* Astrocy-
    toma, 96
Asymbolia
  pain: *supplementary term,* 505. *Di-
    agnose disease*
  supplementary term, 502. *Diagnose*
    disease
Asynergia: *supplementary term,* 502.
    Diagnose disease
Ataxia
  locomotor. *See* Tabes dorsalis, 403
    (1)
  supplementary term, 489. *Diagnose*
    disease
Atelectasis
  congenital, 192 (0)
  due to bronchial tuberculosis, 192
    (1)
  due to compression, 195 (4)
  due to foreign body in bronchus, 196
    (6)
  due to infection, 192 (1)
  due to undetermined cause, 197 (y)
  following operation, 195 (4)
  massive, due to trauma, 195 (4)
Atelomyelia, 421 (0)
Atherocarcinoma. *Diagnose as* Epi-
    dermoid carcinoma, 94
Atheroma cutis. *Diagnose as* Squa-
    mous cell papilloma, 94

Atherosclerosis, 218 (9)
of heart valve, 212 (9)
Athetosis
bilateral
acquired, 502
congenital, 410 (0)
supplementary term, 502. *Diagnose disease*
Athlete's foot. *See* Dermatophytosis, 134 (2)
Athyrea
following operation, 388 (4)
Atonia: *supplementary term,* 489. *Diagnose disease*
Atresia. *See under organ affected*
Atrial abnormalities, 202 (0)
Atrial fibrillation
chronic
due to unknown cause, 213 (x)
supplementary term, 491. *Diagnose disease*
paroxysmal
due to unknown cause, 213 (x)
supplementary term, 491. *Diagnose disease*
Atrial flutter
chronic
due to unknown cause, 213 (x)
supplementary term, 491. *Diagnose disease*
paroxysmal
due to unknown cause, 214 (x)
supplementary term, 491. *Diagnose disease*
Atrial paroxysmal tachycardia
due to unknown cause, 214 (y)
supplementary term, 491. *Diagnose disease*
Atrial premature contractions
due to unknown cause, 214 (x)
supplementary term, 491. *Diagnose disease*
Atrial septal defects, 202 (0)
Atrioventricular block
due to unknown cause, 214 (x)
supplementary term, 491. *Diagnose disease*
Atrioventricular nodal rhythm
due to unknown cause, 214 (x)
supplementary term, 491. *Diagnose disease*
Atrium. *See under* Heart; *and terms beginning with* "Atrial"

Atrophia. *See also* Atrophy
gyrata, of choroid and retina, 441 (5)
of nails, 138 (7)
unguium, 131 (0)
Atrophoderma
macular, 140 (9)
neuritic, 138 (55)
pigmentosum. *See* Xeroderma, pigmented, 132 (0)
Atrophy. *See also* Atrophia; Hemiatrophy; *and under name of specific disease or of organ, region or structure affected*
macular, due to syphilis, 132 (1)
Atropine
conjunctivitis due to, 469 (3)
injury of eyelid by, 462 (3)
Auditory canal, external
abscess, 474 (1)
absence, congenital, 474 (0)
atresia, congenital, 474 (0)
exostosis due to cold, 475 (4)
foreign body in, 475 (4)
furunculosis, 475 (1)
infection of external auditory meatus, 475 (1)
inflammation of external meatus due to chemical irritant, 475 (3)
injury, 476 (4)
mycosis, 475 (2)
narrowing, congenital, 474 (0)
stricture
due to sodium hydroxide, 475 (3)
due to trauma, 476 (4)
following operation, 476 (4)
Auricle
abscess, 474 (1)
absence, congenital, 474 (0)
anthrax, 474 (1)
burn from heat, 475 (4)
calcification, 476 (9)
chemical burn, 475 (3)
deformity
congenital, 474 (0)
due to infection, 475 (1)
displacement (melotus), 474 (0)
fistula, congenital, 474 (0)
frostbite, 475 (4)
gangrene due to infection (noma), 475 (1)
hemangioma, 472 (8)

Auricle—Continued
hematoma, 476 (4)
infection, 475 (1)
injury, 476 (4)
lymphangioma, 472 (8)
neurofibroma, 472 (8)
perichondritis, 475 (1)
preauricular cyst, 474 (0)
preauricular sinus, 474 (0)
prominence, congenital, 474 (0)
pruritus, 476 (55)
sinus, 474 (0)
Auricle of heart. *See under* Heart
Auricular. *See* Atrial
Auriculotemporal nerve syndrome:
supplementary term, 502. *Diagnose disease*
Autodigestion, 125 (3)
Automatism, paroxysmal: *supplementary term,* 485. *Diagnose disease*
Autotopagnosia: *supplementary term,* 502. *Diagnose disease*
Avellis paralysis: *supplementary term,* 506. *Diagnose disease*
Avertin. *See* Tribromethanol, 118 (3)
Avitaminosis. *See* Hypovitaminosis
Axialis extracorticalis congenita, 402 (0)
Azoospermia: *supplementary term,* 498. *Diagnose disease*
Azotemia: *supplementary term,* 493. *Diagnose disease*
Azygos lobe of lung, 192 (0)

B

Babinski-Nageotte paralysis. *See* Paralysis, medullary, tegmental: *supplementary term,* 506
Bacillary dysentery, 276 (1)
Bacilli
infection. *See under name of specific disease or organ, region or structure affected*
list, 57 ff.
Back. *See also* Spine
round
due to senile atrophy, 153 (7)
with wedging of vertebrae, due to unknown cause, 155 (9)
Bacteremia, 114 (1)

Bacteria
infection. *See under name of specific disease or organ, region or structure affected*
list, 57 ff.
Bacterid, 132 (1)
Bacteriuria: *supplementary term,* 498. *Diagnose disease*
Baker's cyst. *See* Ganglion of knee joint, 162 (6)
Balanitis
due to infection, 329 (1)
xerotica obliterans, 331 (9)
Balanoposthitis
due to filth, 330 (4)
Balantidiasis. *See* Colitis, balantidial, 276 (1)
Baldness. *See* Alopecia
Bamberger-Marie disease. *See* Secondary hypertrophic osteoarthropathy, 152 (7)
Bandl's ring. *See* Contraction ring, 375 (55)
Bands, anomalous
constriction by, 122 (0)
Banti's disease. *See* Splenomegaly of undetermined origin, 233 (y); Congestive splenomegaly, 228 (5)
Bar median, 348 (9)
Baragnosis: *supplementary term,* 501. *Diagnose disease*
Barber's itch. *See* Tinea of beard, 135 (2)
Barbital poisoning, 117 (3)
Barcoo disease. *See* Veldt sore, 142 (9)
Barlow's disease. *See* Scurvy, 121 (7)
Barosinusitis, 181 (4)
Barré-Guillain syndrome (virus encephalomyelitis): *supplementary term,* 504. *Diagnose disease*
Bartholin's glands
abscess, 352 (1)
adenitis, 352 (1)
cyst due to unspecified cause, 353 (6)
retention cyst due to infection, 352 (1)
Bartonellosis, 114 (1)
Basal cell tumor
of bronchus. *Diagnose as* Specific tumors of epithelium, 93

Basal cell tumor—Continued
except of bronchus. *Diagnose as*
Basal cell carcinoma, 94
Basal metabolism
depressed or elevated: *supplementary terms, 500. Diagnose disease*
Basedow's disease. See Toxic diffuse goiter, 390 (9)
Basilar impression. See Platybasia, 155 (9)
Basophilic tumor, 94
Basophilism, pituitary, 394 (7)
Baumgarten-Cruveilhier cirrhosis. See Cirrhosis of liver, congenital, 287 (0)
Bazin's disease. See Tuberculosis indurativa (erythema induratum), 134 (1)
Bechterew's disease. See Arthritis, rheumatoid, of spine, 163 (9)
Bedbug infestation, 134 (2)
Bedsore. See Decubitus ulcer, 136 (4)
Bedwetting. See Enuresis, 112 (x)
Beheading. See Decapitation, 126 (4)
Belching. See Eructation: *supplementary term, 496*
Bell's palsy (neuropathy of facial nerve), 429 (4)
Bence-Jones protein in urine: *supplementary term, 498. Diagnose disease*
Bends. See Caisson disease, 118 (4)
Benedikt paralysis. See Paralysis, mesencephalic, tegmental, 506
Benzene
liver degeneration due to derivative, 288 (3)
normocytic hypoplastic anemia due to, 228 (3)
Benzol. See Benzene
von Bergmann's hypopituitarism. *See* Juvenile hypopituitarism, 394 (7)
Beriberi, 120 (7)
heart, 211 (7)
myelopathy due to, 424 (7)
Berlock dermatitis, 135 (3)
Bernard-Horner syndrome. See Horner syndrome
Bernhardt's disease. See Meralgia paresthetica, 429 (4)

Bertolotti's syndrome, 156 (0)
Berylliosis
acute, 194 (3)
chronic (chronic pulmonary granulomatosis in beryllium workers), 194 (3)
Beryllium. See Berylliosis
Besnier-Boeck disease. See Sarcoidosis, generalized, 116 (1)
Best's disease. See Degeneration, macular, congenital, 446 (0)
Bezoar. See Phytobezoar, 265 (6); Hair ball, 265 (6)
Bidermoma. *Diagnose as* Teratoma, 97
Biedl-Laurence-Moon syndrome, 114 (0)
Bielschowsky-Jansky disease. See Amaurotic familial idiocy, late infantile, 403 (7)
Biermer's disease. See Anemia, pernicious, 229 (7)
Bile passages
aberrant
cystic duct, 291 (0)
hepatic duct, 291 (0)
absence, congenital, 291 (0)
accessory hepatic ducts, 291 (0)
adenocarcinoma, 294 (8)
adenoma, 294 (8)
adhesions, 272 (4)
atresia, congenital, 291 (0)
calculus, 293 (6)
carcinoma, epidermoid, 294 (8)
cholangioma, 294 (8)
dilatation of common bile duct, 291 (0)
diseases, 291 ff.
distomiasis, 292 (2)
duplication
of common bile duct, 291 (0)
of cystic duct, 291 (0)
dyskinesia, 293 (55)
elongation
of common bile duct, 291 (0)
of cystic duct, 291 (0)
fistula
due to calculus, 293 (6)
due to infection, 292 (1)
following operation, 293 (4)
between gallbladder and cystic duct, congenital, 291 (0)

Bile passages—Continued
inflammation. *See also* Cholangiolitis, 292 (1); Cholangitis, 292
   (1)
   due to calculus, 293 (6)
injury, 293 (4)
kinking of cystic duct, congenital,
   291 (0)
neoplasms, 294 (8)
obliteration, congenital, 291 (0)
obstruction, due to foreign body, 293
   (6)
parasitic obstruction, 292 (1)
shortening
   of common bile duct, congenital,
      292 (0)
   of cystic duct, congenital, 292 (0)
stenosis
   of common bile duct due to pres-
      sure, 293 (4)
   due to adhesions, 293 (4)
   due to calculus, 293 (6)
   due to infection, 292 (1)
   due to trauma, 293 (4)
   following operation, 293 (4)
tumors, unlisted, 294 (8)
ulceration of common bile duct, due
   to calculus, 293 (6)
variations of common bile duct and
   pancreatic duct openings into
   ampulla of Vater, 292 (0)
Bile pigments in urine: *supplementary term,* 498. *Diagnose disease*
Bilharziasis. *See* Schistosomiasis *under organ affected*
Biliary disease. *See* Bile passages;
   Gallbladder
**Binocular vision, ocular neuro-
   muscular mechanism for**
diseases, 455 ff.
Bird face, 122 (0)
Birth. *See also* Delivery
multiple, 379
premature, 378
term, 378
Birth injury, 122 (0). *See also under organ, region or structure
   affected*
of cerebral vessels, 418 (0)
chronic brain syndrome with birth
   trauma, 108 (4)
encephalopathy due to, 410 (0)

Birth injury—Continued
hematoma due to, 122 (0)
infected, 122 (0)
keratitis due to, 434 (0)
laceration of spinal cord and meninges, 405 (0)
luxation of eyeball due to, 433 (0)
paralysis of extrinsic muscle of eye
   due to, 455 (0)
Birth paralysis. *See* Paralysis, obstetric, 167 (0)
Bite, animal or human, 126 (4)
Blackhead. *See* Comedo, 138 (7)
Bladder
abnormal communication with
   uterus, 306 (0)
abscess
   perivesical, 317 (1)
   of wall, 317 (1)
absence, 317 (0)
adenocarcinoma, 320 (8)
adenoma, 320 (8)
adhesions, perivesical, due to infection, 317 (1)
amebiasis, 317 (1)
amyloidosis, 321 (9)
atony, 320 (7)
calculus, 320 (6)
   acute cystitis due to, 320 (6)
   due to drug, 318 (3)
carcinoma
   epidermoid, 320 (8)
   mucinous, 321 (8)
   papillary, 321 (8)
   transitional cell (papillary), 321
      (8)
chondrosarcoma, 320 (8)
contracture
   of neck following operation, 318
      (4)
   of vesicourethral orifice due to in-
      fection, 317 (1)
   of vesicourethral orifice due to
      trauma, 318 (4)
cyst, mucous, 320 (6)
deformity (acquired), due to unknown cause, 320 (6)
dilatation
   congenital, 317 (0)
   due to unknown cause, 320 (6)
diseases, 317 ff.
displacement, 320 (6)

Bladder—Continued

diverticulitis, 320 (6)

diverticulum

acquired, due to unknown cause, 320 (6)

congenital, 317 (0)

due to stress, 318 (4)

double, 317 (0)

ectopia, 317 (0)

embolism, 319 (5)

embolus, infected, 319 (5)

embryoma. *Diagnose as* Mesenchymal mixed tumor, 98

exstrophy, 317 (0)

fibroma, 320 (8)

fistula

between colon and bladder, 318 (1), 318 (4)

between sigmoid and bladder, due to infection, 318 (1)

due to infection, 318 (1)

due to trauma, 319 (4)

rectovesical, 319 (4)

into seminal vesicle, 318 (1)

vesicoabdominal, following operation, 319 (4)

vesicoenteric, 318 (1)

vesicoperineal, 319 (4)

vesicoureteral, due to infection, 318 (1)

vesicouterine, due to infection, 318 (1)

vesicovaginal, 318 (1)

congenital, 355 (0)

due to trauma, 356 (4)

obstetric, 375 (4)

postoperative, 356 (4)

foreign body in

due to trauma, 319 (4)

not due to trauma, 320 (6)

hemangioma, 320 (8)

hemorrhage

due to trauma, 319 (4)

following operation, 319 (4)

hernia

congenital, 317 (0)

displacement into hernial sac, 320 (6)

prevesical, 320 (6)

hypertrophy of interureteral ridge, congenital, 317 (0)

infestation, 318 (2)

inflammation. *See* Cystitis

Bladder—Continued

inhibition following operation, 319 (55)

injury, 319 (4)

inversion, 320 (6)

leiomyoma, 320 (8)

leiomyosarcoma, 320 (8)

leukoplakia

due to infection, 318 (1)

due to unknown cause, 321 (9)

lichen planus, 321 (9)

lipoma, 320 (8)

lymphangioma, 321 (8)

lymphangiosarcoma, 321 (8)

malacoplakia, 318 (1)

mesenchymal mixed tumor, malignant, 321 (8)

mesothelioma, 321 (8)

myiasis, 318 (2)

myxoma, 321 (8)

myxosarcoma, 321 (8)

neoplasms, 321 (8)

neurofibroma, 321 (8)

osteoma, 321 (8)

pain: *supplementary term,* 499. *Diagnose disease*

paralysis

due to cord injury, 319 (55)

due to trauma, 319 (55)

of external sphincter, 319 (55)

flaccid, 319 (55)

of internal sphincter, 319 (55)

postpartum, 319 (55)

spastic, 319 (55)

paramedial vesicourethral orifice, 317 (0)

paresis, tabetic, 320 (55)

polyp, 321 (8)

simple, 321 (9)

prolapse, 320 (6)

prolapse of mucosa

congenital, 317 (0)

into urethra following operation, 319 (4)

puncture by instrument, 319 (4)

rhabdomyoma, 321 (8)

rhabdomyosarcoma, 321 (8)

rupture

due to trauma, 319 (4)

due to unknown cause, 321 (9)

sacculation due to stress, 319 (4)

sarcoma, 321 (8)

Bladder—Continued
spasm of external sphincter, neurogenic, 320 (55)
strangulation, 319 (5)
stricture of vesicourethral orifice
congenital, 317 (0)
due to calculus, 320 (6)
tenesmus: *supplementary term,* 499. *Diagnose disease*
teratoma, 321 (8)
tumors, unlisted, 321 (8)
ulcer
due to radium burn, 319 (4)
solitary, due to unknown cause, 321 (9)
varix, 320 (6)
zoster, 318 (1)
Blast injury, 118 (4)
Blastoma
lymphoepitheliomatous. *Diagnose as* Epidermoid carcinoma, 94
Blastomycin test reactions: *supplementary term,* 487. *Diagnose disease*
Blastomycosis
North American, 124 (2)
South American, 124 (2), 135 (2)
Bleb. *See also* Blister
subpleural (bullous emphysema), 200 (4)
Bleeding. *See also* Hemorrhage
time
abnormality: *supplementary term,* 493. *Diagnose disease*
increase: *supplementary term,* 494. *Diagnose disease*
Blennorrhea
inclusion, 468 (1)
Blepharitis
squamosa, 463 (7)
ulcerosa, 462 (1)
Blepharochalasis, 464 (9)
Blepharophimosis, 461 (0)
Blepharospasm, 463 (55)
supplementary term. See Eye, extrinsic muscles, spasm, 508
Blindness. *See also* Amaurosis; Amblyopia
color. *See* Color blindness
from loss of blood, 448 (5)
night. *See* Night blindness
psychic: *supplementary term,* 509. *Diagnose disease*

Blindness—Continued
word: *supplementary term,* 510. *Diagnose disease*
Blister
due to trauma, 136 (4)
fever. *See* Herpes simplex of lip, 243 (1)
Blood and blood-forming organs.
See also Coagulation; Erythrocytes; Leukocytes; Plasma
amino acids in blood: *supplementary terms. Diagnose disease*
decrease, 493
increase, 494
bile in blood. *See* Cholemia: *supplementary term,* 493
blood in feces, occult: *supplementary term,* 496. *Diagnose disease*
blood in gastric contents: *supplementary term,* 496. *Diagnose disease*
blood groups: *supplementary terms,* 493. *Diagnose disease*
calcium in blood
decrease. *See* Hypocalcemia, 494
increase. *See* Hypercalcemia, 493
carotene in blood. *See* Carotenemia, 120 (7), 493
cevitamic acid in blood: *supplementary terms. Diagnose disease*
decrease, 493
increase, 494
change in blood volume: *supplementary term,* 493. *Diagnose disease*
change in proportion of blood plasm and cells: *supplementary term,* 493. *Diagnose disease*
chloride in blood
decrease. *See* Hypochloremia, 494
increase. *See* Hyperchloremia, 493
cholesterol in blood
decrease. *See* Hypocholesteremia, 494
increase. *See* Hypercholesteremia, 494
cholesterol esters in blood, decrease: *supplementary term,* 493. *Diagnose disease*
diseases, 227 ff.
donor of blood, 481
Hodgkin's disease, 230 (8)
immature cells in blood, presence of: *supplementary term,* 495. *Diagnose disease*

Blood—Continued
leukemoid blood picture: *supplementary term,* 494. *Diagnose disease*
loss of blood. *See* Hemorrhage
lymphoma, 230 (8)
giant follicular, 230 (8)
lymphosarcoma, 230 (8)
neoplasms, 230 (8)
oxygen deficiency of blood. *See* Anoxemia
phenols in blood: *supplementary terms. Diagnose disease*
decrease, 493
increase, 494
phosphorus in blood
decrease. *See* Hypophosphatemia, 494
increase. *See* Hyperphosphatemia, 494
plasma cell myeloma, 230 (8)
potassium in blood
decrease, *See* Hypopotassemia, 494
increase. *See* Hyperpotassemia, 494
protein in blood
decrease. *See* Hypoproteinemia, 494
increase. *See* Hyperproteinemia, 494
sarcoma, reticulum cell, 230 (8)
spitting of blood. *See* Hemoptysis: *supplementary term,* 490
sugar in blood
decrease. *See* Hypoglycemia, 494
increase. *See* Hyperglycemia, 494
tubercle bacilli in blood: *supplementary term,* 495. *Diagnose disease*
tumors unlisted, 230 (8)
viscosity of blood, abnormal: *supplementary term,* 493. *Diagnose disease*
Blood circulation. *See also* Cardiovascular system; *and under organ or region affected*
congestion due to, 127 (5)
gangrene due to disturbance, 128 (5)
Blood marrow donor, 481
Blood pressure
high. *See* Hypertension
low. *See* Hypotension
Blood transfusion
nephrosis due to hemoglobinemia following, 309 (3)

Blood transfusion—Continued
reaction following, 118 (3)
Blood vessels. *See also* Aorta; Artery; Capillary; Vein
anomalous entry of pulmonary veins into other vessels, 205 (0)
congenital abnormalities of central vessels, 204 (0)
endothelioma. *Diagnose as* Hemangioendothelioma, 96
malignant. *Diagnose as* Lymphangiosarcoma, 96
nevus, not otherwise specified. *Diagnose as* Hemangioma (angioma), 96
sarcoma, endothelial. *Diagnose as* Hemangiosarcoma, 96
transposition of great vessels, 205 (0)
Blue sclera, 438 (9)
Blushing: *supplementary term,* 487. *Diagnose disease*
Boarder, 481
Boas-Oppler bacilli
in gastric contents: *supplementary term,* 496. *Diagnose disease*
Body as a whole
diseases, 114 ff.
Boeck's sarcoid. *See* Sarcoidosis, 123 (1)
Boil. *See* Furuncle, 132 (1)
Bone(s). *See also* Osteitis *and other terms with prefix* "Oste-"; Periosteum; *and under name of specific bone*
abscess, 148 (1)
absence, congenital, 146 (0)
accessory, 146 (0)
navicular, of carpus, 146 (0)
of tarsus, 146 (0)
supernumerary, 146 (0)
amyloid infiltration of, 154 (9)
aneurysm, malignant. *Diagnose as* Osteosarcoma (osteogenic sarcoma), 97
angioendothelioma. *Diagnose as* Ewing's sarcoma, 97
atrophy
due to arteriosclerosis, 152 (5)
due directly to interference with blood supply, 152 (5)
due to disuse, 152 (7)
due to embolism, 152 (5)

Brain—Continued
  vessels—continued
    atypical distribution, 418 (0)
    birth injury, 418 (0)
    calcification, familial arterial, 420 (9)
    diseases, 418 ff.
    embolism, 418 (1), 419 (4), 419 (6)
    hemangioma of intrinsic arteries, 420 (8)
    hemangiosarcoma of intrinsic arteries, 420 (8)
    hemorrhage, 418 (1), 419 (4), 419 (5), 420 (9), 420 (y)
    hypoplasia, 402 (0)
    mycotic aneurysm, 419 (2)
    neoplasms, 420 (8)
    occlusion by malarial parasites, 418 (1)
    thromboangiitis obliterans, 420 (9)
    thrombosis, 418 (1), 419 (5), 419 (6), 420 (9)
    tumors, unlisted, 420 (8)
  wound, 413 (4)
Branchial chondroma. *Diagnose as* Branchioma, 98
Branchial cleft, 255 (0)
  carcinoma, transitional cell. *Diagnose as* Branchioma, 98
  cyst. *Diagnose as* Branchioma, 98
Branchial cyst. *Diagnose as* Branchioma, 98
  congenital, 255 (0)
Branchial inclusion cyst. *Diagnose as* Branchioma, 98
Branchial vestiges, 255 (0)
Branchioma, 98
Breakbone fever. *See* Dengue, 115 (1)
Breast. *See also* Lacteal duct; Nipple
  aberrant, 143 (0)
  absence, 143 (0)
  abscess, 143 (1)
    premammary, 143 (1)
    puerperal, 143 (1)
    retromammary, 143 (1)
  adenocarcinoma, 145 (8)
  adenofibroma, 145 (8)
  adenomatosis, 145 (9)
  carcinoma
    intracystic papillary, 145 (8)

Breast—Continued
  carcinoma—continued
    medullary, with lymphoid stroma, 145 (8)
    sweat gland, 145 (8)
  chemical burn, 144 (3)
  cyst. *See also* Galactocele, 143 (1)
    due to trauma, 144 (4)
    involution, 144 (7)
    retention, due to infection, 143 (1)
  cystic, due to unknown cause, 144 (6)
  cystosarcoma phyllodes, 145 (8)
  diseases, 143 ff.
  fat necrosis, 144 (4)
  fibromyxoma, fibromyxosarcoma or fibrosarcoma. *Diagnose as* Cystosarcoma phyllodes, 97
  fibrosis, due to unknown cause, 145 (9)
  fistula, 143 (1)
    puerperal, 143 (1)
  hemangiosarcoma, 145 (8)
  hematoma due to trauma, 144 (4)
  hypertrophy
    hereditary, 145 (9)
    in male. *See* Gynecomastia, 144 (7)
    in newborn, 144 (7)
  hypoplasia, 143 (0)
  infarction, 144 (4)
  inflammation. *See* Mastitis
  injury, 144 (4)
  lymphosarcoma, 145 (8)
  male, overdevelopment, 143 (0). *See also* Gynecomastia, 144 (7)
  milk. *See* Lactation; Milk
  mixed tumor. *Diagnose as* Cystosarcoma phyllodes, 97
  myxofibroma, myxofibrosarcoma or myxosarcoma. *Diagnose as* Cystosarcoma phyllodes, 97
  neoplasms, 145 (8)
  overdevelopment in female, 144 (7)
  pigeon, congenital, 146 (0)
  pregnancy changes, 144 (7)
  sarcoma, 145 (8)
  supernumerary, 143 (0)
  thrombophlebitis of veins, 144 (1)
  tumors, unlisted, 145 (8)
  varicose veins, 144 (6)

Bronchus(i)—Continued
edema, localized—continued
  due to unknown cause, 190 (6)
epithelioma, adenoid basal cell, or epithelioma adenoides cysti-cum. *Diagnose as* Adenoma, 191 (8)
fibroma, 191 (8)
fistula
  bronchocutaneous
    due to infection, 189 (1)
    due to tuberculosis, 189 (1)
  bronchoesophageal
    due to foreign body, 175 (4)
    due to trauma, 175 (4)
  bronchopleural
    due to infection, 189 (1)
    due to tuberculosis, 189 (1)
  bronchovisceral, 171 (1)
  esophagobronchial
    congenital, 260 (0)
    due to foreign body, 175 (4)
  following operation, 190 (4)
  hepatobronchial, 287 (1)
foreign body in, 190 (4)
injury, 190 (4)
malignant tumor cells in bronchial secretions: *supplementary term,* 490. *Diagnose disease*
myocytic or parasitic infection, 190 (2)
neoplasms, 191 (8)
oncocytoma. *Diagnose as* Adenoma, 191 (8)
spasm: *supplementary term,* 490. *Diagnose disease*
stenosis
  due to infection, 189 (1)
  due to poison, 190 (3)
  due to pressure, 190 (4)
syphilis, 189 (1)
tracheal, 189 (0)
tuberculosis, 190 (1)
tumors
  adenomatoid. *Diagnose as* Adenoma, 191 (8)
  mixed; mixed salivary gland. *Diagnose as* Adenoma, 191 (8)
  unlisted, 191 (8)
ulcer due to unknown cause, 191 (9)
ulceration
  due to foreign body, 190 (4)

Bronchus(i)—Continued
ulceration—continued
  due to trauma, 190 (4)
Brooke-Fordyce disease. *Diagnose as* Neoplastic cyst, 93
Brow presentation, 382 (6)
Brown-Séquard syndrome: *supplementary term,* 502. *Diagnose disease*
Brucellosis, 114 (1)
Bruise. *See* Contusion
Bruxism: *supplementary term,* 484. *Diagnose disease*
Bubo
inguinal, 235 (1)
Buccal cavity. *See also* Cheek; Mouth
cyst, 241 (6)
fistula
  buccal pharyngeal
    due to infection, 241 (1)
    due to trauma, 241 (4)
  postoperative, 241 (4)
Buerger's disease. *See* Thromboan-giitis obliterans, 219 (9)
Bulbar paralysis: *supplementary term,* 506. *Diagnose disease*
Bulbourethral glands (Cowper's)
abscess, 322 (1)
adenitis, 322 (1)
adenocarcinoma, 325 (8)
cyst, 325 (6)
tuberculosis, 323 (1)
Bulimia: *supplementary term,* 496. *Diagnose disease*
Bulla. *See* Blister
Bullet wounds. *See also* Gunshot wounds
multiple, 118 (4)
Bundle branch block. *See also* In-traventricular block
congenital, 203 (0)
due to rheumatic fever, 212 (9)
due to sclerosis of nutrient artery, 210 (5)
due to unknown cause, 214 (x)
supplementary term, 492. *Diagnose disease*
Bunion, 158 (4)
Burn(s). *See also* Incineration, 118 (4); Scald, 127 (4)
chemical, 125 (3)
cicatrix of skin due to, 135 (3)
of cornea, 125 (3)

Burn(s)—Continued
  chemical—continued
    of eyeball, 433 (3)
    gangrene due to, 125 (3)
    of larynx, 183 (3)
    of palate, 250 (3)
    of pharynx, 255 (3)
    of rectum, 281 (3)
    sinus due to, 125 (3)
    staphyloma of cornea due to, 435
      (3)
  duodenal ulcer due to, 273 (4)
  electric, 126 (4)
    gangrene due to, 126 (4)
    of urethra, 324 (4)
  heat
    of auricle, 475 (4)
    cicatrix of skin due to, 136 (4)
    deformity due to, 126 (4)
    of epiglottis, 184 (4)
    of larynx, 184 (4)
    ulceration of trachea due to, 188
      (4)
  inhalation, 175 (4)
  radiation, 127 (4)
  radium, of urethra, 324 (4)
  of skin
    first degree, 136 (4)
    second degree, 136 (4)
    third degree, 126 (4)
Bursa. *See also* Bursitis; Hygroma
  adventitious, 165 (4)
  calcium deposits in, 166 (9)
  chondroma, 165 (8)
  diseases, 165
  fibroma, 165 (8)
  injury, 165 (4)
  myxoma, 165 (8)
  neoplasms, 165 (8)
  pharyngeal
    abscess, 176 (1)
    cyst, 176 (1)
  sarcoma, 165 (8)
  tumors, unlisted, 165 (8)
Bursitis
  acute
    due to infection, 165 (1)
    due to trauma, 165 (4)
    suppurative, 165 (1)
  chronic
    with calcification, 165 (4)
    due to infection, 165 (1)
    due to trauma, 165 (4)

Bursitis—Continued
  due to gout, 165 (7)
  due to unknown cause, 166 (9)
  gluteal, 165 (4)
  olecranon, 165 (4)
  prepatellar, 165 (4)
Buttocks. *See* Gluteal region

C

Cachexia
  hypopituitary, 394 (7)
  myelopathy due to, 424 (7)
  neuropathy due to, 430 (7)
  supplementary term, 484. *Diagnose
    disease*
Caecum. *See* Cecum
Caffey's syndrome. *See* Hyperostosis, cortical, congenital, 147 (0)
Caisson disease, 118 (4)
  of bone or joint, 150 (4)
Calcaneus
  exostosis due to infection, 148 (1)
  osteochondrosis, 155 (9)
Calcification. *See also* Calcinosis;
    Calculus; Ossification; *and under
    organ or structure affected*
  due to unknown cause, 129 (9)
  subperiosteal, due to trauma, 150 (4)
  supplementary term, 498. *Diagnose
    disease*
Calcified tumor. *Diagnose as* Neoplastic cyst, 93
Calcinosis, 120 (7)
Calcium
  deficient absorption, tetany due to,
    120 (7)
Calculosis, intrahepatic, 289 (6)
Calculus(i). *See also under organ,
    region or structure affected*
  in nose. *See* Rhinolith, 178 (6)
  supplementary term, 498. *Diagnose
    disease*
Calf muscles
  weakness, congenital, 167 (0)
Callositas, 136 (4)
Callus, 136 (4)
  compression of peripheral nerve by,
    429 (4)
  compression of spinal cord by, 423
    (4)
  excessive, following fracture, 150 (4)

Calvé-Perthes disease. *See* Osteochondrosis of capital epiphysis of femur, 155 (9)

Calyx, renal. *See* Kidney, calyx

Canal of Cloquet, remains, 444 (0)

Canal of Nuck
cyst, 353 (6)
hydrocele, 354 (9)
patent, 351 (0)

Canaliculus
absence, 465 (0)
displacement due to amniotic deformities, 465 (0)
foreign body in, 466 (4)
granuloma (polyp) in, 465 (1)
stenosis, cicatricial
due to infection, 466 (1)
due to trauma, 466 (4)
wound, 466 (4)

Cancer. *See also* Carcinoma; Sarcoma; *and name of specific neoplasm under organ, region or structure affected*
black. *Diagnose as* Melanoma, 94
mule spinners'. *Diagnose as* Epidermoid carcinoma, 94
tar. *Diagnose as* Carcinoma, not otherwise specified, 94

Cancerophobia: *supplementary term,* 484. *Diagnose disease*

Cancroid. *Diagnose as* Epidermoid carcinoma, 94

Cancrum oris. *See* Stomatitis, gangrenous, 241 (1)

Canities, 138 (7)

Canker sores. *See* Stomatitis, aphthous, 241 (1)

Canthus
abscess, 462 (1)
carcinoma
basal cell, 464 (8)
epidermoid, 464 (8)

Capillary(ies)
diseases, 226
fragility, hereditary, 226 (9)
multiple hemorrhages: *supplementary term,* 495. *Diagnose disease*
purpura
due to allergy or drug reaction, 226 (3)
due to embolism, 226 (5)
due to infection, 226 (1)
due to mechanical cause, 226 (4)

Capillary(ies)—Continued
purpura—continued
due to metabolic disturbance, 226 (7)
generally, 226 (5)

Caput succedaneum, 381 (4)

Car sickness, 119 (55)

Carbohydrate metabolism, disorders of, 120 (7)

Carbolic acid. *See* Phenol

Carbon monoxide
hemorrhage of retina due to, 447 (3)
liver degeneration due to, 288 (3)
poisoning, 117 (3)

Carbon tetrachloride
liver degeneration due to, 288 (3)

Carbuncle, 132 (1)
malignant. *See* Anthrax

Carcinoid
of bronchus. *Diagnose as* Adenoma, 94
malignant, of skin. *Diagnose as* Basal cell carcinoma, 94
not otherwise specified (except of bronchus, intestines, skin, stomach, rectum). *Diagnose as* Carcinoma, not otherwise specified, 94
of skin. *Diagnose as* Basal cell carcinoma, 94

Carcinoma
actinic. *Diagnose as* Carcinoma, not otherwise specified, 94
adenogenous (skin). *Diagnose as* Basal cell carcinoma, 94
adenoid basal cell
of bronchus. *Diagnose as* Adenoma, 94
except of bronchus. *Diagnose as* Basal cell carcinoma, 94
adenoid cystic. *Diagnose as* Basal cell carcinoma, 94
adrenal cortical
except of ovary, testis. *Diagnose as* Adenocarcinoma, 94
of ovary. *Diagnose as* Virilizing tumor, 93
alveolar
except of lung. *Diagnose as* Adenocarcinoma, 94
of lung. *Diagnose as* Bronchiolar carcinoma, 94

Carcinoma—Continued

anaplastic. *Diagnose as* Carcinoma, not otherwise specified, 94

apocrine. *Diagnose as* Sweat gland tumor, 94

appendage cell (skin). *Diagnose as* Adenocarcinoma, 94

argentaffin. *Diagnose as* Argentaffinoma, 95

arising in polyp or polyposis. *Diagnose as* Carcinoma, not otherwise specified, 94

arsenical. *Diagnose as* Carcinoma, not otherwise specified, 94

basal cell, 94 (8)

keratotic. *Diagnose as* Baso-squamous carcinoma, 94

basal clear cell. *Diagnose as* Basal cell carcinoma, 94

basal squamous. *Diagnose as* Baso-squamous carcinoma, 94

basocellulare hyalinicum. *Diagnose as* Sweat gland tumor, 94

baso-squamous, 94

of skin, 139 (8)

branchial. *Diagnose as* Branchioma, 98

branchiogenic. *Diagnose as* Branchioma, 98

bronchial. *Diagnose as* Carcinoma, not otherwise specified, 94

bronchiolar, 94

bronchogenic. *Diagnose as* Carcinoma, not otherwise specified, 94

squamous cell. *Diagnose as* Epidermoid carcinoma, 94

ceruminous. *Diagnose as* Sweat gland tumor, 94

chimney sweeps'. *Diagnose as* Epidermoid carcinoma, 94

chromophobe. *Diagnose as* Chromophobe tumor, 94

clear cell (kidney). *Diagnose as* Adenocarcinoma, 94

colloid. *Diagnose as* Mucinous carcinoma, 93

columnar cell. *Diagnose as* Adenocarcinoma, 94

cylindrical (sweat gland). *Diagnose as* Sweat gland tumor, 94

diffuse bronchiolar. *Diagnose as* Bronchiolar carcinoma, 94

Carcinoma—Continued

diffuse scirrhous (stomach), 94

embryonal, of testis, 98

endometrial, 94

epidermoid, 94

of skin, 139 (8)

follicular (thyroid), 94

functionally active (thyroid). *Diagnose as* Functionally hyperactive thyroid tumor, 93

fungating. *Diagnose as* Papillary or polypoid tumor, not otherwise specified, 93

gelatinous. *Diagnose as* Mucinous carcinoma, 93

giant cell, 94

gill cleft. *Diagnose as* Branchioma, 98

goblet cell. *Diagnose as* Mucinous carcinoma, 93

granular cell (kidney). *Diagnose as* Adenocarcinoma, 94

hair matrix. *Diagnose as* Basal cell carcinoma, 94

hidradenoid. *Diagnose as* Sweat gland tumor, 94

Hürthle cell. *Diagnose as* Hürthle cell tumor, 94

hypernephroid (ovary). *Diagnose as* Virilizing tumor, 93

with hyperparathyroidism. *Diagnose as* Functionally hyperactive thyroid tumor, 93

intermediary or intermediate. *Diagnose as* Baso-squamous carcinoma, 94

intra-epidermal. *Diagnose as* Epidermoid carcinoma, 94

islet cell. *Diagnose as* Nonfunctioning islet cell tumor, 94

juvenile (liver). *Diagnose as* Hepatoblastoma, 98

Kultschitzky's. *Diagnose as* Argentaffinoma, 95

large cell (lung). *Diagnose as* Specific tumors of epithelium, 93

large cellular medullary (ovary). *Diagnose as* Disgerminoma, 97

liver cell. *Diagnose as* Hepatoma, 94

medullary. *Diagnose as* Carcinoma, not otherwise specified, 94

with lymphoid stroma, 94

Carcinoma—Continued
  metatypical. *Diagnose as* Baso-squamous carcinoma, 94
  mixed (skin); mixed baso-squamous. *Diagnose as* Baso-squamous carcinoma, 94
  mucinous, 93
  mucoid. *Diagnose as* Mucinous carcinoma, 93
  multicentric basal cell. *Diagnose as* Basal cell carcinoma, 94
  multiple bronchiolar. *Diagnose as* Bronchiolar carcinoma, 94
  nevus. *Diagnose as* Melanoma, not otherwise specified, 94
  oat cell. *Diagnose as* Carcinoma, not otherwise specified, 94
  with osseous metaplasia (breast), 94
  papillary. *Diagnose as* Papillary or polypoid tumor, not otherwise specified, 93
    intracystic (breast), 93
    serous. *Diagnose as* Serous papillary cystic tumor, 93
    sweat gland. *Diagnose as* Sweat gland tumor, 94
  pleomorphic. *Diagnose as* Carcinoma, not otherwise specified, 94
  polypoid. *Diagnose as* Papillary or polypoid tumor, not otherwise specified, 93
  prickle cell. *Diagnose as* Epidermoid carcinoma, 94
  pseudomucinous. *Diagnose as* Cystic tumor, 93
  radiation. *Diagnose as* Carcinoma, not otherwise specified, 94
  Regaud type. *Diagnose as* Epidermoid carcinoma, 94
  reserve cell (lung). *Diagnose as* Specific tumors of epithelium, 93
  rete cell. *Diagnose as* Rete cell tumor, 94
  round cell. *Diagnose as* Carcinoma, not otherwise specified, 94
  sarcomatodes. *Diagnose as* Carcinosarcoma, 97
  Schmincke type. *Diagnose as* Epidermoid carcinoma, 94
  Schneiderian. *Diagnose as* Transitional cell carcinoma, 94

Carcinoma—Continued
  scirrhous, 94
  sebaceous. *Diagnose as* Sebaceous tumor, 94
  of skin, 140 (8)
  sebaceum basocellulare of Loos. *Diagnose as* Sebaceous tumor, 94
  seminal. *Diagnose as* Disgerminoma, 97
  signet ring cell. *Diagnose as* Mucinous carcinoma, 93
  simple adenoid (skin). *Diagnose as* Basal cell carcinoma, 94
  simplex. *Diagnose as* Carcinoma, not otherwise specified, 94
  in situ of cervix. *Diagnose as* Epidermoid carcinoma, 94
  small cell
    except of lung, thyroid. *Diagnose as* Carcinoma, not otherwise specified, 94
    of lung. *Diagnose as* Specific tumors of epithelium, 93
    of thyroid, 94
  solitary bronchiolar. *Diagnose as* Bronchiolar carcinoma, 94
  spheroidal cell. *Diagnose as* Argentaffinoma, 95
  spindle cell. *Diagnose as* Carcinoma, not otherwise specified, 94
  spinous cell. *Diagnose as* Epidermoid carcinoma, 94
  squamous cell. *Diagnose as* Epidermoid carcinoma, 94
  subepidermal basal cell. *Diagnose as* Basal cell carcinoma, 94
  syncytial. *Diagnose as* Choriocarcinoma, 97
  teratoid
    except of testis. *Diagnose as* Teratoma, 97
    of testis. *Diagnose as* Embryonal carcinoma of testis, 98
  terminal bronchiolar. *Diagnose as* Bronchiolar carcinoma, 94
  transitional cell, 94
    of branchial cleft. *Diagnose as* Branchioma, 98
    of skin. *Diagnose as* Baso-squamous carcinoma, 94
    of tonsil. *Diagnose as* Epidermoid carcinoma, 94

Carcinoma—Continued
tubular. *Diagnose as* Adenocarcinoma, 94
undifferentiated. *Diagnose as* Carcinoma, not otherwise specified, 94
verrucal. *Diagnose as* Epidermoid carcinoma, 94
Carcinomatosis. *Diagnose as* Carcinoma, not otherwise specified, 94
generalized, 121 (8)
abdominal, 129 (8)
Carcinosarcoma, 97
embryonal. *Diagnose as* Nephroblastoma, 98
Carcinosis
miliary. *Diagnose as* Carcinoma, not otherwise specified, 94
Cardia. *See also* Cardiospasm
stenosis, 265 (9)
Cardiac. *See also* Heart
arrest
due to contusion, 209 (4)
due to traumatic interference with innervation, 209 (4)
functional capacity, Classes I, II, III and IV: *supplementary terms,* 492. *Diagnose disease*
insufficiency: *supplementary term,* 491. *Diagnose disease*
tamponade, 209 (4)
thrombosis within chamber: *supplementary term,* 492. *Diagnose disease*
Cardialgia. *See* Pain in epigastrium: *supplementary term,* 497
Cardiochalasia, 261 (55)
Cardiopsychoneurosis. *Supplementary term,* 491. *Diagnose disease*
Cardiospasm
achalasia, 263 (0)
congenital, 263 (0)
dilatation of esophagus due to achalasia, 261 (55)
reflex, 261 (55)
Cardiovascular system. *See also* Arteries; Blood vessels; Heart
diseases, 201 ff.
carcinoid, 206 (7)
due to hypertension of lesser circulation, 206 (5)
hypertensive cardiovascular, 206 (5)
psychophysiologic reaction, 111 (55)

Carditis. *See also* Endocarditis; Pericarditis
acute bacterial, 207 (1)
subacute bacterial, 207 (1)
Caries
of petrous bone, 148 (1)
of teeth, 247 (1)
Carotenemia, 120 (7)
supplementary term, 493. *Diagnose disease*
Carotenosis of skin, 138 (7)
Carotid artery
anomalous left common, 205 (0)
Carotid body tumor, 98
Carotid gland
diseases, 400
neoplasms, 400 (8)
tumors, unlisted, 400 (8)
Carotid sinus syncope (syndrome), 206 (55)
glossopharyngeal neuralgia with, 431 (x)
supplementary term, 491. *Diagnose disease*
Carrier state, 114 (1). *See also under name of specific disease*
Carrións disease. *See* Bartonellosis, 114 (1); Verruga peruana, 134 (1)
Cartilage. *See also* Chondritis *and terms beginning with* "Chondro-"; Joint; Ligament; *and name of specific cartilage*
abscess, 157 (1)
atrophy
due to infection, 157 (1)
due to trauma, 158 (4)
due to unknown cause, 163 (9)
calcification
due to trauma, 158 (4)
undiagnosed, 163 (7)
chondroma, 163 (8)
chondrosarcoma, 163 (8)
costal. *See* Costal cartilage
dyschondroplasia (skeletal enchondromatosis), 147 (0)
ectopic, in lung, 192 (0)
hypertrophy due to unknown cause, 163 (9)
intervertebral. *See* Intervertebral cartilage

Cartilage—Continued
  of joint, injury, 159 (4)
  ossification, senile, 163 (7)
  softening. *See* Chondromalacia
Caruncle, lacrimal
  abscess, 468 (1)
  deformity following operation, 468
    (4)
Caruncle of urethra, 325 (9)
Casoni test, positive reaction to:
  supplementary term, 487. *Diagnose disease*
Castaneda's stain for rickettsia,
  positive: *supplementary term,*
  486. *Diagnose disease*
Casts in urine: *supplementary term,*
  498. *Diagnose disease*
Cat scratch fever, 235 (1)
Cataplexy
  narcolepsy with, 417 (x)
  supplementary term, 502. *Diagnose disease*
Cataract
  with atopic dermatitis, 442 (3)
  cause unknown, 443 (9)
  congenital, 442 (0)
  diabetic, 443 (7)
  due to injury, 442 (4)
  due to physical agent, 442 (4)
  due to radiant injury, 442 (4)
  due to toxic agent, 442 (3)
  due to uveitis, 442 (1)
  in myotonic dystrophy, 443 (9)
  in myxedema, 443 (7)
  secondary, following operation, 442
    (4)
  senile, 443 (7)
  tetany, 443 (7)
Catarrh
  nasal. *See* Rhinitis
  spring (vernal conjunctivitis), 469
    (3)
Catatonia: *supplementary term,* 502.
  Diagnose disease
Caterpillar hairs
  conjunctivitis due to, 469 (3)
Catheter
  ureteritis due to, 314 (4)
Cauda equina
  adhesions due to trauma, 423 (4)
Causalgia
  of arm, 128 (55)

Causalgia—Continued
  of leg, 128 (55)
  supplementary term, 484. *Diagnose disease*
Caustic potash
  conjunctivitis due to, 469 (3)
Caustic soda (sodium hydroxide)
  stricture of external auditory canal
    due to, 475 (3)
Caval veins. *See* Vena cava
Cavernitis. *See* Corpora cavernosa,
  inflammation, 329 (1)
Cavernoma. *Diagnose as* Hemangioma (angioma), 96
Cavernous sinus
  phlebitis, 408 (1)
  thrombosis, marantic, 409 (5)
Cavum septi pellucidi
  cyst, congenital, 410 (0)
  dilatation, 410 (0)
Cecum
  duplication, congenital, with duplication of appendix, 276 (0)
  inflammation. *See* Typhlitis, 277 (1)
  mobile, 276 (0)
  nondescent, 276 (0)
  retrocecal abscess, 298 (1)
  rupture, spontaneous, during birth,
    276 (0)
Celiac disease, 240 (7)
Celioma. *Diagnose as* Mesothelioma,
  97
  malignant. *Diagnose as* Mesothelial
    sarcoma, 97
Cellules epitheliales eruptifs.
  Diagnose as Sweat gland tumor,
  94
Cellulitis, 123 (1), 132 (1). *See also
  under organ, region or structure
  affected*
  dissecting, 133 (1)
  peritonsillar tissue, 258 (1)
  periurethral, 323 (1)
  retroperitoneal, 299 (1)
Celothelioma. *Diagnose as* Mesothelioma, 97
  malignant. *Diagnose as* Mesothelial
    sarcoma, 97
Cementoblastoma. *Diagnose as*
  Odontogenic tumor, benign, 98
Cementoma, 249 (8)
Central nervous system. *See* Nervous system, central

Cephalalgia. *See* Headache: *supplementary term,* 504
Cephalhematoma, 151 (4)
Cephalogyric disturbances. *See* Spinal accessory nerve, paralysis: *supplementary term,* 509
Cephalopelvic disproportion, 382 (6)
Cerebellopontine angle tumor. *Diagnose as* Schwannoma, 95
Cerebellum. *See also* Brain
  abscess, 411 (1)
  aplasia, 410 (0)
  atrophy, 416 (9)
  caudal displacement, 402 (0)
  cyst due to bullet wound, 413 (4)
  hereditary atrophy, 416 (9)
  rubrospinal cerebellar (Claude) syndrome: *supplementary term,* 503. *Diagnose disease*
  sclerosis, 416 (9)
Cerebral. *See also* Brain
  dysrhythmia: *supplementary term,* 502. *Diagnose disease*
  hemorrhage. *See* Brain, hemorrhage
  palsy. *See* Cerebral spastic infantile paralysis, 410 (0)
  paralysis. *See* Paralysis
  spastic infantile paralysis, 410 (0)
  vessels. *See* Brain, vessels
Cerebral thromboangiitis obliterans, 420 (9)
Cerebral thrombosis
  due to arteriosclerosis, 420 (9)
Cerebromacular degeneration, 403 (7)
Cerebrospinal fluid
  abnormal cell count: *supplementary term,* 502. *Diagnose disease*
  decrease in sugar: *supplementary term,* 502. *Diagnose disease*
  increase in globulins: *supplementary term,* 502. *Diagnose disease*
  increase in proteins: *supplementary term,* 502. *Diagnose disease*
  increase in sugar: *supplementary term,* 502. *Diagnose disease*
  increased pressure: *supplementary term,* 502. *Diagnose disease*
  otorrhea: *supplementary term,* 503. *Diagnose disease*

Cerebrospinal fluid—Continued
  reaction to loss of, 403 (4)
  rhinorrhea: *supplementary term,* 503. *Diagnose disease*
  subarachnoid accumulation following operation, 407 (4)
  tumor cells in: *supplementary term,* 507. *Diagnose disease*
Cerebrospinal vessels
  arteriosclerosis, 404 (9)
  diseases, 404
  endarteritis, 404 (9)
  periarteritis nodosa, 404 (9)
  thromboangiitis obliterans, 404 (9)
Cerebrum. *See* Brain
Cerumen, impacted, 476 (6)
Cervical pregnancy, 380 (7)
Cervicitis
  acute, 358 (1)
  chronic
    primarily due to infection, 358 (1)
    primarily due to trauma, 359 (4)
  due to foreign body, 359 (4)
  senile, 359 (7)
Cervix uteri. *See also* Uterus
  abscess of cervical stump, 358 (1)
  absence, 358 (0)
  adhesions, cervicovaginal
    congenital, 358 (0)
    following parturition, 359 (4)
  atresia, congenital, 358 (0)
  atrophy
    at menopause, 359 (7)
    senile, 359 (7)
  calcification, 359 (9)
  carcinoma in situ. *Diagnose as* Epidermoid carcinoma, 94
  cervical os, incompetent, 359 (4)
    congenital, 358 (0)
  cicatrix
    due to trauma, 359 (4), 374 (4)
    following operation, 359 (4), 374 (4)
    following parturition, 359 (4), 374 (4)
    during pregnancy, 373 (1)
  contraction, abnormal, obstetric, 375 (55)
  cyst
    due to trauma, 359 (4)
    embryonal, 358 (0)

Cervix uteri—Continued
cyst—continued
nabothian, 359 (6)
detachment, annular, 359 (4), 374
(4)
diseases, 358 ff.
displacement of cuboidal epithelium
beyond external os, 358 (0)
diverticulum, congenital, 358 (0)
edema, obstetric, acute, 374 (4)
embryoma. *Diagnose as* Mesenchymal mixed tumor, 98
erosion
cause unknown, 359 (9)
due to chemicals, 358 (3)
due to infection, 358 (1)
primarily due to trauma, 359 (4)
eversion (ectropion)
due to infection, 358 (1)
due to lacerations, 359 (4)
external os, division into two openings by frenum, 358 (0)
fetal form, persistence, 358 (0)
hemorrhage following operation, 359
(4)
hyperplasia, basal cell, 359 (9)
hypertrophy
congenital, 358 (0)
primarily due to trauma, 359 (4)
hypoplasia, congenital, 358 (0)
injury, 359 (4)
laceration, 359 (4)
obstetric, 374 (4)
leukoplakia, 359 (9)
metaplasis, 359 (9)
neoplasms, 364 (8)
polyp
due to infection, 358 (1)
simple, 359 (9)
prolapse of cervical stump due to
operation, 359 (4)
prolapse of hypertrophied, congenital, 358 (0)
rigidity during labor, 375 (6)
sarcoma, 364 (8)
squamous epithelium in cervical
canal, 358 (0)
stricture
due to infection, 358 (1)
due to trauma, 359 (4)
following operation, 359 (4)
following parturition, 359 (4)
trichomonas infection, 358 (1)

Cervix uteri—Continued
tumor cells in secretions: *supplementary term,* 499. *Diagnose
disease*
Cestan syndrome: *supplementary
term,* 503. *Diagnose disease*
Cestodes
list, 65
Cevitamic acid in blood: *supplementary terms. Diagnose disease*
decrease, 493
increase, 494
Chafing. *See* Intertrigo, 136 (4)
Chagas' disease. *See* Trypanosomiasis, American, 116 (1)
Chalazion, 463 (7)
Chalcosis
of cornea, 435 (3)
Chancre. *See also* syphilis *under organ affected*
soft. *See* Chancroid
Chancroid, 132 (1). *See also* Ulcus
molle cutis, 132 (1)
of anus, 284 (1)
of penis, 329 (1)
of rectum, 281 (1)
of scrotum, 339 (1)
of urethra, 323 (1)
of vulva, 352 (1)
Charcot joint (neurogenic arthropathy), 162 (55)
Charcot-Leyden crystals in sputum: *supplementary term,* 490.
Diagnose disease
Charcot-Marie-Tooth disease. *See*
Progressive neuropathic (peroneal) muscular atrophy, 425 (9)
Charcot's syndrome. *See* Angiospasm of arteries of leg and foot,
217 (5)
Cheating personality, 112 (x)
Cheek. *See also* Buccal cavity; Mouth
cutaneous horn, 242 (9)
epidermoid carcinoma, 241 (8)
Cheilitis
actinic, 243 (4)
due to infection, 243 (1)
exfoliata, 140 (9)
glandular, 140 (9)
Cheilosis (riboflavin deficiency), 121
(7), 244 (7)
Cheiromegaly: *supplementary term,*
484. *Diagnose disease*

Chemicals
  burns due to. *See* Burns, chemical;
    *and under organ, region or
    structure affected*
  irritant, chronic hypertrophic rhini-
    tis due to, 177 (3)
  poison. *See also* Poison and poison-
    ing
  acute rhinitis due to, 177 (3)
Chemodectoma. *Diagnose as* Carotid
  body tumor, 98
Chest. *See also* Thorax
  deformity, heart disease due to, 211
    (6)
  funnel, congenital, 146 (0)
  wall
    empyema perforating, 198 (1)
    fistula following operation, 126
      (4)
    hydropneumothorax due to injury
      of, 199 (4)
    pneumothorax due to injury of,
      200 (4)
    pyoneumothorax due to injury of,
      200 (4)
    weakness in (flail chest): *supple-
      mentary term, 490. Diagnose
      disease*
    wound, 127 (4)
Chiari's network, 202 (0)
Chiari's syndrome. *See* Endophlebitis of hepatic veins, 304 (9)
Chiari-Arnold syndrome. *See* Caudal displacement of brain stem,
  cerebellum and spinal cord, 402
  (0)
Chickenpox, 114 (1)
Chigger infestation, 134 (2)
Chilblain, 126 (4), 137 (4)
Child
  adjustment reaction, 112 (x)
  feeding problem: *supplementary
    term, 485. Diagnose disease*
  nursing, 482
Childbed fever. *See* Septicemia,
  puerperal, 116 (1)
Childbirth. *See* Birth; Delivery; Labor; Parturition; Puerperium
Chills
  and fever, urethral, 324 (4)
  *supplementary term, 484. Diagnose
    disease*

Chilly sensations: *supplementary
  term, 484. Diagnose disease*
Chilomastix infection
  of intestine, 268 (1)
Chimney sweeps' carcinoma. *Diagnose as* Epidermoid carcinoma, 94
Chin, abnormal smallness. *See* Microgenia, 153 (7)
Chloasma, 138 (7)
  of eyelids, 462 (4), 463 (7)
  due to trauma, 462 (4)
Chloral
  liver degeneration due to, 288 (3)
Chloroform
  liver degeneration due to, 288 (3)
  poisoning
    acute, 117 (3)
    of heart by, 209 (3)
Chloroma; chloromyeloma. *Diagnose as* Leukosarcoma, 95
Chlorosarcoma. *Diagnose as* Leukosarcoma, 95
Choana, atresia, congenital, 176 (0)
Choked disk. *See* Papilledema
Cholangiolitis, 292 (1)
Cholangioma, 94
  of bile passages, 294 (8)
  of liver, 289 (8)
Cholangitis, 292 (1)
  obliterative, cirrhosis of liver with,
    .congenital, 287 (0)
Cholecystitis
  acute, 292 (1)
  chronic, 292 (1)
  due to trauma, 293 (4)
  gangrenous, 292 (1)
  paratyphoidal, 292 (1)
  with perforation, acute, 292 (1)
  typhoidal, 292 (1)
Cholelithiasis, 293 (6). *See also* Calculus in gallbladder, 293 (6)
Cholemia: *supplementary term, 493.
  Diagnose disease*
Cholera, 114 (1)
Cholesterol
  decrease in esters: *supplementary
    term, 493. Diagnose disease*
  deposit in retina, 448 (7)
  imbibition of gallbladder, 294 (9)
Cholesterosis, 129 (9)
Chondritis, 157 (1)
Chondroblastoma, 97, 154 (8)

Chondrocarcinoma, 97
  salivary gland type. *Diagnose as*
    Mixed tumor, salivary gland
    type, 98
Chondrodermatitis nodular
  of ear, 476 (9)
Chondrodysplasia. *See* Dyschondroplasia, 147 (0)
Chondrodystrophia foetalis. *See*
  Achondroplasia, 146 (0)
Chondroendothelioma. *Diagnose as*
  Osteosarcoma (osteogenic sarcoma), 97
Chondrofibroma. *Diagnose as* Chondroblastoma, 97
Chondrofibrosarcoma; chondro-
  liposarcoma. *Diagnose as* Chondrosarcoma, 97
Chondroma, 97, 154 (8)
  branchial. *Diagnose as* Branchioma,
    98
  medullary. *Diagnose as* Giant cell
    tumor of bone, 97
  multiple; multiple ossifying. *Diag-*
    nose as Chondroma, 97
Chondromalacia
  due to trauma, 158 (4)
  due to unknown cause, 129 (9)
  of patella due to trauma, 150 (4)
Chondromyxoma. *Diagnose as* Chondroma, 97
Chondromyxohemangioendothelio-
  sarcoma. *Diagnose as* Mixed tumor, salivary gland type, 98
Chondromyxosarcoma. *Diagnose as*
  Chondrosarcoma, 97
Chondro-osteoma. *Diagnose as* Osteoma, 97
Chondro-osteosarcoma. *Diagnose as*
  Osteosarcoma (osteogenic sar-
  coma), 97
Chondrosarcoma, 154 (8)
Chordae tendineae
  anomalous, 203 (0)
  rupture due to infection, 208 (1)
Chordee, 329 (1)
Chorditis
  due to overstrain, 184 (4)
  fibrinous, due to poisonous gas or
    fumes, 183 (3)
Chordoma, 98
Chorea, 411 (1)

Chorea—Continued
  chronic progressive
    hereditary, 416 (9)
    nonhereditary, 416 (9)
  gravidarum, 412 (3)
  supplementary term, 503. *Diagnose*
    disease
Choreoathetosis: *supplementary*
  term, 503. *Diagnose disease*
Chorioadenoma, 97, 384 (8)
  destruens. *Diagnose as* Chorioade-
    noma, 97
Chorioangioma. *Diagnose as* Hydatiform mole, 97
Choriocarcinoma, 97, 384 (8)
Chorioepithelioma; Chorioepithe-
  lioma malignum. *Diagnose as*
  Choriocarcinoma, 97
Chorioma; Chorioma ectodermale.
  Diagnose as Choriocarcinoma, 97
Chorioncarcinoma. *Diagnose as*
  Choriocarcinoma, 97
Chorioretinitis, 446 (1)
  due to trauma, 447 (4)
  of progressive myopia, 448 (6)
Choristoma. *Diagnose as* Hamartoma, 98
Choroid
  atrophia gyrata of retina and, 441
    (5)
  atrophy, 441 (9)
  coloboma, 441 (0)
    of retina and, 446 (0)
  crescent or conus, congenital, 441
    (0)
  degeneration, 441 (9)
  detachment
    due to hemorrhage, 441 (5)
    due to infection, 441 (1)
    due to trauma, 441 (4)
    following operation, 441 (4)
  diseases, 441 ff.
  drusen, 441 (9)
  hemangioma, 441 (8)
  injury, 441 (4)
  melanoma, malignant, 441 (8)
  neoplasms, 441 (8)
  neurofibroma, 441 (8)
  pigmented nevus, 441 (8)
  rupture, 441 (4)
  tumors, unlisted, 441 (8)

Clouded states, paroxysmal: *supplementary term,* 485. *Diagnose disease*
Clubbed fingers, 128 (7)
Clubfoot. *See also* Talipes
  cogenital paralytic (in spina bifida), 157 (0)
  overlapping fifth toe with, 123 (0)
Clubhand, congenital, 156 (0)
Coagulation
  supplementary terms. Diagnose disease
  decrease, 493
  increase, 494
Coalition, congenital. *See* Segmentation, incomplete (synostosis), 147 (0)
Coarctation of aorta, 204 (0)
Cocaine
  poisoning, 117 (3)
Coccidioidin test reaction
  supplementary term, 487. *Diagnose disease*
Coccidioidomycosis, 124 (2). *See also under organ or region affected*
  generalized, 116 (2)
Coccidiosis
  generalized, 114 (1)
  of liver, 287 (1)
  of peritoneum, 298 (1)
Coccygodynia, 169 (55). *Supplementary term,* 489. *Diagnose disease*
Codeine. *See* Opium, 117 (3)
Codman's tumor. *Diagnose as* Chondroblastoma, 97
Coitus, painful. *See* Dyspareunia
Cold. *See also* Freezing, 118 (4)
  common, 175 (1)
  exhaustion from, 118 (4)
  gangrene due to, 126 (4)
  myositis (mygelosis) due to, 168 (4)
  sensation of: *supplementary terms. Diagnose disease*
    absence, 501
    diminution, 503
    increase, 505
  torticollis, acute, due to, 164 (4)
Coldsore. *See* Herpes of lip, 243 (1)
Colic, renal: *supplementary term,* 499. *Diagnose disease*
Colitis. *See also* Enterocolitis
  acute, 276 (1)
    due to poison, 277 (3)

Colitis—Continued
  amebic, 276 (1)
  balantidial, 276 (1)
  chronic, 276 (1)
    due to poison, 276 (3)
  parasitic, 277 (2)
  regional, 278 (9)
  ulcerative, 278 (9)
    left-sided or universal, 278 (9)
    right-sided or regional, 278 (9)
    sacro-parasympathetic, 278 (55)
Collagen disease, 121 (y)
Collapse: *supplementary term,* 484. *Diagnose disease*
Colles' fracture, 150 (4)
Colliculitis, 323 (1)
  due to poison, 324 (3)
Colliculus seminalis. *See* Verumontanum
Colloid degeneration, 129 (9)
  of eyelid, 464 (9)
  of skin, 140 (9)
Colloidal benzoin test, positive: *supplementary term,* 503. *Diagnose disease*
Colloidal gold test, reactions: *supplementary terms,* 503. *Diagnose disease*
Coloboma
  of choroid, 441 (0)
  of ciliary body, 439 (0)
  of eyelid, congenital, 461 (0)
  of iris, 439 (0)
    following operation, 440 (4)
  of lens, 442 (0)
  of optic nerve, 450 (0)
  of retina, 446 (0)
    and choroid, 446 (0)
Colon. *See also* Colitis; Enterocolitis
  abnormality of opaque enema: *supplementary term,* 496. *Diagnose disease*
  abscess of wall, 276 (1)
  adenocarcinoma, 278 (8)
  adhesions due to infection, 276 (1)
  atony, 278 (55)
  calculus in. *See* Enterolith, 278 (6)
  cyst, 278 (6)
  dilatation, 278 (6)
    congenital, 276 (0)
  diseases, 276 ff.
  diverticulitis, 278 (6)
  diverticulosis, 278 (6)

Colon—Continued
  diverticulum, congenital, 276 (0)
  duplication, congenital, 276 (0)
  fistula
    between bladder and, 318 (1), 318
      (4)
    between gallbladder and, due to
      calculus, 278 (6)
    due to infection, 277 (1)
    gastrocolic, 267 (1)
    gastrojejunocolic, 267 (9)
    postoperative, 277 (4)
  gangrene due to disturbance of cir-
    culation, 277 (5)
  granuloma due to unknown cause,
    278 (9)
  hernia, congenital, 276 (0)
  injury, 277 (4)
  intussusception, 278 (6)
  irritability, 278 (55)
  melanosis: *supplementary term,* 496.
    Diagnose disease
  megacolon, congenital. *See also*
    Colon, dilatation, 276 (0)
  microcolon, congenital, 276 (0)
  neoplasms, 278 (8)
  nondescent, 276 (0)
  obstruction following operation, 277
    (4)
  oxyuriasis, 277 (2)
  polyp, neoplastic, 278 (8)
  ptosis, 278 (6)
  redundancy, congenital, 276 (0)
  rotation, incomplete, 276 (0)
  rupture due to infection, 277 (1)
  spastic. *See* Colon, irritability, 278
    (55)
  strangulation due to hernia, 277 (5)
  stricture
    due to infection, 277 (1)
    due to simple ulcer, 278 (9)
  transposition, congenital, 276 (0)
  trichuriasis, 277 (2)
  triplication, congenital, 276 (0)
  tumors, unlisted, 278 (8)
  ulcer
    granulocytopenic, 277 (5)
    simple, with perforation, 278 (9)
  valve formation, congenital, 276
    (0)
  varix, 278 (6)
  volvulus, 278 (6)

Color blindness
  congenital, 446 (0)
    Hering classification, 446 (0)
  supplementary term, 508. *Diagnose*
    disease
Colorado tick fever, 115 (1)
Colostomy (artificial anus), 277 (4)
  malfunctioning, 277 (4)
  stenosis, 277 (4)
Colpitis. *See also* Pyocolpos; Vagini-
    tis
  adhesive, congenital, 355 (0)
Coma: *supplementary term,* 503. *Di-*
    agnose disease
Comedo, 138 (7)
  mastitis, 145 (9)
Comedocarcinoma; comedocarci-
    noma in situ. *Diagnose as* Duc-
    tal tumor, not otherwise specified,
    93
Common bile duct. *See under* Bile
    passages
Common cold, 175 (1). *See also*
    Nasopharyngitis; Rhinitis
Commotio retinae, 447 (4)
Commotion. *See also* Concussion of
    brain, 413 (4)
  of spinal cord, 424 (4)
Compound presentation, 382 (6)
Compression
  of cranial nerve, 429 (4)
  of spinal cord, 423 (4)
Compulsions: *supplementary term,*
    484. *Diagnose disease*
Compulsive personality, 112 (x)
Compulsive reaction, obsessive,
    112 (x)
Compulsive talking: *supplementary*
    term, 503. *Diagnose disease*
Concretion. *See* Calculus; *and under*
    organ, region or structure af-
    fected
Concussion
  of brain, 413 (4)
  of spinal cord, 424 (4)
  syndrome. *See* Encephalopathy due
    to remote trauma, 412 (1)
Conductive system (cardiac). *See*
    under Heart
Condyloma acuminatum. *See also*
    Verruca acuminata, 134 (1)
  of anus, 284 (1)
  of penis, 329 (1)

Condyloma acuminatum—Continued
  syphilitic, 352 (1)
  of vulva
    due to filth, 353 (4)
    due to infection, 352 (1)
Confabulation: *supplementary term,*
  503. *Diagnose disease*
Congenital defects. *See also under*
  organ, region or structure affected
  list, 55
Congestion. *See also under organ,*
  region or structure affected
  due to disturbance of circulation, 127
    (5)
Conglutination, 375 (6)
Conjunctiva. *See also under organ,*
  region or structure affected
  abscess, 468 (1)
  adhesions, congenital, 468 (0)
  amyloidosis, 471 (9)
  atrophy, senile, 470 (7)
  birth injury, 468 (0)
  burn, 469 (4)
  carcinoma
    basal cell, 470 (8)
    epidermoid, 470 (8)
  concretions in, 471 (9)
  cyanosis, 470 (5)
  cyst, 469 (4)
  diphtheria, 468 (1)
  diseases, 468 ff.
  edema due to Trichinella, 469 (2)
  emphysema, 469 (4)
  fibroma, 471 (8)
  foreign body in, 470 (4)
  granulation following operation, 470
    (4)
  hemangioma, 471 (8)
  hemorrhage
    due to unknown cause, 470 (5)
    subconjunctival, due to remote in-
      jury, 470 (4)
  herpes, 468 (1)
    iris (erythema multiforme), 468
      (1)
  hyaline degeneration, 471 (9)
  hyperemia
    due to eyestrain, 470 (4)
    due to paralysis of sympathetic
      nervous system, 470 (5)
  injury, 470 (4)
  leprosy, 468 (1)
  lipoma, 471 (8)

Conjunctiva—Continued
  lymphangiectasis, 470 (5)
  lymphangioma, 471 (8)
  lymphoma, 471 (8)
  lymphosarcoma, 471 (8)
  melanoma, malignant, 471 (8)
  myiasis, 469 (2)
  neoplasms, 470 (8)
  neurofibroma, 471 (8)
  nevus
    pigmented, 471 (8)
  orbital, necrosis due to foreign body,
    470 (4)
  pemphigus, 471 (9)
  polyp, simple, 471 (9)
  pressure of prosthesis, lesion due to,
    470 (4)
  radium necrosis, 470 (4)
  roentgen ray burn, 470 (4)
  sarcoma, 471 (8)
  syphilis, 468 (1)
  trachomatous contraction, 468 (1)
  tuberculosis, 468 (1)
  tumors, unlisted, 471 (8)
  ulceration due to infection, 468 (1)
  urticaria, 469 (3)
  vaccinia, 469 (1)
  variola, 469 (1)
  xerosis, 470 (7)
  zoster, 469 (1)
Conjunctivitis
  acne rosacea, 470 (5)
  allergic, 469 (3)
  caterpillar, 469 (2)
  chronic, 468 (1)
    due to physical agent, 469 (4)
    due to smoke, 469 (4)
  due to lagophthalmos, 469 (4)
  due to paralysis of fifth nerve, 470
    (55)
  due to poison, 469 (3)
  eczematous, 469 (3)
  follicular, 468 (1)
  hay fever, 469 (3)
  infectious, acute, 468 (1)
  tularensis, 468 (1)
  with urethritis and arthritis
    (Reiter's disease), 116 (1)
  vernal (spring catarrh), 469 (3)
Constipation, 269 (x)
  supplementary term, 496. *Diagnose*
    disease

Constriction
by anomalous bands, 122 (0)
ring, 375 (55)
Constructional apraxia: *supplementary term,* 503. *Diagnose disease*
Contraction. *See also* Contracture
of ligaments, congenital, 156 (0)
ring, 375 (55)
Contracture. *See also* Fascia; Joints;
Muscles; *and under organ or
structure affected*
Dupuytren's, 174 (9)
supplementary term, 489. *Diagnose
disease*
Volkmann's. *See* Contracture due to
ischemia, 169 (5)
Contusion. *See also under organ, region or structure affected*
multiple, 118 (4)
Conus (crescent)
of choroid, congenital, 441 (0)
Conversion reaction, 112 (x)
Convulsions, generalized: *supplementary term,* 503. *Diagnose disease*
Convulsive disorders
non-epileptic, 481
Cooley's anemia, 231 (9)
Copper. *See also* Chalcosis
liver degeneration due to, 288 (3)
Cor biloculare, 203 (0)
Cor pulmonale
due to pulmonary arterial hypertension, 210 (5)
Cor triloculare
biatrium, 203 (0)
biventricularis, 202 (0)
Cord presentation, 385 (6)
Corectopia, 439 (0)
Corn. *See* Clavus, 136 (4)
Cornea. *See also* Descemet's membrane; Keratitis; Limbus
abrasion, 435 (4)
abscess, 434 (1)
argyrosis, 434 (3)
blood staining, 436 (5)
burn, 435 (4)
from radium, 435 (4)
from roentgen rays, 435 (4)
carcinoma, epidermoid, 437 (8)
chalcosis, 435 (3)
changes due to defects in Descemet's
membrane, 434 (0), 436 (4)

Cornea—Continued
chemical burn, 435 (3)
contusion, 436 (4)
degeneration
familial, 437 (9)
lipid, following keratitis, 437 (9)
diseases, 434 ff.
dystrophy
endothelial, 437 (9)
epithelial, 437 (9)
marginal, 437 (9)
ectasia. *See also* Keratectasia, 434
(0)
due to infection, 434 (1)
erosion, recurrent, 436 (4)
fistula
due to infection, 434 (1)
due to trauma, 436 (4)
foreign body in, 436 (4)
guttata (endothelial dystrophy), 437
(9)
herpes, keratitis, 434 (1)
infiltrate, 434 (1)
injury, 436 (4)
by foreign body, 436 (4)
keloid, 437 (8)
keratomycosis, 435 (2)
lead incrustation, 435 (3)
leprosy, 434 (1)
linea corneae senilis, 436 (7)
melanosis, 436 (7)
congenital, 434 (0)
following uveitis, 435 (1)
metallic incrustation, 435 (3)
neoplasms, 437 (8)
neurofibroma, 437 (8)
opacity
congenital (leukoma), 434 (0)
due to aniline, 435 (3)
due to infection, 435 (1)
due to poison, 435 (3)
due to trauma, 436 (4)
perforation due to infection, 435
(1)
plana, 434 (0)
rupture due to increased intraocular
pressure, 436 (4)
scald, 436 (4)
siderosis, 435 (3)
due to unknown cause, 437 (9)
staphyloma, 435 (1)
due to chemical burn, 435 (3)
due to infection, 435 (1)

Cyanosis—Continued

of retina due to intoxication by organic poison, 447 (3)

supplementary term, 487. *Diagnose disease*

Cyclophoria, 457 (x)

Cyclopia, 433 (0)

Cyclothymic personality, 112 (x)

Cyclotropia, 456 (5)

Cylindroma

of bronchus. *Diagnose as* Adenoma, 94

except of bronchus. *Diagnose as* Sweat gland tumor, 94

Cyst

apical, 247 (1)

atheromatous cutaneous. *Diagnose as* Neoplastic cyst, 93

Baker's. *See* Ganglion of knee joint, 162 (6)

bone, malignant hemorrhagic. *Diagnose as* Osteosarcoma (osteogenic sarcoma), 97

branchial; branchial cleft; branchial inclusion. *Diagnose as* Branchioma, 98

calcified. *Diagnose as* Neoplastic cyst, 93

chocolate. *Diagnose as* Adenomyosis, 98

cutaneous. *Diagnose as* Neoplastic cyst, 93

dental. *Diagnose as* Odontogenic tumor, benign, 98

dentigerous, 249 (9)

dermoid

except of tooth. *Diagnose as* Teratoma, 97

with foreign body reaction. *Diagnose as* Teratoma, 97

of tooth. *Diagnose as* Odontogenic tumor, benign, 98

due to undetermined cause, 130 (y)

ectopic endometrial. *Diagnose as* Adenomyosis, 98

epidermal, 131 (0)

epidermoid, 131 (0)

epithelial inclusion. *Diagnose as* Neoplastic cyst, 93

fibrosed. *Diagnose as* Neoplastic cyst, 93

Cyst—Continued

follicular

except of tooth. *Diagnose as* Neoplastic cyst, 93

of tooth. *Diagnose as* Odontogenic tumor, benign, 98

gill cleft. *Diagnose as* Craniopharyngioma, 98

glandular proliferous. *Diagnose as* Cystosarcoma phyllodes, 97

hairy. *Diagnose as* Teratoma, 97

hereditary sebaceous. *Diagnose as* Neoplastic cyst, 93

implantation, due to trauma, 136 (4)

lymphatic. *Diagnose as* Lymphangioma, 96

mixed. *Diagnose as* Teratoma, 97

mucosal; mucosal inclusion. *Diagnose as* Neoplastic cyst, 93

mucous

except of ovary. *Diagnose as* Neoplastic cyst, 93

of ovary. *Diagnose as* Pseudomucinous cystic tumor, 93

multilocular

except of ovary. *Diagnose as* Neoplastic cyst, 93

of ovary. *Diagnose as* Pseudomucinous cystic tumor, 93

multiple; multiple follicular. *Diagnose as* Neoplastic cyst, 93

nabothian, 359 (6)

neoplastic, 93

odontogenic, of tooth. *Diagnose as* Odontogenic tumor, benign, 98

papillary serous. *Diagnose as* Serous papillary cystic tumor, 93

parovarian. *Diagnose as* Neoplastic cyst, 93

pilonidal, 122 (0)

pseudomucinous; pseudomucinous multilocular. *Diagnose as* Pseudomucinous cystic tumor, 93

retention, of Bartholin's gland, due to infection, 352 (1)

Sampson's. *Diagnose as* Adenomyosis, 98

sebaceous. *Diagnose as* Sebaceous tumor, 94

serous. *Diagnose as* Serous papillary cystic tumor, 93

simple dermoid. *Diagnose as* Teratoma, 97

Cyst—Continued
squamous epithelial. *Diagnose as* Neoplastic cyst, 93
synovial. *Diagnose as* Ganglion of tendon sheath, 97
teratoid; teratoid dermoid; teratomatous. *Diagnose as* Teratoma, 97
tracheobronchial, congenital. *Diagnose as* Hamartoma, 98
Cystadenocarcinoma
not otherwise specified. *Diagnose as* Serous papillary cystic tumor, 93
papillary; papillary serous. *Diagnose as* Serous papillary cystic tumor, 93
pseudomucinous; pseudomucinous papillary. *Diagnose as* Mucinous carcinoma, 93
sebaceous. *Diagnose as* Sebaceous tumor, 94
serous. *Diagnose as* Serous papillary cystic tumor, 93
Cystadenoma, 93
epithelial. *Diagnose as* Sweat gland tumor, 94
lymphomatosum; lymphomatosum, papillary. *Diagnose as* Adenolymphoma, 98
mucinous; mucous. *Diagnose as* Pseudomucinous cystic tumor, 93
papillary
except of ovary, salivary gland, thyroid. *Diagnose as* Papillary or polypoid tumor, not otherwise specified, 93
of ovary, thyroid. *Diagnose as* Serous papillary cystic tumor, 93
of salivary gland. *Diagnose as* Adenolymphoma, 98
serous. *Diagnose as* Serous papillary cystic tumor, 93
pseudomucinous. *Diagnose as* Pseudomucinous cystic tumor, 93
malignant. *Diagnose as* Mucinous carcinoma, 93
papillary. *Diagnose as* Pseudomucinous cystic tumor, 93
of salivary gland. *Diagnose as* Adenolymphoma, 98

Cystadenoma—Continued
sebaceous. *Diagnose as* Sebaceous tumor, 94
Cystadenosarcoma (breast). *Diagnose as* Cystosarcoma phyllodes, 97
Cystic duct. *See under* Bile passages
Cysticercosis, 125 (2), 134 (2). *See also under organ, region or structure affected*
Cystinosis, 120 (7)
Cystitis. *See also* Pericystitis, 318 (1)
acute, 317 (1)
due to calculus, 320 (6)
due to obstruction, 320 (6)
exudative, 317 (1)
hemorrhagic, 317 (1)
allergic, 318 (3)
chemical, 318 (3)
chronic, 317 (1)
glandularis, 317 (1)
cystica, 321 (9)
due to infection, 318 (1)
due to trauma, 318 (4)
follicularis, 321 (9)
gangrenous, 318 (1)
interstitial, 321 (9)
with ulceration, 321 (9)
Cystocele, 318 (4)
Cystoepithelioma
chorioectodermale. *Diagnose as* Disgerminoma, 97
epidermal. *Diagnose as* Disgerminoma, 97
Cystofibroma papillare (breast). *Diagnose as* Cystosarcoma phyllodes, 97
Cystoma
pseudomucinous, carcinomatous. *Diagnose as* Mucinous carcinoma, 93
Cystosarcoma. *Diagnose as* Cystosarcoma phyllodes, 97
gelatinous. *Diagnose as* Cystosarcoma phyllodes, 97
phyllodes, 97
miniature. *Diagnose as* Cystosarcoma phyllodes, 97
Cystostomy, opening, 318 (4)
Cytology test, 481
Cytomegalic inclusion disease
generalized, 115 (1)

D

Dacryoadenitis, 465 (1)

Dacryocystitis, 465 (1)

Dacryolith. *See* Lacrimal gland, calculus, 466 (6)

Dacryops, 466 (6)

Dacryostenosis. *See* stenosis *under* Canaliculus; Lacrimal passages; Lacrimonasal duct

Dactylolysis spontanea (ainhum), 129 (9)

Dana-Putnam syndrome. *See* Dorsolateral sclerosis: *supplementary term,* 503

Dandy fever. *See* Dengue, 115 (1)

Darling's disease. *See* Histoplasmosis, 124 (2)

Darwin's tubercle, 474 (0)

Day blindness: *supplementary term,* 508. *Diagnose disease*

Dead on arrival, 481

Deaf-mutism

acquired, 414 (7)

symptomatic: *supplementary term,* 508. *Diagnose disease*

Deafness. *See also* Hearing

acoustic trauma resulting in, 472 (4)

blue sclera and fragility of bone with, 438 (9)

conduction

otosclerosis, with fixation of stapes, 480 (7)

supplementary term, 508. *Diagnose disease*

due to degeneration of acoustic nerve, 480 (9)

due to undetermined cause, 480 (9)

high frequency, 479 (0)

low frequency, 479 (0)

middle ear: *supplementary term,* 509. *Diagnose disease*

nerve

primary, otosclerosis, without stapes fixation, 480 (7)

supplementary term, 509. *Diagnose disease*

sensory, neural

due to drug, 479 (3)

due to otosclerosis, 480 (7)

due to trauma, 480 (4)

unspecified: *supplementary term,* 508. *Diagnose disease*

Deafness—Continued

word development: *supplementary term,* 503, 510. *Diagnose disease*

Debility

amenorrhea due to, 363 (7)

Decapitation, 126 (4)

Decidua

retention of decidual fragment, 383 (6)

Deciduitis, acute, 373 (1)

Deciduoma malignum. *Diagnose as* Chorioadenoma, 97

Decubitus ulcer, 136 (4)

of sacrococcygeal region, 285 (4)

Deer fly fever. *See* Tularemia, 116 (1)

Deficiency

diseases. *See* Hypovitaminosis; *and name of specific disease*

mental. *See* Mental deficiency

moral: *supplementary term,* 484. *Diagnose disease*

Deformity. *See also under organ, region or structure affected, or name of specific disease*

due to burn (from heat), 126 (4)

due to trauma, 126 (4)

following operation, 126 (4)

Degeneration. *See* Fatty degeneration; Hyaline degeneration

Dehydration. *See also* Water, deprivation of, 119 (7)

supplementary term, 484. *Diagnose disease*

Déjerine-Roussy syndrome: *supplementary term,* 503. *Diagnose disease*

Déjerine-Sottas neuropathy. *See* Progressive hypertrophic interstitial neuropathy, 431 (9)

Delayed union following fracture, 151 (4)

Délire de toucher: *supplementary term,* 484. *Diagnose disease*

Delirium: *supplementary term,* 503. *Diagnose disease*

Delirium tremens, 106 (3)

Delivery. *See also* Birth

discharged before, 482

immature, 377

threatened, 377

Delivery—Continued
  premature, 377
    threatened, 377
  term, 378
Delusions: *supplementary term,* 503.
  Diagnose disease
Dementia: *supplementary term,* 503.
  Diagnose disease
Dementia paralytica
  juvenilis, 411 (1)
  without psychosis, 411 (1)
Dementia precox. *See* Schizophrenic
  reactions, 110 (x)
Demetri-Sturge-Weber disease.
  Diagnose as Hemangiomatosis,
  96
DeMorgan spot. *Diagnose as* He-
  mangioma (angioma), 96
Dengue, 115 (1)
Dens in dente, 249 (7)
Dental. *See* Teeth
Dentia precox. *See* Precocious denti-
  tion, 247 (0), 249 (9)
Dentigerous cyst, 249 (9)
Dentin, opalescent, 247 (0)
Dentinogenesis imperfecta, 247 (0)
Dentinoma. *Diagnose as* Odontogenic
  tumor, benign, 98
Dentition
  precocious, 247 (0), 249 (9)
  retarded, 249 (7)
Depersonalization: *supplementary
  term,* 484. *Diagnose disease*
Depression: *supplementary term,* 484.
  Diagnose disease
Depressive reaction, 112 (x)
  psychotic, 110 (x)
Dercum's disease. *See* Adiposis do-
  lorosa, 120 (7)
Dermalipoma. *Diagnose as* Lipoma,
  97
Dermatalgia, 138 (55)
Dermatitis. *See also* Acarodermati-
  tis; Acrodermatitis; Dermatosis;
  Eczema; Neurodermatitis
  actinica
    due to roentgen rays or radioactive
      substance, 136 (4)
    due to ultraviolet radiation, 136
      (4)
  atopic, 141 (9)
    cataract with, 442 (3)
  berlock, 135 (3)

Dermatitis—Continued
  caterpillar, 134 (2)
  chigger, 134 (2)
  demodex, 134 (2)
  of eyelid due to poison, 462 (3)
  due to undetermined cause, 142
    (y)
  escharotica, 135 (3)
  exfoliativa, 140 (9)
    neonatal, 140 (9)
  factitial, 136 (4)
  gangrenous, of newborn, 140 (9)
  herpetiform, 140 (9)
  hypostatica, 137 (5)
  infectious eczematoid, 132 (1)
  medicamentosa, 135 (3)
  papillaris capillitii. *See* Folliculitis,
    keloidal, 132 (1)
  photomelanotic, 135 (3)
  purpuric lichenoid, 137 (5)
  seborrheic, 132 (1)
  vegetative, 132 (1)
  venenata, 135 (3)
Dermatofibroma. *Diagnose as* Fibroma, 96
  progressive and recurring. *Diagnose
    as* Fibrosarcoma, 96
Dermatofibrosarcoma
  protuberans. *Diagnose as* Fibrosar-
    coma, 96
Dermatographia: *supplementary
  term,* 487. *Diagnose disease*
Dermatomegaly (cutis laxa), 131
  (0)
Dermatomycosis, 134 (2)
Dermatomyositis, 170 (9)
Dermatophytid, 135 (3)
Dermatophytosis, 134 (2)
Dermatopolyneuritis. *See* Erythre-
  dema polyneuropathy, 431 (x)
Dermatosis. *See also* Dermatitis;
  Skin, diseases
  papulosa nigra, 141 (9)
  progressive pigmentary, 137 (5)
Dermographia, 137 (5)
Dermoid. *Diagnose as* Teratoma, 97
Dermolipoma. *Diagnose as* Lipoma,
  97
Descemet's membrane
  defect, 436 (4)
    congenital, corneal changes due to,
      434 (0)
Descemetocele, 434 (1)

Desert sore, 142 (9)
Desmoid. *Diagnose as* Fibroma, 96
Destructiveness: *supplementary term,* 484. *Diagnose disease*
Developmental apraxia, 502
Devic's disease. *See* Optic neuroen-cephalomyelopathy, 404 (9)
Devil's grip. *See* Pleurodynia, epidemic, 198 (1)
Dextrocardia
  with situs inversus, 202 (0)
  true, 202 (0)
Dextrose tolerance: *supplementary terms. Diagnose disease*
  decreased, 500
  increased, 500
Diabetes, bronze. *See* Hemochromatosis, 128 (7)
Diabetes insipidus
  due to unknown cause, 394 (7)
  supplementary term, 484. *Diagnose disease*
Diabetes mellitus, 398 (7)
  cataract in, 443 (7)
  change of refraction due to, 454 (7)
  dorsal sclerosis in, 424 (7)
  encephalomyelopathy due to, 403 (7)
  gangrene, 128 (7)
  with hyperadrenalcorticism, 398 (7)
  with hyperfunction of chromaffin tissue, 398 (7)
  with hyperpituitarism, 398 (7)
  with hyperthyroidism, 398 (7)
  with hypoadrenalcorticism, 398 (7)
  with hypopituitarism, 398 (7)
  with hypothyroidism, 398 (7)
  without known cause or structural change, 398 (x)
  melanosis of cornea in, 436 (7)
  myeloradiculopathy due to, 425 (7)
  necrobiosis lipoidica diabeticorum, 139 (7)
  nephrosis due to, 311 (7)
  neuropathy in, 430 (7)
  retinal hemorrhage due to, 448 (7)
  retinopathy in, 448 (7)
  with sclerosis of insular tissue, 398 (9)
  ulcer, 128 (7)
  vulvitis, 453 (7)
  xanthoma diabeticorum, 139 (7)
Diagnosis deferred, 401

Diaper rash. *See* Erythema gluteale, 135 (3)
Diaphragm
  avulsion, peripheral, 171 (4)
  defect
    congenital, 171 (0)
    intrathoracic kidney with, 307 (0)
  diseases, 171 ff.
  elevation, congenital, 171 (0)
  enlargement of normal apertures, congenital, 171 (0)
  eventration, congenital, 171 (0)
  fistula, 171 (1)
  gunshot wound, 171 (4)
  hernia
    congenital, 171 (0)
    due to trauma, 171 (4)
    esophageal hiatus, congenital, 171 (0)
      sliding, 172 (6)
    paraesophageal hiatus, 172 (6)
  infection at congenital abnormal apertures, 171 (1)
  inversion (due to abnormal intrathoracic tension), 171 (4)
  paralysis, flaccid
    due to section of phrenic nerve, 172 (55)
    following poliomyelitis, 172 (55)
  puncture
    by fractured rib, 171 (4)
    by instrument, 171 (4)
  reflex spasm (hiccup), 172 (55)
  rupture, 171 (4)
  stab wound, 171 (4)
  subdiaphragmatic abscess, 298 (1)
Diaphragmitis, 171 (1)
Diarrhea. *See also* Dysentery
  due to undetermined cause, 270 (y)
  epidemic, of newborn, 115 (1)
  fermentative, 269 (7)
  parenteral, 268 (1)
  putrefactive, 269 (7)
  supplementary term, 496. *Diagnose disease*
Diastasis
  of cranial bones, 150 (4)
  of muscle, congenital, 167 (0)
  of rectus abdominis
    due to pregnancy, 168 (4)
    following operation, 168 (4)
Diastematomyelia, 421 (0)

Diverticulosis—Continued
of small intestine, 271 (0), 274 (6)
Diverticulum. *See under organ, region or structure affected*
Meckel's. *See* Meckel's diverticulum, 271 (0)
Donor: of blood; of blood marrow; of bone; of skin, 481
Dorsal sclerosis: *supplementary term,* 503. *Diagnose disease*
Dorsolateral medullary syndrome: *supplementary term,* 503. *Diagnose disease*
Dorsolateral sclerosis: *supplementary term,* 503. *Diagnose disease*
Douglas cul-de-sac
hernia, 371 (4)
Dracunculosis, 124 (2)
Dream states: *supplementary term,* 503. *Diagnose disease*
Dresbach's anemia. *See* Sickle cell anemia, 230 (9)
Dropsy. *See* Ascites; Edema; Hydrops
Drowning. *See also* Submersion, 119 (4)
anoxia due to, 119 (7)
due to trauma, 118 (4)
Drugs
addiction, 112 (x)
agranulocytosis due to, 228 (3)
dermatitis due to. *See* Dermatitis medicamentosa, 135 (3)
extravasated
subcutaneous atrophy due to, 136 (3)
subcutaneous inflammation due to, 136 (3)
hypoprothrombinemia due to, 237 (3)
intoxication
acute brain syndrome, 106 (3)
chronic brain syndrome, 107 (3)
porphyria due to, 237 (3)
use of: *supplementary term,* 486. *Diagnose disease*
Drunkenness. *See* Alcohol; Alcoholism
Drusen
of choroid, 441 (9)
of optic papilla, 452 (9)
Dual personality: *supplementary term,* 485. *Diagnose disease*
Dubin-Johnson syndrome, 290 (x)

Duchenne-Aran muscular atrophy. *See* Myelopathic muscular atrophy, 425 (9)
Duct. *See under name of duct*
Ductal tumors, 93
Ductless glands. *See* Endocrine glands
Ductus arteriosus
absence, 204 (0)
bilateral, 204 (0)
patent, 204 (0)
aneurysm of, 204 (0)
Duhring's disease. *See* Dermatitis herpetiformis, 140 (9)
Duodenitis, 272 (1)
due to unknown cause, 275 (9)
Duodenum
displacement of gastric mucosa into, 271 (0)
diverticulum, congenital, 271 (0)
filling, abnormality of: *supplementary term,* 496. *Diagnose disease*
fistula, 274 (6)
ureteroduodenal, 315 (6)
due to infection, 314 (1)
obstruction, duodenojejunal, due to bands, 274 (6)
polyp, simple, due to unknown cause, 275 (9)
stasis, 273 (55)
due to circulatory disturbance, 273 (5)
ulcer, 275 (9)
due to burns, 273 (4)
Dupuytren's contracture, 174 (9)
Durosarcoma. *Diagnose as* Meningioma, 95
Dust, tracheitis due to, 188 (4)
Dwarfism
achondroplasia, complete or incomplete, 146 (0)
congenital, 114 (0)
infantilism and, 394 (7)
nephrotic glycosuric hypophosphatemic, with rickets: *supplementary term,* 485. *Diagnose disease*
pituitary, 394 (7)
Dysautonomia: *supplementary term,* 503. *Diagnose disease*
Dysbasia: *supplementary term,* 503. *Diagnose disease*
Dyschondroplasia, 147 (0)

Ear—Continued
 fibroma, 472 (8)
 fibrosarcoma, 472 (8)
 glomangioma, 472 (8)
 internal. *See also* Labyrinth; Labyrinthitis
 absence of organ of Corti, 479 (0)
 allergy, 475 (3)
 defect of organ of Corti, 479 (0)
 diseases, 479 ff.
 fracture of osseous labyrinth and,
  480 (4)
 lipoma, 472 (8)
 lobule
  absence, congenital, 474 (0)
  duplication, 474 (0)
  enlargement, 474 (0)
  fissure, congenital, 474 (0)
  rudimentary, 474 (0)
  supernumerary, 474 (0)
 lop, 474 (0)
 macacus, 474 (0)
 middle. *See also* Otitis media
  absence, 477 (0)
  allergy, 478 (3)
  ankylosis of incudostapedial joint,
   477 (1)
  diseases, 477 ff.
  granulations following operation,
   478 (4)
  granuloma, mucous polyp, 477 (1)
  narrowing, congenital, 477 (0)
  tuberculosis, 478 (1)
 neoplasms, 472 (8)
 osseous meatus
  atresia, congenital, 474 (0)
  exostosis, 476 (9)
   congenital, 474 (0)
  fracture, 475 (4)
 ossicles
  absence, 477 (0)
  blast injury, 478 (4)
  deformity, congenital, 477 (0)
  disruption due to trauma, 478 (4)
  fusion, congenital, 477 (0)
  necrosis, 477 (1)
  supernumerary, 477 (0)
 pigmented nevus, 472 (8)
 pointed, 474 (0)
 ridged, 474 (0)
 ringing in. *See* Tinnitus
 sarcoma, 473 (8)

Ear—Continued
 semicircular canals, fistula, 479 (1),
  480 (4), 480 (9)
 supernumerary. *See* Polyotia, 474
  (0)
 tuberculosis, diffuse, 472 (1)
 tumors, unlisted, 473 (8)
Earache. *See* Otalgia
Eardrum. *See* Tympanic membrane
Earwax. *See* Cerumen, 476 (6)
Ebstein's disease (downward displacement of tricuspid valve),
 203 (0)
Eccentro-osteochondrodysplasia,
 147 (0)
Ecchondroma; Ecchondrosis. *Di-
 agnose as* Chondroma, 97
Echinococcosis, 125 (2). *See under
 organ, region or structure affected*
Echinococcus, positive reaction to
 (Casoni test): *supplementary
 term,* 487. *Diagnose disease*
Echolalia: *supplementary term,* 484,
 504. *Diagnose disease*
Eclampsia, 118 (3)
Economo's disease. *See* Encephalitis, epidemic, acute, lethargic
 type, 411 (1)
Ectasia. *See* Cornea, ectasia, 434 (1);
 Sclera, ectasia, 438 (1)
Ecthyma, 132 (1)
Ectodermal defect, congenital, 131
 (0)
Ectodermal dysplasia
 anhydrotic type (hereditary), 142
  (x)
Ectopia; ectopy. *See under organ
 affected*
Ectopic ovarian tumor. *Diagnose as*
 Teratoma, 97
Ectropion
 cicatricial, 462 (1)
  due to trauma, 463 (4)
  following operation, 463 (4)
 paralytic, 463 (55)
 senile, 464 (7)
 spastic, 463 (55)
 uveae, 439 (0)
Eczema, 135 (3)
 allergic, of eyelid, 462 (3)
 eczematous conjunctivitis, 469 (3)
 of scrotum, allergic, 339 (3)

Edema. *See also* Ascites; Hydrops; Lymphedema; *and under name of specific disease or organ or region affected*

angioneurotic. *See* Angioneurotic edema

of cardiovascular origin: *supplementary term,* 484. *Diagnose disease*

due to excessive sodium chloride administration, 119 (7)

due to lymphatic obstruction: *supplementary term,* 484. *Diagnose disease*

due to trauma, 126 (4)

familial or hereditary, 142 (x)

hysterical: *supplementary term,* 484. *Diagnose disease*

inanition with, 119 (7)

localized, due to venous obstruction, 128 (50)

malignant, 123 (1)

neonatorum, 131 (0)

of renal origin: *supplementary term,* 484. *Diagnose disease*

supplementary term, 484. *Diagnose disease*

Effusion. *See under* Hemopericardium; Pericarditis; Pericardium; Pleurisy

in joints. *See* Hydrarthrosis: *supplementary term,* 489

Eggshell nails, 137 (5)

Eisenmenger complex, 203 (0)

Ejaculation of semen, premature: *supplementary term,* 499. *Diagnose disease*

• **Ejaculatory ducts**

absence, congenital, 346 (0)

atresia, congenital, 346 (0)

fibrosis, 346 (1)

stricture, 346 (1)

Elastoma, juvenile. *Diagnose as* Chordoma, 98

Elastosis solar, 136 (4)

Elbow

arthritis

due to fracture involving joint, 158 (4)

due to habitual dislocation, 158 (4)

dislocation, open, 159 (4)

miner's, 165 (4)

Elbow—Continued

tennis, 165 (4)

Electric shock. *See under* Electricity

Electricity. *See also* Electrocution; Lightning stroke

burn, 126 (4)

gangrene due to, 126 (4)

of urethra, 324 (4)

incineration by, 118 (4)

shock, 118 (4)

of brain, 413 (4)

of peripheral nerve, 429 (4)

of spinal cord, 424 (4)

Electrocution, 118 (4)

Electrolytes

metabolism, disorders of, 120 (7)

in urine, abnormal content: *supplementary term,* 498. *Diagnose disease*

Elephantiasis

congenital, 122 (0)

due to venous thrombosis, 128 (50)

of eyelid, 463 (5)

lymphangiectatic, 128 (5)

of external ear, 476 (5)

of external genitalia, 330 (5)

of scrotum, 339 (5)

of vulva, 353 (5)

neuromatosa. *Diagnose as* Schwannoma, 95

nostras, 137 (5)

Embolism. *See also* Thrombosis; *and under name of vessel or organ affected*

air, of artery, 217 (4)

of artery

due to remote infection, 216 (1)

due to remote trauma, 217 (4)

following operation, 217 (4)

capillary purpura due to, 226 (5)

fat, of artery, 217 (1)

gangrene due to, 128 (5)

hemorrhage of pancreas due to, 296 (5)

infarction of liver due to, 288 (5)

infarction of lung due to, 196 (5)

infarction of myocardium due to, 210 (5)

infarction of spleen due to, 232 (5)

pulmonary. *See* Pulmonary artery, embolism

saddle embolus, of aorta, 220 (6)

Embryoma
of bladder, cervix, prostate, uterus, vagina. *Diagnose as* Mesenchymal mixed tumor, 98
of kidney. *Diagnose as* Nephroblastoma, 98
of liver. *Diagnose as* Hepatoblastoma, 98
not otherwise specified, 98
of ovary. *Diagnose as* Disgerminoma, 97
of testis. *Diagnose as* Embryonal carcinoma of testis, 98
Embryonal adenoma (thyroid). *Diagnose as* Undifferentiated adenoma (thyroid), 389 (8)
Embryonal carcinoma of testis, 98
Embryonal cell lipoma; embryonal lipomatosis. *Diagnose as* Fetal fat cell lipoma, 97
Embryonal sarcoma, 98
Embryonal tumor. *See* Embryoma
Embryonic rest, malignant, 98
Emesis. *See* Hematemesis; Vomiting
Emissions, nocturnal: *supplementary term,* 499. *Diagnose disease*
Emmetropia, 454 (6)
Emotional instability. *See also* Personality, emotionally unstable, 112 (x)
supplementary term, 484. *Diagnose disease*
Emphysema, 126 (4)
of conjunctiva, 469 (4)
of eyelid, due to trauma, 463 (4)
of lung
bullous, 196 (6)
compensatory, 196 (6)
congenital, 192 (0)
interstitial
due to infection, 193 (1)
due to trauma, 195 (4)
obstructive, 196 (6)
postural, 195 (4)
senile, 196 (7)
unknown cause, 197 (9)
of mediastinum, 126 (4)
of orbit, 458 (4)
pulmonary. *See* Emphysema of lung
subcutaneous
due to trauma, 137 (4)

Emphysema—Continued
subcutaneous—continued
of trunk, following operation, 137 (4)
Empyema
of gallbladder, 292 (1)
pleural, 198 (1)
due to foreign body, 199 (4)
following operation, 199 (4)
interlobar, 198 (1)
loculated, 198 (1)
perforating chest wall, 198 (1)
tuberculous, 198 (1)
Enamel
hyperplastic, 249 (7)
hypoplastic, 249 (7)
mottled, due to fluorine, 248 (3)
Enameloma. *Diagnose as* Odontogenic tumor, benign, 98
Encephalitis. *See also* Encephalomyelitis; Encephalopathy; Ependymitis; Meningoencephalitis; Polioencephalitis
acute, 411 (1)
chronic, 411 (1)
due to herpetic virus, 411 (1)
epidemic
acute, various types, 411 (1)
chronic, 411 (1)
parasitic, 412 (2)
postinfectious, 411 (1)
post vaccination, 412 (3)
Encephalocele. *See also* Brain, hernia, 413 (4)
Encephalomalacia
due to arteriosclerosis, 414 (5)
due to circulatory disturbance, 414 (5)
due to trauma, 413 (4)
supplementary term, 504. *Diagnose disease*
Encephalomyelitis. *See also* Meningoencephalomyelitis
acute, 402 (1)
chronic, 402 (1)
supplementary term, 504. *Diagnose disease*
Encephalomyelopathy
due to diabetes, 403 (7)
due to pellagra, 403 (7)
due to poison, 403 (3)
due to Rh sensitization, 403 (3)

Encephalopathy
congenital
due to maternal infection, 410 (0)
due to maternal intoxication, 410 (0)
due to anoxemia at birth, 410 (0)
due to anoxia, 413 (4)
due to arterial hypertension, 414 (5)
due to arteriosclerosis, 414 (5)
due to birth injury, 410 (0)
due to cardiac standstill, 414 (5)
due to cerebral anoxia, result of high altitude, 413 (4)
due to depressed fracture, 413 (4)
due to foreign body, 413 (4)
due to heat, 413 (4)
due to hyperinsulinism, 414 (7)
due to hypobaropathy, 413 (4)
due to insolation. *See* due to sunstroke, 413 (4)
due to remote infection, 412 (1)
due to remote trauma, 413 (4)
due to starvation, 414 (7)
due to sunstroke, 413 (4)
due to vitamin deficiency, 414 (7)
progressive subcortical, 416 (9)
toxic
due to poison, 412 (3)
due to thyroid gland extract, 412 (3)

Encephalorrhagia, pericapillary
due to poison, 412 (3)

Enchondroma. *Diagnose as* Chondroma, 97

Enchondromatosis, skeletal, 147 (0)

Enchondrosis, multiple. *Diagnose as* Chondroma, 97

Encopresis: *supplementary term,* 484. *Diagnose disease*

Enclavoma. *Diagnose as* Mixed tumor, salivary gland type, 98

Endarteritis
atrophy of bone due to, 152 (5)
cerebrospinal, 404 (9)

Endocarditis
acute bacterial, 207 (1)
aneurysm of valve due to, 207 (1)
nonbacterial thrombotic, 212 (9)
rheumatic, 213 (9)
subacute bacterial, 207 (1)
  aneurysm of valve due to, 207 (1)
verrucous, atypical, 213 (9)
  heart disease with, 213 (9)
  mural, 213 (9)

Endocardium
adult, fibroelastosis of, 212 (9)

Endocrine glands. *See also names of specific glands*
diseases, 387 ff.
hemorrhage from: *supplementary term,* 500. *Diagnose disease*
pluriglandular atrophy or sclerosis, 389 (9)
psychophysiologic reaction, 111 (55)

Endometrial carcinoma, 94

Endometrioma. *Diagnose as* Adenomyosis, 98

Endometriosis
of bladder, 321 (9)
of broad ligament, 372 (9)
due to unknown cause, 129 (9)
of Fallopian tube, 367 (9)
of kidney, 312 (9)
of lymph node, 236 (9)
of ovary, 370 (9)
of ureter, 316 (9)
of uterus, 364 (9)

Endometritis
acute, 360 (1)
chronic, 361 (1)
decidual. *See* Deciduitis, 373 (1)
during pregnancy, acute, 374 (1)
puerperal, acute, 374 (1)
septic, 361 (1)

Endometrium
atrophy
due to absence, destruction or atrophy of ovary, 363 (7)
due to irradiation, 361 (4)
due to poison, 361 (3)
spontaneous, 365 (9)
dysfunction
due to decrease in estrogenic substance, 364 (7)
due to excessive administration of estrogenic substance, 363 (7)
secondary to eosinophilic hyperpituitarism, 363 (7)
secondary to hyperadrenalism, 363 (7)
secondary to hyperthyroidism, 363 (7)
secondary to hypoadrenalism, 363 (7)
secondary to hypopituitarism, 363 (7)

Endometrium—Continued
dysfunction—continued
secondary to hypothyroidism, 363
(7)
hyperplasia
due to unknown cause, 365 (9)
secondary to basophilic hyperpituitarism, 364 (7)
static, due to continuous ovarian
stimulation, 364 (7)
no disease, 481
obliteration, due to infection, 361 (1)
polyp, due to infection, 361 (1)
sarcoma, 364 (8)
Endophlebitis. *See* Phlebitis; *and
organ or vessel affected*
Endophthalmitis, 439 (1)
allergic, 439 (1)
Endosalpingiosis. *Diagnose as* Adenomyosis, 98
Endothelioangiitis
diffuse, 115 (1)
Endothelioma. *Diagnose as* Mesothelioma, 97
of blood vessel. *Diagnose as* Hemangioendothelioma, 96
malignant. *Diagnose as* Lymphangiosarcoma, 96
of bone. *Diagnose as* Ewing's sarcoma, 97
diffuse
of bone. *Diagnose as* Ewing's sarcoma, 97
of meninges. *Diagnose as* Meningioma, 95
dural. *Diagnose as* Meningioma, 95
of lymph vessel, benign. *Diagnose as*
Lymphendothelioma, 96
of meninges. *Diagnose as* Meningioma, 95
not otherwise specified, of lymph
gland, lymph node. *Diagnose as*
Reticulum cell sarcoma, 95
perithelial. *Diagnose as* Hemangiopericytoma, 96
synovial. *Diagnose as* Synovioma, 97
**Endotheliosis; endotheliosis,
spreading**
of meninges. *Diagnose as* Meningioma, 95
Enema, opaque, abnormality: *supplementary term,* 496. *Diagnose
disease*

Engman's disease. *See* Dermatitis,
infectious eczematoid, 132 (1)
Enophthalmos
due to emaciation, 459 (7)
due to loss of orbital tissue, 458 (4)
due to loss of water, 459 (7)
due to senile atrophy, 459 (7)
following infection of orbital tissue,
458 (1)
following operation, 458 (4)
supplementary term, 508. *Diagnose
disease*
Enteric cyst, 274 (6)
Enteritis
acute, 272 (1)
due to poison, 272 (3)
chronic, 272 (1)
due to poison, 272 (3)
due to unknown cause, 275 (9)
Enterobius vermicularis infection.
See Oxyuriasis
Enterocele, 268 (4)
vaginal, 371 (4)
Enterocolitis
acute, 268 (1)
due to poison, 268 (3)
pseudomembranous, 268 (9)
chronic, 268 (1)
due to poison, 268 (3)
staphylococcic, 268 (1)
tuberculous, 268 (1)
Enterocystoma. *Diagnose as* Hamartoma, 98
Enterolith, 278 (6)
Enteroptosis, 269 (6)
Enterostomy
stenosis of stoma after, 268 (4)
Entropion
cicatricial, 462 (1)
due to trauma, 463 (4)
following operation, 463 (4)
spastic, 463 (55)
Enuresis, 112 (x)
supplementary term, 484. *Diagnose
disease*
Eosinophilia: *supplementary term,*
493. *Diagnose disease*
pulmonary. *See* Pneumonia, allergic,
194 (3)
Eosinophilic granuloma
of bone, 120 (7)
of skin, 120 (7)

Epithelioma—Continued
superficial basal cell. *Diagnose as* Basal cell carcinoma, 94
Epitheliomatosis
multiple superficial. *Diagnose as* Neoplastic cyst, 93
superficial. *Diagnose as* Basal cell carcinoma, 94
Epitheliosarcomatous   neoplasm. *Diagnose as* Epidermoid carcinoma, 94
Epithelium
specific tumors of, 93
Epoophoron cyst, 370 (9)
Epulis
of newborn. *Diagnose as* Granular cell myoblastoma, 96
Equinia. *See* Glanders, 115 (1)
Erb's palsy. *See* Birth injury: laceration of peripheral nerve, 429 (4)
Erb-Goldflam disease. *See* Myasthenia gravis, 169 (55)
Erectile tumor. *Diagnose as* Hemangioma (angioma), 96
Ergot
abnormal contraction of pregnant uterus due to, 374 (3)
gangrene due to, 125 (3)
Erosio interdigitalis blastomycetica, 134 (2)
Erosion. *See under organ or structure affected*
Erotomania: *supplementary term,* 484. *Diagnose disease*
Eructation: *supplementary term,* 496. *Diagnose disease*
Eruption
creeping. *See* Larva migrans, 134 (2)
Kaposi's varicelliform, 115 (1)
Erysipelas, 132 (1)
of scrotum, 339 (1)
Erysipeloid, 132 (1)
Erythema
annulare centrifugum, 141 (9)
caloricum, 136 (4)
elevatum diutinum, 141 (9)
epidemic arthritic (Haverhill fever), 115 (1)
general: *supplementary term,* 487. *Diagnose disease*
gluteale, 135 (3)

Erythema—Continued
induratum, 134 (1)
nodular vasculitis, 141 (9)
tuberculosis indurative, 134 (1)
infectiosum (fifth disease), 115 (1)
local: *supplementary term,* 487. *Diagnose disease*
multiforme, 132 (1)
toxic, 135 (3)
nodose, 132 (1)
scarlatiniform, 135 (3)
toxic, 135 (3)
Erythralgia. *See* Erythromelalgia *supplementary term,* 504
Erythrasma, 134 (2)
Erythredema polyneuropathy, 431 (x)
Erythremia. *Diagnose as* Polycythemia vera, 95
Erythroblastemia. *Diagnose as* Erythroblastoma, 95
Erythroblastoma, 95
Erythroblastosis, fetal. *See* Hemolytic disease of fetus and newborn, 228 (3)
Erythrocyanosis crurum, 137 (5)
Erythrocytes
abnormal sedimentation rate: *supplementary term,* 493. *Diagnose disease*
fragility: *supplementary terms. Diagnose disease*
decreased, 493
increased, 494
stippling: *supplementary term,* 495. *Diagnose disease*
Erythrocythemia. *Diagnose as* Polycythemia vera, 95
Erythrocytosis
due to arterial anoxemia, 229 (7)
megalosplenica. *Diagnose as* Polycythemia vera, 95
Erythroderma
ichthyosiforme congenitum, 131 (0)
psoriatic, 141 (9)
Erythroleukemia;   Erythroleukosis. *Diagnose as* Polycythemia vera, 95
Erythromelalgia, 217 (55)
supplementary term, 504. *Diagnose disease*
Erythroplasia of Queyrat, 141 (9)

Eustachian tube—Continued
stricture due to infection, 478 (1)
Eventration, 268 (4)
of diaphragm, 171 (0)
Eversion. *See* Ectropion
Evisceration, 126 (4)
Ewing's angioendothelioma. *Diagnose as* Ewing's sarcoma, 97
Ewing's sarcoma, 97
of bone, 154 (8)
of bone marrow, 239 (8)
Ewing's tumor. *Diagnose as* Ewing's sarcoma, 97
Examination
none, 481
only, 481
Exanthem
acute rhinitis associated with, 177 (1)
Exanthema subitum, 114 (1)
Excoriations, neurotic: *supplementary term, 505. Diagnose disease*
Exhaustion, 119 (7)
from cold, 118 (4)
from heat. *See* Heat prostration, 118 (4)
Exocrine tumor. *Diagnose as* Sweat gland tumor, 94
Exophoria
cause unknown, 457 (x)
due to error of refraction, 456 (5)
Exophthalmos
congenital, 458 (0)
due to hyperthyroidism, 433 (7)
due to orbital edema, 459 (0)
supplementary term, 508. Diagnose disease
Exostosis(es)
congenital, 147 (0)
due to infection, 148 (1)
due to trauma or pressure, 150 (4)
multiple osteocartilaginous, 147 (0)
of orbit, 460 (9)
solitary. *Diagnose as* Osteoma, 97
Exotropia, 456 (5)
following trauma, 456 (4)
of unknown cause, 457 (x)
Experiment only, 481
Exstrophy of bladder, 317 (0)
Extinction: *supplementary term, 504. Diagnose disease*
Extravasation of lymph, 128 (5)

Extremities
angiospasm of arteries of leg and foot, 217 (5)
cyanosis. *See* Acrocyanosis, 127 (5)
Extrinsic muscles of eye. *See under* Eye, muscles
Eye(s). *See also under names of various structures of eye, as* Cornea
absence, congenital. *See* Anophthalmos, 433 (0)
diseases, 433 ff.
imbalance, torticollis due to, 169 (55)
intra-ocular changes: *supplementary term, 509. Diagnose disease*
muscles
absence of extrinsic, 455 (0)
agenesis of extrinsic, 455 (0)
contracture of extrinsic, following paralysis of antagonist, 456 (55)
diseases, 455 ff.
disturbances of intrinsic: *supplementary term, 509. Diagnose disease*
overaction of inferior oblique, 457 (x)
paralysis, strabismus due to, 456 (55)
paralysis of extrinsic, 455 (0), 456 (55); *supplementary term, 508*
paralysis of intrinsic, *supplementary term, 509*
skew deviation of extrinsic: *supplementary term, 508. Diagnose disease*
spasm of accommodation, 456 (55)
spasm of extrinsic: *supplementary term, 508. Diagnose disease*
spasm of intrinsic: *supplementary term, 509. Diagnose disease*
rudimentary, 433 (0)
spots before. *See* Muscae volitantes, 444 (0)
strain, hyperemia due to, 470 (4)
Eyeball. *See also* Eye; Orbit
absence following operation, 433 (4)
atrophy
cause unknown, 433 (9)
due to infection, 433 (1)
due to trauma, 433 (4)
avulsion, 433 (4)
chemical burn, 433 (3)
diseases, 433 ff.

Eyelids—Continued
xanthelasma, 464 (7)
zoster, 462 (1)

F

Faber's syndrome. *See* Anemia, hypochromic microcytic, 229 (7)
Face
bird, or dish (facies scaphoidea), 122 (0)
clefts, congenital, 122 (0)
dystrophy, congenital, 122 (0)
scaphoid, 122 (0)
Face presentation, 382 (6)
Facetiousness: *supplementary term,* 484. *Diagnose disease*
Facial nerve
disturbances: *supplementary term,* 508. *Diagnose disease*
neuralgia
atypical, 432 (x): *supplementary term,* 505
sympathetic, 432 (x)
neuropathy (Bell's palsy), 429 (4)
paralysis. *See also* Neuropathy of facial nerve, 429 (4)
central: *supplementary term,* 508. *Diagnose disease*
peripheral: *supplementary term,* 508. *Diagnose disease*
Faciocephalalgia
autonomic, 432 (x)
Fahr-Volhard disease. *See* Malignant nephrosclerosis, 310 (5)
Fainting. *See* Syncope: *supplementary term,* 486
Fallopian tube(s). *See also* Salpingitis
abscess, tubo-ovarian, 366 (1)
absence, 366 (0)
adenocarcinoma, 367 (8)
atresia due to infection, 366 (1)
blood in. *See* Hematosalpinx, 367 (6)
convolutions, persistence of, 366 (0)
cyst, congenital, 366 (0)
diseases, 366 ff.
displacement, 367 (6)
displacement of uterine opening, 366 (0)
duplication, 366 (0)

Fallopian tube(s)—Continued
endometriosis, 367 (9)
fibrosis, 367 (7)
fistula, external, following operation, 366 (4)
hematosalpinx, 366 (1)
hemorrhage due to trauma, 366 (4)
hydrosalpinx, 367 (6)
inflammation. *See* Salpingitis; Perisalpingitis
injury, 367 (4)
length, abnormal, 366 (0)
mesothelioma, 367 (8)
neoplasms, 367 (8)
occlusion
congenital, 366 (0)
following operation, 367 (4)
ovarian rest in, 366 (0)
polyp, simple, 367 (9)
pus in. *See* Pyosalpinx, 366 (1)
senile atrophy, 367 (7)
supernumerary, 366 (0)
triplication of ostiums, 366 (0)
tumors, unlisted, 367 (8)
volvulus, 367 (6)
Fallot's tetralogy, 203 (0)
Familial periodic paralysis, 170 (x)
Fanconi-de Toni syndrome: *supplementary term,* 485. *Diagnose disease*
Farcy. *See* Glanders, 115 (1)
Farsightedness. *See* Hypermetropia, 454 (0), 454 (6)
Fascia. *See also* Fasciitis
abscess, 173 (1)
contracture
due to trauma, 174 (4)
due to unknown cause, 174 (9)
diseases, 173 ff.
fat, herniation, 138 (6)
sloughing, 173 (1)
Fasciitis
due to infection, 173 (1)
due to trauma, 174 (4)
palmar, due to trauma, 174 (4)
Fat. *See also* Lipid; Obesity
embolism, 217 (1)
fascial, herniation, 138 (6)
indigestion, 269 (7)
metabolism, disorders of, 120 (7)
necrosis. *See also* Adiponecrosis neonatorum, 136 (4)
of mesentery, 272 (3)

Fat—Continued
 necrosis—continued
  neonatal, 136 (4)
  of peritoneum, 299 (3)
Fat cell tumor, primitive. *Diagnose as* Fetal fat cell lipoma, 97
Fatigue, abnormal: *supplementary term,* 485. *Diagnose disease*
Fatty degeneration
 of heart
  due to anemia, 210 (5)
  due to unknown cause, 212 (9)
Fatty infiltration
 of aorta, 220 (7)
 of heart, 211 (7)
Fatty tumor. *See* Tumors of lipoid tissue, 97
 benign. *Diagnose as* Lipoma, 97
Favism, 117 (3)
Favus
 alopecia due to, 134 (2)
 capitis, 134 (2)
 corporis, 134 (2)
Fear(s). *See also* Acaraphobia, etc.: *supplementary terms,* 484; Phobic reaction, 111 (x)
 mixed: *supplementary term,* 485. *Diagnose disease*
Fecalith. *See also* Enterolith, 278 (6)
 in appendix, 280 (6)
Feces
 blood in, occult: *supplementary term,* 496. *Diagnose disease*
 fat in, undigested: *supplementary term,* 497. *Diagnose disease*
 fecal fistula, 268 (4), 273 (4)
 impacted, 278 (6)
 incontinence of: *supplementary term,* 496. *Diagnose disease*
 pathogenic bacteria in: *supplementary term,* 497. *Diagnose disease*
 protein in, undigested: *supplementary term,* 497. *Diagnose disease*
 starch in, undigested: *supplementary term,* 497. *Diagnose disease*
 yeast and molds in: *supplementary term,* 497. *Diagnose disease*
Feeblemindedness. *See* Mental deficiency
Feeding
 improper, 119 (7)

Feeding—Continued
 problem in children: *supplementary term,* 485. *Diagnose disease*
Feer's disease. *See* Erythredema polyneuropathy, 431 (x)
Feet. *See* Foot
Felon, 173 (1)
Female genital system, diseases, 349 ff.
Feminizing tumor, 93
Femur
 absence, congenital, 146 (0)
 anteversion of neck, congenital, 146 (0)
 avulsion of epiphysis, 150 (4)
 epiphysiolysis of upper end, due to unknown cause, 154 (9)
 epiphysis, slipping due to infection, 148 (1)
 growth arrest due to streptococcic osteomyelitis, 148 (1)
 osteochondrosis of capital epiphysis, 155 (9)
 osteomyelitis of neck due to staphylococcic infection, 148 (1)
 syphilitic osteochondritis of, 149 (1)
Fetal fat cell lipoma, 97
Fetal rickets. *See* Achondroplasia, 146 (0)
Fetor oris. *See* Halitosis: *supplementary term,* 496
Fetus. *See also* Newborn
 amniotic adhesions, 383 (7)
 asphyxia
  due to interference with fetal circulation, 381 (5)
  due to trauma, 381 (4)
 calcified, retained. *See* Lithopedion, 380 (9)
 heart disease, inflammatory, 202 (0)
 hemolytic disease, 228 (3)
 papyraceus, 380 (9)
Fever. *See also* Pyrexia: *supplementary term,* 486
 Colorado tick, 115 (1)
 desert. *See* Coccidioidosis, generalized, 114 (1)
 glandular. *See* Mononucleosis, infectious, 114 (1)
 Haverhill (epidemic arthritic erythema), 115 (1)
 hemoglobinuric (nonmalarial), 115 (1)

Fever—Continued
Malta. *See* Brucellosis, 114 (1)
miliary, 115 (1)
Oroya. *See* Bartonellosis, 114 (1)
pappataci, 115 (1)
parrot. *See* Psittacosis, 116 (1)
pretibial, 116 (1)
Q, 116 (1)
rat bite, 116 (1)
recurrent. *See* Relapsing fever, 116 (1)
relapsing, 116 (1)
rheumatic. *See* Rheumatic fever, 121 (9)
Rocky Mountain spotted, 116 (1)
trench, 116 (1)
tsutsugamushi, 116 (1)
of undetermined origin, 121 (y)
undulant. *See* Brucellosis, 114 (1)
valley. *See* Coccidioidosis, generalized, 114 (1)
yellow, 116 (1)
Fibrillation. *See* Atrial fibrillation; Ventricular fibrillation
Fibrin ball
in pleural sac, 199 (4)
Fibrinogenopenia
associated with pregnancy, 238 (x)
hereditary, 238 (x)
supplementary term, 493. *Diagnose disease*
Fibroadenoma. *Diagnose as* Adenofibroma, 97
diffuse. *Diagnose as* Adenofibroma, 97
fetal. *Diagnose as* Cystosarcoma phyllodes, 97
giant. *Diagnose as* Cystosarcoma phyllodes, 97
intracanalicular fibromatosum; intracanalicular papillary cystic. *Diagnose as* Adenofibroma, 97
pericanalicular. *Diagnose as* Adenofibroma, 97
pleomorphic. *Diagnose as* Adenofibroma, 97
Fibroadenomyxoma
giant intracanalicular. *Diagnose as* Cystosarcoma phyllodes, 97
Fibroangioendothelioma. *Diagnose as* Hemangiosarcoma, 96

Fibroblastoma, 96
arachnoid. *Diagnose as* Meningioma, 95
meninges, or meningeal. *Diagnose as* Meningioma, 95
of nerve sheath. *Diagnose as* Neurofibroma, 95
perineural. *Diagnose as* Neurofibroma, 95
Fibrocarcinoma. *Diagnose as* Carcinoma, not otherwise specified, 94
Fibrochondroma. *Diagnose as* Chondroblastoma, 97
Fibrochondro-osteoma. *Diagnose as* Osteoma, 97
Fibrochondrosarcoma. *Diagnose as* Chondrosarcoma, 97
Fibroendothelioma. *Diagnose as* Fibroma, 96
malignant. *Diagnose as* Fibrosarcoma, 96
Fibroepithelioma
except of ovary. *Diagnose as* Squamous cell papilloma, 94
of ovary. *Diagnose as* Adenofibroma, 97
Fibroglioma
except of nose. *Diagnose as* Neurofibroma, 95
Fibroid
with fibrinoid degeneration. *Diagnose as* Leiomyoma, 96
Fibrolipoma. *Diagnose as* Lipoma, 97
Fibroliposarcoma. *Diagnose as* Liposarcoma, 97
Fibroma, 76
angiomatosum. *Diagnose as* Hemangioma (angioma), 96
dermal. *Diagnose as* Fibroma, 96
giant cell
of bone. *Diagnose as* Giant cell tumor, of bone, 97
except of bone. *Diagnose as* Giant cell tumor except bone, 97
molluscum (nerve sheath). *Diagnose as* Neurofibroma, 95
of nerve sheath. *Diagnose as* Neurofibroma, 95
nonosteogenic (bone). *Diagnose as* Fibroma, 96
odontogenic. *Diagnose as* Odontogenic tumor, benign, 98

Fibroma—Continued

ossifying (bone). *Diagnose as* Fibroma, 96

ovarii adenocysticum. *Diagnose as* Adenofibroma, 97

papillare superficiale. *Diagnose as* Adenofibroma, 97

periosteal. *Diagnose as* Fibroma, 96

polypoid (uterus). *Diagnose as* Leiomyoma, 96

of uterus. *Diagnose as* Leiomyoma, 96

Fibromyoma

except of uterus. *Diagnose as* Myoma, 96

of uterus. *Diagnose as* Leiomyoma, 96

Fibromyxoendothelioma

salivary gland type. *Diagnose as* Mixed tumor, salivary gland type, 98

Fibromyxoma

of breast. *Diagnose as* Cystosarcoma phyllodes, 97

except of breast, nerve sheath, vagina. *Diagnose as* Myxoma, 97

of nerve sheath. *Diagnose as* Neurofibroma, 95

of vagina. *Diagnose as* Mesenchymal mixed tumor, 98

Fibromyxosarcoma

of breast. *Diagnose as* Cystosarcoma phyllodes, 97

except of breast, nerve sheath, vagina. *Diagnose as* Myxosarcoma, 97

of nerve sheath. *Diagnose as* Fibrosarcoma, 96

of vagina. *Diagnose as* Mesenchymal mixed tumor, 98

Fibroneuroma. *Diagnose as* Neurofibroma, 95

Fibro-osteochondroma. *Diagnose as* Osteoma, 97

Fibro-osteoma

of bone. *Diagnose as* Osteoma, 97

except of bone. *Diagnose as* Fibroma, 96

Fibro-osteosarcoma (bone). *Diagnose as* Osteosarcoma (osteogenic sarcoma), 97

Fibroplasia, retrolental, 447 (3)

Fibrosarcoma, 96

of breast. *Diagnose as* Cystosarcoma phyllodes, 97

giant cell

of bone. *Diagnose as* Giant cell tumor of bone, 97

except of bone. *Diagnose as* Fibroblastoma, 96

mucocellulare carcinomatodes. *Diagnose as* Mucinous carcinoma, 93

myxomatodes (nerve sheath). *Diagnose as* Fibrosarcoma, 96

odontogenic. *Diagnose as* Adamantinocarcinoma, 98

periosteal

of bone. *Diagnose as* Osteosarcoma (osteogenic sarcoma), 97

except of bone. *Diagnose as* Fibrosarcoma, 96

phyllodes. *Diagnose as* Cystosarcoma phyllodes, 97

Fibrosis

appendical, noninflammatory, 280 (7)

of breast, due to unknown cause, 145 (9)

diatomite, 196 (4)

of heart, 212 (9)

of lung, 193 (1), 195 (4), 197 (9). *See also* Pneumonia, interstitial, chronic, 193 (1)

of myocardium, 213 (9)

of seminal vesicles, 344 (1)

uteri, 364 (7)

Fibrositis

periarticular, 164 (x)

Fibrosum molluscum. *Diagnose as* Neurofibroma, 95

Fiedler's myocarditis (myocarditis of unknown cause), 213 (9)

Filariasis, 124 (2). *See also under organ, region or structure affected*

Filioma. *Diagnose as* Fibroma, 96

Finger(s)

amputation stump, abnormal, 125 (4)

clubbed, 128 (7)

failure of segmentation of parts (syndactyly), 122 (0)

Finger(s)—Continued
infection of distal closed space
(felon), 173 (1)
spider. *See* Arachnodactyly, 114 (0)
stenosis of tendon sheath, congenital,
173 (0)
supernumerary, 123 (0)
trigger
acquired, 174 (6)
congenital, 173 (0)
webbed, 132 (0)
Fingernails. *See* Nails
Fires, setting. *See* Pyromania: *supplementary term,* 486
Fistula. *See also under organ, region
or structure affected*
arteriovenous, 216 (0)
of chest wall, following operation,
126 (4)
due to infection, 123 (1)
due to radioactive substance, 126 (4)
due to trauma, 126 (4)
fecal, 268 (4), 273 (4)
following operation, 126 (4)
sacrococcygeal. *See* Pilonidal sinus,
122 (0)
Flail chest: *supplementary term,* 490.
Diagnose disease
Flail joint
due to paralysis from poliomyelitis,
162 (55)
Flajani's disease. *See* Toxic diffuse
goiter, 390 (9)
Flatau-Schilder disease. *See* Progressive subcortical encephalopathy, 416 (9)
Flatfoot
congenital, due to paralysis, 157 (0)
due to posture, 164 (x)
fixed type, due to unknown cause,
164 (9)
spastic, due to muscle spasm (not
paralytic), 164 (x)
Flea infestation, 134 (2)
Flexibilitas cerea: *supplementary
term,* 504. *Diagnose disease*
Flexner agglutination, positive:
supplementary term, 496. *Diagnose disease*
Floating kidney. *See* Wandering
kidney, 308 (0)
Floating spleen, 232 (6)
Fluid of reexpansion, 199 (4)

Flukes
list, 65
Fluorine
mottled enamel due to, 248 (3)
poisoning, of bone, 149 (3)
Fluorosis, endemic, 248 (3)
Fogo seluagem, 141 (9)
Folie du doute: *supplementary term,*
485. *Diagnose disease*
Folliculitis
cheloidalis. *See* Folliculitis, keloidal,
132 (1)
decalvans, 132 (1)
due to undetermined cause, 142 (y)
keloidal, 132 (1)
pyodermal, 132 (1)
ulerythematosus reticulated, 141 (9)
Folliculoma
lipidique. *Diagnose as* Granulosa cell
tumor, 93
malignum ovarii. *Diagnose as* Teratoma, 97
of ovary. *Diagnose as* Granulosa cell
tumor, 93
Food. *See also* Feeding
allergy, 117 (3)
ball. *See* Phytobezoar, 265 (6)
poisoning due to Salmonella, 115 (1)
Foot. *See also* Talipes; Toes; etc.
abnormal division, 122 (0)
angiospasm of arteries, 217 (5)
athlete's. *See* Dermatophytosis, 134
(2)
circulatory disturbance due to previous poliomyelitis, 217 (55)
clawfoot, cause unknown, 163 (9)
clubfoot, 134 (0). *See also* Talipes
congenital paralytic (in spina bifida), 157 (0)
flatfoot
due to posture, 164 (x)
due to unknown cause, 164 (9)
spastic, due to muscle spasm (not
paralytic), 164 (x)
hypertrophy, congenital, 122 (0)
lime (quicklime) burn, 125 (3)
Madura, 124 (2)
strained, due to constant or intermittent trauma, 160 (4)
ulcer, neurogenic, 138 (55)
Foramen ovale, patent, 202 (0)
Forced crying: *supplementary term,*
503. *Diagnose disease*

Frontal sinus. *See* Sinuses, accessory; Sinusitis
Frostbite, 126 (4), 136 (4)
    of auricle, 475 (4)
    of nose, 178 (4)
    of penis, 330 (4)
    of scrotum, 339 (4)
Fructosuria: *supplementary term,* 498. *Diagnose disease*
Fugue: *supplementary term,* 485. *Diagnose disease*
Fungus(i). *See* Mycosis; *and under specific name of disease or organ or region affected*
Fungus hematodes. *Diagnose as* Neuroepithelioma, 95
Funiculitis
    acute, 342 (1)
    chronic, 342 (1)
    endemic, 342 (1)
Funnel chest, congenital, 146 (0)
Furor, paroxysmal: *supplementary term,* 485. *Diagnose disease*
Furuncle, 132 (1)
    of nose, 177 (1)
Furunculosis, 132 (1)
    of external auditory canal, 475 (1)
Fused kidney, 307 (0)
Fusion. *See under organ or structure affected*

G

Gain in weight: *supplementary term,* 485. *Diagnose disease*
Galactemia: *supplementary term,* 493. *Diagnose disease*
Galactocele
    due to infection, 143 (1)
    due to trauma, 144 (4)
    due to undetermined cause, 145 (y)
Galactorrhea, 145 (x)
Galactosemia
    idiopathic, 120 (7)
    supplementary term, 493. *Diagnose disease*
Galactosuria: *supplementary term,* 498. *Diagnose disease*
Galacturia: *supplementary term,* 498. *Diagnose disease*
Galea aponeurotica, abscess under. *See* Subgaleal abscess, 123 (1)

Gall ducts. *See* Bile passages
Gallbladder. *See also* Bile passages; Cholecystitis
    abnormality after administration of dye: *supplementary term,* 496. *Diagnose disease*
    abscess, pericholecystic, 292 (1)
    absence, congenital, 291 (0)
    adhesions, pericholecystic, 292 (4)
        due to infection, 292 (1)
        due to trauma, 293 (4)
        following operation, 292 (4)
    bifurcation, congenital, 291 (0)
    calcification, 294 (9)
    calculus, 293 (6)
        congenital, 291 (0)
    cholesterol imbibition, 294 (9)
    displacement, congenital, 291 (0)
    duplication, 291 (0)
    empyema, 292 (1)
    fistula
        between colon and, due to calculus, 278 (6)
        between cystic duct and, congenital, 291 (0)
        cholecystogastric
            due to calculus, 293 (6)
            following operation, 293 (4)
        cholecystointestinal, 292 (1)
            due to calculus, 293 (6)
            due to infection, 292 (1)
            following operation, 293 (4)
    hernia in femoral ring, congenital, 291 (0)
    hourglass, congenital, 291 (0)
    hydrops, 293 (6)
    inclusion in liver, congenital, 287 (0)
    inflammation. *See also* Cholecystitis, 292 (1)
        congenital, 291 (0)
    injury, 293 (4)
    mucocele, 294 (9)
    torsion
        due to unknown cause, 293 (6)
        with long mesentery, congenital, 292 (0)
    ulceration due to calculus, 293 (6)
Gallop rhythm: *supplementary term,* 492. *Diagnose disease*
Gallstones. *See also* Bile passages, calculus; Gallbladder, calculus

Gallstones—Continued
obstruction of small intestine, 274 (6)
Ganglia. *See* Ganglion
Ganglioblastoma
except of nose. *Diagnose as* Ganglioneuroma, 95
malignant. *Diagnose as* Malignant ganglioneuroma, 95
Ganglioglioma, 96
Ganglioma. *Diagnose as* Ganglioneuroma, 95
malignant. *Diagnose as* Malignant ganglioneuroma, 95
Ganglion. *See also under name of specific ganglion*
injury, 432 (4)
of joint, 162 (6)
of tendon sheath, 97
Ganglioneuroma, 95
of adrenal medulla, 397 (8)
malignant, 95
retroperitoneal, 301 (8)
of vegetative nervous system, 432 (8)
Ganglionitis, 421 (1). *See also* Zoster
chronic, 421 (1)
of gasserian ganglion, 428 (1)
of geniculate ganglion, 428 (1)
Ganglioschwannospongioblastoma.
Diagnose as Glioma, not otherwise specified, 96
Gangosa, 177 (1)
Gangrene. *See also under organ, region or structure affected*
diabetic, 128 (7)
due to angiitis, 128 (5)
due to arteriosclerosis, 128 (5)
due to chemical burn, 125 (3)
due to cold, 126 (4)
due to disturbance of circulation, 128 (5)
due to electric burn, 126 (4)
due to embolism, 128 (5)
due to ergot, 125 (3)
due to heat, 126 (4)
due to infection, 123 (1)
due to phenol (carbolic acid), 125 (3)
due to poison, 125 (3)
due to Raynaud's disease, 128 (5)

Gangrene—Continued
due to section or constriction of artery, 128 (5)
due to thromboangiitis obliterans, 128 (5)
due to thrombosis, 128 (5)
due to trauma, 126 (4)
of skin
due to infection, 132 (1)
due to physical agent, 136 (4)
due to trauma, 136 (4)
due to undetermined cause, 142 (y)
Gargoylism. *See* Lipochondrodystrophy, 114 (0)
Garré's disease. *See* Osteitis, sclerotic, nonsuppurative, 148 (1)
Gas. *See also under name of gas*
anesthetic, poisoning by, 117 (3)
conjunctivitis due to, 469 (3)
illuminating, poisoning, 117 (3)
irritant, pharyngitis due to, 255 (3)
poisonous
acute rhinitis due to, 177 (3)
bronchiolitis due to, 190 (3)
bronchitis due to, 190 (3)
fibrinous chorditis due to, 183 (3)
laryngitis due to, 183 (3)
pneumonia, chronic interstitial, due to, 194 (3)
rhinitis, acute, due to, 177 (3)
suffocation by nonpoisonous, 119 (4)
war, poisoning, 118 (3)
Gasserian ganglion
ganglionitis, 428 (1)
Gastric. *See also* Gastritis; Gastro-; Stomach
crisis: *supplementary term,* 496. *Diagnose disease*
Gastritis. *See also* Perigastritis, 263 (1)
acute
corrosive, 264 (3)
infectious, 263 (1)
ulcerative, 263 (1)
chronic, 263 (1)
atrophic, 265 (9)
following operation, 264 (4)
hypertrophic, 265 (9)
nonspecific, 265 (9)
erosive, 265 (9)

Gastrocarcinoma. *Diagnose as* Carcinoma, not otherwise specified, 94
Gastroduodenitis
acute, catarrhal jaundice due to, 293 (6)
due to infection, 267 (1)
due to poison, 267 (3)
Gastroenteric stoma
malfunction, 267 (4)
stenosis, 267 (4)
Gastroenteritis
due to infection, 267 (1)
due to naturally toxic foods, 267 (3)
due to poison, 267 (3)
due to Salmonella paratyphi B (food poisoning), 267 (1)
due to staphylococcus toxin, 267 (1)
due to unknown cause, 267 (9)
Gastroileostomy, 267 (4)
Gastrointestinal tract. *See also* Intestines; Stomach
allergy, 267 (3)
diseases, 267
psychophysiologic reaction, 111 (55)
Gastroptosis, 265 (6)
Gastrostomy opening, 264 (4)
Gaucher's disease (lipid histiocytosis of kerasin type), 229 (7)
Gaze paralysis, lateral (Foville syndrome) : *supplementary term,* 504. *Diagnose disease*
Gee's disease. *See* Celiac disease, 240 (7)
Gélineau's syndrome. *See* Narcolepsy, 417 (x)
Gemmanoma. *Diagnose as* Hemangioma (angioma), 96
Geniculate ganglion
ganglionitis, 428 (1)
neuralgia, 418 (x)
Genital organs. *See* Genital system; Genitalia
Genital system. *See also* Genitalia
anomalies, with anomalies of other organs, 327 (0)
congenital defects, 327 (0)
diseases, 327 ff.
female
acute diffuse inflammation of internal organs, 349 (1)

Genital system—Continued
female—continued
chronic diffuse inflammation of internal organs, 349 (1)
diseases, 349 ff.
distortion or displacement of pelvic organs, sterility due to, 349 (6)
obstruction following infection, sterility due to, 349 (1)
male, diseases, 328 ff.
Genitalia
absence, complete, of internal and external, 327 (0)
female
internal, inflammation, 349 (1)
pain referable to: *supplementary term,* 499. *Diagnose disease*
infantile, 327 (7)
lymphangiectatic elephantiasis of external, 330 (5)
lymphatic reticuloendothelioma. *Diagnose as* Mesothelioma, 97
male, pain referable to: *supplementary term,* 499. *Diagnose disease*
Genitourinary system. *See* Urogenital system
Genu. *See also* Knee
recurvatum
congenital, 156 (0)
due to paralysis, 162 (55)
valgum
congenital, 156 (0)
due to rickets, 163 (7)
due to unknown cause, 164 (9)
varum
congenital, 156 (0)
due to rickets, 153 (7)
Geographic tongue, 246 (9)
Geotrichosis, 124 (2)
German measles. *See* Rubella, 116 (1)
Germinoma
except of pineal. *Diagnose as* Disgerminoma, 97
of pineal. *Diagnose as* Pinealoma, 98
Gerstmann's syndrome: *supplementary term,* 504. *Diagnose disease*
Gestation. *See* Pregnancy
Ghon tubercle. *See* Tuberculosis of lung, primary complex, 194 (1)
Giant cell tumor, 97
of bone, 154 (8)

Gliosis
of brain, due to trauma, 413 (4)
of cerebral aqueduct, 416 (9)
of spinal cord, due to trauma, 424
(4)
Glisson's disease. *See* Rickets, 121
(7)
Globe. *See* Eyeball
Glomangioma, 96, 129, 139 (8)
Glomerulonephritis
acute (acute hemorrhagic nephritis),
308 (1)
chronic or subacute, 308 (1)
embolic, 308 (1)
focal, 308 (1)
Glomerulosclerosis, intercapillary,
310 (7)
Glomus tumor. *Diagnose as* Glomangioma, 96
Glossitis
acute, 245 (1)
chronic, due to infection, 245 (1)
median rhomboidal, 246 (9)
Glossopharyngeal nerve
disturbances: *supplementary term,*
508. *Diagnose disease*
neuralgia, 431 (x)
Glottis
edema, obstructive
due to chemical changes in blood,
185 (5)
due to infection, 183 (1)
due to poison, 183 (3)
due to trauma, 184 (4)
spasm
due to lesion of central nervous
system, 185 (55)
reflex, through recurrent laryngeal nerve, 185 (55)
supplementary term, 507. *Diagnose disease*
Glucose tolerance. *See* Dextrose
tolerance: *supplementary term,*
500
Gluteal region
bursitis, 165 (4)
Glycogen
infiltration of myocardium (in von
Gierke's disease), 211 (7)
Glycogenosis, 120 (7)
hepatic, 289 (7)

Glycosuria
renal, 312 (x)
supplementary term, 498. *Diagnose
disease*
Goiter. *See also* Hyperthyroidism
"benign" metastasizing. *Diagnose as*
Functionally hyperactive thyroid tumor, 93
congenital, 388 (0)
diffuse, with hyperthyroidism, 390
(9)
exophthalmic. *See* Toxic diffuse goiter, 390 (9)
hyperfunctioning adenomatous. *Diagnose as* Functionally hyperactive thyroid tumor, 93
juvenile or adolescent, due to iodine
deficiency, 389 (7)
nodular, with hyperthyroidism, 390
(9)
nontoxic diffuse, 389 (9)
nontoxic nodular, 390 (9)
toxic diffuse, 390 (9)
toxic nodular, 390 (9)
Goldflam-Erb disease. *See* Myasthenia gravis, 169 (55)
Gonads. *See also* Hypergonadism;
Hypogonadism; Ovary; Testis
agenesis, 399 (0)
diseases, 399
dysplasia, 399 (0)
Gonococcic infections, 123 (1)
abscess
of bulbourethral gland
(Cowper's), 322 (1)
of ovary, 268 (1)
periurethral, 322 (1)
prostatic, 346 (1)
of seminal vesicle, 344 (1)
of urethral gland, 322 (1)
adenitis
of Bartholin's gland, 323 (1)
of bulbourethral gland, 322 (1)
arthritis, 157 (1)
balanitis, 329 (1)
cervicitis, 358 (1)
chordee, 329 (1)
conjunctivitis, 468 (1)
endometritis, 360 (1)
epididymitis, 335 (1)
exostosis of calcaneus, 148 (1)
lymphangitis of penis, 329 (1)
oophoritis, 368 (1)

Gonococcic infections—Continued
  prostatitis, 346 (1)
  pyelitis, 308 (1)
  pyosalpinx, 366 (1)
  stricture
    of urethra, 323 (1)
    of vagina, 355 (1)
  ureteritis, 314 (1)
  urethritis, 323 (1)
  vaginitis, 355 (1)
  vulvitis, 352 (1)
Gonorrhea. *See* Gonococcic infections
Goundou, 154 (9)
Gout, 120 (7)
  arthritis due to, 163 (7)
  bursitis due to, 165 (7)
Gower's syndrome. *See* Paroxysmal
  vasovagal attacks, 417 (x)
Graafian follicle
  cyst, 369 (7)
  hemorrhage of ovary from rupture
    of, 369 (7)
Gradenigo syndrome: *supplementary term,* 504. *Diagnose disease*
Graft. *See* Bones, graft
Grain itch (acarodermatitis), 134 (2)
Grand mal, 417 (x)
  and petit mal, 417 (x)
Granular cell myoblastoma, 96
Granulocytic myelosis. *Diagnose as*
  Granulocytic leukemia, 94
Granulocytopenia. *See also* Agranulocytosis, 228 (3), 228 (5)
  generally and unspecified, 229 (7)
  necrosis of larynx in, 185 (5)
  necrosis of pharynx in, 256 (5)
  necrosis of tonsil in, 259 (5)
  necrosis of vagina in, 356 (50)
  supplementary term, 493. *Diagnose
    disease*
  ulcer of colon in, 277 (5)
  ulcer of skin in, 137 (5)
Granuloma
  annulare, 141 (9)
  apical, 247 (1)
  due to infection, 123 (1)
  eosinophilic. *See* Histiocytosis, 120
    (7)
    of bone, 153 (7)
  foreign body, 126 (4)
  fungoides. *Diagnose as* Lymphosarcoma, 95

Granuloma—Continued
  Hodgkin's. *Diagnose as* Hodgkin's
    disease, 95
  inguinale, 133 (1)
  malignant. *Diagnose as* Hodgkin's
    disease, 95
  multiplex hemorrhagicum. *Diagnose
    as* Multiple hemorrhagic hemangioma of Kaposi, 139 (8)
  pyogenicum, 133 (1)
  telangiectaticum, 133 (1)
  umbilical, 123 (1)
Granulomatosis
  chronic pulmonary, in beryllium
    workers, 194 (3)
Granulosa cell tumor, 93
  diffuse. *Diagnose as* Granulosa cell
    tumor, 93
Granulosis rubra nasi, 138 (7)
Grasping and groping, forced: *supplementary term,* 504. *Diagnose
  disease*
Graves' disease. *See* Toxic diffuse
  goiter, 390 (9)
Grawitz tumor
  except of ovary. *Diagnose as* Adenocarcinoma, 94
  of ovary. *Diagnose as* Virilizing
    tumor, 93
Ground itch, 134 (2)
Growth. *See also* Dwarfism; Gigantism; Infantilism
  arrest, of bones, 148 (1), 151 (4).
    See also Retardation of ossification of epiphysis: *supplementary term,* 489
  disorders. *See under organ, region
    or structure affected*
Gubler-Millard syndrome: *supplementary term,* 505. *Diagnose disease*
Guillain-Barré syndrome: *supplementary term,* 504. *Diagnose disease*
Guinea worm infection. *See* Dracunculosis, 124 (2)
Gull's disease. *See* Atrophy of thyroid gland with myxedema, 389
  (9)
Gull and Sutton's disease. *See* Arteriosclerosis, general, 218 (9)

Gumma, 123 (1). *See also* Syphiloma; *and under organ or region affected*
Gums. *See* Gingiva
Gunshot wounds. *See* Bullet wounds, 118 (4); *and under organ, region or structure affected*
Gynandroblastoma, 94
Gynecomastia, 144 (7). *See also* Overdevelopment of breast in male, 143 (0)
due to estrogen administration, 144 (7)
Gyrate scalp, 131 (0)

H

Habit spasm: *supplementary term,* 504. *Diagnose disease*
Hadfield-Clarke syndrome. *See* Pancreatic infantilism, 295 (0)
Haemangioma. *See* Hemangioma
Haff disease. *See* Arsenic poisoning, 117 (3)
Hair
avulsion, 136 (4)
ball in stomach, 265 (6)
breaking off. *See* Trichokryptomania: *supplementary term,* 486
excessive growth. *See* Hypertrichosis, 131 (0), 138 (7), 461 (0); *See also* Hirsutism: *supplementary term,* 487
follicle. *See under* Skin, 131 ff.
gray or white. *See* Canities, 138 (7)
loss of. *See also* Alopecia *supplementary term,* 487. *Diagnose disease*
matrix carcinoma. *Diagnose as* Basal cell carcinoma, 94
piedra, 135 (2)
pubic, abnormal growth, 353 (7)
pulling out one's own. *See* Trichotillomania: *supplementary term,* 486
ringed. *See* Thrix annulata, 139 (7)
Halitosis: *supplementary term,* 496. *Diagnose disease*
Hallucinations: *supplementary terms,* 509. *Diagnose disease*
of hearing, 509
of smell, 509

Hallucinations—Continued
of taste, 509
of vision, 509
Hallucinosis
acute, 106 (3)
general: *supplementary term,* 504. *Diagnose disease*
hypnagogic: *supplementary term,* 504. *Diagnose disease*
hypnopompic: *supplementary term,* 504. *Diagnose disease*
Hallux
rigidus
due to infection, 158 (1)
due to trauma, 159 (4)
due to unknown cause, 164 (9)
valgus
congenital, 157 (0)
due to acute trauma, 159 (4)
due to nonpoliomyelitic paralysis, 161 (55)
due to pressure, 159 (4)
due to unknown cause, 164 (9)
following poliomyelitis, 161 (55)
varus
congenital, 157 (0)
due to scar tissue, 159 (4)
Hamartoblastoma
except of kidney. *Diagnose as* Hamartoma, 98
of kidney. *Diagnose as* Nephroblastoma, 98
Hamartoma, 98, 139 (8)
of liver. *Diagnose as* Hepatoblastoma, 98
pilo sebaceum; sebaceous. *Diagnose as* Neoplastic cyst, 93
tubular (ovary). *Diagnose as* Virilizing tumor, 93
vascular. *Diagnose as* Hemangioma (angioma), 96
Hamman-Rich syndrome, 197 (9)
Hammer toe
congenital, 156 (0)
due to unknown cause, 164 (9)
following poliomyelitis, 161 (55)
Hamstring muscles
contracture, congenital, 167 (0)
Hand. *See also* Fingers
abnormal division, 122 (0)
claw
due to spastic paralysis, 161 (55)
syringomyelic, 162 (55)

Hand—Continued
club, congenital, 156 (0)
elephantiasis, congenital, 122 (0)
sulfuric acid burn, 125 (3)
Hand-Schüller-Christian disease,
120 (7)
Handwriting disability. *See*
Agraphia, 501
Hanot's cirrhosis (hypertrophic
cirrhosis), 289 (9)
Hansen's disease. *See* Leprosy
Harelip. *See also* Lip(s), cleft
flattening of nose with, 176 (0)
Hashimoto's disease. *See* Chronic
thyroiditis, lymphomatous, 389
(9)
Hatred. *See* Misanthropy; Misogyny;
supplementary terms, 485
Haverhill fever (epidemic arthritic
erythema), 115 (1)
Hay fever (allergic rhinitis), 177 (3)
conjunctivitis, 469 (3)
Headache
supplementary term, 504. *Diagnose
disease*
Hearing. *See also* Deafness
disturbances: 112 (x) ; *supplementary term,* 508. *Diagnose disease*
hallucinations of: *supplementary
term,* 509. *Diagnose disease*
Heart. *See also* Cardiovascular system; Coronary artery; Endocardium; Myocardium; Pericardium
aberrant ventricular conduction, 213
(x)
absence. *See* Acardia, hemicardia,
201 (0)
absence of atrial septum (cor triloculare biventricularis), 202
(0)
absence of interatrial and interventricular septa, 203 (0)
absence of ventricular septum, 203
(0)
air embolism, 209 (4)
amyloidosis due to unknown cause,
212 (9)
anemia due to blood disease, 209 (5)
aneurysm
due to infarction, 210 (5)
due to infection, 207 (1)
due to reduced coronary blood
flow, 209 (5)
of ventricular septum, 203 (0)

Heart—Continued
anomalies, 201 (0)
anomalous atrial band, 202 (0)
anomalous atrial fold, 202 (0)
anomalous atrial septum, 202 (0)
anomalous coronary sinus, 202 (0)
anomalous eustachian valve, 202 (0)
anomalous muscle bundle between
atrium and ventricle, 202 (0)
anomalous ventricular band, 203 (0)
anomalous ventricular fold, 203 (0)
anomalous ventricular septum, 203
(0)
arrhythmia. *See* Arrhythmia
atrial abnormalities, 202 (0)
atrial septal defects, 202 (0)
with mitral stenosis and dilatation
of pulmonary artery, 202 (0)
atrophy
due to inanition, 211 (7)
due to unknown cause, 212 (9)
senile, 211 (7)
beats, premature, unspecified: *supplementary term,* 492. *Diagnose
disease*
beriberi, 211 (7)
bifid apex, 202 (0)
block
atrioventricular, due to unknown
cause, 214 (x)
bundle branch
congenital, 203 (0)
due to rheumatic fever, 212 (9)
due to sclerosis of nutrient artery, 210 (5)
due to unknown cause, 214 (x)
congenital, 203 (0)
intraventricular, due to unknown
cause, 214 (x)
sino-atrial, due to unknown cause,
214 (x)
calcification due to unknown cause,
212 (9)
conduction system, syphilis, 208 (1)
congenital defects. *See under* Cardiovascular system, 201
congestion, passive, 210 (5)
contractions, premature
atrial, due to unknown cause, 214
(x)
originating in atrioventricular
node, due to unknown cause, 214
(x)

Heart—Continued

Heart—Continued

Heart—Continued
valves—continued
fibrosis or calcification due to unknown cause, 213 (9)
perforation
due to acute bacterial endocarditis, 207 (1)
due to subacute bacterial endocarditis, 208 (1)
due to syphilis, 208 (1)
valvular disease, undiagnosed, 215 (y)
valvulitis
rheumatic, 213 (9)
syphilitic, 208 (1)
ventricular abnormalities, 203 (0)
ventricular septal defects, 203 (0)
with dextroposition of aorta, 203 (0)
localized, 203 (0)
with levoposition of pulmonary artery, 203 (0)
with pulmonary stenosis, dextroposition of aorta, hypertrophy of right ventricle, 203 (0)
Heartburn. *See* Pain in epigastrium: *supplementary term, 497*
Heat. *See also* Burn
abnormality of elimination: *supplementary term, 487. Diagnose disease*
cramps, 168 (4)
encephalopathy due to, 413 (4)
gangrene due to, 126 (4)
prostration, 118 (4)
rash (miliaria rubra), 137 (4)
sensation of: *supplementary terms. Diagnose disease*
absence, 501
diminution, 503
increase, 505
Heatstroke. *See* Heat prostration, 118 (4) ; Sunstroke, 119 (4)
Hebephrenia. *See* Schizophrenic reaction, hebephrenic type, 110 (x)
Heberden's nodes. *See* Degenerative joint disease, multiple, due to unknown cause, 164 (9)
Hebra's disease. *See* Erythema multiforme exudative, 141 (9)
Heel. *See* Calcaneus ; Foot ; Tendons

Helminthiasis. *See also specific parasitic infection under organ affected*
obstruction of appendix due to, 279 (2)
obstruction of small intestine due to, 272 (2)
Hemangioblastoma. *Diagnose as* Hemangiosarcoma, 96
Hemangioendothelioblastoma. *Diagnose as* Hemangiosarcoma, 96
Hemangioendothelioma, 96, 129 (8), 139 (8)
of bone. *Diagnose as* Ewing's sarcoma, 97
tubersum multiplex. *Diagnose as* Hemangiomatosis, 96
Hemangioendotheliosarcoma. *Diagnose as* Hemangiosarcoma, 96
Hemangiolipoma. *Diagnose as* Mesenchymoma, 98
malignant. *Diagnose as* Mesenchymal mixed tumor, 98
Hemangioma (angioma), 96, 129 (7)
ameloblastic. *Diagnose as* Odontogenic tumor, benign, 98
arterial ; arterial racemose. *Diagnose as* Hemangioma (angioma), 96
arteriovenous. *Diagnose as* Hemangioma (angioma), 96
benign "metastasizing." *Diagnose as* Hemangiomatosis, 96
capillare varicosum ; capillary. *Diagnose as* Hemangioma (angioma), 96
cavernous. *Diagnose as* Hemangioma (angioma), 96
hereditary hemorrhagic. *Diagnose as* Hemangiomatosis, 96
multiple hemorrhagic, 96
of Kaposi, 96, 129 (8), 140 (8)
papillary. *Diagnose as* Hemangioma (angioma), 96
pigmentosum atrophicum (pigmented atrophic). *Diagnose as* Hemangioma (angioma), 96
plexiform. *Diagnose as* Hemangioma (angioma), 96
racemose. *Diagnose as* Hemangioma (angioma), 96

Hemangioma—Continued
senile. *Diagnose as* Hemangioma (angioma), 96
serpinginosum. *Diagnose as* Hemangioma (angioma), 96
simplex. *Diagnose as* Hemangioma (angioma), 96
spider. *Diagnose as* Hemangioma (angioma), 96
telangiectoides (telangiectatic). *Diagnose as* Hemangioma (angioma), 96
venous. *Diagnose as* Hemangioma (angioma), 96
Hemangiomatosis, 96, 129 (8)
of retina, 449 (8)
of vessels of nervous system, 404 (8)
Hemangiomyolipoma. *Diagnose as* Mesenchymoma, 98
malignant. *Diagnose as* Mesenchymal mixed tumor, 98
Hemangiopericytoma, 96, 129 (8)
Hemangiosarcoma, 96
of skin, 139 (8)
Hemarthrosis
due to trauma, 159 (4)
Hematemesis
due to undetermined cause, 266 (y)
Hematoblastoma. *Diagnose as* Hemangiosarcoma, 96
Hematocele
pelvic, 372 (5)
of spermatic cord, due to unknown cause, 343 (9)
of tunica vaginalis, 337 (0)
due to trauma, 337 (4)
due to unknown cause, 338 (9)
induced during delivery, 337 (0)
Hematocolpos, 357 (6)
Hematoma
compression of spinal cord by, 423 (4)
due to birth injury, 122 (0)
due to hemophilia, 128 (5)
due to trauma, 126 (4)
following operation, 126 (4)
of retina. *Diagnose as* Hemangiomatosis, 96
subcutaneous, 136 (4)
subdural
due to trauma, 407 (4)
due to unknown cause, 407 (9)

Hematoma—Continued
subperiosteal, 151 (4)
Hematometra, 362 (6)
Hematomyelia, 424 (4)
Hematoporphyria. *See* Porphyria
Hematosalpinx, 367 (6)
due to infection, 366 (1)
Hematuria
renal, due to unknown cause, 312 (x)
supplementary term, 498. *Diagnose disease*
Hemendothelioma
of bone. *Diagnose as* Ewing's sarcoma, 97
except of bone. *Diagnose as* Hemangioendothelioma, 96
Hemeralopia. *See* Day blindness: *supplementary term,* 508
Hemianalgesia: *supplementary term,* 504. *Diagnose disease*
Hemianencephaly, 410 (0)
Hemianesthesia: *supplementary term,* 504. *Diagnose disease*
Hemianopsia: *supplementary terms. Diagnose disease*
binasal, 509
bitemporal, 509
homonymous, 509
macular involving, 509
macular sparing, 509
quadrantic, 509
Hemiathetosis: *supplementary term,* 504. *Diagnose disease*
Hemiatrophy
of face, 152 (55)
Hemiballismus: *supplementary term,* 504. *Diagnose disease*
Hemic and lymphatic systems
diseases, 227 ff.
psychophysiologic reaction, 111 (55)
Hemicardia, 201 (0)
Hemichorea: *supplementary term,* 504. *Diagnose disease*
Hemicrania (simple migraine), 417 (x)
Hemihypalgesia: *supplementary term,* 504. *Diagnose disease*
Hemihypertrophy, congenital, 114 (0)
Hemihypesthesia: *supplementary term,* 504. *Diagnose disease*
Hemimelus anomaly, 114 (0)

Hemiparesis: *supplementary term,* 504. *Diagnose disease*
Hemiplegia: *supplementary term,* 504. *Diagnose disease*
Hemispasm facialis: *supplementary term,* 507. *Diagnose disease*
Hemisporosis, 124 (2)
Hemivertebra
  absence, congenital, 146 (0)
Hemochromatosis, 128 (7)
  chloasma of eyelid in, 463 (7)
  of liver, 289 (7)
  of myocardium, 211 (7)
Hemocytoblastoma. *Diagnose as* Leukosarcoma, 95
Hemoglobin
  diseases of, 230 (9)
Hemoglobin pigment
  disturbance due to poison, 237 (3)
Hemoglobinemia
  following blood transfusion, nephrosis due to, 309 (3)
Hemoglobinopathy, 230 (9)
Hemoglobinuria
  paroxysmal
    due to cold, 237 (4)
    due to exertion, 237 (7)
    nocturnal, 238 (x)
  supplementary term, 498. *Diagnose disease*
Hemoglobinuric fever (nonmalarial), 115 (1)
Hemolymphangioma. *Diagnose as* Hemangioma (angioma), 96
Hemolysis: *supplementary term,* 493. *Diagnose disease*
  transfusion, 228 (3)
Hemolytic disease of fetus and newborn, 228 (3)
Hemopericardium
  due to rupture of adjacent structures, 210 (5)
  due to ruptured aneurysm, 210 (5)
  due to trauma, 209 (4)
Hemoperitoneum
  due to infection, 298 (1)
  due to trauma, 300 (4)
  due to undetermined cause, 302 (y)
  following operation, 299 (4)
Hemophilia, 238 (x)
  hematoma due to, 128 (5)
  vascular, 226 (9)

Hemopneumothorax
  due to rupture of adhesion, due to infection, 198 (1)
  due to unknown cause, 200 (9)
  produced by rupture of adhesion due to trauma, 199 (4)
  spontaneous, 200 (6)
Hemoptysis: *supplementary term,* 490. *Diagnose disease*
Hemorrhage. *See also* Epistaxis; *and under organ, region or structure affected*
  from artery
    compression of nerve by, 429 (4)
    due to essential polyangiitis, 218 (9)
    due to infection, 216 (1)
  due to trauma, 126 (4)
  following operation, 126 (4)
  from gastrointestinal tract or peritoneum: *supplementary term,* 496. *Diagnose disease*
  from lung (terminal): *supplementary term,* 490. *Diagnose disease*
  postpartum. *See* Uterus, hemorrhage
  from respiratory tract: *supplementary term,* 490. *Diagnose disease*
  visual disturbances (blindness) from loss of blood, 448 (5)
Hemorrhoids, 286 (6)
  prolapsed, 286 (6)
  thrombophlebitis of hemorrhoidal vein, 285 (1)
  thrombosed, 286 (6)
Hemospermia: *supplementary term,* 498. *Diagnose disease*
Hemothorax
  due to infection, 198 (1)
  due to rupture of blood vessel, 200 (5)
  due to trauma, 199 (4)
Henpue. *See* Goundou, 154 (9)
Hepaptosis. *See* Liver, ptosis, 289 (6)
Heparlobatum (syphilitic cirrhosis of liver), 288 (1)
Hepatic artery
  aneurysm due to trauma, 303 (4)
  embolic, 303 (1)
  arteriosclerosis, 304 (9)
  diseases, 303 ff.

Hepatic artery—Continued
  embolism
    due to trauma, 303 (4)
    due to unspecified cause, 303 (6)
    following operation, 303 (4)
  periarteritis nodosa, 304 (9)
  thrombosis due to unknown cause,
    304 (9)
Hepatic duct. *See under* Bile passages
Hepatic veins
  diseases, 303 ff.
  endophlebitis
    due to unknown cause, 304 (9)
    syphilitic, 303 (1)
  phlebitis, 303 (1)
  thrombosis
    due to infection, 303 (1)
    due to obstruction, 303 (6)
    due to unknown cause, 304 (9)
Hepatitis
  acute, due to infection, 287 (1)
  amebic, 287 (1)
  chronic, 287 (1)
  due to diphtheria, 289 (55)
  due to poison, 288 (3)
  following serum or blood transfusion, 287 (1)
  infectious (epidemic), 287 (1)
  syphilitic, secondary stage, 288 (1)
Hepatoblastoma, 98
  with heterotopic tissue. *Diagnose as*
    Hepatoblastoma, 98
Hepatolenticular degeneration, 414
  (7). *See also* Lenticular degeneration
Hepatoma, 94
  congenital. *Diagnose as* Hepatoblastoma, 98
  teratoid. *Diagnose as* Hepatoblastoma, 98
Hepatomegaly: *supplementary term,*
  496. *Diagnose disease*
  of undetermined origin, 290 (y)
Hepatoptosis. *See* Liver, ptosis, 289
  (6)
Hepatopleural fistula. *See* Liver,
  fistula
Hepatopulmonary fistula. *See* Liver,
  fistula
Hepatorenal syndrome, 290 (y)

**Hering classification of color
  blindness,** 446 (0)
Hermaphroditism, 327 (0). *See also*
  Pseudohermaphroditism
Hernia. *See also under organ, region
  or structure affected*
  diaphragmatic (esophageal hiatus),
    congenital, 171 (0)
    sliding, 172 (6)
  diaphragmatic (paraesophageal hiatus), 172 (6)
  epigastric, 300 (6)
  femoral, 300 (6)
    congenital, 298 (0)
  incarcerated, 300 (*footnote*)
  incision
    following operation, 126 (4)
    strangulated, 126 (4)
  inguinal, 300 (6)
    congenital, 298 (0)
    direct, 300 (4)
    indirect, 300 (6)
    interstitial, 300 (6)
  internal, 300 (6)
  irreducible, nonstrangulated, 300
    (*footnote*)
  ischiatic, 301 (6)
  ischiorectal, 301 (6)
  intestinal obstruction due to, 274 (6)
  lumbar, 301 (6)
  obturator, 301 (6)
  pannicular lumbosacroiliac, 174 (4)
  posterior vaginal, 371 (4)
  spigelian, 300 (4)
  strangulated, 300 (*footnote*)
  strangulation of colon due to, 277
    (5)
  umbilical, 301 (6)
    congenital, 298 (0)
  ventral
    congenital, 298 (0)
    due to trauma, 300 (4)
    postoperative, 300 (4)
    recurrent, due to trauma, 300 (4)
    strangulated, 300 (4)
Herniation, 128 (6)
  of fascial fat, 138 (6)
  of gastric mucosa, 265 (6)
  of nucleus pulposus
    due to trauma, 159 (4)
    due to unknown cause, 164 (9)
Heroin. *See* Opium, 117 (3)

Herpes
of eyelid, 462 (1)
iris, of conjunctiva, 468 (1)
keratitis of cornea, 434 (1)
simplex, 133 (1)
of conjunctiva, 468 (1)
of larynx, 183 (1)
of lip, 243 (1)
of mouth, 241 (1)
of penis or prepuce, 329 (1)
of scrotum, 339 (1)
systemic, 115 (1)
of vulva, 352 (1)
zoster. *See* Zoster
Herrick's anemia. *See* Anemia, sickle
cell, 230 (9)
Heterochromia iridis, 439 (0)
Heterophil antibody test, positive:
supplementary term, 495. *Diag-*
nose disease
Heterotopia
cerebralis, 410 (0)
spinalis, 421 (0)
Hexapods
list, 66
Hibernation: *supplementary term,*
500. *Diagnose disease*
Hibernoma. *Diagnose as* Lipoma, 97
Hiccup, 172 (55)
supplementary term, 496. *Diagnose*
disease
Hidradenitis suppurativa, 133 (1)
Hidradenocarcinoma. *Diagnose as*
Sweat gland tumor, 94
Hidradenoides, apocrine. *Diagnose*
as Sweat gland tumor, 94
Hidradenoma, 140 (8)
intracanaliculare. *Diagnose as* Sweat
gland tumor, 94
papillary or papilliferum. *Diagnose*
as Sweat gland tumor, 94
tubular. *Diagnose as* Sweat gland
tumor, 94
Hidrocystadenoma. *Diagnose as*
Sweat gland tumor, 94
Hidrocystoma. *Diagnose as* Sweat
gland tumor, 94
Hidrosadenitis. *See* Hidradenitis, 133
(1)
Hilus cell tumor (ovary). *Diagnose*
as Virilizing tumor, 93
Hip. *See also* Coxa valga; Coxa vara

Hip—Continued
contracture
abduction, following poliomyelitis,
160 (55)
adduction
due to trauma, 158 (4)
following poliomyelitis, 160 (55)
due to flaccid paralysis, following
poliomyelitis, 161 (55)
extension, following poliomyelitis,
160 (55)
external rotation, following poliomyelitis, 160 (55)
flexion
due to trauma, 158 (4)
following poliomyelitis, 160 (55)
internal rotation, following paralysis, 161 (55)
dislocation, 159 (4)
congenital, 157 (0)
deformity of pelvis due to, 385
(4)
snapping, 174 (6)
Hippel's *or* **Hippel-Lindau disease.**
Diagnose as Hemangiomatosis, 96
Hirschsprung's disease. *See* Dilatation of colon, congenital; Megacolon, congenital, 276 (0)
Hirsutism. *See also* Hypertrichosis
supplementary term, 487. *Diagnose*
disease
Histiocytosis, lipid, 229 (7)
kerasin type (Gaucher's disease),
229 (7)
phosphatide type (Niemann-Pick
disease), 229 (7)
Histiocytosis X, 120 (7), 128 (7)
Histoplasmin test reaction: *supple-*
mentary term, 487. *Diagnose dis-*
ease
Histoplasmosis, 124 (2). *See also*
under organ, region or structure
affected
generalized, 116 (2)
Hives. *See* Urticaria
Hoarseness: *supplementary term,*
490. *Diagnose disease*
Hodgkin's disease, 95, 129 (8), 236
(8)
of blood, 230 (8)
of bone marrow, 239 (8)
of skin, 139 (8)
of spleen, 233 (8)

Hodgkin's granuloma *or* granulomatous lymphoma. *Diagnose as* Hodgkin's disease, 95

Hodgkin's lymphoblastoma *or* lymphoma. *Diagnose as* Hodgkin's disease, 95

Hodgkin's lymphoreticuloma. *Diagnose as* Reticulum cell sarcoma, 95

Hodgkin's paragranuloma. *Diagnose as* Hodgkin's disease, 95

Hodgkin's pseudoleukemia. *Diagnose as* Hodgkin's disease, 95

Hodgkin's sarcoma. *Diagnose as* Reticulum cell sarcoma, 95

Homatropine
mydriasis due to, 439 (3)

Homologous serum jaundice, 287 (1)

Homosexual panic, acute: *supplementary term,* 485. *Diagnose disease*

Homosexual personality, 112 (x)

Homosexuality: *supplementary term,* 485. *Diagnose disease*

Hookworm infection. *See* Ancylostomiasis, intestinal 272 (2)

Hordeolum
externum, 462 (1)
internum, 462 (1)

Hormonal glands. *See* Endocrine glands; *and name of specific gland*

Horn, cutaneous, 140 (9)
of mouth, 242 (9)

Horner's syndrome. *See also* Cervical sympathetic paralysis, 432 (4) *supplementary term,* 504. *Diagnose disease*

Horseshoe kidney, 307 (0)

Hourglass gallbladder, 291 (0)

Hourglass stomach
congenital, 263 (0)
due to ulcer, 265 (9)

Hugier's disease. *Diagnose as* Leiomyoma, 96

Humerus
fracture due to syphilis, 148 (1)
periostitis due to streptococcic infection, 149 (1)

Humpback. *See* Kyphosis

Hunner's ulcer. *See* Interstitial cystitis with ulceration, 321 (9)

Huntington's chorea. *See* Hereditary chronic progressive chorea with mental deterioration, 416 (9)

Hurler's disease. *See* Lipochondrodystrophy, 114 (0)

Hürthle cell tumor, 94
salivary gland. *Diagnose as* Adenolymphoma, 98

Hutchinson's teeth, 247 (0)

Hutchinson-Boeck disease. *See* Sarcoidosis, generalized, 116 (1)

Hutchinson-Gilford disease. *See* Progeria, 121 (7)

Hyaline degeneration
of conjunctiva, 471 (9)

Hyaline membrane
of lung, 197 (9)

Hyalinosis cutis, 139 (7)

Hyaloid artery, persistent, 444 (0)

Hydatid of Morgagni, 366 (0)

Hydatiform mole, 97, 384 (8)

Hyde's disease. *See* Prurigo nodularis, 142 (9)

Hydradenoma. *See* Hidradenoma

Hydramnios. *See* Polyhydramnios, 384 (x)

Hydrarthrosis
intermittent, 164 (9)
supplementary term, 489. *Diagnose disease*

Hydrencephalomeningocele, 402 (0)

Hydroa vacciniform, 138 (7)

Hydrocele
of canal of Nuck, 354 (9)
of round ligament, 372 (9)
of spermatic cord
congenital, 342 (0)
due to unknown cause, 343 (9)
of tunica vaginalis
acute, due to infection, 337 (1)
acute suppurative, 337 (1)
chronic, due to infection, 337 (1)
congenital, 337 (0)
due to trauma, 337 (4)
senile, 337 (7)

Hydrocephalus
congenital
communicating, 410 (0)
obstructive type, 410 (0)
due to inadequate absorption following operation, 406 (4)
due to sclerosis of foramen, 412 (1)

Hydrocephalus—Continued
ependymitis with, 412 (1)
external: *supplementary term,* 504.
Diagnose disease
supplementary term, 504. *Diagnose*
disease
Hydroma, solid. *Diagnose as* Sweat
gland tumor, 94
Hydromicrocephaly, 411 (0)
Hydromyelia, 421 (0)
Hydronephrosis, 310 (6)
congenital, 307 (0)
due to pressure of aberrant vessel,
309 (4)
hydroureter with, congenital, 313
(0)
infected, 310 (6)
Hydropericardium
due to heart failure, 210 (5)
due to unknown cause, 213 (9)
Hydroperitoneum: *supplementary*
term, 496. *Diagnose disease*
Hydrophobia. *See* Rabies, 116 (1)
Hydrophthalmos
due to lesions of early life, 453 (6)
infantile glaucoma, 453 (0)
Hydropneumopericardium, 208 (1)
Hydropneumothorax
due to infection, 198 (1)
due to injury
of chest wall, 199 (4)
of lung, 199 (4)
due to spontaneous pneumothorax,
200 (9)
due to tuberculosis, 198 (1)
following operation, 199 (4)
supplementary term, 490. *Diagnose*
disease
Hydrops. *See also* Edema
hypertensive meningeal, 407 (x)
of labyrinth, 480 (9)
Hydrorrhea
due to unknown cause, 179 (x)
gravidarum, 384 (x)
nasal, due to vasomotor disturbance,
178 (5)
Hydrosalpinx, 367 (6)
Hydrothorax
due to neoplasm, 200 (4)
due to passive congestion, 200 (5)
supplementary term, 490. *Diagnose*
disease

Hydroureter
congenital (with hydronephrosis),
313 (0)
due to obstruction, 315 (6)
Hygroma
of neck, 234 (0)
subdural, due to infection, 405 (1)
due to trauma, 407 (4)
Hymen
absence, 351 (0)
atresia
congenital, 351 (0)
due to infection, 352 (1)
due to undetermined cause, 354
(y)
blood supply, excessive, 351 (0)
cyst, 353 (6)
due to lacerations, 353 (4)
embryonal, 351 (0)
displacement upward, 351 (0)
division into two parts, 351 (0)
hypertrophy, congenital, 351 (0)
injury, 353 (4)
supernumerary, 351 (0)
thickening, 354 (9)
variations in form, 351 (0)
Hyoid bone
abnormal union with thyroid cartilage, 182 (0)
fracture, 184 (4)
Hypalgesia: *supplementary term,* 504.
Diagnose disease
Hyperadrenalcorticism
with diabetes mellitus, 398 (7)
Hyperadrenalism
endometrial dysfunction secondary
to, 363 (7)
Hyperalgesia: *supplementary term,*
504. *Diagnose disease*
Hyperbilirubinemia
constitutional, 237 (x)
infantile constitutional, 238 (x)
Hypercalcemia: *supplementary term,*
493. *Diagnose disease*
Hypercementosis, 249 (7)
Hyperchloremia: *supplementary*
term, 493. *Diagnose disease*
Hyperchlorhydria: *supplementary*
term, 496. *Diagnose disease*
Hypercholesteremia: *supplementary*
term, 494. *Diagnose disease*
familial, 230 (9)

Hypertension—Continued
arterial—continued
encephalopathy due to, 414 (5)
cerebral hemorrhage due to, 419 (5)
essential vascular, 219 (x)
intraocular. *See* Intraocular pressure
of lesser circulation, 222 (5)
cardiovascular disease due to, 206
(5)
due to arteriovenous shunt, 222
(5)
due to obstruction of blood flow,
222 (5)
portal, 288 (5)
Hypertensive cardiovascular disease, 206 (5)
Hypertensive vascular disease, 217
(5)
Hyperthermia. *See* Pyrexia: *supplementary term,* 486
Hyperthyroid heart, 211 (7)
Hyperthyroidism. *See also* Goiter
chloasma of eyelid in, 463 (7)
diabetes mellitus with, 398 (7)
diffuse goiter with, 390 (9)
endometrial dysfunction secondary
to, 363 (7)
without evident goiter, 389 (7)
exophthalmos due to, 433 (7)
factitious, due to chronic ingestion
of thyroid hormone, 388 (3)
nodular goiter with, 390 (9)
secondary to hyperpituitarism, 389
(7)
Hypertrichosis. *See also* Hirsutism
acquired, 138 (7)
congenital, 131 (0)
of eyelids
acquired, 464 (7)
congenital, 461 (0)
Hypertrophy. *See also under organ,*
region or structure affected
congenital, 122 (0)
due to increased blood supply, 128
(5)
of nail, 141 (9)
Hypertropia
due to error of refraction, 456 (5)
of unknown cause, 457 (x)
Hyperuricemia: *supplementary term,*
498. *Diagnose disease*

Hyperventilation, tetany due to:
supplementary term, 486. *Diagnose disease*
Hypervitaminosis, 119 (7)
Hypesthesia: *supplementary term,*
505. *Diagnose disease*
Hyphemia, 433 (50)
Hypoadrenalcorticism
diabetes mellitus with, 398 (7)
Hypoadrenalism
endometrial dysfunction secondary
to, 363 (7)
Hypoalderstonism. *See* Adrenal cortical hyperfunction, 397 (7)
Hypobaropathy, 118 (4)
Hypocalcemia: *supplementary term,*
494. *Diagnose disease*
Hypochloremia: *supplementary term,*
494. *Diagnose disease*
Hypochlorhydria: *supplementary*
term, 496. *Diagnose disease*
Hypocholesteremia: *supplementary*
term, 494. *Diagnose disease*
Hypochondriasis: *supplementary*
term, 485. *Diagnose disease*
Hypochromasia: *supplementary term,*
494. *Diagnose disease*
Hypocupremia: *supplementary term,*
494. *Diagnose disease*
Hypogammaglobulinemia: *supplementary term,* 494. *Diagnose disease*
Hypoglobulinemia: *supplementary*
term, 494. *Diagnose disease*
Hypoglossal nerve
atrophy: *supplementary term,* 509.
Diagnose disease
disturbances: *supplementary term,*
508. *Diagnose disease*
paralysis: *supplementary term,* 509.
Diagnose disease
Hypoglycemia: *supplementary term,*
494. *Diagnose disease*
Hypogonadism
ovarian, 369 (7)
testicular, 333 (7)
Hyponatremia: *supplementary term,*
494. *Diagnose disease*
Hyponitremia: *supplementary term,*
494. *Diagnose disease*
Hypoparathyroidism
due to operation, 391 (4)
due to radiation injury, 391 (4)

Hypophosphatasia, 152 (7)
Hypophosphatemia: *supplementary term*, 494. *Diagnose disease*
Hypophysis cerebri. *See* Pituitary gland
Hypopituitarism
anterior hypofunction, 394 (7)
decreased function of ovary in, 369 (7)
diabetes mellitus with, 398 (7)
due to postpartum hemorrhage, 393 (5)
endometrial dysfunction secondary to, 363 (7)
juvenile, 394 (7)
secondary to adrenal cortical hypofunction, 397 (7)
sterility due to, 349 (7)
Hypopituitary cachexia, 394 (7)
Hypoplasia. *See also under organ, region or structure affected*
congenital, 122 (0), 147 (0)
erythroid
due to unknown cause, 231 (9)
secondary to anemia, 229 (5)
thrombocytic, 229 (7)
unguinal, congenital, 131 (0)
Hypopotassemia: *supplementary term*, 494. *Diagnose disease*
Hypoproteinemia: *supplementary term*, 494. *Diagnose disease*
with reversed albumin-globulin ratio, 494
Hypoprothrombinemia
due to drugs, 237 (3)
familial, 238 (x)
supplementary term, 494. *Diagnose disease*
Hyposalivation. *See* Xerostomia, 497 *supplementary term. Diagnose disease*
Hyposomnia: *supplementary term*, 505. *Diagnose disease*
Hypospadias
female, 351 (0)
frenular, 322 (0)
glandular, 322 (0)
penile, 322 (0)
penoscrotal, 322 (0)
perineal, 322 (0)
scrotal, 322 (0)

Hypotension
arterial
constitutional, 217 (5)
due to disease of adrenal glands, 218 (7)
intraocular. *See* Intraocular pressure
orthostatic, 219 (x)
Hypothermia: *supplementary term*, 485. *Diagnose disease*
Hypothyroidism
adult, due to unknown cause, 389 (7)
anemia, normocytic, due to, 229 (7)
congenital (cretinism), 388 (0)
diabetes mellitus with, 398 (7)
due to action of goitrogens, 388 (3)
endometrial dysfunction secondary to, 363 (7)
juvenile, due to unknown cause, 389 (7)
with roentgen ray injury, 388 (4)
secondary to hypopituitarism, 389 (7)
Hypotony, intraocular. *See under* Intraocular pressure
Hypotrichosis of eyelids
congenital, 461 (0)
due to infection, 462 (1)
Hypovitaminosis
multiple or undefined, 121 (7)
Hypsarhythmia: *supplementary term*, 505. *Diagnose disease*
Hysterical personality, 112 (x)

I

Ichthyosis, 131 (0)
of eyelid, 461 (0)
Icterus index, high: *supplementary term*, 493. *Diagnose disease*
Ideational apraxia: *supplementary term*, 502. *Diagnose disease*
Ideomotor apraxia: *supplementary term*, 502. Diagnose disease
Idiocy
amaurotic familial, 403 (7)
retinal atrophy in, 449 (9)
Mongolian. *See* Mongolism, 114 (0)
Ileitis, regional, 275 (9)
Ileocolitis
progressive caudal, 278 (9)

Ileocolitis—Continued
progressive cephalic, 278 (9)
Ileostomy
stenosis, 273 (4)
Ileum. *See also* Intestine, small, fistula, ileorectal, 268 (1)
Ileus
due to meconium, 271 (0)
paralytic
due to remote infection, 272 (1)
following operation, 273 (4)
neurogenic, 274 (55)
Iliac artery(ies)
arteriosclerosis, 218 (9)
common, and ureter, fistula, 314 (1)
Ilium
osteochondrosis, 155 (9)
Illuminating gas
poisoning, 117 (3)
Illusions: *supplementary term,* 505. *Diagnose disease*
Immature delivery, 377
Immature personality, 112 (x)
Immaturity, sexual: *supplementary term,* 486. *Diagnose disease*
Immersion, 118 (4)
cold water, exostosis of external auditory canal due to, 475 (4)
cramps, general muscular, due to, 168 (4)
syndrome, 126 (4)
Impacted cerumen, 476 (6)
Impacted feces, 278 (6)
Impetigo, 133 (1)
bullous, 133 (1)
herpetiform, 141 (9)
localized, 133 (1)
neonatal, 133 (1)
Implantation cyst
due to trauma, 136 (4)
Impotence, sexual
due to unknown cause, 328 (x)
neurogenic, 328 (55)
supplementary term, 498. *Diagnose disease*
Inadequate personality, 112 (x)
Inanition, 119 (7). *See also* Malnutrition; Starvation
with edema, 119 (7)
heart atrophy due to, 211 (7)

Incendiarism. *See* Pyromania: *supplementary term,* 486
Incineration, 118 (4)
by electricity, 118 (4)
Incision, hernia of, 126 (4)
Inclusion, dermoid *or* **epidermal.** *Diagnose as* Neoplastic cyst, 93
Incontinence. *See* Feces, incontinence; Urine, incontinence
Incoordination. *See* Ataxia: *supplementary term,* 489
Incudostapedial joint
ankylosis due to infection, 477 (1)
Indigestion. *See also* Digestive system, diseases; *and name of specific disease*
fat, 269 (7)
Induration
due to phlebitis, 137 (5)
Infantile genitalia, 327 (7)
Infantile uterus, 364 (7)
Infantilism
dwarfism and, 394 (7)
pancreatic, 295 (0)
renal. *See* Osteodystrophy, renal, 152 (7)
sex, 394 (7)
Infants
immature birth, 380 (0)
multiple births, 380 (0)
premature, 380 (0)
newborn. *See* Newborn
postmature birth, 380 (0)
premature birth, 380 (0)
term birth, 380 (0)
triplets, 380 (0)
premature, 380 (0)
twin birth, 380 (0)
double ovum, 380 (0)
single ovum, 380 (0)
twin birth, premature, 380 (0)
double ovum, 380 (0)
single ovum, 380 (0)
Infarction, 128 (5). *See also under organ affected*
Infection
diseases due to, 114 ff. *See also under name of specific disease or organ, region or structure affected*
prenatal maternal, chronic brain syndrome due to, 107 (0)

Infection—Continued
organisms causing, list, 57 ff.
Infestation
with insects, 134 (2)
with parasites, 134 (2)
Influenza, 115 (1)
myocarditis due to, 207 (1)
Infrapatellar fat pad. *See* Retropatellar fat pad
Infundibular stenosis: *supplementary term, 492. Diagnose disease*
Infusion reaction, 117 (3)
Inguinal ring
relaxation, 301 (6)
Inhalation burn, 175 (4)
Injuries, 126 (4). *See also* Fracture; Trauma; Wounds; *and under organ, region or structure affected*
Innervation, disturbance of
diseases due to. *See under organ, region or structure affected*
Inoculation, 481
serum sickness due to, 118 (3). *See also under* Serum
types, 115 (1)
Insanity. *See* Mental disorders; Psychotic disorders
Insects
in larynx, 183 (2)
list, 66
Insolation. *See also* Heat; Sunstroke
encephalopathy due to. *See* Encephalopathy due to sunstroke, 413 (4)
Insomnia: *supplementary term, 505. Diagnose disease*
Instability, emotional. *See* Emotional instability
Insular tissue
adenocarcinoma, 398 (8)
islet cell, 398 (8)
adenoma, 398 (8)
islet cell, 398 (8)
diseases, 398
inclusion in wall of small intestine, 271 (0)
inclusion in wall of stomach, 263 (0)
neoplasms, 398 (8)
sclerosis due to unknown cause, 398 (9)
tumors, unlisted, 398 (8)
Insulin
shock, 117 (3)

Insulin—Continued
subcutaneous atrophy due to injection of, 136 (3)
Insuloma
functioning. *Diagnose as* Functioning islet cell tumor, 93
not otherwise specified. *Diagnose as* Non-functioning islet cell tumor, 94
Integumentary system
diseases, 131 ff.
Intention tremor. *See* Asynergia: *supplementary term, 502*
Intercourse, painful. *See* Dyspareunia, 498
Internal ear. *See* Ear, internal
Internal secretion, glands of. *See* Endocrine glands
Intersexuality. *See* Hermaphroditism, 327 (0); Pseudohermaphroditism, 327 (0)
Interstitial cell tumor, 93
Interstitioma. *Diagnose as* Interstitial cell tumor, 93
Intertrigo, 136 (4)
Intervertebral cartilage. *See also* Nucleus pulposus
calcification due to infection, 157 (1)
chondritis, 157 (1)
chondroma, 163 (8)
tuberculosis, 157 (1)
Intestine(s). *See also* Colon; Gastrointestinal tract; Rectum; etc.
abnormality of filling: *supplementary term, 496. Diagnose disease*
adenocarcinoma, 274 (8)
adhesions
due to infection, 268 (1)
due to trauma, 273 (4)
following operation, 273 (4)
postoperative, 268 (4)
amyloid disease, due to infection, 272 (1)
ancylostomiasis, 272 (2)
argentaffinoma, 274 (8)
ascariasis, 272 (2)
calculus. *See* Enterolith, 278 (6)
carcinoma, epidermoid, 274 (8)
Chilomastix infection, 268 (1)
contents, tubercle bacilli in: *supplementary term, 497. Diagnose disease*

Intestine(s)—Continued
  diseases, 268 ff.
  distomiasis, 272 (2)
  diverticulosis, general, 269 (6)
  enteric cyst, 274 (6)
  eventration, 268 (4)
  fibroma, 274 (8)
  fistula
    cholecystointestinal, 292 (1)
      due to calculus, 293 (6)
    vesicoenteric, 318 (1)
  foreign body in, not due to trauma,
    269 (6)
  Giardia infection, 268 (1)
  hemangioma, 274 (8)
  hemorrhage
    due to trauma, 273 (4)
    due to undetermined cause, 270
      (y)
  hypermotility: *supplementary term,*
    496. *Diagnose disease*
  hypomotility: *supplementary term,*
    496. *Diagnose disease*
  infarction, 269 (5)
  injury, 268 (4)
  intussusception, 269 (6)
  lipodystrophy, 269 (7)
  lipoma, 274 (8)
  lymphosarcoma, 269 (8), 274 (8)
  neoplasms, 274 (8)
  obstruction
    due to congenital peritoneal adhe-
      sions and bands, 298 (0)
    due to foreign body, 269 (6)
    due to hernia, 274 (6)
    due to infarction, 269 (5)
    due to postoperative adhesions, 273
      (4)
    due to ulcer, 275 (9)
    due to undetermined cause, 270
      (y)
    supplementary term, 496. Diag-
     nose disease
  oxyuriasis, 268 (2)
  passive congestion, 269 (5)
  polyp, neoplastic, 274 (8)
  ptosis. *See* Enteroptosis, 269 (6)
  sarcoma, 274 (8)
    reticulum cell, 274 (8)
  small. *See also* Duodenum; Ileum;
    Jejunum
    abscess, 272 (1)
    adhesions, due to infection, 272 (1)

Intestine(s)—Continued
  small—continued
    anthrax, 272 (1)
    atresia, congenital, 271 (0)
    diseases, 271 ff.
    diverticulitis, 271 (0), 274 (6)
    diverticulosis, 271 (0), 274 (6)
    gallstone obstruction, 274 (6)
    gangrene due to circulatory dis-
      turbance, 273 (5)
    granuloma due to unknown cause,
      275 (9)
    hernia into omental sac or fossae,
      274 (6)
    inclusion of pancreatic tissue in
      wall, 271 (0)
    infarction, 273 (5)
    infection, parasitic, 272 (2)
    injury, 273 (4)
    neoplasms, 274 (8)
    obstruction due to helminthiasis,
      272 (2)
    perforation
      due to infection, 272 (1)
      due to poison, 273 (3)
    redundancy, congenital, 271 (0)
    rupture due to trauma, 273
      (4)
    stenosis, congenital, 271 (0)
    strangulation, congenital, 271 (0)
    stricture
      due to infection, 272 (1)
      following operation, 273 (4)
    tumors, unlisted, 274 (8)
    ulcer, granulocytopenic, 273 (5)
    volvulus, congenital, 271 (0)
  stasis: *supplementary term, 496. Di-*
    agnose disease
  stoma, stenosis after enterostomy,
    268 (4)
  strangulation, 273 (5)
  strongyloidiasis, 268 (2), 272 (2)
  tuberculosis
    primary, 268 (1)
    secondary, 268 (1)
  tumors, unlisted, 274 (8)
  volvulus, 269 (6)
Intoxication. *See also* Poisons and
  poisoning
  alcohol, 481. *See also* Alcohol; Al-
    coholism

Islet cell tumor—Continued
non-functioning, 94
not otherwise specified. *Diagnose as*
Non-functioning islet cell tumor,
94
Isoimmunization
due to ABO factor incompatibility,
117 (3)
due to Rh factor incompatibility, 117
(3)
Itch
grain (acarodermatitis), 134 (2)
ground, 134 (2)
Itching. *See* Pruritus
Ivory bones. *See* Osteopetrosis, 147
(0)

J

Jackson's veil *or* **membrane.** *See*
Peritoneal adhesions and bands,
congenital, 298 (0)
Jacksonian seizures (cortical), 416
(x)
supplementary term, 505. *Diagnose*
disease
Jacob's ulcer. *Diagnose as* Basal cell
carcinoma, 94
Jadassohn's nevus. *Diagnose as* Pigmented nevus, 94
Jansky-Bielschowsky disease. *See*
Amaurotic familial idiocy, late
infantile, 403 (7)
Japanese river fever. *See* Tsutsugamushi fever, 116 (1)
Jargon aphasia. *See* Agrammatism
aphasia: *supplementary term,* 501
Jaundice
catarrhal
acute, due to undetermined cause,
290 (y)
due to acute gastroduodenitis, 293
(6)
chronic idiopathic, 290 (x)
familial nonhemolytic, 290 (x)
homologous serum, 287 (1)
of newborn, physiologic, 290 (x)
spirochetal, 115 (1)
supplementary term, 485. *Diagnose*
disease
Jaw(s). *See also* Mandible
lower, marked projection, 154 (7)

Jaw(s)—Continued
meniscus, dislocation (snapping
jaw), 162 (6)
micrognathism, 153 (7)
prognathism, 154 (7)
Jejunum. *See also* Intestine, small
fistula
gastrojejunocolic, 267 (9)
obstruction, duodenojejunal, due to
bands, 274 (6)
petechiae of: *supplementary term,*
497. *Diagnose disease*
ulcer, 275 (9)
due to trauma, 273 (4)
gastrojejunal, 267 (9)
with perforation, 275 (9)
Jensen's disease. *See* Retinochoroiditis juxtapapillaris, 447 (1)
Johnson-Dubin syndrome, 290 (x)
Joint(s). *See also* Cartilage; Ligament; *and under name of specific*
joint or disease
actinomycosis of, 124 (2)
adhesions due to trauma, 158 (4)
ankylosed, fracture of, 159 (4)
ankylosis, bony or fibrous
due to trauma, 158 (4)
following operation, 158 (4)
caisson disease, 150 (4)
calcification due to unknown cause,
164 (y)
capsule, tear of, 160 (4)
Charcot (neurogenic arthropathy),
162 (55)
contracture
due to flaccid paralysis
following poliomyelitis, 160 (55)
nonpoliomyelitic, 161 (55)
due to infection, 157 (1)
due to spastic paralysis, 161 (55)
due to trauma, 158 (4)
deformity
congenital multiple, 156 (0)
congenital paralytic, 157 (0)
due to hemophilia, 164 (x)
due to hemorrhage, 164 (x)
due to infection, 158 (1)
due to osteomalacia, 163 (7)
due to rickets, 163 (7)
due to trauma, 158 (4)

Joint(s)—Continued
degenerative disease, multiple, due
    to unknown cause, 164 (9)
diseases, 157 ff.
dislocation
  congenital, 157 (0)
  due to flaccid paralysis, nonpolio-
      myelitic, 162 (55)
  due to infection, 158 (1)
  due to paralysis following polio-
      myelitis, 162 (55)
  due to spastic paralysis, 162 (55)
  due to spina bifida, 162 (55)
fistula into, due to infection, 158 (1)
flail, due to paralysis from polio-
    myelitis, 162 (55)
foreign body in, 159 (4)
ganglion, 162 (6)
hemorrhage into. *See* Hemarthrosis,
    159 (4)
injury, 159 (4)
instability
  due to trauma, 159 (4)
  following operation, 159 (4)
loose bodies in, 162 (6)
mice, 162 (6)
myxoma, 163 (8)
neoplasms, 163 (8)
neurogenic arthropathy, 162 (55)
osteochondritis dissecans, 164 (9)
pain, general (arthralgia) : *supple-
    mentary term,* 489. *Diagnose
    disease*
relaxation
  due to flaccid paralysis, nonpolio-
      myelitic, 162 (55)
  due to paralysis following polio-
      myelitis, 162 (55)
septic. *See* Arthritis due to infec-
    tion, 157 (1)
sprain of ligament, 159 (4)
stiffness
  due to trauma, 159 (4)
  following operation, 160 (4)
swelling: *supplementary term,* 489.
    Diagnose disease
synovioma, 163 (8)
tabetic arthropathy of knee, 162
    (55)
tumors, unlisted, 163 (8)
xanthoma, 163 (7)

Joint, contiguous
compression of nerve by, 429 (4)
Jokes, mania for playing. *See* Mo-
    ria: *supplementary term,* 485
Jugular vein
acute septic phlebitis, 224 (1)
thrombosis, due to infection, 224 (1)
Junctional paroxysmal tachycar-
    dia: *supplementary term,* 492.
    Diagnose disease
Juxta-articular nodules
due to syphilis, 133 (1)

K

Kahler's disease. *Diagnose as*
    Plasma cell myeloma, 95
Kala-azar, 115 (4). *See also* Leish-
    maniasis
Kaposi's disease. *See* Xeroderma
    pigmented, 132 (0)
Kaposi's multiple hemorrhagic he-
    mangioma, 96, 139 (8)
Kaposi's sarcoma. *Diagnose as* Mul-
    tiple hemorrhagic hemangioma of
    Kaposi, 96
Kaposi's varicelliform eruption,
    115 (1)
Kast's syndrome. *Diagnose as* Hem-
    angiomatosis, 129 (8)
Keloid, 96, 139 (8)
acne. *See* Folliculitis keloidal, 132
    (1)
of cornea, 437 (4)
Keratectasia, 434 (0)
Keratitis
band, 437 (9)
bullosa, due to unknown cause, 437
    (9)
deep, 434 (1)
disciformis, postvaccinulosa, 434 (1)
due to birth injury, 434 (0)
due to lagophthalmos, 436 (4)
lipid degeneration of cornea follow-
    ing, 437 (9)
neuroparalytica, 436 (55)
parenchymatous, 434 (1)
phlyctenular, 434 (1)
punctata leprosa, 434 (1)
punctata profunda, 434 (1)
pustuliformis profunda, 434 (1)

Keratitis—Continued
  syphilitic, 434 (1)
    congenital, 434 (0)
  tuberculous, 435 (1)
Keratocanthoma, 141 (9)
Keratocele, 434 (1)
Keratoconjunctivitis sicca, 436 (7)
Keratoconus, 434 (0), 437 (9)
Keratolysis exfoliativa, 141 (9)
Keratomalacia, 436 (7)
Keratomycosis, 435 (2)
Keratosis
  arsenical, 135 (3)
  congenital, 131 (0)
  due to unknown cause, 129 (9)
  folliculosis, 141 (9)
  nigricans. *See* Acanthosis nigricans,
    140 (9)
  palmar and plantar, 131 (0)
    acquired, 135 (3)
  pharyngeus, 259 (9)
  pilaris, 141 (9)
  punctate, 131 (0)
  seborrheic, 139 (7)
  senile, 139 (7)
Kerion, 134 (2)
Ketosis: *supplementary term,* 494.
  Diagnose disease
Kidney(s)
  abscess, 308 (1)
    perirenal, 308 (1)
  absence, 307 (0)
  adenocarcinoma, 311 (8)
  adenoma, 311 (8)
  adenomyosarcoma. *Diagnose as*
    Nephroblastoma, 98
  adhesions, perirenal, due to infec-
    tion, 308 (1)
  amyloid degeneration
    due to infection, 308 (1)
  amyloidosis, due to unknown cause,
    312 (9)
  atrophy due to pressure, 309 (4)
  blood vessels. *See also* Renal artery;
    Renal vein
    accessory, 307 (0)
    anomalous connection with kid-
      ney, 307 (0)
    anomalous origin, 307 (0)
  calcification, 312 (9)
  calculus, 310 (6)
    congenital, 307 (0)

Kidney(s)—Continued
  calyx
    calculus encysted in, 310 (6)
    carcinoma, transitional cell, 311
      (8)
    dilatation due to obstruction, 310
      (6)
    diverticulum, congenital, 307 (0)
  carcinoma, 311 (8)
    basal cell, 311 (8)
  carcinosarcoma, 311 (8)
  cholesteatoma, 311 (8)
  concentrating power: *supplementary
    terms. Diagnose disease*
    decreased, 498
    increased, 498
  contracted, due to pyelonephritis, 308
    (1)
  cyst
    congenital, 307 (0)
    due to trauma, 309 (4)
    multiple, 310 (6)
    solitary, 310 (6)
  cystic, congenital, 307 (0)
  diseases, 307 ff. *See also* Glomeru-
    lonephritis; Hydronephrosis;
    Nephritis; Nephrosclerosis;
    Nephrosis; Perinephritis; Pye-
    litis; Pyelonephritis; Pyone-
    phrosis
  displacement, 310 (6)
  double, with double renal pelvis, 307
    (0)
  ectopic, 307 (0)
  embolism, due to unspecified cause,
    310 (6)
  embryoma; embryonal adenomyosar-
    coma. *Diagnose as* Nephroblas-
    toma, 98
  endometriosis, 312 (9)
  fibroma, 311 (8)
  fibrosarcoma, 311 (8)
  fistula
    due to infection, 308 (1)
    due to trauma, 309 (4)
    following operation, 309 (4)
  floating. *See* Wandering kidney, 308
    (0)
  foreign body in, due to trauma, 309
    (4)
  fused, 307 (0)
  gumma, congenital, 308 (0)

Kidney(s)—Continued
hamartoblastoma. *Diagnose as* Nephroblastoma, 98
hemangioma, 311 (8)
hemangiosarcoma, 311 (8)
hematoma
  due to trauma, 309 (4)
  perirenal, due to trauma, 309 (4)
hemorrhage following operation, 309 (4)
herniation
  due to unknown cause, 309 (4)
  following operation, 309 (4)
horseshoe, 307 (0)
hydronephrotic contracted, 310 (6)
hyperplasia (giant kidney), 307 (0)
hypertrophy, 307 (0)
hypoplasia, 307 (0)
infarction
  due to embolism, 310 (5)
  due to thrombosis, 310 (5)
  due to uric acid, 310 (7)
infection due to trauma, 309 (4)
injury, 309 (4)
intrathoracic, with defect in diaphragm, 307 (0)
leiomyoma, 311 (8)
leiomyosarcoma, 311 (8)
lipoma, 311 (8)
  of hilus, 311 (8)
  perirenal, 311 (8)
liposarcoma, perirenal, 311 (8)
lobulation, fetal, 307 (0)
lone: *supplementary term,* 499. *Diagnose disease*
luxation due to trauma, 309 (4)
myxoma of hilus, 311 (8)
myxosarcoma of hilus, 311 (8)
necrosis of cortex due to ischemia (bilateral cortical necrosis), 310 (5)
neoplasms, 311 (8)
nephroblastoma, 311 (8)
passive congestion, 310 (5)
pelvis. *See also* Pyelitis; Pyelonephritis
  bifurcation, 307 (0)
  calculus, 310 (6)
  carcinoma
    epidermoid, 311 (8)
    papillary, 311 (8)

Kidney(s)—Continued
pelvis—continued
  double, with double ureter, 313 (0)
  foreign body in (exogenous), 309 (4)
  leukoplakia, due to infection, 308 (1)
  leukoplakia of ureter and, due to unknown cause, 316 (9)
  liposarcoma, 311 (8)
  malacoplakia, 308 (1)
  myoma, 311 (8)
  ramifying, 307 (0)
periarteritis nodosa, 312 (9)
poisoning, 309 (3)
polycystic, 307 (0)
ptosis. *See* Nephroptosis, 310 (6)
rotation, insufficient, 307 (0)
rupture
  during delivery, 308 (0)
  due to trauma, 309 (4)
  indirect, 309 (4)
  spontaneous, 312 (9)
sarcoma, 311 (8)
sclerotic capsulitis, 312 (9)
secretion of dye, abnormal: *supplementary term,* 498. *Diagnose disease*
senile atrophy, 311 (7)
serous papillary cystic tumor, 311 (8)
shield, 307 (0)
supernumerary, 308 (0)
syphilis, congenital, 308 (0)
teratoma, 311 (8)
thrombosis due to unspecified cause, 310 (6)
torsion of pedicle, 310 (6)
triple, 308 (0)
tumor cells in secretions: *supplementary term,* 499. *Diagnose disease*
tumors, unlisted, 311 (8)
wandering, congenital, 308 (0)
varix of renal papilla, 310 (6)
Kienböck's disease. *See* Osteochondrosis of lunate bone, 155 (9)
Kleptomania: *supplementary term,* 485. *Diagnose disease*
Klinefelter's syndrome, 332 (0)

Knee

arthritis
  due to contusion, 158 (3)
  due to gonococcic infection, 157
    (1)
bursitis, prepatellar, 165 (4)
contracture due to flaccid paralysis,
  161 (55)
  following poliomyelitis, 161 (55)
  nonpoliomyelitic, 161 (55)
dislocation, habitual, 159 (4)
ganglion of joint, 162 (6)
genu recurvatum
  congenital, 156 (0)
  due to paralysis, 162 (55)
genu valgum
  congenital, 156 (0)
  due to unknown cause, 164 (9)
genu varum, congenital, 156 (0)
hernia of joint, 162 (6)
ligament
  calcification of medial collateral,
    due to trauma, 158 (4)
  congenital relaxation, 157 (0)
  loose bodies in (joint mice), 162
    (6)
  sprain, 159 (4)
meniscus
  congenital hypertrophy, 157 (0)
  cyst (snapping knee), 162 (6)
  lateral, tear, 159 (4)
  medial, detachment, 159 (4)
retropatellar fat pad, hypertrophy,
  due to trauma, 151 (4)
tabetic arthropathy, 162 (55)

Knock knees. *See* Genu valgum, 164
  (9)
Köhler's bone disease. *See* Osteochondrosis of navicular, 155 (9)
Koilonychia, 141 (9)
Korsakoff's psychosis. *See* Chronic
  brain syndrome associated with
  alcohol intoxication, 107 (3)
Kraepelin-Morel disease (dementia
  precox). *See* Schizophrenic reactions, 110 (x)
Kraft-Weber-Demetri disease. *Diagnose as* Hemangiomatosis, 96,
  129 (8)
Kraurosis, 141 (9)
  of penis, 331 (9)
  of vagina, 357 (9)

Kraurosis—Continued
  of vulva, 354 (9)
Kraus's gland. *See* Gland of Kraus
Krukenberg tumor, 93
  of ovary, 370 (8)
Kümmel's disease (compression
  fracture of vertebra). *See* Fracture, compression, 150 (4)
Kultschitzky's carcinoma. *Diagnose
  as* Argentaffinoma, 95
Kussmaul's disease. *See* Periarteritis
  nodosa, 218 (9)
Kwashiorkor, 119 (7)
Kyphosis
  due to trauma, 158 (4)
  due to tuberculosis, 158 (1)
  following poliomyelitis, 161 (55)
  supplementary term, 489. *Diagnose
    disease*
  thoracic, osteochondrosis of vertebra
    with, 155 (9)

L

Labia

fistula, rectolabial, due to infection,
  352 (1)
majora
  abscess, 352 (1)
  absence (with ectopia vesicae),
    351 (0)
  adhesion, 351 (0)
  cyst, 353 (6)
  fusion of, congenital, with uro-
    genital sinus, 351 (0)
  hypertrophy, congenital, 351 (0)
minora
  absence (with epispadias), 351 (0)
  adhesion, congenital, 351 (0)
  elongation, 353 (4)
Labium frenum
  abnormality, congenital, 243 (0)
Labor. *See also* Parturition
  abnormal, 482
  false, 380 (7)
  missed, 380 (7)
  obstructed
    abnormal contraction of uterus
      due to, 375 (6)
    rupture of uterus due to, 375 (6)
  rigidity
    of cervix during, 375 (6)
    of perineum during, 375 (6)

Labyrinth
aplasia, congenital, 479 (0)
blast injury, 480 (4)
congestion, 480 (5)
dead, due to previous infection. *See*
    Labyrinthitis, chronic diffuse,
    479 (1)
degeneration of saccule, congenital,
    479 (0)
dilatation of saccule, congenital, 479
    (0)
fracture of osseous labyrinth and in-
    ternal ear, 480 (4)
hemorrhage, 480 (5)
hydrops (Ménière's syndrome), 480
    (9)
ischemia, 480 (5)
membranous
    collapse, congenital, 479 (0)
    degeneration (epithelial meta-
        plasia), congenital, 479 (0)
Labyrinthine syndrome. *See*
    Ménière's syndrome
Labyrinthitis
acute diffuse, 479 (1)
chronic diffuse, 479 (1)
diffuse serous, 479 (1)
due to poison, 479 (3)
due to trauma, 480 (4)
due to unknown cause, 480 (9)
Lacrimal gland(s)
achroacytosis
    due to infection, 465 (1)
    due to unknown cause, 467 (9)
adenocarcinoma, 466 (8)
calculus, 466 (6)
carcinoma, epidermoid, 466 (8)
dislocation, 466 (4)
epithelioma, multiple benign cystic,
    467 (8)
fistula
    due to infection, 465 (1)
    due to trauma, 466 (4)
hypersecretion, epiphora due to, 467
    (x)
luxation
    due to infection, 465 (1)
    due to trauma, 466 (4)
lymphosarcoma, 466 (8)
neoplasms, 466 (8)
retention cyst, 466 (6)
supernumerary, 465 (0)
tuberculosis, 465 (1)

Lacrimal gland(s)—Continued
tumors
    mixed, salivary gland type, 466
        (8)
    unlisted, 467 (8)
wound, 466 (4)
Lacrimal passages
atresia, congenital, 465 (0)
infection, 465 (1)
stenosis
    congenital, 465 (0)
    following operation, 466 (4)
Lacrimal sac
fistula
    due to infection, 465 (1)
    due to trauma, 466 (4)
foreign body in, 466 (4)
granuloma (polyp) in, 465 (1)
rhinoscleroma, 466 (1)
wound, 466 (4)
Lacrimal tract. *See also* Canaliculus;
    Lacrimal gland; Lacrimal pas-
    sages; Lacrimal sac; Lacrimo-
    nasal duct; Punctum lacrimale
diseases, 465 ff.
Lacrimonasal duct
atresia, congenital, 465 (0)
fistula
    due to infection, 465 (1)
    due to trauma, 466 (4)
stenosis
    cicatricial
        due to infection, 466 (1)
        due to trauma, 466 (4)
    congenital, 465 (0)
supernumerary, 465 (0)
    cyst due to, 465 (0)
Lactation
abnormal secretion of milk, 145 (x)
absence of milk secretion. *See* Aga-
    lactia, 145 (x)
disorders, 145 (x)
excessive milk secretion. *See* Galac-
    torrhea, 145 (x)
Lacteal duct(s)
carcinoma. *See* Breast, carcinoma,
    145 (8)
occlusion due to infection, 144 (1)
Lactic acid in gastric contents:
    supplementary term, 496. *Diag-
    nose disease*
Laennec's cirrhosis, 289 (9)

Lagleyze's disease. *Diagnose as*
Hemangiomatosis, 96
Lagophthalmos, 463 (55)
conjunctivitis due to, 469 (4)
keratitis due to, 436 (4)
Lambliasis. *See* Giardiasis, 268 (1)
Landouzy-Déjerine atrophy
Landry's paralysis. *See* Myelitis, ascending, acute, 422 (1)
de Lange's syndrome. *See* Dystrophia myotonica, 170 (9)
Langerhans' islands. *See* Insular
tissue
Langhans' tumor. *Diagnose as*
Hürthle cell tumor, 94
Lanois syndrome. *See* Hypophysial
gigantism, 393 (7)
Larva migrans, 134 (2)
Laryngismus stridulus
congenital, 182 (0)
Laryngitis
acute, 183 (1)
atrophic
due to infection, 183 (1)
due to unknown cause, 186 (9)
chronic
due to infection, 183 (1)
due to unknown cause, 186 (9)
due to vocal overstrain, 184 (4)
due to Borrelia vincenti, 183 (1)
due to parasitic infection, 183 (2)
due to poison, 183 (3)
infiltrative
due to infection, 183 (1)
due to unknown cause, 186 (9)
subglottic, due to unknown cause,
186 (9)
Laryngocele
ventricular, congenital, 182 (0)
Laryngoplegia: *supplementary term,*
508. *Diagnose disease*
Laryngoptosis, 185 (6)
Laryngotracheitis
acute, 183 (1)
chronic, due to infection, 183 (1)
Larynx. *See also* Epiglottis; Glottis;
Laryngitis; Vocal cords
abnormal union with trachea, 182
(0)
abscess, 182 (1)
absence, congenital, 182 (0)
acromegaly affecting, 185 (7)
adenoma, 186 (8)

Larynx—Continued
adenocarcinoma of ventricle, 186 (8)
articulation
cricoarytenoid
ankylosis, 182 (1)
arthritis, 182 (1)
dislocation, 184 (4)
atresia, congenital, 182 (0)
burn
chemical, 183 (3)
from heat, 184 (4)
by radium, 184 (4)
by roentgen rays, 184 (4)
calcification, 186 (9)
carcinoma, epidermoid, 186 (8)
chondroma, 186 (8)
constriction, congenital, 182 (0)
cyst, 185 (6)
congenital, 182 (0)
diphtheria, 182 (1)
diseases, 182 ff.
edema, cause unknown, 186 (9)
fibroma, 186 (8)
fistula, 183 (1)
due to trauma, 184 (4)
following operation, 184 (4)
foreign body in, 184 (4)
granuloma, 183 (1)
gunshot wound, 184 (4)
hematoma, 184 (4)
herpes simplex, 183 (1)
hyperesthesia due to reflex action of,
185 (55)
injury, 184 (4)
insects in, 183 (2)
leprosy, 183 (1)
lipoma, 186 (8)
necrosis in granulocytopenia, 185 (5)
neoplasms, 186 (8)
nodules, 184 (4)
obstruction due to foreign body, 185
(6)
paralysis
due to diphtheria toxin, 185 (55)
due to lead poisoning, 183 (3)
due to pressure, 185 (55)
supplementary term, 490. *Diagnose*
disease
perichondritis
due to infection, 183 (1)
due to trauma or following operation, 184 (4)
polyp, 186 (9)

Larynx—Continued
ptosis. *See* Laryngoptosis, 185 (6)
radiation injury of perichondrium,
184 (4)
sarcoidosis, 183 (1)
serum diseases of, 183 (3)
spasm. *See also* Laryngismus stridulus, 182 (0)
  due to foreign body, 184 (4)
  due to poison, 183 (3)
stab wound, 184 (4)
stenosis
  cicatricial, due to intubation, 184
  (4)
  due to abductor paralysis, 185 (55)
  due to infection, 183 (1)
  due to trauma, 184 (4)
  following radiation, 184 (4)
stricture
  due to acromegaly, 185 (7)
  due to poison, 184 (3)
syphilitis perichondritis, 183 (1)
thyroid (aberrant) tissue in (laryngeal struma), 182 (0)
tuberculosis, 183 (1)
tumors, unlisted, 186 (8)
ulcer, aphthous, 186 (9)
urticaria, 184 (3)
ventricle, prolapse, 185 (6)
  due to trauma or strain, 184 (4)
ventricular laryngocele, congenital,
182 (0)
ventricular sacculation, intralaryn-
geal, congenital, 182 (0)
web, congenital, 182 (0)
Lashes. *See* Eyelashes
Lateral gaze paralysis (Foville syndrome) : *supplementary term,*
504. *Diagnose disease*
Lateral sclerosis: *supplementary
term,* 505. *Diagnose disease*
Lateral sinus
phlebitis, 408 (1)
thrombosis due to infection, 408 (1)
Lateropulsion: *supplementary term,*
505. *Diagnose disease*
Latosuria: *supplementary term,* 498.
Diagnose disease
Laughter, forced: *supplementary
term,* 505. *Diagnose disease*
Laurence-Moon-Biedl syndrome,
114 (0)

Lead
arteriosclerosis, 217 (3)
incrustation of cornea, 435 (3)
myelopathy due to, 422 (3)
optic neuritis due to, 450 (3)
osteosclerosis, 149 (3)
paralysis of larynx due to poisoning,
183 (3)
paralysis of uvula due to, 250 (3)
poisoning, 117 (3)
Leather bottle (stomach). *Diagnose
as* Diffuse scirrhous carcinoma,
94
Leber's optic atrophy. *See* Hereditary atrophy of optic nerve, 452
(9)
Leg(s). *See also* Foot ; Knee ; etc.
angiospasm of arteries, 217 (5)
causalgia, 128 (55)
lymphedema precox, 234 (9)
milk. *See* Phlegmasia alba dolens,
128 (5)
phlebitis, induration due to, 137 (5)
shortening, congenital, 122 (0)
varicose veins, 225 (6)
Legg-Calvé-Perthes disease. *See*
Osteochondrosis of capital epiphysis of femur, 155 (9)
Leiofibromyoma. *Diagnose as* Leiomyoma, 96
Leiomyoadenosarcoma. *Diagnose as*
Nephroblastoma, 98
Leiomyofibroma. *Diagnose as* Leiomyoma, 96
Leiomyoma, 96, 139 (8)
cutis. *Diagnose as* Leiomyoma, 96
pedunculated. *Diagnose as* Leiomyoma, 96
retroperitoneal, 301 (8)
submucous. *Diagnose as* Leiomyoma, 96
subserous. *Diagnose as* Leiomyoma,
96
Leiomyosarcoma, 96
Leishmaniasis, 133 (1). *See also*
Kala-azar
americana (mucocutaneous), 115
(4)
of eyelid, 462 (1)
of skin (oriental sore), 133 (1)
Lens, crystalline
absence. *See* Aphakia, 442 (0)
coloboma, 442

Lip(s)—Continued
adenocarcinoma, 244 (8)
carcinoma
   basal cell, 244 (8)
   epidermoid, 244 (8)
chemical burn, 243 (3)
chondroma, 244 (8)
cleft, 243 (0)
cyst of glands, 244 (6)
deformity
   cicatricial, following operation,
      243 (4)
   congenital, 243 (0)
   due to trauma, 243 (4)
   due to unknown cause, 244 (6)
diseases, 243 ff.
fibroma, 244 (8)
fissure, cause unknown, 244 (9)
fistula, congenital, 243 (0)
hemangioma, 244 (8)
herpes, 243 (1)
hypertrophy, congenital, 243 (0)
injury, 243 (4)
lipoma, 244 (8)
lymphangioma, 244 (8)
myoblastoma, granular cell, 244 (8)
neoplasms, 244 (8)
neurofibroma, 244 (8)
split, congenital, 243 (0)
tumors
   mixed, salivary gland type, 244
      (8)
   unlisted, 244 (8)
ulcer due to unknown cause, 244 (9)
Lipemia
retinal, 448 (7)
supplementary term, 494. *Diagnose
   disease*
Lipid. *See also* Fat
pneumonia, 195 (4)
proteinosis, 139 (7)
Lipid cell tumor (ovary). *Diagnose
   as* Virilizing tumor, 93
Lipoblastoma. *Diagnose as* Fetal fat
   cell lipoma, 97
Lipochondrodystrophy, 114 (0)
Lipodystrophy
intestinal, 269 (7)
progressive, 139 (7)
Lipofibroma. *Diagnose as* Lipoma, 97
Lipofibrosarcoma. *Diagnose as* Liposarcoma, 97
Lipoid. *See* Lipid

Lipoma, 97, 139 (8)
embryonal cell. *Diagnose as* Fetal
   fat cell lipoma, 97
fetal fat cell, 97
lipoblastic. *Diagnose as* Fetal fat
   cell lipoma, 97
primitive cell. *Diagnose as* Fetal fat
   cell lipoma, 97
retroperitoneal, 301 (8)
subcutaneous. *Diagnose as* Lipoma,
   97
Lipomatosis
embryonal. *Diagnose as* Fetal fat
   cell lipoma, 97
not otherwise specified. *Diagnose as*
   Lipoma, 97
Lipomyohemangioma. *Diagnose as*
   Mesenchymoma, 98
malignant. *Diagnose as* Mesenchymal mixed tumor, 98
Lipomyoma. *Diagnose as* Mesenchymoma, 98
malignant. *Diagnose as* Mesenchymal mixed tumor, 98
Lipomyxoma. *Diagnose as* Fetal fat
   cell lipoma, 97
Lipomyosarcoma. *Diagnose as* Mesenchymal mixed tumor, 98
Lipomyxosarcoma. *Diagnose as*
   Liposarcoma, 97
Liponeurilemmoblastoma. *Diagnose
   as* Schwannoma, 95
Liposarcoma, 97
retroperitoneal, 301 (8)
Lissencephalia. *See* Brain, hypoplasia
Lithopedion, 380 (9)
Littré's glands. *See* Urethral glands
Livedo reticularis, 137 (5)
Liver. *See also* Hepatitis *and terms
   with prefix* "Hepato-"
abnormal function of: *supplementary
   term,* 496. *Diagnose disease*
abscess, 287 (1)
   due to trauma, 288 (4)
absence, congenital, 287 (0)
accessory, 287 (0)
adenocarcinoma, 289 (8)
adenoma, 289 (8)
amebic abscess, 287 (1)
amyloid degeneration due to infection, 287 (1)

Liver—Continued
amyloidosis due to unknown cause, 289 (9)
calculosis, intrahepatic, 289 (6)
cholangioma, 289 (8)
cirrhosis
  alcoholic. *See* Laennec's cirrhosis, 289 (9)
  coarse nodular, 289 (9)
  congenital, 287 (0)
  due to passive congestion, 288 (5)
  hypertrophic (Hanot's), 289 (9)
  Laennec's, 289 (9)
  in lenticular nuclear degeneration, 289 (9)
  with obliterative cholangiitis, congenital, 287 (0)
  obstructive biliary, 289 (6)
  syphilitic (heparlobatum), 288 (1)
coccidiosis, 287 (1)
cyst
  due to calculus, 289 (6)
  inflammatory, of falciform ligament, 289 (6)
cystic disease, congenital, 287 (0)
cysticercosis, 288 (2)
degeneration, diffuse, due to poison, 288 (3)
diseases, 287 ff.
distomiasis, 288 (2)
echinococcosis, 288 (2)
embryoma. *Diagnose as* Hepatoblastoma, 98
enlargement. *See* Hepatomegaly, 290 (y); *supplementary term,* 496
fatty
  due to alcohol poisoning, 288 (3)
  with malnutrition, 289 (7)
  with obesity, 289 (7)
fibroma, 289 (8)
fistula
  due to abscess, 287 (1)
  hepatoabdominal wall, 287 (1)
  hepatobronchial, 287 (1)
  hepatopleural, 287 (1)
  hepatopulmonary, 287 (1)
granuloma due to infection, 287 (1)
hamartoma. *Diagnose as* Hepatoblastoma, 98
hemangioma, 289 (8)
hemochromatosis, 289 (7)

Liver—Continued
hepatoblastoma, 289 (8)
hepatoma, 289 (8)
hernia, congenital, 287 (0)
hypoplasia of one lobe with hyperplasia of others, congenital, 287 (0)
inclusion of gallbladder in, congenital, 287 (0)
infarction
  due to embolism, 288 (5)
  due to periarteritis nodosa, 288 (5)
  due to thrombosis, 288 (5)
injury, 288 (4)
lobulation, abnormal, congenital, 287 (0)
necrosis, acute diffuse, 289 (9)
neoplasms, 289 (8)
passive congestion, 288 (5)
porocephaliasis, 288 (2)
ptosis, 289 (6)
Riedel's lobe, 287 (0)
sarcoidosis, 288 (1)
subhepatic abscess, 298 (1)
tumors, unlisted, 289 (8)
yellow atrophy, acute or subacute, 289 (9)
Loa loa. *See* Filariasis
Lobstein's disease. *See* Fragilitas ossium, 147 (0)
Lobster claw foot, 122 (0)
Lobster claw hand, 122 (0)
Localization sense, loss of: *See* Agnosia, localization: *supplementary term,* 501
Lockjaw. *See* Tetanus, 116 (1)
Locomotor ataxia. *See* Tabes dorsalis, 403 (1)
Loeffler's syndrome, 194 (3)
Longitudinal sinus, superior
diseases, 408
Lop ear, 474 (0)
Lorain syndrome. *See* Dwarfism and infantilism, 394 (7)
Lordosis
due to poliomyelitis, 161 (55)
supplementary term, 489. *Diagnose disease*
Ludwig's angina. *See* Cellulitis of floor of mouth, 241 (1)
Lues. *See* Syphilis

Lumbago: *supplementary term,* 489.
Diagnose disease
Lumbosacral joint
transitional (incomplete sacralization), 156 (0)
unstable, 156 (0)
with posterior displacement, 156
(0)
Lumbosacral pain: *supplementary
term,* 489. *Diagnose disease*
Lunate bone
osteochondrosis, 155 (9)
Lung(s). *See also* Pleura; Pneumonia; Pneumonitis; Pneumoconiosis, etc.
abscess, 192 (1)
due to aspiration of foreign body,
195 (4)
due to foreign body, 195 (4)
due to fungus, 194 (2)
due to pneumococcus, 192 (1)
due to trauma, 195 (4)
due to undetermined cause, 197
(y)
absence of fissures, 192 (0)
absence of lobe with blind bronchus,
189 (0)
accessory, 192 (0)
accessory lobe, 192 (0)
actinomycosis, 194 (2)
adenocarcinoma, 196 (8)
agenesis, 192 (0)
alveolar microlithiasis, 197 (9)
alveolar proteinosis, 197 (9)
amebiasis, 192 (1)
anthrax, 192 (1)
aplasia, 192 (0)
with aplasia of bronchus, 189 (0)
ascariasis, 194 (2)
atrophy, 192 (0)
azygos lobe, 192 (0)
blastomycosis, 194 (2)
calcification
due to infection, 193 (1)
due to unknown cause, 197 (9)
carcinoma, 196 (8)
alveolar cell (bronchiolar), 196
(8)
epidermoid, 197 (8)
undifferentiated, 197 (8)
coccidioidomycosis, 194 (2)
collapse. *See also* Atelectasis; Pneumothorax

Lung(s)—Continued
collapse—continued
massive, due to undetermined
cause, 197 (y)
congestion
due to blast injury, 195 (4)
due to hot or cold air, 195 (4)
hypostatic, 196 (5)
passive, 196 (5)
cyst
acquired, 196 (6)
congenital, 192 (0)
parasitic, 194 (2)
pulmonary hydatid, 194 (2)
cystic disease, congenital, 192 (0)
associated with intralobular
sequestration, 192 (0)
diseases, 192 ff.
heart enlargement due to, 210 (5)
division, abnormal, 192 (0)
echinococcosis, 194 (2)
ectopic bone and cartilage in, 192 (0)
edema
acute, due to trauma or physical
agent, 195 (4)
due to infection, 193 (1)
due to poisoning, 194 (3)
due to undetermined cause, 197
(y)
following operation, 195 (4)
supplementary term, 490. *Diagnose disease*
emphysema. *See* Emphysema
fibrosis. *See also* Pneumonia, interstitial, chronic, 193 (1)
diffuse interstitial, 197 (9)
due to foreign body, 195 (4)
due to roentgen rays, 195 (4)
due to unknown cause, 197 (9)
following tuberculosis, 193 (1)
fistula
hepatopulmonary, 287 (1)
pulmonoperitoneal, 171 (1)
foreign body in, 195 (4)
gangrene
due to circulatory disturbance, 196
(5)
due to embolus, 196 (5)
due to infection, 193 (1)
due to trauma, 195 (4)
granuloma, 193 (1)
due to fungus, 194 (2)
due to tuberculosis, 193 (1)

Lung(s)—Continued
granuloma—continued
due to undetermined cause, 197
(y)
hamartoma, 197 (8)
hemorrhage
due to undetermined cause, 197
(y)
secondary to pulmonary hypertension, 196 (5)
supplementary term, 490. *Diagnose disease*
hernia
congenital, 192 (0)
due to trauma, 195 (4)
subcutaneous, due to trauma, 195
(4)
transmediastinal, 195 (4)
histoplasmosis, 194 (2)
hyaline membrane, 197 (9)
hypoplasia, 192 (0)
infarction, 196 (5)
infection, due to atypical mycobacte-
rium, 193 (1)
infection, parasitic, 194 (2)
with cavitation, 194 (2)
due to fungus, 194 (2)
injury, 195 (4)
laceration by fractured rib, 195 (4)
neoplasms, 197 (8)
nocardiosis, 194 (2)
peripheral air leak following operation, 195 (4)
poisoning by chemical (congestion),
195 (3)
radiopaque body in: *supplementary
term,* 490. *Diagnose disease*
rales: *supplementary term,* 490. *Diagnose disease*
sclerosis. *See* Pneumonia, interstitial, chronic, 193 (1)
syphilis, 193 (1)
tuberculosis. *See* Tuberculosis of
lung, 193 (1), 194 (1)
tumors, unlisted, 197 (8)
Lupus
erythematosus
discoid, 133 (1)
disseminatus, 121 (9)
of skin, 133 (1)
systemic, 133 (1)

Lupus—Continued
vulgaris (tuberculosis luposa), 134
(1)
Luteinoma. *Diagnose as* Thecoma
(Theca cell tumor), 93
Lutembacher syndrome, 202 (0)
Lutenoma. *Diagnose as* Thecoma
(Theca cell tumor), 93
Luteoblastoma. *Diagnose as* Thecoma (Theca cell tumor), 93
Luteoma. *Diagnose as* Thecoma
(Theca cell tumor), 93
Luxation: *See* Dislocation, *and under
bone, joint, or organ affected*
Lymph node(s)
abscess, 235 (1)
calcification
due to infection, 235 (1)
due to tuberculosis, 235 (1)
diseases, 235 ff.
endometriosis, 236 (9)
endothelioma, not otherwise specified. *Diagnose as* Reticulum cell
sarcoma, 95
enlargement: *supplementary term,*
493. *Diagnose disease*
foreign body, 235 (4)
hyperplasia due to unknown cause,
236 (9)
lymphoma, 236 (8)
giant follicular, 236 (8)
lymphosarcoma, 236 (8)
myeloma, plasma cell, 236 (8)
neoplasms, 236 (8)
polyp, benign lymphoid, 236 (8)
sarcoma, reticulum cell, 236 (8)
tumors, unlisted, 236 (8)
Lymph vessels. *See* Lymphatic channels
Lymphadenia, aleukemic. *Diagnose
as* Lymphocytic leukemia, 230 (8)
Lymphadenitis
acute, due to infection, 235 (1)
aleukemic. *Diagnose as* Lymphocytic leukemia, 230 (8)
chronic, due to infection, 235 (1)
due to irritation by foreign body,
235 (4)
due to trauma, 235 (4)
nonbacterial, regional, 235 (1)
purulent, 235 (1)
toxic, due to exogenous poison, 235
(3)

Lymphadenoma
malignant, not otherwise specified. *Diagnose as* Lymphoma, type not specified, 230 (8)
multiple, not otherwise specified. *Diagnose as* Lymphoma, type not specified, 230 (8)
salivary gland. *Diagnose as* Adenolymphoma, 98
Lymphadenopathy. *See also* Lymph nodes, diseases
due to undetermined cause, 236 (y)
Lymphangiectasis. *See also* Elephantiasis, lymphangiectatic
of conjunctiva, 470 (5)
due to infection, 234 (1)
Lymphangio-endothelioma. *See* Lymphendothelioma, 96
malignant. *Diagnose as* Lymphangiosarcoma, 96
Lymphangioma, 96, 129 (8), 140 (8), 234 (8)
Lymphangiosarcoma, 96, 140 (8), 234 (8)
Lymphangitis
acute, 234 (1)
chronic, 234 (1)
due to tuberculosis, 234 (1)
of penis, 329 (1)
Lymphatic channels
diseases, 234
endothelioma, benign. *Diagnose as* Lymphendothelioma, 96
filariasis, 234 (2)
injury, 234 (4)
lymphangioma, 234 (8)
lymphangiosarcoma, 234 (8)
lymphendothelioma, 234 (8)
neoplasms, 234 (8)
nevus, not otherwise specified. *Diagnose as* Lymphangioma, 96
occlusion
due to infection, 234 (1)
due to trauma, 234 (4)
following operation, 234 (4)
rupture due to infection, 234 (4)
Lymphatism, 121 (x)
Lymphedema. *See also* Elephantiasis; Lymphatic channels, occlusion
precox, of leg, 234 (9)
Lymphendothelioma, 96, 234 (8)
malignant. *Diagnose as* Lymphangiosarcoma, 96

Lymph-haemangioma. *Diagnose as* Hemangioma (angioma), 96
Lymphoblastoma
giant follicular. *Diagnose as* Giant follicular lymphoma, 95
Hodgkin's. *Diagnose as* Hodgkin's disease, 95
not otherwise specified. *Diagnose as* Lymphosarcoma, 95
scirrhous. *Diagnose as* Hodgkin's disease, 95
Lymphochloroma. *Diagnose as* Leukosarcoma, 95
Lymphocytes, increase in. *See* Lymphocytosis
Lymphocythemia. *Diagnose as* Lymphocytic leukemia, 230 (8)
Lymphocytoma. *Diagnose as* Lymphoma, type not specified, 230 (8)
Lymphocytomatosis
aleukemic. *Diagnose as* Lymphocytic leukemia, 230 (8)
Lymphocytosis
infectious, 115 (1)
supplementary term, 494. *Diagnose disease*
Lymphoendothelioma, 96
benign. *Diagnose as* Lymphoendothelioma, 96
malignant. *Diagnose as* Lymphangiosarcoma, 96
Lymphoepithelioma. *Diagnose as* Epidermoid carcinoma, 94
Lymphoepitheliomatous blastoma. *Diagnose as* Epidermoid carcinoma, 94
Lymphogranuloma
malignant. *Diagnose as* Hodgkin's disease, 95
Lymphogranulomatosis
eosinophilic. *Diagnose as* Hodgkin's disease, 95
not otherwise specified. *Diagnose as* Hodgkin's disease, 95
Lymphoid polyp, benign, 95
Lymphoma, 95
aleukemic, aleukemic malignant. *Diagnose as* Hodgkin's disease, 95
benign
except of orbit. *Diagnose as* Giant follicular lymphoma, 95
of orbit, 459 (8)
compound, 95

Lymphoma—Continued
giant follicular, 95, 139 (8), 230 (8)
granulomatous. *Diagnose as* Hodgkin's disease, 95
Hodgkin's. *Diagnose as* Hodgkin's disease, 95
Hodgkin's granulomatous. *Diagnose as* Hodgkin's disease, 95
and leukemia, 95
malignancy code (behavior), 99
nodular. *Diagnose as* Giant follicular lymphoma, 95
ocular. *Diagnose as* Lymphoma of orbit, 459 (8)
type not specified, 230 (8)
Lymphomatosis
chronic malignant. *Diagnose as* Hodgkin's disease, 95
not otherwise specified
of orbit. *Diagnose as* Lymphoma of orbit, 459 (8)
Lymphopathia, venereal, 133 (1), 235 (1)
of pelvis, 371 (1)
of vagina, 355 (1)
Lymphoreticuloma, Hodgkin's. *Diagnose as* Reticulum cell sarcoma, 95
Lymphoreticulosis. *Diagnose as* Giant follicular lymphoma, 95
Lymphosarcoma, 95, 230 (8)
giant follicular. *Diagnose as* Giant follicular lymphoma, 95
pleomorphic. *Diagnose as* Hodgkin's disease, 95
reticulum cell. *Diagnose as* Reticulum cell sarcoma, 95
retroperitoneal, 301 (8)
Lymphosarcomatosis
not otherwise specified. *Diagnose as* Lymphosarcoma, 95
Lyssa. *See* Rabies, 116 (1)

M

Macrocheilia, 243 (0)
Macrocytosis: *supplementary term,* 494. *Diagnose disease*
Macrofolliculoid granulosa cell tumor. *Diagnose as* Granulosa cell tumor, 93
Macrogenitosomia precox male
virilizing with, 396 (0)

Macroglobulinemia
idiopathic, 238 (x)
supplementary term, 494. *Diagnose disease*
Macroglossia, 245 (0)
acquired, 246 (9)
Macrogyria, 410 (0)
Macrostomia, 243 (0)
Macrotia, 474 (0)
Macula
of cornea, 435 (1)
degeneration, 449 (9)
congenital, 446 (0)
senile, 448 (7)
heredodegeneration, 449 (9)
Maculae ceruleae, 134 (2)
Madelung's deformity. *See* Radius, idiopathic progressive curvature of, 146 (0)
Madura foot, 124 (2)
Maduromycosis, 124 (2)
Majocchi's disease. *See* Purpura annularis telangiectodes, 137 (5)
Malacoplakia
of bladder, 318 (1)
of pelvis of kidney, 308 (1)
of ureter, 314 (1)
of urethra, due to infection, 323 (1)
Maladjustment. *See* Personality disorders, transient stress, 113 (x)
Malaria, 115 (1)
anemia due to, 228 (1)
splenomegaly due to, 232 (1)
Male climacteric: *supplementary term,* 500. *Diagnose disease*
Male genital system, diseases, 328 ff.
Malformations. *See* Deformities; *and specific malformations under organ, region or structure affected*
Malherbe's epithelioma. *Diagnose as* Neoplastic cyst, 93
Malingerer, 481
Malingering. *See* Simulation; *supplementary term,* 486
Malnutrition. *See also* Inanition; Starvation
in child under 2 years, 119 (7)
osteoporosis due to prolonged, 152 (7)
in person over 2 years, 119 (7)
Malocclusion, 249 (6)
Malta fever. *See* Brucellosis, 114 (1)

Malunion following fracture, 151 (4)

Mammary glands. *See also* Breast; Mastitis; Mastopathy
hypertrophy in male. *See* Gynecomastia, 144 (7)

Mammillitis. *See* Thelitis, 144 (1)

Mandible. *See also* Jaws
marked projection of lower jaw, *see* Prognathism, 153 (7)
phosphorus poisoning, 149 (3)
torus mandibulare, 249 (9)

Mania: *supplementary term,* 485. *Diagnose disease*

Manic depressive reactions, 110 (x)

Manometric block: *supplementary term,* 505. *Diagnose disease*

Marasmus, 119 (7)

Marble bones. *See* Osteopetrosis, 147 (0)

Marble skin, 137 (4)

Marfan's syndrome. *See* Arachnodactyly, 114 (0)

Marginal ulcer, 273 (4)

Marie's syndrome. *See* Acromegaly, 394 (7)

Marie-Bamberger disease. *See* Secondary hypertrophic osteoarthropathy, 152 (7)

Marie-Strümpell arthritis. *See* Arthritis, rheumatoid, of spine, 163 (9)

Marie-Tooth disease. *See* Progressive neuropathic (peroneal) muscular atrophy, 425 (9)

Marrow. *See* Bone marrow

Masculinizing tumor. *Diagnose as* Virilizing tumor, 93

Masculinovoblastoma. *Diagnose as* Virilizing tumor, 93

Mass movements: *supplementary term,* 505. *Diagnose disease*

Mastic test, reactions: *supplementary terms. Diagnose disease*
cerebrospinal syphilitic, 505
paretic, 505
tabetic, 505

Mastitis
acute, 143 (1)
of adolescence, 144 (7)
chronic, 143 (1)

Mastitis—Continued
comedo, 145 (9)
interstitial, 143 (1)
with mumps, 143 (1)
plasma cell, 145 (9)
puerperal, 143 (1)
suppurative, 144 (1)

Mastocytosis, 132 (0)

Mastoid. *See also* Mastoiditis
fistula following operation, 478 (4)
foreign body in, 478 (4)
fracture of petrous pyramid and, 478 (4)
tuberculosis, 478 (1)

Mastoiditis
acute, 477 (1)
coalescent, 477 (1)
hemorrhagic, 477 (1)
necrotic, 477 (1)
chronic, 477 (1)
recurrent, 477 (1)

Mastopathy
of ovarian origin, 144 (7)

Masturbation: *supplementary term,* 485. *Diagnose disease*

Maxilla. *See* Jaws

Maxillary sinus. *See* Sinuses, accessory; Sinusitis

Measles, 114 (1)
German. *See* Rubella, 116 (1)

Meatitis, urethral, 323 (1)

Meatus urinarius
double, 322 (0)
prolapse, acquired, 325 (6)
stricture
congenital, 322 (0)
due to infection, 323 (1)
ulcer, 326 (9)

Meckel's diverticulitis, 271 (0), 272 (1)

Meckel's diverticulum, 271 (0)
dilatation, congenital, 271 (0)
displacement of gastric mucosa into, 271 (0)
hernia, congenital, 271 (0)
hypertrophy, congenital, 271 (0)
incarceration, congenital, 271 (0)
rupture during birth, 273 (4)
small diverticulations on end of, 271 (0)
torsion, congenital, 271 (0)

Meckel's ganglion. *See* Sphenopalatine ganglion

Median bar, 348 (9)
Mediastinitis
nonsuppurative, 123 (1)
suppurative, 123 (1)
Mediastinopericarditis
due to unknown cause, 213 (9)
rheumatic, 213 (9)
tuberculous, 208 (1)
Mediastinum
bronchogenic cyst, 122 (0)
depression, 126 (4)
emphysema, 126 (4)
teratoma, 129 (8)
tuberculosis, 123 (1)
Medical induction, 481
Medulla oblongata
syringobulbia, 416 (9)
Medulloblastoma, 95
of brain, 415 (8)
Medulloepithelioma. *Diagnose as* Neuroepithelioma, 95
Megacolon. *See also* Colon, dilatation
congenital, 276 (0)
Megalocornea
without hypertension, 434 (0)
Megalogastria, congenital, 263 (0)
Megaloureter, 313 (0)
due to unknown cause, 315 (6)
Meibomian gland(s)
adenoma, 464 (8)
hypersecretion, 464 (x)
infarct, 463 (6)
Melancholia. *See* Involutional psychotic reaction, 110 (x)
Melanoameloblastoma. *Diagnose as* Ameloblastoma, 98
Melanoblast, tumors of, 94
Melanoblastoma, 94
Melanocarcinoma. *Diagnose as* Melanoma, 94
Melanocytoblastoma. *Diagnose as* Melanoblastoma, 94
Melanoepithelioma. *Diagnose as* Melanoma, 94
Melanoma, 94, 140 (8)
amelanotic, 94, 139 (8)
malignant. *Diagnose as* Melanoma, 94
Melanosarcoma. *Diagnose as* Melanoma, 94

Melanosis
of colon: *supplementary term,* 496. *Diagnose disease*
of cornea
congenital, 434 (0)
following uveitis, 435 (1)
senile, 436 (7)
neoplastic, not otherwise specified. *Diagnose as* Pigmented nevus, 94
of sclera, congenital, 438 (0)
supplementary term, 487. *Diagnose disease*
Melanotic tumor, malignant. *Diagnose as* Melanoma, 94
Melasma, 138 (7)
Melena. *See* Blood in feces, occult: *supplementary term,* 496
Melioidosis, 114 (1)
Melorheostosis, 155 (9)
Melotus (displacement of auricle), 474 (0)
Membrana capsularis lentis posterior, 444 (0)
Membrana epipapillaris, 450 (0)
Membrana tympani. *See* Tympanic membrane
Membranes, birth. *See also* Amnion; Chorion
inflammation, acute, 383 (1)
premature rupture, 383 (6)
retention, 383 (6)
Memory, loss of. *See* Amnesia: *supplementary term,* 501
Mendacity, pathologic: *supplementary term,* 485. *Diagnose disease*
Menge's adenoma. *Diagnose as* Adenomyosis, 98
Ménière's syndrome, 480 (9)
supplementary term, 509. *Diagnose disease*
Meningeal vessels
aneurysm
arteriovenous, 409 (4)
due to trauma, 409 (4)
due to unknown cause, 409 (9)
birth injury, 408 (0)
dilatation, congenital, 408 (0)
diseases, 408 ff.
embolism by infected thrombus, 408 (1)
hemangioma, 409 (8)
injury, 409 (4)

Meningeal vessels—Continued
neoplasms, 409 (8)
sinus pericranii, 408 (0)
subarachnoid hemorrhage
due to congenital arterial hypoplasia with rupture, 408 (0)
due to vascular disease with hypertension, 409 (5)
thrombosis, 409 (6)
due to infection, 408 (1)
marantic, 409 (5)
progressive, due to unknown
cause, 409 (9)
tumors, unlisted, 409 (8)
Meninges. *See also* Epidural space;
Meningitis; Meningo-; Subdural
space
adhesions
compression of cranial nerve by,
429 (4)
compression of spinal cord by, 423
(4)
congenital, 405 (0)
due to infection, 406 (1)
due to trauma, 406 (4)
upper sacral, due to crushing, 406
(4)
anomaly of dural sinus, 405 (0)
bands or folds, constriction by, 402
(0)
birth injury (laceration), 405 (0)
calcification due to unknown cause,
407 (9)
congenital dermal sinus, 405 (0)
diseases, 405 ff.
endothelioma; endothelioma, diffuse.
Diagnose as Meningioma, 95
foreign body in, 406 (4)
fungal infection, 406 (2)
hypertensive meningeal hydrops, 407
(x)
injury, 406 (4)
lipoma, 407 (8)
melanoma, 407 (8)
meningioma, 407 (8)
mesothelioma. *Diagnose as* Meningioma, 95
moniliasis, 406 (2)
neoplasms, 407 (8)
parasitic infection, 406 (2)
sarcomatosis; sarcomatosis, diffuse.
Diagnose as Meningioma, 95
tumors, unlisted, 407 (8)

**Meningioblastoma; Meningiofibro-
blastoma.** *Diagnose as* Meningioma, 95
Meningioma, 95
angioblastic. *Diagnose as* Hemangiosarcoma, 96
of brain, 415 (8)
of meninges, 407 (8)
mesenchymal. *Diagnose as* Meningioma, 95
Meningiomatosis. *Diagnose as* Meningioma, 95
diffuse. *Diagnose* as Meningioma,
95
diffuse leptomeningeal. *Diagnose as*
Meningioma, 95
diffuse pial. *Diagnose as* Meningioma, 95
Meningiosarcoma. *Diagnose as* Meningioma, 95
Meningiothelioma. *Diagnose as* Meningioma, 95
Meningismus
due to serum, 406 (3)
due to vaccine, 406 (3)
supplementary term, 505. *Diagnose
disease*
Meningitis. *See also* Arachnoiditis;
Leptomeningitis; Pachymeningi-
tis
acute, 405 (1)
lymphocytic, 406 (1)
serous, 406 (1)
aseptic
due to serum, 406 (3)
due to vaccine, 406 (3)
chronic, 405 (1)
serous, 406 (1)
due to hepatic virus, 405 (1)
due to mumps, 406 (1)
hypertrophic, 406 (1)
nonsuppurative, 405 (1)
Meningocele, 405 (0). *See also* Hydrencephalomeningocele, 402 (0)
radiculopathy by pressure of, 421
(0)
Meningococcemia, 114 (1)
Meningoencephalomyelitis
acute, 402 (1)
chronic, 403 (1)
due to toxoplasma, 402 (1)
Meningoencephalomyelopathy
due to poison, 403 (3)

Meningoencephalopathy
due to poison, 403 (3)
due to trauma, 403 (4)
Meningomyelitis
acute, 422 (1)
chronic, 422 (1)
mycotic, 422 (2)
parasitic, 422 (2)
syphilitic, 422 (1)
Meniscus
of jaw, dislocation (snapping jaw), 162 (6)
of knee
congenital hypertrophy, 157 (0)
cyst (snapping knee), 162 (6)
lateral, tear, 159 (4)
medial, detachment, 159 (4)
Menopause
artificial
due to radium, 369 (4)
due to roentgen rays, 369 (4)
atrophy of cervix at, 359 (7)
post-menopausal osteoporosis, 153 (7)
premature, due to unknown cause, 349 (7)
syndrome: *supplementary term,* 500. *Diagnose disease*
Menorrhagia
due to acute infection, 361 (1)
due to anemia, 362 (5)
due to distortion or displacement of uterus, 362 (6)
functional, 365 (x)
supplementary term, 499. *Diagnose disease*
Menstruation. *See also* Amenorrhea; Dysmenorrhea; Menorrhagia; Metrorrhagia
delayed
due to unknown cause, 349 (x)
supplementary term, 498. *Diagnose disease*
infrequent, due to unknown cause, 350 (x)
premenstrual tension, 364 (7)
vicarious, nasal, 178 (7)
Mental deficiency
familial or hereditary, 110 (x)
idiopathic, 110 (x)
supplementary term, 505. *Diagnose disease*

Mental deterioration
chorea, chronic progressive, with, 416 (9)
supplementary term, 505. *Diagnose disease*
Mental disorders. *See also* Personality disorders; Psychogenic disorders; Psychoneurotic disorders; Psychotic disorders
none, 481
undiagnosed, 481
Meralgia paresthetica, 429 (4)
Mercury
poisoning, 117 (3)
salts, injury of eyelid by, 462 (3)
Merycism. *See* Rumination: *supplementary term,* 497
Mesarteritis, syphilitic, 216 (1)
Mesenchymal mixed tumor, 98
Mesenchymal tumor, benign. *Diagnose as* Mesenchymoma, 98
Mesenchymoblastoma (gonad). *Diagnose as* Disgerminoma, 97
Mesenchymoma, 98
embryonale angioblasticum (genital organs). *Diagnose as* Mesenchymal mixed tumor, 98
feminizing (ovary). *Diagnose as* Feminizing tumor, 93
fibromyoma angiomatosum. *Diagnose as* Mesenchymal mixed tumor, 98
Mesenteric artery
arteriosclerosis, 305 (9)
embolism
due to trauma, 305 (4)
due to unspecified cause, 305 (6)
following operation, 305 (4)
intestinal infarction due to, 273 (5)
injury, 305 (4)
narrowing due to arteriosclerosis, 305 (9)
periarteritis nodosa, 305 (9)
thrombosis
due to arteriosclerosis, 305 (9)
due to periarteritis nodosa, 305 (9)
due to unspecified cause, 305 (6)
intestinal infarction due to, 273 (5)
Mesenteric veins
phlebitis due to infection, 305 (1)
phlebosclerosis, 305 (9)

Mesenteric veins—Continued
  thrombosis
    due to infection, 305 (1)
    due to unknown cause, 305 (9)
    due to unspecified cause, 305 (6)
Mesentery
  adhesions
    due to infection, 272 (1)
    following operation, 273 (4)
  cysts
    gas, 275 (9)
    simple, 274 (6)
  diseases, 271 ff.
  extravasation of chyle into, 273 (5)
  fat necrosis, 272 (3)
  fibroma, 274 (8)
  hemangioma, 274 (8)
  hematoma, 273 (4)
  injury, 273 (4)
  leiomyoma, 274 (8)
  lipoma, 274 (8)
  lymphangioma, 274 (8)
  sarcoma, 274 (8)
  torsion, 274 (6)
Mesodermal mixed tumor. *Diagnose as* Mesenchymal mixed tumor, 98
Mesoglioma. *Diagnose as* Oligodendroma, 96
Mesonephroma, 98
  of ovary, 370 (8)
Mesothelial sarcoma, 97
Mesothelioma, 97
  except of meninges, malignant. *Diagnose as* Mesothelial sarcoma, 97
  of meninges. *Diagnose as* Meningioma, 95
Metabolism
  basal, depressed or elevated: *supplementary terms,* 500. *Diagnose disease*
  disorders, diseases due to. *See under name of specific disease or organ, region or structure affected*
Metaphysial aclasis, 147 (0)
Metaphysitis. *See* Bone, necrosis, aseptic, 155 (9)
Metaplasia
  agnogenic myeloid, 239 (9)
Metastases. *See* Neoplasms, metastatic, 129 (8)

Metatarsus
  adductus, 157 (0)
  osteochondrosis of head of metatarsal bone (infraction), 155 (9)
  sesamoid bone of first metatarsal, fusion defect, 147 (0)
  short first segment, 147 (0)
  varus, congenital, 157 (0)
Methemoglobinemia
  hereditary, 237 (7)
  supplementary term, 494. *Diagnose disease*
Methyl alcohol
  poisoning, 117 (3)
Metritis. *See also* Endometritis; Parametritis
  acute, 361 (1)
  chronic, 361 (1)
  during pregnancy, 374 (1)
  puerperal, 374 (1)
Metrorrhagia
  due to distortion or displacement of uterus, 362 (6)
  due to infection, 361 (1)
  functional, 365 (x)
  supplementary term, 499. *Diagnose disease*
Microcephaly, 411 (0)
Microcolon, 276 (0)
Microcornea, 434 (0)
Microcytosis: *supplementary term,* 494. *Diagnose disease*
Microfolliculoid granulosa cell tumor. *Diagnose as* Granulosa cell tumor, 93
Microgastria, congenital, 263 (0)
Microgenia, 153 (7)
Microglossia, 245 (0)
Micrognathism, 153 (7)
Microgyria, 411 (0)
  acquired, 414 (5)
Micromyelia, 421 (0)
Microorganisms
  list, 57 ff.
Microphakia, 442 (2)
Microphthalmos, 443 (0)
Microstomia, 243 (0)
Microtia, 474 (0)
Micturition, frequency: *supplementary term,* 498. *Diagnose disease*
Middle ear. *See* Ear, middle

Midtarsal joints
dislocation, congenital, 157 (0)
subluxation due to trauma, 160 (4)
Migraine
abdominal, 417 (x)
cause unknown, 417 (x)
cerebellar, 417 (x)
migrainous equivalents, 417 (x)
ophthalmic, 417 (x)
ophthalmoplegic, 417 (x)
simple (hemicranial), 417 (x)
supplementary term, 505. *Diagnose disease*
Mikulicz's disease. *See* Hypertrophy of salivary gland, 254 (9) ; Achroacytosis of lacrimal gland due to infection, 465 (1)
Miliaria (prickly heat), 137 (4)
crystallina, 137 (4)
rubra, 137 (4)
Miliary fever, 115 (1)
Miliary tuberculosis
acute, 116 (1)
of lung, 194 (1)
Milium, 138 (6)
of eyelid, 463 (6)
Milk
abnormal quality, 145 (x)
abnormal secretion, 145 (x)
absence of secretion. *See* Agalactia, 145 (x)
excessive flow. *See* Galactorrhea, 145 (x)
Milk leg. *See* Phlegmasia alba dolens, 128 (5)
Milkman's syndrome (osteomalacia due to unknown cause), 155 (9)
Millard-Gubler syndrome: *supplementary term,* 505. *Diagnose disease*
Milroy's edema. *See* Familial or hereditary edema, 142 (x)
Miner's elbow, 165 (4)
Miosis
due to diminished sympathetic innervation, 440 (55)
due to lesion of central nervous system, 440 (55)
due to opium or derivative, 439 (3)
due to physostigmine, 439 (3)
due to pilocarpine, 439 (3)
Misanthropy: *supplementary term,* 485. *Diagnose disease*

Miscarriage. *See* Abortion, 378
Misogyny: *supplementary term,* 485. *Diagnose disease*
Mitchell's disease. *See* Erythromelalgia, 217 (55)
Mitral valve
accessory leaflet, 203 (0)
double orifice, 203 (0)
incompetency: *supplementary term,* 492. *Diagnose disease*
insufficiency, congenital, 204 (0)
stenosis
congenital atresia or, 204 (0)
dilatation of pulmonary artery due to, 223 (6)
not congenital: *Supplementary term,* 492. *Diagnose disease*
Mittelschmerz (ovulation pain): *supplementary term,* 499. *Diagnose disease*
Mixed tumor
embryonal. *Diagnose as* Mesenchymal mixed tumor, 98
mesenchymal, 98
mesodermal. *Diagnose as* Mesenchymal mixed tumor, 98
of pharynx. *Diagnose as* Epidermoid carcinoma, 94
of testis. *Diagnose as* Embryonal carcinoma of testis, 98
not otherwise specified, 98
salivary gland type, 98
Moebius-Leyden dystrophy. *See* Progressive muscular dystrophy, 170 (9)
Molds and yeasts
in feces ; *supplementary term,* 497. *Diagnose disease*
in sputum ; *supplementary term,* 490. *Diagnose disease*
Mole. *See also* Nevus
blue black. *Diagnose as* Pigmented nevus, 94
common. *Diagnose as* Pigmented nevus, 94
destructive (placenta). *Diagnose as* Chorioadenoma, 97
hydatid or hydatidiform. *Diagnose as* Hydatiform mole, 97
malignant. *Diagnose as* Chorioadenoma, 97
hydatiform, malignant. *Diagnose as* Chorioadenoma, 97

Mole—Continued
invasive (placenta). *Diagnose as*
Chorioadenoma, 97
malignant (placenta). *Diagnose as*
Chorioadenoma, 97
of melanin forming tissue. *Diagnose
as* Pigmented nevus, 94
melanotic. *Diagnose as* Pigmented
nevus, 94
pigmented. *Diagnose as* Pigmented
nevus, 94
of placenta. *Diagnose as* Hydatiform
mole, 97
Moll's gland. *See* Gland of Moll
Mollities ossium. *See* Osteomalacia,
153 (7)
Molluscum, 133 (1)
Mönckeberg's arteriosclerosis. *See*
Arteriosclerosis, medial, especially with calcification, 218 (9)
Mongolism, 114 (0)
chronic brain syndrome with, 107
(0)
Monilethrix, 131 (0)
Moniliasis, 124 (2), 277 (2)
of skin, 134 (2)
*See also under organ, region, or
structure affected*
Monocellular tumor (testis). *Diagnose as* Disgerminoma, 97
Monocytes, increase in. *See* Monocytosis
Monocytosis: *supplementary term,*
495. *Diagnose disease*
Mononucleosis, infectious, 114 (1)
Monoplegia: *supplementary term,*
505. *Diagnose disease*
Monsters
absence of alimentary tract in
marked fetal malformations,
239 (0)
composite, 114 (0)
double, 114 (0)
duplication of respiratory organs in,
192 (0)
rudimentary respiratory organs in
thoracopagus, 192 (0)
Monteggia's fracture, 151 (4)
Moon-Laurence-Biedl syndrome,
114 (0)
Moral deficiency: *supplementary
term,* 484. *Diagnose disease*

Morel's syndrome: *See* Stewart-
Morel syndrome, 155 (9)
Morel-Kraepelin disease (dementia
precox). *See* Schizophrenic reac-
tions, 110 (x)
Morgagni, crypts of. *See* Anus,
crypts; Cryptitis
Morgagni, hydatid of, 366 (0)
Morgagni's syndrome. *See* Stewart-
Morel syndrome, 155 (9)
Moria (Witzelsucht): *supplementary
term,* 485. *Diagnose disease*
Morphea (localized scleroderma), 142
(9)
Morphine. *See* Opium, 117 (3)
Morquio's disease: *See* Eccentro-
osteochondrodysplasia, 147 (0)
Morton's disease. *See* Osteochondrosis of head of metatarsal bone,
159 (9)
Morvan's disease. *See* Syringomyelia, 425 (9)
Motion sickness, 119 (55)
air, 119 (55)
car, 119 (55)
sea, 119 (55)
Motor apraxia: *supplementary term,*
502. *Diagnose disease*
Mottled enamel due to fluorine,
248 (3)
Mouches volantes. *See* Muscae volitantes, 444 (0)
Mountain sickness. *See* Hypobaropathy, 118 (4)
Mouth. *See also* Buccal cavity;
Cheek; Lips; Stomatitis; Teeth
abscess, 241 (1)
acanthomia, 242 (8)
cellulitis of floor of, 241 (1)
cutaneous horn, 242 (9)
diseases, 241 ff.
epithelioma adenoides cysticum of
mucous membrane, 242 (8)
erythroplasia of Queyrat, 141 (9)
fibroma, 242 (8)
fibrosarcoma, 242 (8)
gunshot wound, 241 (4)
herpes, 241 (1)
injury, 241 (4)
lymphangioma, 242 (8)
neoplasms, 242 (8)
sinus
due to infection, 241 (1)

Mouth—Continued
sinus—continued
due to trauma, 241 (4)
stab wound, 241 (4)
thrush, 241 (2)
tumors
mixed, salivary gland type, 242 (8)
unlisted, 242 (8)
ulcer due to unknown cause, 242 (9)
varix, 241 (6)
Vincent's infection, 241 (1)
Movement
dystonic: *supplementary term, 504. Diagnose disease*
loss or diminution of sense of position and: *supplementary term, 505. Diagnose disease*
mass: *supplementary term, 505. Diagnose disease*
Mucinoid degeneration, 129 (9)
Mucinous degeneration, 129 (9)
Mucocele
of appendix due to obstruction, 280 (6)
of gallbladder, 294 (9)
of middle turbinate, 178 (6)
of sinus, 180 (1)
Mucocutaneous junction
sebaceous glands, aberrant, 131 (0)
of anus, 284 (0)
of lips, 243 (0)
Mucoepidermoid tumor. *Diagnose as* Myoepithelial tumor, 98
Mucormycosis, 124 (2)
Mucous membrane. *See also under organ or region, as* Mouth
superficial, diseases, 131
Mucoviscidosis, 295 (0)
Mule spinner's cancer. *Diagnose as* Epidermoid carcinoma, 94
Müllerianoma; müllerianoma, ectopic. *Diagnose as* Adenomyosis, 98
Multiple sclerosis, 404 (9)
optic neuritis (retrobulbar neuritis) in, 452 (9)
Mumps (epidemic parotitis), 115 (1), 253 (1)
epididymitis due to, 335 (1)
mastitis with, 143 (1)
oophoritis of, 168 (1)
orchitis due to, 332 (1)

Muscae volitantes, 444 (0)
Muscles. *See also* Myasthenia gravis; Myositis; Tendons
abscess, 167 (1)
absence, 167 (0)
accessory, 167 (0)
atrophy
due to disuse, 169 (7)
familial spinal muscular infantile, 425 (9)
myelopathic, 425 (9)
progressive neuropathic (peroneal), 425 (9)
contracture
congenital, 167 (0)
due to infection, 167 (1)
due to ischemia, 169 (5)
due to trauma, 167 (4)
of hamstring, congenital, 167 (0)
contusion, 167 (4)
cramps. *See* Cramp
diastasis, congenital, 167 (0)
diseases, 167 ff.
dystrophy
dystrophia myotonica, 170 (9)
progressive, 170 (9)
reflex type, 169 (55)
fibroma (desmoid), 169 (8)
fibrosarcoma, 169 (8)
foreign body reaction, 168 (4)
hemangioma, 169 (8)
hematoma, 168 (4)
hernia, 168 (4)
lipoma, 170 (8)
liposarcoma, 170 (8)
myoblastoma, granular cell, 170 (8)
neoplasms, 170 (8)
neurofibroma, 170 (8)
ocular. *See* Eye, muscles
pain. *See* Myalgia
paralysis, 147 (55)
obstetric, 167 (0)
rhabdomyoma, 170 (8)
rhabdomyosarcoma, 170 (8)
rupture, 168 (4)
scar
due to trauma, 168 (4)
following operation, 168 (4)
supernumerary, 167 (0)
tone. *See* Amyotonia congenita; Atonia; Dystonia musculorum deformans; Myotonia
tumors, unlisted, 170 (8)

Muscles—Continued
weakness of calf (gastrocnemius and soleus), congenital, 167 (0)
wound, 168 (4)
infected, 168 (4)

Musculoskeletal system
diseases, 146
psychophysiologic reaction, 111 (55)

Musical sounds, inability to recognize. *See* Amusia: *supplementary term,* 501

Myalgia
epidemic. *See* Pleurodynia, epidemic, 198 (1)
supplementary term, 489. *Diagnose disease*

Myalgic encephalomyelitis, benign, 115 (1)

Myasthenia gravis, 169 (55)
thymoma with. *Diagnose as* Thymoma, malignant, 392 (8)

Mycetoma
of leg, 124 (2)

Mycosis: *See also* Actinomycosis; Blastomycosis; Coccidioidomycosis, etc. *under organ, region or structure affected*
fungoides. *Diagnose as* Lymphosarcoma, 95
generalized, 116 (2)

Mydriasis
due to lesion of central nervous system, 440 (55)
due to plant or animal poison, 439 (3)

Myelemia. *Diagnose as* Granulocytic leukemia, 94

Myelitis. *See also* Encephalomyelitis; Meningoencephalomyelitis; Meningomyelitis; Poliomyelitis
acute, 422 (1)
ascending, acute, 422 (1)
chronic, 422 (1)
disseminated, 421 (1)
transverse, 422 (1)

Myeloblastic myelosis. *Diagnose as* Granulocytic leukemia, 94

Myelochloroma. *Diagnose as* Leukosarcoma, 95

Myelocythemia. *Diagnose as* Granulocytic leukemia, 94

Myelocytoma. *Diagnose as* Plasma cell myeloma, 95

Myelodysplasia, 421 (0)

Myelofibrosis
idiopathic, 239 (9)
myeloid metaplasia of spleen due to, 233 (9)

Myelogenous myelosis. *Diagnose as* Granulocytic leukemia, 94

Myeloid myelosis. *Diagnose as* Granulocytic leukemia, 230 (8)

Myeloid tumor. *Diagnose as* Plasma cell myeloma, 95

Myelolipoma (adrenal). *Diagnose as* Mesenchymoma, 98

Myeloma
endothelial. *Diagnose as* Ewing's sarcoma, 97
hemic. *Diagnose as* Plasma cell myeloma, 95
lymphocytic. *Diagnose as* Plasma cell myeloma, 95
multiple. *Diagnose as* Plasma cell myeloma, 95
not otherwise specified. *Diagnose as* Plasma cell myeloma, 95
plasma cell, 95, 230 (8)
plasmocytic. *Diagnose as* Plasma cell myeloma, 95

Myelomatosis. *Diagnose as* Plasma cell myeloma, 95

Myelomeningocele, 421 (0)

Myelopathy
due to anoxemia, 424 (7)
due to arteriosclerosis, 424 (5)
due to arteritis or phlebitis, 424 (5)
due to cachexia, 424 (7)
due to circulatory disturbance, 424 (5)
due to decompression disease, 424 (4)
due to embolism, 424 (5)
due to hemorrhage, 424 (5)
due to poison, 422 (3)
due to starvation, 424 (7)
due to thrombosis, 424 (5)
due to vitamin deficiency, 424 (7)
muscular atrophy in, 425 (9)
toxic, 422 (3)
transverse, due to poison, 422 (3)

Myelophthisis
thrombocytopenic purpura due to, 231 (9)

Myeloplaxic tumor. *Diagnose as* Giant cell tumor of bone, 97
Myeloradiculitis virus, 422 (1)
Myeloradiculopathy due to diabetes, 425 (7) due to poison, 423 (3)
Myelosarcoma. *Diagnose as* Plasma cell myeloma, 95
Myelosis. *Diagnose as* Granulocytic leukemia, 230 (8)
Myiasis of bladder, 318 (2) of conjunctiva, 469 (2) of ear, 475 (2) of sinus, 180 (2)
Myiodesopsia, 444 (0)
Myoblastoma embryonal. *Diagnose as* Mesenchymal mixed tumor, 98 granular. *Diagnose as* Granular cell myoblastoma, 96 granular cell, 139 (8) not otherwise specified. *Diagnose as* Granular cell myoblastoma, 96
Myocarcinoma. *Diagnose as* Carcinosarcoma, 97
Myocardial ischemia: *supplementary term,* 491. *Diagnose disease*
Myocarditis acute bacterial, 207 (1) acute isolated, due to unknown cause, 213 (9) due to diphtheria toxin, 211 (55) due to influenza, 207 (1) due to scarlet fever, 208 (1) due to typhoid bacillus, 208 (1) due to virus, 208 rheumatic, 213 (9) subacute bacterial, 208 (1) of unknown cause, 213 (9)
Myocardium. *See also* Myocarditis abscess, 208 (1) fibrosis
  due to degeneration and replacement fibrosis, 210 (5)
  due to infarction, 210 (5)
  due to rheumatic fever, 213 (9)
  due to unknown cause, 213 (9) glycogen infiltration (in von Gierke's disease), 211 (7) hemochromatosis, 211 (7)

Myocardium—Continued infarction
  due to arteriosclerotic coronary thrombosis, 210 (5)
  due to embolism, 210 (5)
  due to unknown cause, 213 (9)
  from coronary thrombosis due to arteritis, 210 (5)
  pericarditis due to, 210 (5) myxoma, 211 (8) rhabdomyoma, 211 (8) rhabdomyosarcoma, 211 (8) sarcoidosis, 208 (1) tuberculosis, 208 (1)
Myoclonus: *supplementary term,* 505. *Diagnose disease*
Myoepidermoid tumor. *Diagnose as* Myoepithelial tumor, 98
Myoepithelial tumor, 98, 140 (8)
Myoepithelioma. *Diagnose as* Myoepithelial tumor, 98
Myofibroma. *Diagnose as* Myoma, 96 of uterus. *Diagnose as* Leiomyoma, 96
Myofibrosarcoma. *Diagnose as* Leiomyosarcoma, 96
Myogelosis chronic (chronic myositis), 167 (1) due to cold, 168 (4) due to occupation, 168 (4)
Myoglobinuria due to crush syndrome, 237 (4) idiopathic, 169 (7) recurrent, 169 (7)
Myoidema: *supplementary term,* 489. *Diagnose disease*
Myokymia: *supplementary term,* 505. *Diagnose disease*
Myolipoma. *Diagnose as* Mesenchymoma, 98 malignant. *Diagnose as* Mesenchymal mixed tumor, 98
Myoma, 96 myoblastic. *Diagnose as* Granular cell myoblastoma, 96 striocellulare. *Diagnose as* Rhabdomyoma, 96 of uterus. *Diagnose as* Leiomyoma, 96
Myometrium, hyperplasia due to unknown cause, 365 (9) static, due to continuous ovarian stimulation, 364 (7)

Myopia
axial, 454 (6)
chorioretinitis of, 446 (6)
congenital, 454 (0)
curvature, 454 (6)
due to displacement of lens, 454 (6)
due to increased refraction of nucleus of lens, 454 (6)
progressive, 454 (6)
Myosarcoma, 96
granular cell. *Diagnose as* Granular cell myoblastoma, 96
of infant's prostate, or vagina. *Diagnose as* Mesenchymal mixed tumor, 98
Myoschwannoma. *Diagnose as* Schwannoma, 95
Myositis
acute, 167 (1)
chronic, 167 (1)
due to cold, 168 (4)
due to occupation, 168 (4)
due to overstrain, 168 (4)
due to trauma, 168 (4)
due to unknown cause, 170 (9)
epidemic. *See* Pleurodynia, epidemic, 198 (1)
multiple. *See* Dermatomyositis, 170 (9)
ossificans, 168 (4)
progressive ossifying, 169 (7)
Myosteoma. *Diagnose as* Osteoma, 97
Myotonia
acquisita, 170 (x)
atrophica. *See* Dystrophia myotonica, 170 (9)
congenita, 167 (0)
intermittens, 167 (0)
supplementary term, 489. *Diagnose disease*
Myringitis
due to infection, 475 (1)
due to trauma, 476 (4)
Mysophobia: *supplementary term,* 485. *Diagnose disease*
Myxadenitis labialis. *See* Cheilitis glandularis, 140 (9)
Myxedema. *See also* Hypothyroidism
atrophy of thyroid gland with, 389 (9)
cataract in, 443 (7)

Myxedema—Continued
heart, 211 (7)
of skin, 139 (7)
Myxocarcinoma
salivary gland type. *Diagnose as* Mixed tumor, salivary gland type, 98
Myxochondroadenosarcoma. *Diagnose as* Mixed tumor, salivary gland type, 98
Myxochondrocarcinoma
salivary gland type. *Diagnose as* Mixed tumor, salivary gland type, 98
Myxochondroma. *Diagnose as* Chondroma, 97
Myxochondrosarcoma. *Diagnose as* Chondrosarcoma, 97
Myxofibrochondroma. *Diagnose as* Chondroma, 97
Myxofibroma. *Diagnose as* Myxoma, 97
of breast. *Diagnose as* Cystosarcoma phyllodes, 97
of nerve sheath. *Diagnose as* Neurofibroma, 95
of vagina. *Diagnose as* Mesenchymal mixed tumor, 98
Myxofibrosarcoma. *Diagnose as* Myxosarcoma, 97
of breast. *Diagnose as* Cystosarcoma phyllodes, 97
of nerve sheath. *Diagnose as* Fibrosarcoma, 96
of vagina. *Diagnose as* Mesenchymal mixed tumor, 98
Myxolipoma. *Diagnose as* Fetal fat cell lipoma, 97
Myxoliposarcoma. *Diagnose as* Liposarcoma, 97
Myxoma, 97
chorii. *Diagnose as* Hydatiform mole, 97
giant (breast). *Diagnose as* Cystosarcoma phyllodes, 97
intracanalicular. *Diagnose as* Cystosarcoma phyllodes, 97
odontogenic. *Diagnose as* Odontogenic tumor, benign, 98
of vagina. *Diagnose as* Mesenchymal mixed tumor, 98
Myxomatous degeneration, 129 (9)

Myxosarcoma, 97
of breast. *Diagnose as* Cystosarcoma phyllodes, 97
of nerve sheath. *Diagnose as* Fibrosarcoma, 96
of vagina. *Diagnose as* Mesenchymal mixed tumor, 98

N

Nabothian cyst, 359 (6)
Nageotte-Babinski paralysis. *See* Paralysis, medullary, tegmental: *supplementary term,* 506
Nägele's pelvis, 385 (4)
Nail(s)
absence, congenital. *See* Anonychia, 131 (0)
atrophy, 138 (7)
biting: *supplementary term,* 485. *Diagnose disease*
brittleness. *See* Onychorrhexis, 141 (9)
displacement, congenital, 131 (0)
dystrophy, 138 (55)
eggshell, 137 (5)
fungus infection. *See* Onychomycosis, 135 (2)
hypertrophy, 141 (9)
infection surrounding. *See* Paronychia, 133 (1)
inflammation of bed. *See* Onychia, 133 (1)
ingrowing. *See* Unguis incarnatus, 137 (4)
injury, 137 (4)
malformation, congenital, 131 (0)
onychomycosis, 135 (2)
overgrowth. *See* Onychauxis, 141 (9)
spoon. *See* Koilonychia, 141 (9)
subungual hemorrhage
in blood dyscrasia, 137 (5)
due to trauma, 137 (4)
supernumerary. *See* Polyunguia, 131 (0)
thickening. *See* Pachyonychia, 131 (0)
transverse furrowing, 139 (7)
whitish discoloration. *See* Leukonychia, 141 (9)
Najjer-Crigler disease, 290 (x)

Narcolepsy, 417 (x)
with cataplexy, 417 (x)
supplementary term, 505. *Diagnose disease*
Narcotic addiction. *See* Drugs, addiction, 112 (x)
Nares. *See* Choana; Nostrils
Nasal sinuses. *See* Sinuses, accessory
Nasopharyngitis, 177 (1)
Nasopharynx
abscess, 176 (1)
cyst, 178 (6)
fistula due to fungus, 177 (2)
stenosis following operation, 178 (4)
Nausea: *supplementary term,* 497. *Diagnose disease*
Navel. *See* Umbilicus
Navicular. *See also* Scaphoid, 155 (9)
osteochondrosis, 155 (9)
Nearsightedness. *See* Myopia
Neck. *See also* Spine, cervical portion
hygroma, 234 (0)
islands of glandular tissue in, 252 (0)
Stensen's duct, opening in, 252 (0)
wryneck. *See* Torticollis
Necrobiosis lipoidica diabeticorum, 139 (7)
Necrosis. *See also* Adiponecrosis neonatorum, 136 (4) ; *and under organ, region or structure affected*
due to radioactive substance, 127 (4)
Necrospermia: *supplementary term,* 499. *Diagnose disease*
Negativism: *supplementary term,* 485. *Diagnose disease*
Nelaton's tumor. *Diagnose as* Teratoma, 97
Nematode disease, 124 (2)
Nematodes
list, 64
in vitreous, 444 (2)
Neonatal death, 482
Neoplasm(s). *See* Etiological classification, 93 ff. *See also* Tumors *in Index and name of specific neoplasm in category 8 under organ, region or structure affected. If not found, see* "Unlisted tumor of . . ." *and complete code by specifying appropriate site and neoplasm.*

Neoplasm(s)—Continued
generalized neoplastic disease, 121 (7)
list, 93 ff.
malignancy code (behavior), 99
metastatic, 129 (8)
structural and functional changes due to, 98
of unknown primary site, 481
Neoplastic cyst, 93
Nephritis. *See also* Glomerulonephritis; Perinephritis; Pyelonephritis
acute hemorrhagic (glomerulonephritis), 308 (1)
congenital, 307 (0)
interstitial
acute (acute exudative), 308 (1)
chronic, 308 (1)
congenital, 308 (0)
nonsuppurative excretory. *See* Glomerulonephritis, focal, 308 (1)
suppurative, acute, 308 (1)
tetany of, 120 (7)
Nephroblastoma, 98
Nephroma
embryonal. *Diagnose as* Nephroblastoma, 98
mesoblastic. *Diagnose as* Nephroblastoma, 98
Nephroptosis, 310 (6)
Nephrosclerosis
arteriolar, 310 (5)
malignant, 310 (5)
senile arteriosclerotic, 310 (5)
Nephrosis
of alkalosis, 311 (7)
amyloid. *See* Amyloid disease of kidney, 308 (1), 312 (9)
due to diabetes, 311 (7)
due to diphtheria, 310 (55)
due to disorders of metabolism, 311 (7)
due to disturbance of acid-base balance, 311 (7)
due to exogenous poison, 309 (3)
due to hemoglobinemia following blood transfusion, 309 (3)
due to obstruction, 310 (6)
due to remote infection, 308 (1)
due to syphilis, 308 (1)
due to tuberculosis, 308 (1)
lower nephron, 312 (x)
toxic, due to burn, 309 (4)

Nephrotic syndrome
due to undetermined cause, 312 (x)
Nerve(s). *See also under name of nerves, as* Cranial nerves; Facial nerves
agenesis, 428 (0)
atypical distribution, 428 (0)
avulsion, 429 (4)
birth injury, 428 (0)
compression, 429 (4)
contusion, 429 (4)
electrical shock, 429 (4)
injury, 429 (4)
irritation by scar tissue, 429 (4)
laceration, 429 (4)
neoplasms, 430 (8)
paralysis, flaccid, due to lesion of, 169 (55)
roots. *See also* Radiculitis; Radiculopathy
avulsion, 423 (4)
compression, 424 (4)
contusion, 429 (4)
diseases, 421 ff.
laceration, 424 (4)
neoplasms, 425 (8)
tumors, unlisted, 425 (8)
wound, 424 (4)
sheath
fibroblastoma; fibroma. *Diagnose as* Neurofibroma, 95
fibromyxoma. *Diagnose as* Neurofibroma, 95
fibromyxosarcoma. *Diagnose as* Fibrosarcoma, 96
myxofibroma. *Diagnose as* Neurofibroma, 95
myxosarcoma; myxofibrosarcoma. *Diagnose as* Fibrosarcoma, 96
sarcoma, not otherwise specified. *Diagnose as* Fibrosarcoma, 96
specific nerve sheath tumor. *Diagnose as* Schwannoma, 95
stretching, 430 (4)
Nervous system. *See also* Brain; Nerves; Spinal cord
autonomic. *See* Nervous system, vegetative
caudal displacement of brain stem, cerebellum, and spinal cord, 402 (0)

Nervous system—Continued
  central, paralysis, flaccid, due to le-
    sion of, 169 (55)
  cerebrospinal syphilis, congenital, 402
    (0)
  classification of diseases, 401
  diseases, 402 ff.
  dysplasia, general, 402 (0)
  hyperplasia, congenital, 402 (0)
  hypoplasia, 402 (0)
  infection, 403 (2), 406 (2)
  injury, diffuse, 403 (4)
  neoplasms, 404 (8)
  parasympathetic. *See* Nervous sys-
    tem, vegetative
  paroxysmal disorders, 417 (x)
  sympathetic. *See also* Nervous sys-
    tem, vegetative
    paralysis, hyperemia of conjunc-
      tiva due to, 470 (5)
  syphilis
    cerebrospinal, 403 (1)
    congenital, 402 (0)
    meningovascular, 403 (1)
  trypanosomiasis, 403 (1)
  undiagnosed disease, 401
  vegetative
    diseases, 432
    ganglioneuroma, 432 (8)
    neoplasms, 432 (8)
    neuroepithelioma, 432 (8)
    paraganglioma, 432 (8)
    pheochromocytoma, 432 (8)
    sympathicoblastoma, 432 (8)
    tumors, unlisted, 432 (8)
  vessels
    diseases, 404
    hemangiomatosis, 404 (8)
Nesidoblastoma
  functioning. *Diagnose as* Function-
    ing islet cell tumor, 93
  nonfunctioning. *Diagnose as* Non-
    functioning islet cell tumor, 94
  not otherwise specified. *Diagnose as*
    Nonfunctioning islet cell tumor,
    94
Neumann's disease. *See* Pemphigus
  vegetans, 141 (9)
Neuralgia
  due to trauma, 429 (4)
  facial, 431 (x)
    atypical, 431 (x) : *supplementary
      term,* 505

Neuralgia—Continued
  geniculate, 431 (x)
  glossopharyngeal, 431 (x)
    with carotid sinus syndrome, 431
      (x)
  sphenopalatine, 431 (x)
  toxic
    due to infection, 430 (5)
    due to poison, 428 (3)
  trigeminal, 431 (x)
Neurilemoblastoma. *Diagnose as*
  Schwannoma, 95
Neurilemoblastosis. *Diagnose as*
  Neurofibromatosis, 95
Neurilemoma. *Diagnose as* Schwannoma, 95
Neurilemosarcoma. *Diagnose as*
  Schwannoma, 95
Neurinoma. *Diagnose as* Schwannoma, 95
Neurinomatosis. *Diagnose as* Neurofibromatosis, 95
Neuritis. *See also* Neuropathy
  acute, 428 (1)
  multiple, 428 (1)
  chronic, due to infection, 428 (1)
  optic. *See* Optic neuritis
  retrobulbar. *See under* Optic neuritis
Neuroastrocytoma. *Diagnose as* Astrocytoma, 96
Neuroblastoma
  except of retina. *Diagnose as* Sym-
    pathicogonioma, 95
  of retina. *Diagnose as* Neuroepithe-
    lioma, 95
  sympathetic. *Diagnose as* Sympathi-
    cogonioma, 95
Neuroblastomatosis. *Diagnose as*
  Neurofibromatosis, 95
Neurocirculatory asthenia: *supplementary term,* 491. *Diagnose disease*
Neurocytoma. *Diagnose as* Sympathicoblastoma, 95
Neurodermatitis
  disseminata (dermatitis atopic), 141
    (9)
  localized (lichen chronicus sim-
    plex), 141 (9)
Neuroencephalomyelopathy
  optic, 404 (9)
Neuro-epithelioma, 95

Neurofibroma, 95, 140 (8), 430 (8)
multiple. *Diagnose as* Neurofibromatosis, 95
plexiform. *Diagnose as* Plexiform neuroma, 95
sheath. *Diagnose as* Neurofibroma, 95
solitary. *Diagnose as* Neurofibroma, 95
Neurofibromatosis, 95, 140 (8), 404 (8), 430 (8)
multiple. *Diagnose as* Neurofibromatosis, 95
Neurofibromyxoma. *Diagnose as* Neurofibroma, 95
Neurofibrosarcoma. *Diagnose as* Fibrosarcoma, 96
Neuroglioma. *Diagnose as* Glioma, 96
Neurolemoblastoma. *Diagnose as* Schwannoma, 95
Neurolemoma. *Diagnose as* Schwannoma, 95
Neuroma
acoustic. *Diagnose as* Schwannoma, 95
due to trauma, 429 (4)
fibrillare. *Diagnose as* Neurofibroma, 95
multiple. *Diagnose as* Neurofibromatosis, 95
not otherwise specified, 96
plexiform, 95, 430 (8)
Neuromatosis. *Diagnose as* Neurofibromatosis, 95
Neuromuscular mechanism, ocular diseases, 455 ff.
Neuronevus. *Diagnose as* Pigmented nevus, 94
Neuropathy. *See also* Neuritis
of cranial nerve following premature closure of cranial sutures, 429 (4)
diabetic, 430 (7)
diphtheritic, of abducens nerve, 430 (5)
due to cachexia, 430 (7)
due to hemorrhage, 430 (5)
due to hypercortisonism, 430 (7)
due to hyperinsulinism, 430 (7)
due to porphyria, 430 (7)
due to vitamin deficiency, 430 (7)

Neuropathy—Continued
of facial nerve (Bell's palsy), due to pressure, 429 (4)
ischemic, due to circulatory disturbance, 430 (5)
peripheral, due to pernicious anemia, 430 (7)
progressive hypertrophic interstitial, 431 (9)
progressive muscular atrophy, 425 (9)
toxic
due to poison, 428 (3)
due to remote infection, 430 (5)
Neurosarcoma. *Diagnose as* Fibrosarcoma, 96
Neurosis. *See also* Psychoneurotic disorders, 111 (x)
Neurosyphilis. *See* Nervous system, syphilis
tabetic. *See* Tabes dorsalis, 403 (1)
Neurotic excoriations: *supplementary term,* 505. *Diagnose disease*
Neurovisceral central syndrome: *supplementary term,* 485. *Diagnose disease*
Neuroxanthoma. *Diagnose as* Schwannoma, 95
Neutropenia. *See* Granulocytopenia
Neutrophilia: *supplementary term,* 495. *Diagnose disease*
Neutrophilic myelosis. *Diagnose as* Granulocytic leukemia, 230 (8)
Neutrophils, toxic: *supplementary term,* 495. *Diagnose disease*
Nevocarcinoma. *Diagnose as* Melanoma, 94
Nevolipoma. *Diagnose as* Lipoma, 97
Nevus(i)
acneiformis. *Diagnose as* Neoplastic cyst, 93
anemicus. *Diagnose as* Hemangioma (angioma), 96
apocrine. *Diagnose as* Sweat gland tumor, 94
arachnoideus. *Diagnose as* Hemangioma (angioma), 96
araneus. *Diagnose as* Hemangioma (angioma), 96
arterial. *Diagnose as* Hemangioma (angioma), 96
bathing trunk. *Diagnose as* Pigmented nevus, 94

Newborn—Continued
  hemolytic disease of, 228 (3)
  odor in gastric contents in: *supplementary term,* 497. *Diagnose disease*
  tetany, 120 (7)
Nicotine
  poisoning of heart by, 209 (3)
Niemann-Pick disease (lipid histiocytosis of phosphatide type), 229 (7)
Night blindness
  congenital, 446 (0)
  due to xerophthalmia, 448 (7)
  supplementary term, 509. *Diagnose disease*
Night sweats: *supplementary term,* 487. *Diagnose disease*
Nipple
  fissure, 145 (9)
  inflammation. *See* Thelitis, 144 (1)
  inversion, 143 (0)
  supernumerary, 143 (0)
  thrush, 144 (1)
Nitrogen metabolism, disorders, 120 (7)
Nocardiosis, 124 (2). *See also* Streptotrichosis *under organ or region affected*
  generalized, 116 (2)
Nocturnal emissions: *supplementary term,* 499. *Diagnose disease*
Nodding spasm. *See* Spasmus nutans: *supplementary term,* 507
Nodular granulomatous perifolliculitis, 134 (2)
Nodular nonsuppurative panniculitis, 133 (1)
Nodular vasculitis, 141 (9)
Nodules
  cutaneous: *supplementary term,* 487. *Diagnose disease*
  juxta-articular
    due to syphilis, 133 (1)
    not due to syphilis or yaws, 141 (9)
Noma
  gangrene of auricle due to infection, 475 (1)
  gangrenous stomatitis, 241 (1)
Nondiagnostic terms, 481
Nonunion following fracture, 151 (4)

Nose. *See also* Nasopharynx; Rhinitis
  absence, congenital, 176 (0)
  adenocarcinoma, 178 (8)
  adenoma, 178 (8)
  adhesions
    due to infection, 176 (1)
    due to trauma, 177 (4)
    following operation, 177 (4)
  bifid, 176 (0)
  calculus. *See* Rhinolith, 178 (6)
  carcinoma
    epidermoid, 178 (8)
    transitional cell, 179 (8)
  deformity
    congenital, 176 (0)
    developmental, 178 (7)
    due to infection, 176 (1)
    due to syphilis, 176 (1)
    due to trauma, 177 (4)
  diseases, 176 ff.
  dislocation, 177 (4)
  fibrosarcoma, 178 (8)
  flattening, congenital (with harelip), 176 (0)
  foreign body in, 177 (0)
  frostbite, 178 (4)
  furuncle, 177 (1)
  glanders, 177 (1)
  hemangioma, 178 (8)
  hematoma due to trauma, 178 (4)
  hemorrhage. *See* Epistaxis, 177 (4); Vicarious menstruation, 178 (7)
  hydrorrhea
    due to unknown cause, 179 (x)
    due to vasomotor disturbance, 178 (5)
  injury, 178 (4)
  leprosy, 177 (1)
  lymphosarcoma, 178 (8)
  myeloma, plasma cell, 179 (8)
  neoplasms, 179 (8)
  neurofibroma, 179 (8)
  notching of tip, congenital, 176 (0)
  obstruction due to foreign body, 178 (6)
  overdevelopment of nasal bones, 154 (7)
  papilloma, squamous cell, 179 (8)
  polyp
    due to infection, 177 (1)
    simple, 179 (9)

Nose—Continued
septum
abscess, 176 (1)
deflection
congenital, 176 (0)
due to infection, 176 (1)
due to trauma, 177 (4)
due to unknown cause, 178 (6)
exostosis, 179 (9)
perforation
due to infection, 177 (1)
due to repeated trauma, 178
(4) ,
due to syphilis, 177 (1)
due to tuberculosis, 177 (1)
following operation, 178 (4)
spur due to trauma, 178 (4)
varicose ulcer, 178 (5)
varicose veins, 178 (6)
tuberculosis, 177 (1)
tumors, unlisted, 179 (8)
ulcer
due to infection, 177 (1)
due to trauma, 178 (4)
due to unknown cause, 179 (9)
vestibule, furuncle, 177 (1)
Nostrils
atresia of choana, 176 (0)
stenosis, congenital, 176 (0)
Nuck's canal. *See* Canal of Nuck
Nucleus pulposus
extrusion
compression of nerve roots by, 423
(4)
compression of spinal cord by, 423
(4)
herniation
due to trauma, 159 (4)
due to unknown cause, 164 (9)
Nutrition. *See also* Malnutrition
general, disorders, 119 (7)
Nyctalopia. *See* Night blindness
Nymphomania: *supplementary term,*
485. *Diagnose disease*
Nystagmus
of amblyopia, 456 (5)
congenital, 455 (0)
due to fatigue of nucleus, 457 (7)
supplementary term, 509. *Diagnose
disease*

O

Obesity, 128 (7). *See also* Adiposis
dolorosa; Adiposity
amenorrhea due to, 363 (7)
constitutional, 120 (7)
due to excess of food, 119 (7)
due to undetermined cause, 119 (7)
with pituitary disturbance, 394 (x)
sex infantilism with, 394 (7)
supplementary term, 485. *Diagnose
disease*
Observation, 481
Obsessive compulsive reaction, 112
(x)
Obstetric conditions, 373 ff. *See
also* Abortion; Birth; Fetus;
Labor; Parturition; Pregnancy;
Puerperium
Obstipation: *supplementary term,*
497. *Diagnose disease*
Obstruction. *See under organ
affected*
Occlusion. *See under organ affected*
Occupation spasm *or* tic: *supplementary term,* 505. *Diagnose disease*
Ochronosis, 120 (7), 139 (7)
chloasma in, 464 (7)
Ocular neuromuscular mechanism
diseases, 455 ff.
Oculogyric disturbances: *supplementary terms,* 509. *Diagnose
disease*
Odontoamelosarcoma. *Diagnose as*
Adamantinocarcinoma, 98
Odontogenic cyst of tooth. *Diagnose as* Odontogenic tumor, benign, 98
Odontogenic tumor
benign, 98
malignant. *Diagnose as* Adamantinocarcinoma, 98
of tooth, 249 (8)
Odontoma. *Diagnose as* Odontogenic
tumor, benign, 98
ameloblastic. *Diagnose as* Odontogenic tumor, benign, 98
amorphous. *Diagnose as* Odontogenic tumor, benign, 98
calcified; calcified mixed. *Diagnose
as* Odontogenic tumor, benign, 98

Odontoma—Continued

complex. *Diagnose as* Odontogenic tumor, benign, 98

compound. *Diagnose as* Odontogenic tumor, benign, 98

cystic. *Diagnose as* Odontogenic tumor, benign, 98

gemminate. *Diagnose as* Odontogenic tumor, benign, 98

soft. *Diagnose as* Odontogenic tumor, benign, 98

Oguchi's disease. *See* Night blindness, congenital (Japanese), 446 (0)

Oidiomycosis. *See* Moniliasis *under organ or region affected*

Oil

bronchopneumonia due to aspiration of, 195 (4)

Old age. *See* Senility

Olecranon bursitis, 165 (4)

Oleothorax, 199 (4)

Olfactory nerve

disturbances: *supplementary term,* 508. *Diagnose disease*

Olfactory sense, loss of. *See* Anosmia, 176 (1)

Oligocythemia: *supplementary term,* 495. *Diagnose disease*

Oligodendroblastoma. *Diagnose as* Oligodendroma, 96

Oligodendrocytoma. *Diagnose as* Oligodendroma, 96

Oligodendroglioma. *Diagnose as* Oligodendroma, 96

Oligodendroma, 96

of brain, 415 (8)

Oligodontia, 247 (0)

Oligohydramnios, 384 (x)

Oligomenorrhea: *supplementary term,* 499. *Diagnose disease*

Oligospermia: *supplementary term,* 499. *Diagnose disease*

Oliguria: *supplementary term,* 499. *Diagnose disease*

Olivopontocerebellar atrophy, 416 (9)

Omentum

abscess, 298 (1)

adhesions, anomalous, 298 (0)

diseases, 298 ff.

Omentum—Continued

hernia, 301 (6)

of small intestine into omental sac or fossae, 274 (6)

idiopathic spontaneous infarction, 302 (9)

lymphosarcoma, 301 (8)

neoplasms, 301 (8)

strangulation, 300 (5)

torsion, 301 (6)

tumors, unlisted, 301 (8)

Omphalitis

acute, 299 (1)

chronic, 299 (1)

Omphalocele. *See* Umbilicus, hernia, 298 (0), 301 (6)

Omphalomesenteric duct, patent, 381 (0)

Onkocytoma

except of bronchus. *Diagnose as* Adenolymphoma, 98

of bronchus. *Diagnose as* Adenoma, 94

Onychauxis, 141 (9)

Onychia, 133 (1)

Onychomadesis, 141 (9)

Onychomycosis, 135 (2)

Onychorrhexis, 141 (9)

Oophoritis

acute, 368 (1)

chronic

due to infection, 368 (1)

interstitial, 370 (9)

fetal, 368 (0)

perioophoritis, 368 (1)

Oophoroma. *Diagnose as* Adenofibroma, 97

folliculare. *Diagnose as* Adenofibroma, 97

Opacity

abnormal, in peritoneal cavity: *supplementary term,* 496. *Diagnose disease*

of lens. *See* Cataract

of vitreous. *See* Vitreous, opacity

Opaque enema, abnormality

supplementary term, 496. *Diagnose disease*

Ophthalmia

Egyptian. *See* Trachoma, 468 (1)

electrica, 470 (0)

Ophthalmia—Continued
neonatorum. *See* Conjunctivitis, infectious, acute, 468 (1)
nodosa, 469 (3)
strumous. *See* Keratitis, phlyctenular, 434 (1)
Ophthalmoplegia. *See* Eye, muscles, paralysis
Opisthognathism, 153 (7)
Opium
miosis due to, 439 (3)
poisoning, 117 (3)
Oppenheim's disease. *See* Amyotonia congenita, 421 (0)
Oppenheim-Urbach disease. *See* Necrobiosis lipoidica diabeticorum, 139 (7)
Optic nerve. *See also* Optic neuritis
atrophy
due to circulatory disturbance, 451 (5)
due to infection, 450 (1)
due to low intraocular tension, 451 (4)
due to poison, 450 (3)
due to pressure, 451 (4)
due to pressure of arteriosclerotic arteries (senile), 451 (4)
due to syphilis, 450 (1)
due to trauma, 451 (4)
due to unknown cause, 452 (9)
hereditary, 452 (9)
postretinal, 451 (7)
primary, nonfamilial, 431 (9)
supplementary term, 509. *Diagnose disease*
avulsion, 451 (4)
coloboma, 450 (0)
crushing from fracture of bone, 451 (4)
diseases, 450 ff.
disturbances: *supplementary term,* 508. *Diagnose disease*
foreign body in, 451 (4)
glioma, 451 (8)
injury, 451 (4)
neoplasms, 451 (8)
neurofibroma, 452 (8)
tumors, unlisted, 452 (8)
wound, 451 (4)
Optic neuritis, 450 (1)
due to lead, 450 (3)
due to unknown cause, 452 (9)

Optic neuritis—Continued
meningococcic, 450 (1)
in multiple sclerosis, 452 (9)
retrobulbar neuritis
due to infection, 450 (1)
due to pressure, 451 (4)
supplementary term, 509. *Diagnose disease*
Optic neuroencephalomyelopathy, 404 (0)
Optic papilla. *See also* Papilledema
anomaly of vessels, 450 (0)
cavity, 450 (0)
cup, large physiologic, 450 (0)
drusen, 452 (9)
inversion, 450 (0)
membrana epipapillaris, 450 (0)
pigmentation, 450 (0)
pseudoneuritis, 450 (0)
Optochin
toxic amblyopia due to, 451 (3)
Oral cavity. *See* Buccal cavity; Mouth
Orbit
abscess, 458 (1)
absence, partial, of bony wall, 458 (0)
aneurysm
arteriovenous, retro-orbital due to unknown cause, 460 (9)
due to arteriosclerosis, 460 (9)
due to trauma, 458 (4)
cellulitis, 458 (1)
cyst, 459 (6)
deformity
due to infection, 458 (1)
following operation, 458 (4)
diseases, 458 ff.
edema
circulatory, 459 (5)
due to trauma, 458 (4)
exophthalmos due to, 459 (5)
emphysema, 458 (4)
exostosis, 460 (9)
fibroma, 459 (8)
fibrosarcoma, 459 (8)
fistula due to infection, 458 (1)
foreign body in, 458 (4)
fracture of bone, 458 (4)
granuloma, 458 (1)
hemangioma, 459 (8)
hematoma due to trauma, 458 (4)

Orbit—Continued
  hemorrhage due to disturbance of circulation, 459 (5)
  infection of tissue, enophthalmos following, 458 (1)
  inflammation, chronic, 458 (1)
  injury, 458 (4)
  leiomyoma, 459 (8)
  leiomyosarcoma, 459 (8)
  lipoma, 459 (8)
  lymphoma, 459 (8)
  lymphomatosis, not otherwise specified. *Diagnose as* Lymphoma of orbit, 459 (8)
  lymphosarcoma, 458 (8)
  melanoma, malignant, 459 (8)
  neoplasms, 459 (8)
  neurofibroma, 459 (8)
  osteoma of orbital bone, 458 (8)
  passive congestion, 459 (5)
  periostitis, 458 (1)
  pigmented nevus, 459 (8)
  protrusion of fat due to senile atrophy, 459 (7)
  rhabdomyoma, 459 (8)
  tissue, loss of, enophthalmos due to, 458 (4)
  tumors, unlisted, 459 (8)
  varix, 459 (6)
    congenital, 458 (0)
Orchitis
  acute, 332 (1)
  chronic, 332 (1)
  due to trauma, 333 (4)
  suppurative, acute, 332 (1)
Oriental sore (leishmaniasis of skin), 133 (1)
Ornithosis (psittacosis), 116 (1)
Oroya fever. *See* Bartonellosis, 114 (1)
Orthopnea: *supplementary term,* 490. *Diagnose disease*
Orthostatic hypertension, 219 (x)
Os calcis. *See* Calcaneus
Os uteri. *See under* Cervix uteri
Osgood-Schlatter disease. *See* Osteochondrosis of tuberosity of tibia, 155 (9)
Osler's disease. *Diagnose as* Polycythemia vera, 230 (8)
Osler-Rendu disease. *Diagnose as* Hemangiomatosis, 96

Osler-Rendu-Weber syndrome, 219 (9)
Osler-Vaquez disease. *Diagnose as* Polycythemia vera, 230 (8)
Osseous meatus. *See under* Ear
Ossicles. *See* Ear, ossicles
Ossification. *See also* Calcification; *and under organ or structure affected*
  defective. *See* Dysostosis
  due to trauma, 127 (4)
  of epiphysis, retardation: *supplementary term,* 489. *Diagnose disease*
  progressive ossifying myositis, 169 (7)
  senile, of cartilage, 163 (7)
Osteitis
  deformans, 155 (9)
  fibrosa cystica, generalized, 153 (7)
    coxa vara due to, 153 (7)
    fracture due to, 153 (7)
  sclerotic nonsuppurative, 148 (1)
Osteoarthritis, 164 (9)
  compression of spinal cord by, 423 (4)
Osteoarthropathy
  secondary hypertrophic, 152 (7)
Osteoblastoma, 97
Osteocarcinoma. *Diagnose as* Cystosarcoma phyllodes, 97
Osteochondritis
  dissecans, 164 (9)
  of rib due to trauma, 151 (4)
  syphilitic, 149 (1)
Osteochondrocarcinoma. *Diagnose as* Mixed tumor, salivary gland type, 98
Osteochondroma. *Diagnose as* Osteoma, 97
Osteochondromatosis, 97
Osteochondromyxoma. *Diagnose as* Osteoma, 97
Osteochondromyxosarcoma. *Diagnose as* Osteosarcoma (osteogenic sarcoma), 97
Osteochondrosarcoma. *Diagnose as* Osteosarcoma (osteogenic sarcoma), 97
Osteochondrosis, 155 (9)
  fracture due to, 154 (9)
Osteoclastoma. *Diagnose as* Giant cell tumor of bone, 97

Osteodystrophy
renal, 152 (7)
Osteofibrochondroma. *Diagnose as*
Osteoma, 97
Osteofibroma
of bone. *Diagnose as* Osteoma, 97
except of bone. *Diagnose as* Fibroma
Osteofibrosarcoma (bone). *Diagnose as* Osteosarcoma (osteogenic sarcoma), 97
Osteogenesis imperfecta. *See* Fragilitas ossium, 147 (0)
Osteogenic tumor. *Diagnose as* Osteoma, 97
malignant. *Diagnose as* Osteosarcoma (osteogenic sarcoma), 97
Osteoma, 97
ivory. *Diagnose as* Osteoma, 97
myosteal. *Diagnose as* Osteoma, 97
periosteal. *Diagnose as* Osteoma, 97
Osteomalacia, 153 (7)
associated with pregnancy or puerperium, 153 (7)
deformity of joint due to, 163 (7)
due to unknown cause (Milkman's syndrome), 155 (9)
juvenile, bone changes associated with, 153 (7)
senile, 153 (7)
Osteomyelitis
acute, 148 (1)
chronic, 149 (1)
chronic hemorrhagic. *Diagnose as* Giant cell tumor of bone, 97
due to infection, 148 (1)
due to trauma, 151 (4)
streptococcic, arrest of growth of femur due to, 148 (1)
Osteomyxochondroma. *Diagnose as* Osteoma, 97
Osteopathia condensans disseminata. *See* Osteopoikilosis, 147 (0)
Osteopetrosis (marble bones), 147 (0)
myeloid metaplasia due to, 233 (9)
Osteopoikilosis, 147 (0)
Osteoporosis
due to endocrine disorders, 153 (7)
due to prolonged malnutrition, 152 (7)
due to trauma, 151 (4)
idiopathic, 155 (9)

Osteoporosis—Continued
postmenopausal, 153 (7)
senile, 153 (7)
supplementary term, 489. *Diagnose disease*
Osteosarcoma, 97
fibrosing. *Diagnose as* Osteosarcoma (osteogenic sarcoma), 97
sclerosing. *Diagnose as* Osteosarcoma (osteogenic sarcoma), 97
telangiectatic. *Diagnose as* Osteosarcoma (osteogenic sarcoma), 97
Osteosclerosis
fragilis generalista. *See* Osteopoikilosis, 147 (0)
Osteosis, ivory. *Diagnose as* Osteoma, 97
Ostium primum
with cleft mitral valve, 202 (0)
with localized ventricular septal defect, 203 (0)
persistent, 202 (0)
Ostium secundum. *See* Foramen ovale
Otalgia
due to malocclusion of temporomandibular joint, 472 (6)
reflex, 472 (55)
supplementary term, 509. *Diagnose disease*
Otitis
media
mucopurulent, 477 (1)
nonsuppurative, acute, due to rapid change in air pressure, 478 (4)
serous, 477 (1)
suppurative, acute, 477 (1)
chronic, 478 (1), 478 (9)
panotitis, 472 (1)
Otomycosis, 475 (2)
Otorrhagia: *supplementary term,* 509. *Diagnose disease*
Otorrhea: *supplementary term,* 509. *Diagnose disease*
cerebrospinal: *supplementary term,* 503. *Diagnose disease*
Otosclerosis
conduction deafness, with fixation of stapes, 480 (7)
without impaired hearing, 480 (7)

Otosclerosis—Continued
  primary nerve deafness, without
    stapes fixation, 480 (7)
  with round window closure, 480 (7)
Ovalocytosis, hereditary, 230 (9)
Ovarian tumor, compound. *Diag-
    nose as* Teratoma, 97
Ovary(ies). *See also* Oophoritis
  abscess, 368 (1)
    tubo-ovarian, 366 (1)
  absence, 368 (0)
    sterility due to, 349 (7)
  accessory, 368 (0)
  adhesions, 368 (0)
  arrhenoblastoma, 370 (8)
  Brenner tumor, 370 (8)
  calcification, 370 (9)
  cyst
    due to failure of involution, 369
      (7)
    mucous; multilocular. *Diagnose
      as* Pseudomucinous cystic tu-
      mor, 93
  cystadenocarcinoma, 370 (8)
    pseudomucinous, 370 (8)
    serous papillary, 370 (8)
  cystadenoma, 370 (8)
    pseudomucinous, 370 (8)
    serous papillary, 370 (8)
  cystic, congenital, 368 (0)
  cystic degeneration, 370 (9)
  cystic disease with hirsutism, 369
    (7)
  decreased function in hypopituita-
    rism, 369 (7)
  diseases, 368 ff.
  disgerminoma, 370 (8)
  displacement, 369 (6)
    free in peritoneal cavity, 368 (0)
    into hernial sac, 369 (6)
  dysfunction due to surgery, 369 (4)
  embryoma. *Diagnose as* Disgermi-
    noma, 97
  endometriosis, 370 (9)
  fibroepithelioma. *Diagnose as* Ade-
    nofibroma, 97
  fibroma, 370 (8)
  folliculoma. *Diagnose as* Granulosa
    cell tumor, 93
  granulosa cell tumor, 370 (8)
  Grawitz tumor. *Diagnose as* Viriliz-
    ing tumor, 93

Ovary(ies)—Continued
  hematoma, nontraumatic, 369 (5)
  hemorrhage
    due to remote infection, 368 (1)
    due to trauma, 368 (4)
    due to venous obstruction, 369
      (5)
    from rupture of graafian follicle,
      369 (7)
  hernia, 368 (0)
  hypergonadism, 369 (7)
  hypertrophy, 368 (0)
  hypofunction
    due to radium, 369 (4)
    due to roentgen rays, 368 (4)
    due to unknown cause, 370 (x)
    hypoplasia of uterus due to, 364
      (7)
  hypogonadism, 369 (7)
  hypoplasia, 368 (0)
  inflammation. *See* Oophoritis
  injury, 368 (4)
  Krukenberg tumor, 370 (8)
  mesonephroma, 370 (8)
  necrosis due to circulatory disturb-
    ance, 369 (5)
  neoplasms, 370 (8)
  ovarian rest in tube, 366 (0)
  ovotestis, 368 (0)
  polycystic, 369 (7)
  sclerosis due to infection, 368 (1)
  senile involution, 369 (7)
  stimulation
    static endometrial hyperplasia due
      to, 364 (7)
    static myometrial hyperplasia due
      to, 364 (7)
  strangulation, 369 (5)
  supernumerary, 368 (0)
  teratoma, 370 (8)
    cystic, 370 (8)
  thecoma, 370 (8)
  thyroid teratoma; thyroid tumor.
    Diagnose as Teratoma, 97
  torsion of ovarian pedicle, 369 (6)
    congenital, 368 (0)
  transplants, 369 (4)
  tumors, unlisted, 370 (8)
Overactivity: *supplementary term,*
    485. *Diagnose disease*
Oviducts. *See* Fallopian tubes
Ovotestis, 368 (0)

Ovulation
  bleeding: *supplementary term,* 499.
    Diagnose disease
  pain (Mittelschmerz): *supplementary term,* 499. *Diagnose disease*
Oxalate metabolism
  inborn error of, 120 (7)
Oxalosis, 120 (7)
Oxaluria: *supplementary term,* 499.
    Diagnose disease
Oxycephalia, 122 (0)
Oxygen
  deficiency. *See* Anoxemia; Anoxia
    toxicity, 117 (3)
Oxyuriasis
  of intestine, 268 (2)

P

Pacemaker, wandering
  due to unknown cause, 214 (x)
Pachydermoperiostosis, 121 (9)
Pachymeningitis
  acute, 405 (1)
  chronic
    adhesive, 406 (1)
    due to infection, 405 (1)
  nonsuppurative, 406 (1)
Pachymeningopathy
  internal hemorrhagic, 407 (4)
Pachyonychia congenital, 131 (0)
Paget's disease
  of bone. *See* Osteitis deformans,
    155 (9)
  except bone, 93
Pain
  in abdomen: *supplementary term,*
    497. *Diagnose disease*
  asymbolia: *supplementary term,* 505.
    Diagnose disease
  in epigastrium: *supplementary term,*
    497. *Diagnose disease*
  general: *supplementary term,* 485.
    Diagnose disease
  loss of sensitivity. *See* Analgesia:
    supplementary term, 501
  ovulation (Mittelschmerz): *supplementary term,* 499. *Diagnose disease*
  referable to female genital organs:
    supplementary term, 499. *Diagnose disease*

Pain—Continued
  referable to male genital organs:
    supplementary term, 499. *Diagnose disease*
  referable to urinary system: *supplementary term,* 499. *Diagnose disease*
  in thorax (noncardiac): *supplementary term,* 490. *Diagnose disease*
Palate
  abscess, 250 (1)
  carcinoma
    basal cell, 251 (8)
    epidermoid, 251 (8)
    transitional cell, 251 (8)
  chemical burn, 250 (3)
  chondroma, 251 (8)
  cleft, 250 (0)
  craniopharyngioma, 251 (8)
  cyst, anterior nasopalatine, 250 (0)
  deformity
    due to unknown cause, 251 (6)
    following operation, 250 (4)
  diseases, 250 ff.
  fibroma, 251 (8)
  hemangioma, 251 (8)
  injury, 250 (4)
  lymphosarcoma, 251 (8)
  neoplasms, 251 (8)
  osteoma, 251 (8)
  pigmented nevus, 251 (8)
  plasma cell myeloma, 251 (8)
  sarcoma, 251 (8)
  shortening, congenital, 250 (0)
  syphilis, 250 (1)
  syphilitic perforation, 250 (1)
  torus palatinus, 249 (9)
  tumors
    mixed, salivary gland type, 251
      (8)
    unlisted, 251 (8)
  ulcer due to unknown cause, 251 (9)
Palatoplegia: *supplementary term,*
  508. *Diagnose disease*
Palilalia: *supplementary term,* 505.
    Diagnose disease
Palindromic rheumatism, 164 (9)
Pallor: *supplementary term,* 487. *Diagnose disease*
Palmar abscess, 173 (1)
Palmar fasciitis, 174 (4)

Palpebra. *See* Eyelid
Palpitation: *supplementary term,*
491. *Diagnose disease*
Palsy. *See also* Paralysis
Bell's (neuropathy of facial nerve),
429 (4)
bulbar, 416 (9)
Pancreas. *See also* Insular tissue;
Pancreatic artery; Pancreatic
duct; Pancreatitis
aberrant, 295 (0)
abscess, 295 (1)
accessory, congenital, 295 (0)
adenocarcinoma, 296 (8)
adenoma, 296 (8)
annular, 295 (0)
atrophy
due to malnutrition, 296 (7)
due to obstruction of duct, 296 (6)
senile, 296 (7)
bifurcation, congenital, 295 (0)
calcification due to unknown cause,
297 (9)
cyst due to obstruction, 296 (6)
diseases, 295 ff.
dysfunction (steatorrhea), 296 (7)
fibrocystic disease, 295 (0)
fibrosis due to unknown cause, 297
(9)
fistula, 295 (4)
hemorrhage
due to blood dyscrasia, 296 (5)
due to embolism, 296 (5)
due to scurvy, 296 (7)
infantilism, 295 (0)
injury, 295 (4)
islet cell tumor
functioning, 296 (8)
non-functioning, 296 (8)
necrosis
due to infection, 295 (1)
due to trauma, 296 (4)
ischemic, 296 (5)
neoplasms, 296 (8)
pseudocyst
due to infection, 295 (1)
due to obstruction, 296 (6)
due to traumatic necrosis, 296 (4)
rupture due to trauma, 296 (4)
tissue, islands of. *See* Insular tissue
tumors, unlisted, 296 (8)
Pancreatic artery
aneurysm, 297 (9)

Pancreatic artery—Continued
arteriosclerosis, 297 (9)
ischemic necrosis of pancreas due
to, 296 (5)
embolism, 296 (6)
Pancreatic duct
calculus, 296 (6)
parasitic obstruction, 295 (1)
stricture, congenital, 295 (0)
Pancreatitis
acute, 295 (1)
due to poison, 295 (3)
hemorrhagic, 295 (1)
interstitial, due to unknown cause,
296 (9)
suppurative, 295 (1)
chronic
due to infection, 295 (1)
due to obstruction, 296 (6)
due to poison, 295 (3)
interstitial, 297 (9)
Pancytopenia. *See* Anemia, normocytic hypoplastic
Panic: *supplementary term,* 485. *Diagnose disease*
acute homosexual: *supplementary
term,* 485. *Diagnose disease*
Panniculitis
nodular nonsuppurative, 133 (1)
Pannus
allergic (eczematous), 435 (3)
degenerativus, 437 (9)
trachomatosus, 435 (1)
Panophthalmitis, 433 (1)
Panotitis, 472 (1)
Pansinusitis, 180 (1)
Papillary muscle
anomalous, 203 (0)
rupture due to infection, 208 (1)
**Papillary tumor, not otherwise
specified,** 93
Papilledema
due to abnormally low intraocular
tension, 451 (4)
due to blood dyscrasia, 451 (5)
due to hematoma of orbit, 451 (5)
due to increased intracranial pressure, 451 (5)
due to pressure, 451 (4)
due to tower skull, 451 (4)
due to trauma, 451 (4)
supplementary term, 509. *Diagnose
disease*

Papilloma

angiomatous. *Diagnose as* Papillary tumor, not otherwise specified, 93

basal cell. *Diagnose as* Basal cell carcinoma, 94

carcinomatous. *Diagnose as* Papillary or polypoid tumor, not otherwise specified, 93

choroidal. *Diagnose as* Ependymoma, 96

cutaneous. *Diagnose as* Squamous cell papilloma, 94

dyskeratotic. *Diagnose as* Squamous papilloma, 94

hyperkeratotic. *Diagnose as* Squamous cell papilloma, 94

malignant. *Diagnose as* Papillary or polypoid tumor, not otherwise specified, 93

parakeratotic. *Diagnose as* Squamous cell papilloma, 94

skin. *Diagnose as* Squamous cell papilloma, 94

squamous. *Diagnose as* Squamous cell papilloma, 94

squamous cell, 94

Pappataci fever, 115 (1)

Paracoccidioidomycosis
of skin, 135 (2)

Paraganglioma, 95

Parageusia. *See* Hallucinations of taste: *supplementary term,* 509

Paragrammatism: *supplementary term,* 505. *Diagnose disease*

Paragranuloma, Hodgkin's. *Diagnose as* Hodgkin's disease, 95

Paralysis. *See also* Hemiplegia; Palsy; Paraplegia; Paresis

abducens

alternating, hemiplegic: *supplementary term,* 505. *Diagnose disease*

facial, hemiplegic, alternating (Millard-Gubler syndrome): *supplementary term,* 505. *Diagnose disease*

abductor, laryngeal stenosis due to, 185 (55)

of accommodation: *supplementary term,* 505. *Diagnose disease*

Paralysis—Continued

agitans, 416 (9)

supplementary term, 485. *Diagnose disease*

alternating: *supplementary terms. Diagnose disease*

facial, lateral gaze, hemiplegic, 505

hypoglossal, hemiplegic, 505

oculomotor, hemiplegic (Webber paralysis), 506

ambiguoaccessorius: *supplementary term,* 506. *Diagnose disease*

ambiguoaccessorius-hypoglossal: *supplementary term,* 506. *Diagnose disease*

ambiguo-hypoglossal: *supplementary term,* 506. *Diagnose disease*

ambiguospinothalamic (Avellis): *supplementary term,* 506. *Diagnose disease*

birth. *See* Paralysis, obstetric, 167 (0)

of bladder. *See* Bladder, paralysis

brachial plexus, upper or lower: *supplementary term,* 506. *Diagnose disease*

bulbar: *supplementary term,* 506. *Diagnose disease*

cerebral: *supplementary terms. Diagnose disease*

diplegic, infantile, 506

hemiplegic, infantile, 506

hereditary, spastic, 506

infantile, 506

ataxic, 506

choreoathetoid, 506

cerebrocerebellar, diplegic, infantile: *supplementary term,* 506. *Diagnose disease*

cerebrospinal, hereditary: *supplementary term,* 506. *Diagnose disease*

cervical sympathetic, 432 (4)

due to pressure, 432 (4)

following operation, 432 (4)

of cranial nerve following operation, 430 (4)

cruciate, hemiplegic: *supplementary term,* 506. *Diagnose disease*

divers'. *See* Caisson disease, 118 (4)

of eyes. *See under* Eye, muscles

familial periodic, 170 (x)

Paralysis—Continued
flaccid
contracture of spine due to, 161
(55)
of diaphragm, 172 (55)
due to central nervous system lesion, 169 (55)
due to nerve lesion, 169 (55)
due to poison, 169 (55)
following poliomyelitis, contractures due to, 160 (55)
nonpoliomyelitic
contractures due to, 161 (55)
dislocation of joint due to, 162
(55)
relaxation of joint due to, 162
(55)
from spina bifida, contracture of
spine from, 161 (55)
of larynx. *See* Larynx, paralysis
lateral gaze (Foville syndrome) :
supplementary term, 504. *Diagnose disease*
medullary, tegmental (Babinski-
Nageotte) : *supplementary term,*
506. *Diagnose disease*
mesencephalic, tegmental (Benedikt) : *supplementary term,* 506.
Diagnose disease
obstetric, 167 (0)
oculogyric : *supplementary term,* 509.
Diagnose disease
oculomotor : *supplementary terms.*
Diagnose disease
external, bilateral, 506
tetraplegic, 506
pseudobulbar : *supplementary term,*
506. *Diagnose disease*
residual, following poliomyelitis, 169
(55)
spastic, 169 (55)
contractures due to, 169 (55)
spinal, hereditary, spastic : *supplementary term,* 506. *Diagnose
disease*
of uvula : *supplementary term,* 497.
Diagnose disease
of vocal cord due to nerve lesion, 185
(55)
Parametritis, 361 (1)
Parametrium
leiomyoma, 372 (8)
neoplasms, 372 (8)

Paramyoclonus
multiplex, 170 (x)
supplementary term, 506. *Diagnose
disease*
Paramyotonia congenita, 167 (0)
Paranoia
personality, 112 (x)
reactions, 110 (x)
trends : *supplementary term,* 485. *Diagnose disease*
Paraphasia : *supplementary term,* 506.
Diagnose disease
Paraphimosis, 330 (6)
Paraplegia
congenital spastic, chronic brain syndrome with, 107 (0)
supplementary term, 506. *Diagnose
disease*
Parapsoriasis, 141 (9)
Parasites
animal, in sputum : *supplementary
term,* 490. *Diagnose disease*
list, 63 ff.
Parasitic infection, 124 (2)
Parasympathetic nervous system.
See Nervous system, vegetative
Parathyroid gland(s)
adenocarcinoma, 391 (8)
adenoma, 391 (8)
diseases, 391
hemorrhage, spontaneous, into, 391
(5)
hyperplasia, 391 (7)
adenomatous, 391 (9)
with hyperparathyroidism, 391
(9)
injury, 391 (4)
neoplasms, 391 (8)
radiation injury, 391 (4)
tumors
functionally hyperactive, 93
unlisted, 391 (8)
Paratrophy. *See* Adiposis dolorosa,
120 (7)
Paratyphoid, 115 (1)
cholecystitis, 292 (1)
Paraurethral ducts. *See under* Urethra
Parauterine. *See under* Uterus
Paravaginitis. *See* Vaginitis
**Parenchymatous cortical cerebel-
lar atrophy,** 416 (9)

Parenchymatous granulosa cell tumor. *Diagnose as* Granulosa cell tumor, 93
Parenteral diarrhea, 268 (1)
Paresis. *See also* Paralysis
of bladder, tabetic, 320 (55)
general. *See* Dementia paralytica, 411 (1)
Paresthesia: *supplementary term,* 506. *Diagnose disease*
Parinaud syndrome: *supplementary term,* 506. *Diagnose disease*
Parkinson's disease. *See* Paralysis agitans, 416 (9)
Paronychia, 133 (1)
Paroophoron cyst, 370 (9)
Parosmia: *supplementary term,* 509. *Diagnose disease*
Parotid gland and duct. *See also* Salivary glands and ducts
absence, congenital, 252 (0)
accessory, 252 (0)
adenolymphoma, 253 (8)
diseases, 252 ff.
displacement of gland over masseter or buccinator muscle, 252 (0)
hypoplasia, 252 (0)
islands of parotid tissue in neck structures or lymph nodes, 252 (0)
neoplasms, 253 (8)
Parotitis
epidemic (mumps), 253 (1)
following operation, 253 (4)
Paroxysmal automatism: *supplementary term,* 485. *Diagnose disease*
Paroxysmal clouded states: *supplementary term,* 485. *Diagnose disease*
Paroxysmal disorders. *See also* Atrial fibrillation; Atrial flutter; Tachycardia
mixed, 417 (x)
of nervous system, due to unknown cause, 417 (x)
vasovagal attacks, 417 (x)
Paroxysmal dyspnea: *supplementary term,* 490. *Diagnose disease*
Paroxysmal furor: *supplementary term,* 485. *Diagnose disease*

Paroxysmal psychic equivalents: *supplementary term,* 485. *Diagnose disease*
Parrot fever. *See* Psittacosis, 116 (1)
Parry's disease. *See* Toxic diffuse goiter, 390 (9)
Parturition. *See also* Labor
adhesions, cervicovaginal, following, 359 (4)
displacement of uterus following, 361 (4)
fistula, urethrovaginal, following, 324 (4)
laceration of urethra following, 324 (4)
parauterine adhesions following, 360 (1)
relaxation of pelvic floor due to, 372 (4)
vaginocutaneous fistula following, 356 (4)
Passive-aggressive personality, 112 (x)
Passive-dependent personality, 112 (x)
Pasteurella pseudotuberculosis infection, 115 (1)
Patella
biparta, 147 (0)
dislocation
congenital, 146 (0)
recurrent, 151 (4)
retropatellar fat pad, hypertrophy
due to infection, 149 (1)
due to trauma, 151 (4)
Pediculosis
capitis, 135 (2)
corporis, 135 (2)
palpebrarum, 135 (2)
pubis, 135 (2)
of vulva, 352 (2)
Pel-Ebstein disease. *Diagnose as* Hodgkin's disease, 95
Pellagra, 120 (7)
myelopathy due to, 425 (7)
Pellegrini-Stieda disease. *See* Calcification of medial collateral ligament of knee due to trauma, 158 (4)
Pelvis
abscess, 298 (1), 371 (1)
during pregnancy, 373 (1)

Pelvis—Continued
  abscess—continued
    peritoneal, 298 (1)
  acetabulum, protrusion of, 154 (9)
  android, 386 (7)
  anthropoid, 386 (6)
  assimilation, 385 (0)
  cellulitis, 371 (1)
    in male, 328 (1)
    during pregnancy, 373 (1)
    during puerperium, 373 (1)
  contracted, generally, due to un-
    known cause, 386 (6)
  contracture
    due to flaccid paralysis, 161 (55)
    due to spastic paralysis, 169 (55)
  coxalgic, 385 (4)
  cretin, 386 (7)
  deformity
    due to congenital dislocation of
      hip, 385 (4)
    due to fracture, 385 (4)
    due to tuberculosis, 385 (1)
    due to unequal strain, 385 (4)
  flat, due to unknown cause, 386 (6)
  floor
    laceration, 371 (4)
      obstetric, 374 (4)
    relaxation, 372 (4)
  funnel
    due to unspecified cause, 386 (6)
    tuberculous, 385 (1)
  hematocele, 372 (5)
  infantile, due to unknown cause, 386
    (6)
  kyphotic, 385 (1)
  masculine, 386 (7)
  Nägele's, 385 (4)
  obliquely contracted, due to unspeci-
    fied cause, 386 (6)
  obliquity, 161 (55)
  osteomalacic, 386 (7)
  peritoneum. See Peritoneum, pelvic
  peritonitis, 299 (1)
  platypelloid, 386 (6)
  rachitic, 386 (7)
  Robert's, 386 (9)
  scoliotic, 385 (1)
    following poliomyelitis, 385 (55)
  spondylolisthetic, 385 (4)
  supporting structures
    diseases, 371 ff.

Pelvis—Continued
  supporting structures—continued
    mesothelioma, 372 (8)
    neoplasms, 372 (8)
    tumors, unlisted, 372 (8)
  thrombophlebitis, 374 (1)
  tilt (in sagittal plane), 161 (55)
  transversely contracted, due to un-
    specified cause, 386 (6)
Pelvis of kidney. See under Kidney
Pemphigus, 133 (1)
  benign of Hailey and Hailey, 141
    (9)
  of conjunctiva, 471 (9)
  erythematosus, 141 (9)
  foliaceus, 141 (9)
  pemphigoid, 141 (9)
  South American, 141 (9)
  vegetans, 141 (9)
Penis. See also Balanitis; Balanopos-
    thitis; Corpora cavernosa; Pre-
    puce
  abscess, 329 (1)
  absence, 329 (0)
  adhesion to scrotum, 329 (0)
  carcinoma
    basal cell, 331 (8)
    epidermoid, 331 (8)
    of glans, 331 (8)
  cellulitis, 329 (1)
  chancre (syphilis), 330 (1)
  chancroid (Ducrey's bacillus), 329
    (1)
  cleft, 329 (0)
  concealed, 329 (0)
  deformity, acquired, due to unknown
    cause, 330 (6)
  diseases, 329 ff.
  dorsal fibrosis. See Corpora caver-
    nosa, induration, 331 (9)
  double, 329 (0)
  double glans penis, 329 (0)
  embolism of penile vessels due to un-
    specified cause, 330 (6)
  fibroma, 331 (8)
  frostbite, 330 (4)
  gangrene due to trauma, 330 (4)
  gumma (syphilis), 330 (1)
  hemangioma, 331 (8)
  hematoma due to trauma, 330 (4)
  hemorrhage due to trauma, 330 (4)
  herpes simplex, 329 (1)
  injury, 330 (4)

Penis—Continued
  leiomyoma, 331 (8)
  leukoplakia
    due to infection, 329 (1)
    due to trauma, 330 (4)
  lipoma, 331 (8)
  luxation, 330 (4)
  lymphangitis
    acute, 329 (1)
    chronic, 330 (1)
  lymphopathia venereum, 330 (1)
  melanoma, malignant, 331 (8)
  neoplasms, 331 (8)
  ossification due to trauma, 330 (4)
  osteoma, 331 (8)
  pigmented nevus, 331 (8)
  rupture, 330 (4)
  sarcoma, 331 (8)
  scabies, 330 (2)
  strangulation, 330 (4)
  syphilis, 330 (1)
  thrombosis of penile vessels due to
    unspecified cause, 330 (6)
  torsion
    congenital, 329 (0)
    not due to trauma, 330 (6)
  tumors, unlisted, 331 (8)
Pentosuria, 120 (7)
Peptic ulcer. *See* Duodenum, ulcer;
    Esophagus, ulcer; Stomach, ulcer
Periappendicitis, 279 (1)
Periarteritis nodosa (essential poly-
    angiitis), 218 (9)
  aneurysm of artery due to, 218 (9)
  hemorrhage from artery due to, 218
    (9)
  of hepatic artery, 304 (9)
  infarction of liver due to, 288 (5)
  of kidney, 312 (9)
  of mesenteric artery, 305 (9)
  of skin, 141 (9)
  thrombosis of artery due to, 218 (9)
Pericarditis. *See also* Mediastino-
    pericarditis
  acute bacterial, 208 (1)
    with effusion, 208 (1)
  acute benign, 213 (9)
  due to myocardial infarction, 210
    (5)
  rheumatic, 213 (9)
  subacute bacterial, 208 (1)
  tuberculous, 208 (1)
  uremic, 209 (3)

Pericardium. *See also* Hemopericar-
    dium; Hydropericardium; Pneu-
    mopericardium; Pyopneumoperi-
    cardium
  abnormalities, 202 (0)
  absence, 202 (0)
  adherent, due to unknown cause, 212
    (9)
  adhesions due to trauma, 209 (4)
  calcification due to unknown cause,
    212 (9)
  defect, 202 (0)
  diverticulum (or cyst), 202 (0)
  effusion
    due to scarlet fever, 208 (1)
    due to typhoid, 208 (1)
  foreign body in, 209 (4)
  rheumatic adherent, 213 (9)
  sarcoma, 211 (8)
Pericementitis. *See* Periodontitis,
    248 (4)
Pericholecystic. *See under* Gallblad-
    der
Perichondritis
  of auricle, 475 (1)
  of larynx
    due to infection, 183 (1)
    due to trauma or following opera-
      tion, 184 (4)
Perichondrium. *See also* Perichon-
    dritis
  laryngeal, radiation injury, 184 (4)
Pericoronal abscess. *See* Abscess of
    gum, 247 (1)
Pericoronitis
  of eruption, 249 (6)
Pericystitis, 318 (1)
Periendothelioma. *Diagnose as* He-
    mangiopericytoma, 96
Perifolliculitis capitis abscedens.
    See Perifolliculitis of scalp, dis-
    secting, 133 (1)
**Perigastric abscess; Perigastric
    adhesions.** *See under* Stomach
Perigastritis, 263 (1)
Perihepatitis, 288 (1)
Perilabyrinthitis, 479 (1)
Perinephritis, 308 (1)
Perineum
  abscess, 371 (1)
  cellulitis, 371 (1)
  contracture, congenital, 371 (0)

Perineum—Continued
fistula
due to infection, 371 (1)
following operation, 371 (4)
urethroperineal
due to infection, 323 (1)
following operation, 324 (4)
vesicoperineal, following operation, 319 (4)
rigidity during labor, 375 (6)
wound, 372 (4)
Periodic disease
familial, 121 (9)
Periodontal abscess, 247 (1)
Periodontal traumatism, 248 (4)
Periodontitis
due to filth, 248 (4)
Periodontosis, 249 (7)
Periosteum. *See also* Bones
changes due to scurvy, 153 (7)
subperiosteal calcification due to
trauma, 150 (4)
subperiosteal hematoma, 151 (4)
Periostitis
acute, 149 (1)
chronic, 149 (1)
due to trauma, 151 (4)
orbital, 458 (1)
Peripheral nerves
agenesis, 428 (0)
atypical distribution, 428 (0)
avulsion, 429 (4)
birth injury, 428 (0)
compression
acute, 429 (4)
by aneurysm, 429 (4)
by arteriosclerotic vessel, 429 (4)
by callus, 429 (4)
by dislocation of contiguous joint,
429 (4)
due to displacement or distortion,
429 (4)
by foreign body, 429 (4)
by fracture of contiguous bone,
429 (4)
by hemorrhage or clot, 429 (4)
by meningeal adhesions, 429 (4)
by scar tissue, 429 (4)
contusion, 429 (4)
diseases, 428 ff.
electrical shock, 429 (4)
irritation by scar tissue, 429 (4)
laceration, 429 (4)

Peripheral nerves—Continued
neoplasms, 430 (8)
neurofibroma, 430 (8)
neurofibromatosis, 430 (8)
neuroma, plexiform, 430 (8)
sarcoma, not otherwise specified. *Diagnose as* Fibrosarcoma, 96
schwannoma, malignant, 431 (8)
stretching, 430 (4)
tumors, unlisted, 431 (8)
Periprostatic. *See under* Prostate
Perirectal. *See under* Rectum
Perirenal. *See under* Kidney
Perisalpingitis, 366 (1)
Perithelioma. *Diagnose as* Hemangiopericytoma, 96
multiplex nodulosum; multiplex
nodulosum cavernosum. *Diagnose as* Multiple hemorrhagic
hemangioma of Kaposi, 96
Peritoneum. *See also* Hemoperitoneum; Mesentery; Omentum;
Peritonitis
abnormal opacity in peritoneal cavity: *supplementary term,* 496.
Diagnose disease
abscess, 298 (1)
adhesions
and bands, congenital, 298 (0)
due to infection, 298 (1), 371 (1)
due to trauma, 299 (4)
following operation, 299 (4), 371
(4)
coccidiosis, 298 (1)
cyst, 301 (6)
chylous, 300 (5)
diseases, 298 ff.
fat necrosis, 299 (3)
fistula
pleuroperitoneal, 171 (1)
pulmoperitoneal, 171 (1)
granuloma
due to foreign body, 299 (4)
due to nematodes, 299 (2)
due to ova of helminths, 299 (2)
hemangioma, 301 (8)
hemangiosarcoma, 301 (8)
injury, 300 (4)
lymphosarcoma, 301 (8)
mesothelioma, 301 (8)
neoplasms, 301 (8)
sarcoma, 301 (8)

Peritoneum—Continued
    tumor cells in peritoneal fluid: *supplementary term, 497. Diagnose disease*
    tumors, unlisted, 301 (8)
Peritonitis
    acute, 299 (1)
    adenoides. *Diagnose as* Adenomyosis, 98
    chemical, 299 (3)
    chronic, 299 (1)
    chronic adhesive, due to unknown cause, 302 (9)
    due to extravasated contents of viscera, 299 (3)
    due to remote injury, 300 (4)
    pelvic, 299 (1)
        in pregnancy, 299 (1)
        puerperal, 299 (1)
    subdiaphragmatic, 299 (1)
    tuberculous, 299 (1)
Peritonsillar tissue. *See* Tonsils
Periureteral abscess, 314 (1)
Periureteritis, 314 (1)
Perivesiculitis. *See under* Seminal vesicles
Perleche, 133 (1)
Pernicious anemia, 229 (7)
Pernio (chilblain), 126 (4), 137 (4)
Perseveration: *supplementary term, 506. Diagnose disease*
Personality
    aggressive, 112 (x)
    compulsive, 112 (x)
    cyclothymic, 112 (x)
    disorders, 112
        transient stress, 113 (x)
    dissociated: *supplementary term, 485. Diagnose disease*
    dual: *supplementary term, 485. Diagnose disease*
    emotionally unstable, 112 (x)
    hypochondriacal; *supplementary term, 485. Diagnose disease*
    hysterical, 112 (x); *supplementary term, 485*
    immature, 112 (x)
    inadequate, 112 (x)
    paranoid, 112 (x)
    passive-aggressive, 112 (x)
    passive-dependent, 112 (x)
    schizoid, 112 (x)

Personality—Continued
    special symptom disturbance
        enuresis, 112 (x)
        hearing, 112 (x)
        somnambulism, 112 (x)
        speech, 112 (x)
    sociopathic
        addiction, 112 (x)
        alcohol addiction, 112 (x)
        antisocial, 112 (x)
        cheating type, 112 (x)
        drug addiction, 112 (x)
        dyssocial, 112 (x)
        homosexual, 112 (x)
        sexual deviation, 112 (x)
        stealing type, 112 (x)
        violent type, 112 (x)
        voyeur-exhibitionist, 112 (x)
    syntonic: *supplementary term, 485. Diagnose disease*
Perspiration. *See* Sweat
Perthes' disease. *See* Osteochondrosis of capital epiphysis of femur, 155 (9)
Pertussis (whooping cough), 115 (1)
Perversion, sexual: *supplementary term, 486. Diagnose disease*
Pes planovalgus. *See* Flatfoot
Petechiae: *supplementary term, 487. Diagnose disease*
Petiolus, elongation of, 182 (0)
Petit mal, 417 (x)
    and grand mal, 417 (x)
    supplementary term, 506. Diagnose disease
Petrositis, 478 (1)
Petrous bone
    caries, 148 (1)
    fracture of petrous pyramid and mastoid, 478 (4)
Peyronie's disease. *See* Induration of corpora cavernosa, 331 (9)
Pfeiffer's disease. *See* Mononucleosis, infectious, 114 (1)
Phakoma; phakomatosis. *Diagnose as* Hamartoma, 98
Phantom limb (autotopagnosia): *supplementary term, 502. Diagnose disease*
Pharyngitis
    acute, 255 (1)
        due to poison, 255 (3)
        due to unknown cause, 257 (9)

Phlegmasia alba dolens, 128 (5)

Phlyctenulosis. *See also* Keratitis, phlyctenular, 434 (1)
allergic, nontuberculous, 469 (3)

Phobias: *supplementary terms,* 484. *Diagnose disease*

Phobic reaction, 111 (x)

Phoria. *See* Cyclophoria; Esophoria; Excyclophoria; Exophoria; Heterophoria; Hyperphoria; Incyclophoria

Phosphaturia: *supplementary term,* 499. *Diagnose disease*

Phosphorus
liver degeneration due to, 288 (3)
necrosis of bone, 149 (3)
osteosclerosis, 149 (3)
poisoning
of heart, 209 (3)
of mandible, 149 (3)

Photophobia: *supplementary term,* 509. *Diagnose disease*

Photophthalmia
due to ultraviolet rays, 470 (4)

Photosensitive porphyria, 237 (4)

Phthisiophobia: *supplementary term,* 485. *Diagnose disease*

Phthisis of eyeball. *See* Eyeball atrophy

Physostigmine
miosis due to, 439 (3)
poisoning, 118 (3)

Phytobezoar, 265 (6). *See also* Hair ball, 265 (6)

Pica: *supplementary term,* 497. *Diagnose disease*

Pick's (Friedel Pick) **disease.** *See* Polyserositis, 302 (9)

Pick-Niemann disease (lipid histiocytosis of phosphatide type), 229 (7)

Piedra, 135 (2)

Pigeon breast, congenital, 146 (0)

Pigmentary degeneration of retina, 449 (9)

Pigmentation
arsenic, of eyelid, 462 (3)
loss of. *See* Albinism; Leukoderma; Vitiligo
of retina, grouped (nevoid), 446 (0)
silver. *See* Argyria

Pigmentation—Continued
of skin, increased, not abnormal: *supplementary term,* 487. *Diagnose disease*

Pigmented nevus, 94

Pigmented spots (mongolism), 131 (0)

Pilocarpine
miosis due to, 439 (3)
poisoning of heart by, 209 (3)

Pilomotor disturbances: *supplementary term,* 487. *Diagnose disease*

Pilonidal sinus (or cyst), 122 (0)

Pineal gland
calcification due to unknown cause, 395 (9)
diseases, 395
germinoma. *Diagnose as* Pinealoma, 98
glioma, 395 (8)
injury, 395 (4)
neoplasms, 395 (8)
pinealoma, 395 (8)
teratoma, 395 (8)
tumor
premature puberty due to, 395 (7)
unlisted, 395 (8)

Pineal tumor. *Diagnose as* Pinealoma, 98

Pinealoma, 98
of pineal gland, 395 (8)

Pineoblastoma. *Diagnose as* Pinealoma, 98

Pinguecula, 471 (9)

Pinta, 133 (1)

Pituitary extract
abnormal contraction of pregnant uterus due to, 374 (3)

Pituitary gland
abscess, 393 (1)
adenocarcinoma, 394 (8)
adenoma, 394 (8)
basophilic, 394 (8)
chromophobe, 394 (8)
eosinophilic, 394 (8)
anterior
hyperfunction, 393 (7)
hypofunction, 394 (7)
arterial hypertension due to disease of, 218 (7)

Pleura—Continued
  mesothelioma, 200 (8)
  neoplasms, 200 (8)
  neurofibroma, 200 (8)
  sac, fibrin ball in, 199 (4)
  sarcoma, 200 (8)
  shock, 199 (4)
  subpleural bleb, 200 (6)
  tumors, 200 (8)
Pleurisy. *See also* Pleura
  acute, 198 (1)
  chronic, 198 (1)
  due to fungus, 199 (1)
  due to trauma, 199 (4)
  tuberculous
    chronic, 198 (1)
    with effusion, 198 (1)
    inactive, 198 (1)
Pleurodynia, epidemic, 198 (1)
Pleuroma
  benign. *Diagnose as* Mesothelioma,
    97
  malignant. *Diagnose as* Mesothelial
    sarcoma, 97
Plummer-Vinson syndrome. *See*
    Anemia, hypochromic microcytic,
    due to deficient intake, absorp-
    tion or metabolism of iron, 229
    (7)
Pneumatosis intestinalis, 272 (1)
Pneumocephalus, 413 (4)
Pneumoencephalitis, avian, 116 (1)
Pneumoconiosis, 196 (4)
Pneumonia. *See also* Bronchopneu-
    monia
  allergic, 194 (3)
  anthrax, 192 (1)
  atypical, primary, 193 (1)
  due to aspiration of amniotic fluid,
    196 (4)
  influenzal, 192 (1)
  interstitial
    acute, 193 (1)
    chronic, 193 (1)
    due to poisonous gas, 194 (3)
  lipid (bronchopneumonia due to as-
    piration of oil), 195 (4)
  lobar, 193 (1)
    pneumococcic, 193 (1)
    streptococcic, 193 (1)
    unresolved, 193 (1)
  virus. *See* Virus bronchopneumonia,
    193 (1)

Pneumonitis
  due to rheumatic fever, 197 (9)
  due to roentgen rays, 195 (4)
  eosinophilic (Loeffler's syndrome),
    194 (3)
Pneumonoconiosis. *See* Pneumo-
    coniosis
Pneumopericardium
  due to infection, 208 (1)
  due to trauma, 209 (4)
Pneumothorax. *See also* Hemopneu-
    mothorax; Hydropneumothorax;
    Pyopneumothorax
  due to fungus, 199 (1)
  due to injury of chest wall, 200 (4)
  due to injury of lung, 200 (4)
  induced, 199 (4)
    of chest wall following operation,
      200 (4)
    of lung following operation, 200
      (4)
  spontaneous, 200 (9)
    due to infection, 198 (1)
    due to rupture of emphysematous
      or subpleural bleb, 199 (4)
    due to tuberculosis, 198 (1)
    due to unknown cause, 200 (9)
    hydropneumothorax due to, 200
      (9)
  tense valvular
    due to infection, 199 (1)
    due to trauma, 200 (4)
    due to tuberculosis, 199 (1)
  therapeutic, collapse of lung due to,
    200 (4)
Poikilocytosis
  supplementary term, 495. *Diagnose
    disease*
Poikiloderma, 139 (7)
Poisons and poisoning
  diseases due to. *See under name of
    specific disease or substance*
  general, 117 (3)
  intoxication
    acute brain syndrome, 106 (3)
    chronic brain syndrome, 107 (3)
  list of poisons, 67
  sensitivity to, 118 (3)
Poliodystrophia cerebri progres-
    siva (infantilis), 416 (9)
Polioencephalopathy
  superior, hemorrhagic, due to lack of
    vitamin B complex, 414 (7)

Poliomyelitis
abortive, non-paralytic, 422 (1)
anterior
  acute, 422 (1)
  chronic, 422 (1)
bulbo-spinal, acute, 403 (1)
circulatory disturbance in foot due
  to, 217 (55)
contracture following, 160 (55)
deformities due to. *See under* Bones,
  152 (55); Joints, 160 (55);
  Muscles, 147 (55)
lateral, acute, 422 (1)
residual paralysis following, 169
  (55)
scoliotic pelvis following, 385 (55)
spinal, acute. *See* Poliomyelitis, anterior, acute, 422 (1)
Poliosis. *See also* Canities, 138 (7)
of eyebrow, 461 (0), 464 (7)
of lashes, 461 (0), 464 (7)
Polyangiitis, essential (periarteritis
nodosa), 218 (9)
aneurysm of artery due to, 218 (9)
of cerebrospinal vessels, 404 (9)
hemorrhage from artery due to, 218
  (9)
of hepatic artery, 304 (9)
infarction of liver due to, 288 (5)
of kidney, 312 (9)
of mesenteric artery, 305 (9)
Polyarteritis nodosa. *See* Polyangiitis, essential
Polyarthritis
due to sickle cell anemia, 164 (9)
Polychromatophilia: *supplementary
term,* 495. *Diagnose disease*
Polycoria, 439 (0)
Polycythemia
myelopathic. *Diagnose as* Polycythemia vera, 95
rubra. *Diagnose as* Polycythemia
  vera, 95
splenomegalic. *Diagnose as* Polycythemia vera, 95
supplementary term, 495. *Diagnose
disease*
thrombosis of cerebral vessels due
  to, 419 (5)
thrombosis of vein due to, 225 (5)
vera, 95, 230 (8)
  primary. *Diagnose as* Polycythemia vera, 95

Polydactyly. *See* Supernumerary fingers and toes, 123 (0)
supplementary term, 487. *Diagnose
disease*
Polydipsia. *See* Thirst, excessive:
supplementary term, 497
Polyhydramnios, 384 (x)
Polyneuropathy erythredema, 431
(x)
Polyonychia. *See* Polyungia, 131 (0)
Polyorchism, 332 (0)
Polyostatic fibrous dysplasia, 147
(0)
Polyotia, 474 (0)
Polyp. *See also under organ, region
or structure affected*
adenomatous. *Diagnose as* Papillary
  tumor, not otherwise specified,
  93
angiomatous. *Diagnose as* Papillary
  tumor, not otherwise specified,
  93
benign lymphoid, 95
carcinoma arising in. *Diagnose as*
  Carcinoma, not otherwise specified, 94
cystic (endometrium). *Diagnose as*
  Papillary tumor, not otherwise
  specified, 93
fibroangiomatous (skin). *Diagnose
as* Hemangioma (angioma), 96
fibrolipomatous. *Diagnose as* Lipoma, 97
fibromatous; fibrosed; fibrous. *Diagnose as* Fibroma, 96
formation, simple, 129 (9)
glandular. *Diagnose as* Papillary
  tumor, not otherwise specified,
  93
mucosal. *Diagnose as* Papillary tumor, not otherwise specified, 97
not otherwise specified. *Diagnose as*
  Papillary or polypoid tumor, not
  otherwise specified, 93
Polypoid tumor, not otherwise specified, 93
Polyposis
carcinoma arising in. *Diagnose as*
  Carcinoma, not otherwise specified, 94
Polyradiculoneuropathy, 422 (1)
Polyserositis, 302 (9)

Polyunguia, 131 (0)
Polyuria: *supplementary term,* 499.
  Diagnose disease
Pompholyx, 142 (9)
Pontine syndrome. *See* Cestan syndrome: *supplementary term,* 503
Porencephaly
  congenital, 411 (0)
  due to trauma, 413 (4)
Porocephaliasis
  of liver, 288 (2)
Porokeratosis, 142 (9)
Porphyria
  acquired, due to unknown cause, 120
    (7)
  acute toxic (intermittent), 238 (x)
  cutanea tarda, 135 (3)
  due to drugs, 237 (3)
  generally, 237 (7)
  photosensitive, 237 (4)
Porphyrinuria: *supplementary term,*
  499. *Diagnose disease*
Portal vein
  anomaly (in situs transversus), 224
    (0)
  diseases, 303 ff.
  injury, 303 (4)
  obstruction, passive congestion of
    spleen due to, 232 (5)
  phlebitis, 224 (1)
  phlebosclerosis, 304 (9)
  thrombosis, 303 (1)
    due to compression, 303 (4)
    due to infection, 224 (1)
    due to phlebosclerosis, 304 (9)
    due to thrombocytosis, 303 (5)
    due to unknown cause, 304 (9)
    recanalized thrombus, 303 (1)
Position and movement
  loss or diminution of sense of: *sup-
    plementary term,* 505. *Diagnose
    disease*
**Posterior lacerated (jugular) for-
  amen syndrome**: *supplementary
  term,* 506. *Diagnose disease*
Postpartum admission, 482
Postpericardiotomy   syndrome:
  supplementary term, 491. *Diagnose disease*
Posture
  abnormal, 119 (6)

Posture—Continued
  cataleptic retention of. *See* Flexi-
    bilitas cerea: *supplementary
    term,* 504
  hysterical: *supplementary term,* 489.
    Diagnose disease
  maintenance of fixed. *See* Catato-
    nia: *supplementary term,* 502
Potassium hydroxide
  conjunctivitis due to, 469 (3)
Pott's disease. *See* Tuberculosis of
  vertebra, 149 (1)
Preachers' node. *Diagnose as* Fibroma, 96
Precordial pain
  of cardiac origin: *supplementary
    term,* 491. *Diagnose disease*
Preeclampsia, 118 (3)
Pregnancy. *See also* Fetus; Labor;
  Puerperium
  abdominal, 380 (7)
    ruptured, 380 (7)
  abnormal, 380
  abscess of pelvis during, 373 (1)
  alopecia due to, 135 (3)
  breast changes, 144 (7)
  cellulitis of pelvis during, 373 (1)
  cervical, 380 (7)
  chorea gravidarum, 412 (3)
  cicatrix of cervix during, 373 (1)
  cornual, 380 (7)
  delivered, 377 (0)
    antepartum death, 377 (0)
    immaturely, ante or intrapartum
      death, 377 (0)
    immaturely living child, 377 (0)
    intrapartum death, 377 (0)
  delivered, multiple birth, 379 (0)
    ante or intrapartum death, 379 (0)
    one (or more) living child, 379
      (0)
    prematurely, 379 (0)
      ante or intrapartum death, 379
        (0)
      one (or more) living child, 379
        (0)
  delivered, postmaturely, 377 (0)
    antepartum death, 377 (0)
    intrapartum death, 377 (0)
  delivered, prematurely, 377 (0)
    antepartum death, 377 (0)
    intrapartum death, 377 (0)
    threatened, 377 (0)

Pregnancy—Continued
 delivered, triplets, 379 (0)
  one (or two) living child, 379 (0)
   ante or intrapartum death, 379 (0)
  prematurely, 379 (0)
   ante or intrapartum death, 379 (0)
   one (or two) living child, 379 (0)
 delivered, twins, 378 (0)
  antepartum death, 378 (0)
   double ovum, 378 (0)
   single ovum, 378 (0)
  double ovum, 378 (0)
  intrapartum death, 378 (0)
   double ovum, 378 (0)
   single ovum, 378 (0)
  one living child
   double ovum, 378 (0)
   single ovum, 378 (0)
  prematurely, 378 (0)
   antepartum or intrapartum death, 378 (0)
    double ovum, 379 (0)
    single ovum, 378 (0)
  prematurely, double ovum, 378 (0)
   one living child, 379 (0)
    double ovum, 379 (0)
    single ovum, 379 (0)
  prematurely, single ovum, 378 (0)
   single ovum, 378 (0)
 endometritis during, 374 (1)
 hematoma of vulva during, 374 (4)
 hyperemesis gravidarum, 118 (3)
 intraligamentous, 380 (7)
 metritis during, 374 (1)
 not delivered, 380 (7)
 osteomalacia associated with, 153 (7)
 ovarian, 380 (7)
 oviducal. *See* Pregnancy, tubal, 380 (7)
 pelvic peritonitis in, 299 (1)
 retinitis gravidarum, 447 (3)
 in rudimentary horn, 380 (7)
 spasm of retinal artery due to, 447 (3)
 toxemia of, 118 (3)
 tubal, 380 (7)
  with abortion, 380 (7)
  with rupture, 380 (7)

Pregnancy—Continued
 varix of vulva due to, 375 (4)
 vomiting, pernicious, in, 118 (3)
Pregnant, not, 482
Premammary tissue, abscess, 143 (1)
Premature ejaculation of semen: *supplementary term,* 499. *Diagnose disease*
Prematurity. *See* Infants, premature, 380 (0)
Premenstrual tension, 364 (7)
Prenatal influence, diseases due to. *See under name of specific disease or organ, region or structure affected*
Prepuce. *See also* Penis; Phimosis
 adhesions due to infection, 329 (1)
 carcinoma, epidermoid, 331 (8)
 concretion in, 330 (6)
 cyst, congenital, 329 (0)
 herpes simplex, 329 (1)
 redundant, 331 (7)
Presbycusis, 480 (7)
Presbyopia, 454 (7)
Presentation of fetus, 382
 breech, 382 (6)
 brow, 382 (6)
 compound, 382 (6)
 cord, 385 (6)
 face, 382 (6)
 shoulder position, 382 (6)
 transverse, 382 (6)
 undetermined, 382 (6)
 vertex, 382 (6)
Pretibial fever, 116 (1)
Priapism, 330 (55)
 supplementary term, 499. *Diagnose disease*
Prickly heat (miliaria rubra), 137 (4)
Procidentia, internal, 269 (6)
Proctalgia: *supplementary term,* 497. *Diagnose disease*
 fugax, 283 (x)
Proctitis
 acute, 281 (1)
 amebic, 281 (1)
 chronic, 281 (1)
 gonococcic, 281 (1)
  stricture of rectum due to, 281 (1)
 radiation, 282 (4)
Progeria, 121 (7)

Progesterone
   sterility due to decrease in, 349 (7)
Prognathism, 154 (7)
Progonoma. *Diagnose as* Hamar-
      toma, 98
Proptosis: *supplementary term,* 506.
      Diagnose disease
Prostate. *See also* Ejaculatory ducts;
      Prostatitis; Verumontanum
   abscess, 346 (1)
      periprostatic, 346 (1)
   absence, congenital, 346 (0)
   accumulation of secretion in, 347 (6)
   adenocarcinoma, 347 (8)
   adenofibroma, 347 (8)
   adenoma, 347 (8)
   adhesions, periprostatic, due to in-
      fection, 346 (1)
   amebiasis, 346 (1)
   atrophy due to unknown cause, 348
      (9)
   calculus in, 347 (6)
   carcinoma, mucinous, 347 (8)
   chondrosarcoma, 347 (8)
   congestion
      active, 347 (5)
      passive, 347 (5)
   cyst, simple, 347 (6)
   diseases, 346 ff.
   embryoma. *Diagnose as* Mesenchy-
      mal mixed tumor, 98
   fibroma, 347 (8)
   fibrosis due to infection, 346 (1)
   fistula
      due to infection, 346 (1)
      due to trauma, 346 (4)
   granuloma, 346 (1)
   hemorrhage following operation, 346
      (4)
   hypertrophy, benign, 347 (7)
   infarction
      due to embolus, 347 (5)
      due to thrombus, 347 (5)
   injury, 347 (4)
   lack of development, congenital, 346
      (0)
   leiomyoma, 347 (8)
   leiomyosarcoma, 347 (8)
   lymphosarcoma, 347 (8)
   median bar, 348 (9)
   mesenchymal mixed tumor, 347 (8)
   myosarcoma. *Diagnose as* Mesen-
      chymal mixed tumor, 98
   neoplasms, 348 (8)

Prostate—Continued
   overdevelopment, congenital, 346 (0)
   puncture, 347 (4)
   rhabdomyosarcoma, 347 (8)
   rupture, 347 (4)
   sarcoma, 348 (8)
   trichomonas infection, 346 (1)
   tumors, unlisted, 348 (8)
   varix, 347 (6)
Prostatic utricle. *See* Utriculus mas-
      culinus
Prostatitis
   acute, 346 (1)
   chronic, 346 (1)
   due to coccidioides, 346 (2)
   due to trauma, 347 (4)
Prostatorrhea, 347 (55)
Prosthesis, pressure of
   lesion of conjunctiva due to, 470 (4)
Prostration. *See also* Exhaustion,
      119 (7)
   heat, 118 (4)
Protein
   deficiency, normocytic anemia due
      to, 229 (7)
   deprivation of, 119 (7)
   sickness, 118 (3)
Proteinosis, lipid, 139 (7)
Prurigo
   mitis, 142 (9)
   nodularis, 142 (9)
Pruritus, 138 (55)
   ani, 285 (55)
   of auricle, 476 (55)
   of scrotum, neurogenic, 340 (55)
   supplementary term, 488. *Diagnose
      disease*
   vulvae, neurogenic, 353 (55)
Psammocarcinoma (ovary). *Diag-
      nose as* Papillary or polypoid tu-
      mor, not otherwise specified, 93
Psammoma
   of meninges. *Diagnose as* Menin-
      gioma, 95
   of ovary. *Diagnose as* Papillary tu-
      mor, not otherwise specified, 93
**Pseudoadenomatous granulosa cell
   tumor.** *Diagnose as* Granulosa
      cell tumor, 93
Pseudoarthrosis, 155 (9)
   deformity due to, 155 (9)
   following fusion (or arthrodesis),
      159 (4)

Pseudoarthrosis—Continued
fracture due to, 155 (9)
Pseudohemophilia, 231 (x)
Pseudohemophilia "A," 226 (9)
Pseudohemophilia "B," 226 (9)
Pseudohermaphroditism
cleft scrotum in, 339 (0)
female
due to increase in progesterone,
327 (7)
with ovaries present, 327 (0)
virilizing with, 396 (0)
male
due to decrease in progesterone,
327 (7)
with testes present, 327 (0)
sex undetermined, 327 (0)
Pseudohypoparathyroidism, 391
(x)
Pseudoleukemia. *Diagnose as* Hodgkin's disease, 95
Hodgkin's. *Diagnose as* Hodgkin's
disease, 95
Pseudomucinous cystic tumor, 93
Pseudomyxoma peritonei, 94
Pseudoneuritis
of optic papilla, 450 (0)
Pseudopelade (alopecia cicatrisata),
132 (1)
Pseudopterygium, 471 (9)
Pseudoptosis of lid, 463 (55)
Pseudorabies, 116 (1)
Pseudorickets. *See* Osteodystrophy,
renal, 152 (7)
Pseudosarcoma (breast). *Diagnose
as* Cystosarcoma phyllodes, 97
Pseudosclerosis, 416 (9)
Pseudotrichinosis. *See* Dermatomy-
ositis, 170 (9)
Pseudotumor, inflammatory (or-
bit). *Diagnose as* Lymphoma of
orbit, 459 (8)
Pseudoxanthoma, elastic, 142 (9)
Psittacosis (ornithosis), 116 (1)
bronchopneumonia, 193 (1)
Psoriasis, 142 (9)
exfoliative, 142 (9)
flexural, 142 (9)
generalized, 142 (9)
guttate, 142 (9)
pustular, 142 (9)
Psychic blindness: *supplementary
term,* 509. *Diagnose disease*

Psychic disturbance
diseases due to. *See under organ,
region or structure affected*
Psychic equivalents, paroxysmal:
supplementary term, 485. *Diagnose disease*
Psychobiologic unit, diseases,
105 ff.
Psychogenic disorders, 105 ff.
Psychomotor attacks, 416 (x)
Psychoneurotic disorders, 111 (x)
Psychophysiologic disorders
cardiovascular reaction, 111 (55)
endocrine reaction, 111 (55)
gastrointestinal reaction, 111 (55)
genito-urinary reaction, 111 (55)
hemic and lymphatic reaction, 111
(55)
musculoskeletal reaction, 111 (55)
nervous system reaction, 111 (55)
reaction of organs of special sense,
111 (55)
respiratory reaction, 111 (55)
skin reaction, 111 (55)
Psychoses. *See* Psychobiologic unit,
diseases, 105 ff.
Psychotic disorders
depressive reaction, 110 (x)
involutional psychotic reaction, 110
(x)
Pterygium, 471 (9). *See also* Pseudopterygium, 471 (9)
following operation, 470 (4)
Ptosis. *See* Enteroptosis, 269 (6);
Gastroptosis, 265 (6); Splanchnoptosis, 128 (6); *and under organ or structure affected*
Ptyalism: *supplementary term,* 497.
Diagnose disease
Puberty, premature
adrenal cortical hyperfunction with,
397 (7)
anterior pituitary hyperfunction, 394
(7)
due to pineal tumor, 395 (7)
Pubic hair, abnormal growth, 353
(7)
Puente's disease. *See* Cheilitis glandularis, 140 (9)
Puerperal. *See under* Puerperium
Puerperium
breast abscess in, 143 (1)
cellulitis of pelvis during, 373 (1)

Puerperium—Continued
endometritis in, 374 (1)
lactation atrophy of uterus, 375 (7)
mammary fistula in, 143 (1)
mastitis in, 143 (1)
metritis in, 374 (1)
osteomalacia associated with, 153
(7)
pelvic peritonitis in, 299 (1)
phlebitis in, 224 (1)
septicemia in, 116 (1)
thelitis in, 144 (1)
Pulmonary artery(ies)
accessory, 205 (0)
aneurysm
due to arteriosclerosis, 223 (9)
due to infection, 222 (1)
anomalous origin from aorta, 205
(0)
anomalous origin of coronary arteries from, 205 (0)
atresia, 205 (0)
dilatation, 205 (0)
with atrial septal defect and mitral
stenosis, 203 (0)
due to stenosis of mitral valve, 223
(6)
due to unknown cause, 223 (6)
diseases, 222
embolism
due to amniotic fluid, 195 (4)
due to circulatory disturbance, 196
(5)
due to operative trauma, 222 (4)
due to remote infection, 193 (1)
due to remote trauma, 195 (4)
due to unknown cause, 196 (6),
223 (6)
due to venous stasis and thrombosis, 222 (5)
fat, due to remote trauma, 195 (4)
following operation (intrinsic vessels), 195 (4)
hypertension, cor pulmonale due to,
210 (5)
injury, 222 (4)
levoposition, with ventricular septal
defect, 203 (0)
narrowing, 205 (0)
stenosis in tetralogy of Fallot, 203
(0)
thrombosis
due to unknown cause, 223 (6)

Pulmonary artery(ies)—Continued
thrombosis—continued
due to venous stasis, 222 (5)
transposition, 205 (0)
tuberculosis, 222 (1)
Pulmonary conus. *See* Infundibular
stenosis, 492
Pulmonary edema. *See* Lungs,
edema
Pulmonary tuberculosis. *See* Tuberculosis of lung, 193 (1), 194
(1)
Pulmonary valve
bicuspid, 203 (0)
fenestration of pulmonic cusps, 204
(0)
fusion or defect of pulmonic cusps,
204 (0)
incompetency: *supplementary term,*
492. Diagnose disease
stenosis, not congenital: *supplementary term, 492. Diagnose disease*
supernumerary pulmonic cusps, 204
(0)
Pulmonary vein(s)
anomalous entry into other vessels,
205 (0)
anomalous entry into right atrium,
205 (0)
diseases, 222
thrombosis
due to unknown cause, 223 (6)
due to venous stasis, 222 (5)
Pulmonic valve. *See* Pulmonary
valve
Pulp, dental
exposed
due to infection, 247 (1)
due to operation, 248 (4)
hyperplasia, 249 (7)
necrotic, 247 (1)
nodule, 249 (7)
putrescent, 247 (1)
Pulpitis, 247 (1)
Pulsus alternans: *supplementary*
term, 492. Diagnose disease
Pulsus deletus: *supplementary term,*
492. Diagnose disease
Punctum lacrimale
absence, 465 (0)
eversion
due to infection, 465 (1)

Punctum lacrimale—Continued
eversion—continued
due to trauma or following operation, 466 (4)
senile, 466 (7)
Pupil
changes due to disturbance of sympathetic innervation, 440 (55)
contraction. *See* Miosis
dilatation. *See* Mydriasis
occlusion (papillary membrane), 439 (1)
supernumerary. *See* Polycoria, 439 (0)
Pupillary membrane
occlusion of pupil, 439 (0)
persistent, 439 (0)
Purpura
annularis telangiectodes, 137 (5)
capillary
due to allergy or drug reaction, 226 (3)
due to embolism, 226 (5)
due to infection, 226 (1)
due to mechanical cause, 226 (4)
due to metabolic disturbance, 226 (7)
generally, 226 (5)
hemorrhagic. *See also* Purpura, thrombocytopenic
hemorrhage of retina due to, 448 (5)
supplementary term, 488. *Diagnose disease*
thrombocytopathic, 231 (x)
thrombocytopenic, 229 (7)
due to drugs or toxic agents, 228 (3)
due to infection, 228 (1)
due to myelophthisis, 231 (9)
idiopathic, 229 (7)
Purpuric lichenoid dermatitis, 137 (5)
Pustule, malignant. *See* Anthrax of skin, 132 (1)
Putnam-Dana syndrome. *See* Dorsolateral sclerosis: *supplementary term,* 503
Pyarthrosis. *See* Arthritis due to infection, 157 (1)
Pyelitis
cystica, 312 (9)
due to infection, 308 (1)

Pyelitis—Continued
due to poison, 309 (3)
Pyelonephritis
acute, necrotizing, 309 (1)
chronic, necrotizing, 309 (1)
contracted kidney due to, 308 (1)
Pyknocytoma. *Diagnose as* Adenolymphoma, 98
Pyknolepsy, 417 (x)
supplementary term, 506. *Diagnose disease*
Pylephlebitis
suppurative, 224 (1)
Pyloric. *See* Pylorus
Pylorospasm
congenital, 263 (0)
reflex, 264 (55)
Pylorus
obstruction: *supplementary term,* 497. *Diagnose disease*
spasm. *See* Pylorospasm
stenosis
acquired, 265 (9)
following operation, 264 (4)
hypertrophic, congenital, 263 (0)
Pyocolpos, 355 (1)
Pyoderma gangrenosum, 133 (1)
Pyometra, 361 (1)
Pyonephrosis, 309 (1)
Pyopneumopericardium, 208 (1)
Pyopneumothorax
due to fungus, 199 (1)
due to infection, 199 (1)
following injury to chest wall, 200 (4)
due to injury of chest wall, 200 (4)
due to injury of lung, 200 (4)
due to operative injury of chest wall, 200 (4)
due to operative injury of lung, 200 (4)
due to tuberculosis, 199 (1)
Pyosalpinx, 366 (1)
ruptured, 366 (1)
Pyoureter, 314 (1)
Pyrexia: *supplementary term,* 486. *Diagnose disease*
Pyromania: *supplementary term,* 486. *Diagnose disease*
Pyrosis. *See* Pain in epigastrium: *supplementary term,* 497
Pyuria: *supplementary term,* 499. *Diagnose disease*

Q

Q fever, 116 (1)
Quadriceps femoris
  myositis ossificans of, 168 (4)
Quadrilateral fever. See Q fever,
  116 (1)
Quadriplegia. See Tetraplegia: *sup-
  plementary term,* 507
Quarrelsomeness: *supplementary
  term,* 486. *Diagnose disease*
Queensland fever. See Q fever, 116
  (1)
Queyrat's erythroplasia, 141 (9)
Quicklime
  burn of foot, 125 (3)
Quincke's disease. See Angioneu-
  rotic edema
Quinine
  poisoning of heart by, 209 (3)
Quinsy. See Abscess of peritonsillar
  tissue, 258 (1)

R

Rabbit fever. See Tularemia, 116 (1)
Rabies, 116 (1)
Rachitis. See Rickets
Radiation. See also Radioactive substances; Radium; Roentgen rays;
  Ultraviolet rays
  anemia, normocytic hypoplastic, due
    to, 228 (4)
  atrophy of endometrium due to ir-
    radiation, 361 (4)
  burn, 127 (4)
  carcinoma. *Diagnose as* Carcinoma,
    not otherwise specified, 94
  injury of laryngeal perichondrium,
    184 (4)
  stenosis of larynx following, 184
    (4)
Radiculitis. See also Myeloradiculitis; Radiculoneuritis; Radiculo-
  neuropathy; Radiculopathy
  due to unspecified infection, 422 (1)
Radiculomyelopathy. See Myeloradiculopathy
Radiculopathy
  due to poison, 423 (3)
  due to pressure

Radiculopathy—Continued
  due to pressure—continued
    of congenital malformation, 421
      (0)
    of meningocele, 421 (0)
Radioactive substances. See also
  Radium
  anemia, normocytic hypoplastic, due
    to, 228 (4)
  fistula due to, 126 (4)
  general effects, 119 (4)
  injury by, 127 (4)
  late effect, 126 (4)
  necrosis due to, 127 (4)
    of bone, 151 (4)
  poisoning by, 118 (4)
  remote effect, 127 (4)
Radiodermatitis. See Dermatitis actinica, 136 (4)
Radiopaque body in lung: *supplementary term,* 490. *Diagnose disease*
Radium. See also Radioactive substances
  burn
    of cornea, 435 (4)
    of larynx, 184 (4)
    ulcer of bladder due to, 319 (4)
    of urethra, 324 (4)
  cataract from, 442 (4)
  injury, 127 (4)
  late effect, 127 (4)
  necrosis. *See also* Necrosis due to
    radioactive substance, 127 (4)
    of conjunctiva, 470 (4)
  ovarian hypofunction due to, 369 (4)
  rectovaginal fistula due to, 356 (4)
  remote effect, 127 (4)
Radius
  idiopathic progressive curvature of,
    146 (0), 154 (9)
  synostosis of ulna and, 147 (0)
Rales in lung: *supplementary term,*
  490. *Diagnose disease*
Ranula, 253 (6)
  congenital, 252 (0)
Rash, diaper. See Erythema gluteale,
  135 (3)
Rat bite fever, 116 (1)
Rathke's pouch
  cyst
    neoplastic. *Diagnose as* Cranio-
      pharyngioma, 98

Rectum—Continued
  rupture, 282 (4)
    due to infection, 281 (1)
  stricture
    due to chemical burn, 281 (3)
    due to gonococcic proctitis, 281 (1)
    due to infection, 281 (1)
    due to lymphopathia venereum, 281 (1)
    due to trauma, 282 (4)
    following operation, 282 (4)
  tumors, unlisted, 282 (8)
  ulcer
    due to infection, 281 (1)
    due to unknown cause, 283 (9)
  ulceration
    due to poison, 282 (3)
    due to trauma, 282 (4)
    stercoraceous, 282 (6)
    varicose, 282 (5)
  undescended, 281 (0)
Rectus abdominis, diastasis
  congenital, 167 (0)
  due to pregnancy, 168 (4)
  following operation, 168 (4)
Red blood cells. *See* Erythrocytes
Reed-Sternberg disease. *Diagnose as* Hodgkin's disease, 95
Reflex arrhythmia, 211 (55)
Refraction
  change due to diabetes, 454 (7)
  errors, 454 ff.
Regurgitation, gastric. *See* Vomiting
Regional diseases, 122 ff.
Reiter's disease, 116 (1)
Relapsing fever, 116 (1)
Ren mobilis. *See* Wandering kidney, 308 (0)
Renal artery
  arteriosclerosis, 312 (9)
  thrombosis
    due to arteriosclerosis, 312 (9)
    due to infection, 309 (1)
    due to trauma, 309 (4)
Renal colic: *supplementary term,* 499. *Diagnose disease*
Renal osteodystrophy, 152 (7)
Renal vein
  phlebitis due to infection, 308 (1)
Rendu-Osler-Weber syndrome, 219 (9)

Respiratory insufficiency: *supplementary term,* 490. *Diagnose disease*
Respiratory system. *See also* Bronchi; Lungs; Pleura; etc.
  acute diffuse upper respiratory infection, 175 (1)
  diseases, 175 ff.
  hemorrhage from respiratory tract: *supplementary term,* 490. *Diagnose disease*
  psychophysiologic reaction, 111 (55)
  rudimentary organs (in thoracopagus), 192 (0)
  upper respiratory virus infection, 175 (1)
Rest, malignant embryonic, 98
Rete cell adenoma. *Diagnose as* Rete cell tumor, 94
Rete cell tumor, 94
Reticulocytosis: *supplementary term,* 495. *Diagnose disease*
Reticuloendothelioma
  lymphatic
    except of genital organs. *Diagnose as* Reticulum cell sarcoma, 95
    of genital organs. *Diagnose as* Mesothelioma, 97
  not otherwise specified. *Diagnose as* Reticulum cell sarcoma, 95
Reticuloendotheliosis. *Diagnose as* Lymphoma, type not specified, 230 (8)
Reticulosarcoma, syncytial. *Diagnose as* Reticulum cell sarcoma, 95
Reticulosis
  lymphoid follicular. *Diagnose as* Giant follicular lymphoma, 95
Reticulum cell sarcoma, 95, 140 (8)
Retina
  arteriosclerotic disease, 447 (5)
  arteriovenous aneurysm, congenital, 446 (0)
  atrophia gyrata of choroid and, 441 (5)
  atrophy
    in amaurotic familial idiocy, 449 (9)
    due to circulatory disturbance, 447 (5)
    due to infection, 446 (1)

Retina—Continued
atrophy—continued
  infantile type, 446 (0)
  progressive, 449 (9)
cholesterol deposit in, 448 (7)
coloboma, 446 (0)
commotio retinae, 447 (4)
cyanosis due to intoxication by organic poison, 447 (3)
cysts in, 446 (0)
degeneration due to trauma, 447 (4)
detachment
  due to atrophy, 446 (1)
  due to hemorrhage, 448 (5)
  due to infection of uveal tract, 447 (1)
  due to progressive atrophy, 449 (9)
  due to retinitis exudativa, 448 (5)
  due to subretinal cysticercosis, 447 (2)
  due to trauma, 447 (4)
  due to unknown cause, 449 (9)
  following operation, 447 (4)
diseases, 446 ff.
glioblastoma. *Diagnose as* Neuroepithelioma, 95
hemangioma, 449 (8)
hemangiomatosis, 449 (8)
hematoma. *Diagnose as* Hemangiomatosis, 96
hemorrhage
  due to arteriosclerosis, 449 (9)
  due to blood dyscrasia, 448 (5)
  due to carbon monoxide poisoning, 447 (3)
  due to diabetes, 448 (7)
  due to endophlebitis, 449 (9)
  due to hemorrhagic purpura, 448 (5)
  due to infection, 447 (1)
  due to scurvy, 448 (7)
  due to thrombosis, 448 (6)
hole due to trauma, 447 (4)
infarction, 448 (5)
injury, 447 (4)
ischemia due to arteriosclerosis, 448 (5)
lipemia, 448 (7)
medullated nerve fibers in, 448 (7)
neuroblastoma. *Diagnose as* Neuroepithelioma, 95

Retina—Continued
neuroepithelioma (retinoblastoma), 449 (8)
pigmentary degeneration, primary, 449 (9)
pigmentation, grouped (nevoid), 446 (0)
sarcoma, round cell. *Diagnose as* Neuroepithelioma, 95
syphilis
  congenital and delayed, 447 (1)
  neurorecidive, 447 (1)
tuberculosis, 447 (1)
tumors, unlisted, 449 (8)
vessels
  anastomosis of choroidal vessels and, 446 (0)
  arteriosclerosis, 449 (9)
  embolism of retinal artery, 448 (6)
  endophlebitis of retinal veins
    due to infection, 447 (1)
    due to unknown cause, 449 (9)
  intrinsic, hypertensive vascular disease, 448 (5)
  periphlebitis, 447 (1)
  spasm of retinal artery, 448 (55)
    due to pregnancy, 447 (3)
  thrombosis, 448 (6)
  tortuous veins, 446 (0)
wound, gunshot, 447 (4)
Retinal artery; retinal veins. *See* Retina, vessels
Retinitis, 447 (1)
disciformis, 449 (9)
exudativa, 448 (5)
gravidarum, 447 (3)
pigmentosa. *See* Retina, primary pigmentary degeneration, 449 (9)
proliferans, 448 (5)
Retinoblastoma, 449 (8)
Retinochoroiditis juxtapapillaris, 447 (1)
Retinocytoma. *Diagnose as* Neuroepithelioma, 95
Retinopathy
circinata, 448 (7)
diabetic, 448 (7)
Retrobulbar neuritis
due to infection, 450 (1)
due to pressure, 451 (4)
in multiple sclerosis, 452 (9)
Retrolental fibroplasia, 447 (3)

Retromammary tissue, abscess, 143 (1)

Retroparotid space syndrome: *supplementary term,* 506. *Diagnose disease*

Retropatellar fat pad, hypertrophy
due to infection, 149 (1)
due to trauma, 151 (4)

Retroperitoneal abscess, 298 (1)

Retroperitoneal neoplasms, 301 (8)

Retropharyngeal. *See under* Pharynx

Retropulsion: *supplementary term,* 506. *Diagnose disease*

Rh blood groups: *supplementary terms,* 493. *Diagnose disease*

Rh-Hr sensitization: *supplementary term,* 495. *Diagnose disease*

Rhabdoblastoma. *Diagnose as* Rhabdomyosarcoma, 96

Rhabdomyoadenosarcoma. *Diagnose as* Mesenchymal mixed tumor, 98

Rhabdomyoblastic mixed tumor. *Diagnose as* Mesenchymal mixed tumor, 98

Rhabdomyoblastoma
embryonal. *Diagnose as* Mesenchymal mixed tumor, 98
not otherwise specified. *Diagnose as* Rhabdomyosarcoma, 96

Rhabdomyolysis
recurrent
exertional, 169 (7)
nonexertional, 169 (7)

Rhabdomyoma, 96
embryonal. *Diagnose as* Mesenchymal mixed tumor, 98

Rhabdomyosarcoma, 96
embryonal. *Diagnose as* Mesenchymal mixed tumor, 98

Rhabdosarcoma. *Diagnose as* Rhabdomyosarcoma, 96

Rheostosis. *See* Melorheostosis, 155 (9)

Rheumatic aortitis, 221 (9)

Rheumatic arteritis, 218 (9)

Rheumatic fever, 121 (9)
arthritis due to, 163 (9)
fibrosis of myocardium due to, 213 (9)
pneumonitis due to, 197 (9)

Rheumatic heart disease, 213 (9)

Rheumatism. *See also* Arthritis
acute articular. *See* Rheumatic fever, 121 (9)
palindromic, 164 (9)
psychogenic. *See* Psychophysiologic musculoskeletal reaction, 111 (55)

Rheumatoid arthritis, 163 (9)

Rhinitis
acute, 177 (1)
due to chemical poison, 177 (3)
due to foreign body, 178 (4)
due to poisonous gas, 177 (3)
with exanthem, 177 (1)
allergic (hay fever), 177 (3)
atrophic, 179 (9)
chronic, due to foreign body, 178 (4)
hypertrophic
due to chemical irritant, 177 (3)
due to infection, 177 (1)
due to unknown cause, 179 (9)
vasomotor. *See* Hydrorrhea, nasal, due to vasomotor disturbance, 178 (5)

Rhinolith, 178 (6)
in sinus, 181 (6)

Rhinopharyngitis mutilans. *See* Gangosa, 177 (1)

Rhinophyma, 137 (5)

Rhinorrhea, cerebrospinal: *supplementary term,* 503. *Diagnose disease*

Rhinoscleroma, 133 (1), 177 (1)
of eyelid, 462 (1)
of lacrimal sac, 466 (1)

Rhinosporidiosis, 124 (2), 177 (2)

Rib(s)
cervical, supernumerary, 146 (0)
deformity, congenital, 124 (0)
fracture
laceration of lung by, 195 (4)
laceration of pleura by, 199 (4)
puncture of diaphragm by, 171 (4)
osteochondritis due to trauma, 154 (9)
slipping, 152 (6)

Riboflavin deficiency (cheilosis), 121 (7)

Rickets, 121 (7)
bone changes associated with rachitis tarda, 153 (7)
deformity of bone due to, 153 (7)

Rickets—Continued
deformity of joint due to, 163 (7)
fetal. *See* Achondroplasia, 146 (0)
fracture due to, 153 (7)
nephrotic glycosuric hypophosphatemic dwarfism with: *supplementary term,* 485. *Diagnose disease*
renal, 307 (0)
tetany associated with, 121 (7)
Rickettsia. *See also* Rocky Mountain
spotted fever, 116 (1); Typhus,
116 (1)
positive Castaneda's stain for: *supplementary term,* 486. *Diagnose
disease*
Rickettsialpox, 116 (1)
Rider's bone, 168 (4)
myositis ossificans of, 168 (4)
Riedel's lobe, 287 (0). *See* Lobulation of liver, abnormal, congenital,
287 (0)
Riedel's struma. *See* Chronic thyroiditis, 389 (9)
Ringworm. *See* Dermatophytosis;
Epidermophytosis; Tinea
of beard. *See* Tinea of beard, 135
(2)
of body. *See* Tinea of groin, 135 (2)
honeycomb. *See* Favus
of scalp. *See* Tinea capitis, 135 (2)
Ritter's disease. *See* Dermatitis exfoliative, 140 (9)
Robert's pelvis, 386 (9)
Rocky Mountain spotted fever, 116
(1)
Roentgen rays
anemia, normocytic hypoplastic, due
to, 228 (4)
asymmetry of ventricles demonstrable by: *supplementary term,* 502.
Diagnose disease
burn
of conjunctiva, 470 (4)
of cornea, 435 (4)
of larynx, 184 (4)
cataract from, 442 (4)
dermatitis actinica due to, 136 (4)
general effects, 119 (4)
injury, 127 (4)
of thyroid gland, 388 (4)
late effect, 127 (4)

Roentgen rays—Continued
ovarian hypofunction due to, 368 (4)
remote effect, 127 (4)
Roentgenogram
characteristic of tuberculosis: *supplementary terms,* 490. *Diagnose
disease*
Roger's disease. *See* Ventricular
septal defect, localized, 203 (0)
Rokitansky's disease. *See* Acute
yellow atrophy of liver, 289 (9)
Root of tooth
retained, 248 (4)
Rosacea, 137 (5)
with acne, 137 (5)
of eyelid, 463 (5)
Roseola infantum. *See* Exanthema
subitum, 114 (1)
Round back
due to senile atrophy of vertebra,
153 (7)
with wedging of vertebrae, due to
unknown cause, 155 (9)
Round ligament
hydrocele, 372 (9)
leiomyoma, 372 (8)
neoplasms, 372 (8)
Roundworms. *See* Ascariasis; Nematodes; Strongyloidiasis
Roussy-Déjerine syndrome. *See*
Déjerine-Roussy syndrome, 503
Rubella, 116 (1)
congenital, 381 (1)
Rubeola. *See* Measles, 114 (1)
Rudimentary part, 122 (0). *See also
under organ, region or structure
affected*
Rumination: *supplementary term,*
497. *Diagnose disease*
Rupture. *See under organ or structure affected; see also* Hernia

S

Saccule of ear
degeneration, congenital, 479 (0)
dilatation, congenital, 479 (0)
Sachs-Tay disease. *See* Amaurotic
familial idiocy, infantile, 403 (7);
Atrophy, retinal, in infantile amaurotic familial idiocy, 449 (9)
Sacrococcygeal region
decubitus ulcer, 285 (4)

Sacrococcygeal region—Continued
   fistula. *See* Pilonidal sinus, 122 (0)
   teratoma, 129 (8)
Sacrouterine ligament
   leiomyoma, 372 (8)
   neoplasms, 372 (8)
Sailor's skin, 137 (4)
St. Vitus' dance. *See* Chorea, 411 (1)
Salivary glands and ducts
   abscess, 253 (1)
   absence, congenital, 252 (0)
   adenocarcinoma, 253 (8)
   adenoma, 253 (8)
   calculus of gland, 253 (6)
   cyst, 253 (6)
   cystadenoma. *Diagnose as* Adeno-
      lymphoma, 98
   diseases, 252 ff.
   fistula
      due to infection, 253 (1)
      due to trauma, 253 (4)
   hypertrophy of gland, 254 (9)
   inflammation. *See* Sialadenitis, 253
      (1)
   injury, 253 (4)
   myoepithelial tumor, 253 (8)
   neoplasms, 253 (8)
   oxyphilic or oxyphylic granular cell
      adenoma. *Diagnose as* Adeno-
      lymphoma, 98
   papillary cystadenoma. *Diagnose as*
      Adenolymphoma, 98
   poisoning by iodide, 253 (3)
   sarcoma, not otherwise specified. *Di-
      agnose* as Mixed tumor, salivary
      gland type, 98
   stenosis of duct due to infection, 253
      (1)
   tumors
      mixed, salivary gland type, 98, 253
         (8)
      unlisted, 253 (8)
Salivation
   insufficient. *See* Xerostomia, 497
   supplementary term, 497. *Diagnose
      disease*
Salmonella
   food poisoning due to, 115 (1)
Salpingitis
   acute, 366 (1)
   chronic, 366 (1)
   Eustachian, 478 (1)

Salpingitis—Continued
   isthmica nodosa. *Diagnose as* Ade-
      nomyosis, 98
   nodular, 367 (9)
Salpinx. *See* Fallopian tube
Sampson's cyst *or* **tumor.** *Diagnose
   as* Adenomyosis, 98
Sandfly fever. *See* Pappataci fever,
   115 (1)
Sarcocarcinoma. *Diagnose as* Carcinosarcoma, 97
Sarcoendothelioma. *Diagnose as*
   Synovioma, 97
Sarcoid
   Spiegler-Fendt. *Diagnose as* Hodg-
      kin's disease, 95
Sarcoidosis, 123 (1)
   generalized, 116 (1)
   of larynx, 183 (1)
   of lung, 193 (1)
   of myocardium, 208 (1)
   of skin, 133 (1)
   of spleen, 232 (1)
Sarcoma
   adenoid telangiectatic. *Diagnose as*
      Mesenchymal mixed tumor, 98
   alveolar
      except of pharynx. *Diagnose as*
         Disgerminoma, 97
      of pharynx. *Diagnose as* Epider-
         moid carcinoma, 94
   alveolar round cell. *Diagnose as*
      Disgerminoma, 97
   ameloblastic. *Diagnose as* Adaman-
      tinocarcinoma, 98
   anaplastic. *Diagnose as* Sarcoma,
      not otherwise specified, 97
   angioblastic. *Diagnose as* Heman-
      giosarcoma, 96
      of genital organs. *Diagnose as*
         Mesenchymal mixed tumor, 98
   botryoid. *Diagnose as* Mesenchymal
      mixed tumor, 98
   capillary. *Diagnose as* Hemangio-
      sarcoma, 96
   colli uteri hydropicum papillare. *Di-
      agnose as* Mesenchymal mixed
      tumor, 98
   cutaneum telangiectaticum multiplex.
      Diagnose as Multiple hemor-
      rhagic hemangioma of Kaposi,
      96

Sarcomatosis
of brain, meninges. *Diagnose as* Meningioma, 95
diffuse, of brain, meninges. *Diagnose as* Meningioma, 95
except of brain, meninges. *Diagnose as* Sarcoma, not otherwise specified, 97
primary diffuse
of brain, meninges. *Diagnose as* Meningioma, 95
except of brain, meninges. *Diagnose as* Sarcoma, not otherwise specified, 97
spreading. *Diagnose as* Sarcoma, not otherwise specified, 97
Sarcomatous. *Diagnose as* Sarcoma, not otherwise specified, 97
Scabies, 135 (2). *See also* Itch
of penis, 330 (2)
of vulva, 352 (2)
Scald, 127 (4)
of cornea, 436 (4)
pharyngitis due to, 256 (4)
Scalenus anticus syndrome. *See* Compression of brachial plexus (medial cord) due to displacement, 429 (4)
Scalp. *See also* Alopecia; Hair
abscess under. *See* Subgaleal abscess, 123 (1)
chronic folliculitis. *See* Folliculitis decalvans, 132 (1)
ringworm. *See* Tinea capitis, 135 (2)
Scaphocephalia, 122 (0)
Scaphoid
navicular. *See* Navicular, 155 (9)
Scaphoid face, 122 (0)
Scapula
elevation, congenital, 147 (0)
slipping, 152 (6)
snapping, 152 (6)
Scar. *See also* Cicatrix; *and under organ, region or structure affected*
due to infection, 123 (1)
due to trauma, 127 (4)
fibroastrial, due to trauma, 413 (4)
following operation, 127 (4)
hernia, ventral in, 300 (4)
of skin
due to infection, 133 (1)
due to trauma, 137 (4)

Scar—Continued
tissue
compression of brain by, 413 (4)
compression of peripheral nerve by, 429 (4)
compression of spinal cord by, 423 (4)
irritation of brain by, 413 (4)
irritation of peripheral nerve by, 429 (4)
Scarlet fever (scarlatina), 116 (1)
myocarditis due to, 208 (1)
pericardial effusion due to, 208 (1)
Schamberg's disease. *See* Dermatosis, progressive pigmentary, 137 (5)
Scheuermann's disease. *See* Osteochondrosis of vertebra with thoracic kyphosis, 155 (9)
Schick test, reactions to: *supplementary terms,* 487. *Diagnose disease*
Schilder-Flatau disease. *See* Progressive subcortical encephalopathy, 416 (9)
Schimmelbusch's disease. *See* Cystic breast due to unknown cause, 144 (6)
Schistosomiasis, 124 (2). *See under organ, region or structure affected*
Schizoid personality, 112 (x)
Schizophrenic reactions, 110 (x)
acute undifferentiated type, 110 (x)
catatonic type, 110 (x)
childhood type, 110 (x)
chronic undifferentiated type, 110 (x)
hebephrenic type, 110 (x)
paranoid type, 110 (x)
residual type, 110 (x)
schizo-affective type, 110 (x)
simple type, 110 (x)
Schlatter-Osgood disease. *See* Osteochondrosis of tuberosity of tibia, 155 (9)
Schmorl's disease. *See* Herniation of nucleus pulposus due to unknown cause, 146 (9)
Schneeberg tumor. *Diagnose as* Carcinoma, not otherwise specified, 94

Schneiderian carcinoma. *Diagnose as* Transitional cell carcinoma, 94
Schönberg-Albers disease. *See* Osteopetrosis, 147 (0)
Schwannoglioma. *Diagnose as* Schwannoma, 95
Schwannoma, 95
of nervous system, 431 (8)
Schwannosarcoma. *Diagnose as* Schwannoma, 95
Sciatica. *See also* Neuritis; Neuropathy
with sacralization of fifth lumbar vertebra (Bertolotti's syndrome), 156 (0)
Sclera. *See also* Episcleritis; Scleritis
blue, 438 (9)
diseases, 438 ff.
ectasia, 438 (1)
foreign body in, 438 (4)
injury, 438 (4)
melanosis, congenital, 438 (0)
neoplasms, 438 (8)
rupture
due to increased intraocular pressure (glaucoma), 438 (4)
due to trauma, 438 (4)
staphyloma due to infection, 438 (1)
tumors, unlisted, 438 (8)
wound, 438 (4)
Sclerema neonatorum, 131 (0)
Scleritis
annular, 438 (1)
anterior, due to infection, 438 (1)
rheumatoid, 438 (9)
Scleroderma, 121 (9)
of eyelid, 464 (7)
generalized
progressive, 142 (9)
of skin and mucous membranes, 142 (9)
localized (morphea), 142 (9)
Scleroma. *See* Rhinoscleroma
Sclerosis. *See also* Arteriosclerosis; Atherosclerosis; Phlebosclerosis; *and under organ, region or structure affected*
amyotrophic lateral, 404 (9)
arteriolar, generalized, 219 (9)
diabetic dorsal, 424 (7)
dorsal
due to unknown cause, 425 (9)

Sclerosis—Continued
dorsal—continued
supplementary term, 503. *Diagnose disease*
dorsolateral: *supplementary term,* 503. *Diagnose disease*
lateral, 404 (9)
primary, 404 (9)
supplementary term, 505. *Diagnose disease*
multiple, 404 (9)
optic neuritis (retrobulbar neuritis) in, 452 (9)
posterior spinal. *See* Tabes dorsalis, 403 (1)
progressive muscular, 404 (9)
renal. *See* Nephrosclerosis
systemic, progressive, 121 (9)
venous. *See* Phlebosclerosis
Scoliosis
congenital, 156 (0)
due to hemivertebra, 146 (0)
due to thoracic disease, 159 (4)
due to trauma, 159 (4)
due to unknown cause, 164 (9)
following poliomyelitis, 161 (55)
with sacralization of fifth lumbar vertebra (Bertolotti's syndrome), 156 (0)
supplementary terms, 489. *Diagnose disease*
Scopolamine poisoning, 118 (3)
Scorbutus. *See* Scurvy
Scotoma: *supplementary term,* 509. *Diagnose disease*
Scrofuloderma (tuberculosis colliquativa), 134 (1)
of eyelid, 462 (1)
Scrotum
abscess, 339 (1)
absence of half, 333 (0)
adhesion of penis to, 329 (0)
carcinoma
basal cell, 340 (8)
epidermoid, 340 (8)
cellulitis, 339 (1)
chancroid, 339 (1)
cleft (in pseudohermaphroditism), 339 (0)
diseases, 339 ff.
eczema, allergic, 339 (3)
elephantiasis, lymphangiectatic, 330 (5)

Scrotum—Continued
    epidermophytosis, 339 (2)
    erysipelas, 339 (1)
    fibroma, 340 (8)
    fistula, 339 (1)
        urethroscrotal, due to infection,
            323 (1)
    frostbite, 339 (4)
    gangrene, 339 (1)
    hemangioma, 340 (8)
    hemorrhage due to trauma, 339 (4)
    herpes simplex, 339 (1)
    infection, 339 (1)
    injury, 339 (4)
    leiomyoma, 340 (8)
    lipoma, 340 (8)
    lymphangioma, 340 (8)
    melanoma, malignant, 340 (8)
    neoplasms, 340 (8)
    papilloma, squamous cell, 340 (8)
    pigmentation, abnormal, 339 (0)
    pigmented nevus, 340 (8)
    pruritus, neurogenic, 340 (55)
    redundant, 340 (7)
    sarcoma, 340 (8)
    teratoma, 340 (8)
    tumors, unlisted, 340 (8)
Scrub typhus. *See* Tsutsugamushi
    fever, 116 (1)
Scurvy, 121 (7)
    changes in periosteum due to, 153
        (7)
    hemorrhage due to
        of pancreas, 296 (7)
        of retina, 448 (7)
Seasickness, 119 (55)
Sebaceous cyst. *Diagnose as* Seba-
    ceous tumor, 94
Sebaceous glands
    aberrant, at junction of vagina and
        vulva, 351 (0)
    aberrant, of mucocutaneous junction,
        131 (0)
        of anus, 284 (0)
        of lips, 243 (0)
        of penis, 329 (0)
Sebaceous tumor, 94
Sebocystomatosis. *Diagnose as* Neo-
    plastic cyst, 93
Seborrhea
    nigricans. *See* Chromhidrosis of lid,
        464 (7)

Seborrhea—Continued
    sicca. *See* Dermatitis seborrheic, 132
        (1)
**Secretory and vasomotor nerves,
    disturbances:** *supplementary
    term,* 508. *Diagnose disease*
Secundines, retained
    hemorrhage, uterine, due to, 375 (6)
Segmentation
    failure of, 122 (0). *See also* Webbed
        fingers and toes, 122 (0)
    incomplete (synostosis), 147 (0)
Seizures. *See also* Grand mal; Petit
    mal; Pyknolepsy
    akinetic, 417 (x)
    cortical (Jacksonian), 416 (x)
    focal visceral, 416 (x)
    temporal lobe, 416 (x)
Semen, premature ejaculation: *sup-
    plementary term,* 499. *Diagnose
    disease*
Semicircular canals
    fistula, 480 (9)
        due to infection, 479 (1)
        following operation, 480 (4)
Semilunar bone
    osteochondrosis, 155 (9)
Semilunar cartilage. *See* Meniscus
Seminal vesicles
    abscess, 344 (1)
    adenocarcinoma, 344 (8)
    adenoma, 344 (8)
    adhesions due to infection, 344 (1)
    amebiasis, 344 (1)
    calculus in, 344 (6)
    carcinoma, epidermoid, 344 (8)
    cyst, 344 (6)
    diseases, 344 ff.
    distention due to obstruction, 344
        (6)
    fibroma, 344 (8)
    fibrosis due to infection, 344 (1)
    fistula, vesical, into, 318 (1)
    leiomyoma, 345 (8)
    mesothelioma, 345 (8)
    myoma, 345 (8)
    neoplasms, 345 (8)
    perivesicular adhesions due to infec-
        tion, 344 (1)
    perivesiculitis, 344 (1)
    sarcoma, 345 (8)
    spermatorrhea, 344 (55)
    teratoma, 345 (8)

Siderosis—Continued
transfusion, 120 (7)
of vitreous, 444 (3)
Sigmoid colon. *See also* Colon; Sigmoiditis, 277 (1)
fistula, ureterosigmoid, 315 (6)
fistula between bladder and, due to infection, 318 (1)
Sigmoid sinus
thrombosis due to remote pneumococcic infection, 408 (1)
Sigmoiditis, 277 (1)
Silicosis, 196 (4)
lymphadenitis due to, 235 (4)
Silicotuberculosis, 196 (4)
Silver
conjunctivitis due to, 469 (3)
laryngitis due to, 183 (1)
pigmentation. *See* Argyria
poisoning, 118 (3)
Simmonds' disease. *See* Hypopituitary cachexia, 394 (7)
Simulation: *supplementary term,* 486. *Diagnose disease*
Simultanagnosia: *supplementary term,* 507. *Diagnose disease*
Singers' node. *Diagnose as* Fibroma, 96
Singultus. *See* Hiccup: *supplementary term,* 496; Reflex spasm of diaphragm, 172 (55)
Sinoatrial block
due to unknown cause, 214 (x)
supplementary term, 492. *Diagnose disease*
Sinus. *See also* Sinuses, accessory; Sinusitis
cardiac. *See* Heart, sinus
carotid. *See* Carotid sinus
cavernous. *See* Cavernous sinus
cranial. *See* Cranial sinus
due to chemical burn, 125 (3)
lateral. *See* Lateral sinus
pericranii, 408 (1)
pilonidal. *See* Pilonidal sinus
superior longitudinal. *See* Longitudinal sinus, superior
urogenital
congenital fusion of labia majora, 351 (0)
with vagina communicating, 327 (0)
urogenitalis, persistence, 306 (0)

Sinus—Continued
of Valsalva, 204 (0)
Sinuses, accessory. *See also* Sinusitis
absence, partial, 180 (0)
anomalous, 180 (0)
clouded on transillumination or x-ray: *supplementary term,* 490. *Diagnose disease*
cystic degeneration, 181 (9)
diseases, 180 ff.
duplication, 180 (0)
fetal form, persistence of, 180 (0)
fistula
buccomaxillary, 180 (1)
due to infection, 180 (1)
of maxillary following operation, 181 (4)
granuloma
due to infection, 180 (1)
due to trauma, 181 (4)
hyperplasia, 180 (0)
injury, 181 (4)
mucocele, 180 (1)
myiasis, 180 (2)
polyp formation, simple, 181 (9)
rhinolith in, 181 (6)
tuberculosis, 180 (1)
vacuum in, 181 (6)
Sinusitis
acute (including subacute), 180 (1)
chronic, 180 (1)
due to chemical irritant, 181 (3)
nonpurulent, chronic, 180 (1)
pansinusitis, 180 (1)
due to chemical irritant, 181 (3)
purulent, 180 (1)
Siringohamartoma annulare. *Diagnose as* Sweat gland tumor, 94
Situs inversus, 114 (0)
dextrocardia with, 202 (0)
Situs transversus, 114 (0)
transposition of appendix in, 279 (0)
Skeleton. *See* Bone; Musculoskeletal system
Skene's glands
adenitis, acute, 323 (1)
Skin. *See also* Dermatitis; Dermatosis; *and under name of specific disease*
abrasion, 136 (4)
acromegaly, 138 (7)
amebiasis, 132 (1)

Smallpox vaccination, reactions to: *supplementary terms. Diagnose disease*
intermediate, 487
negative, 487
no-take, 487
positive, 488
successful, 488
Smell
hallucinations of: *supplementary term, 509. Diagnose disease*
loss of sense of. *See* Anosmia, 176 (1)
Smoke
conjunctivitis, chronic, due to, 469 (4)
suffocation by, 119 (4)
Snapping hip, 174 (6)
Snapping jaw, 162 (6)
Snapping knee, 162 (6)
Sneezing, intractable: *supplementary term, 490. Diagnose disease*
Sociopathic personality. *See* Personality, sociopathic
Sodium chloride
edema due to excessive administration, 119 (7)
Sodium hydroxide
stricture of external auditory canal due to, 475 (3)
Solenoma. *Diagnose as* Adenomyosis, 98
Somnambulism, 112 (x)
supplementary term, 486. Diagnose disease
Somniloquism: *supplementary term, 486. Diagnose disease*
Somnolence: *supplementary term, 500. Diagnose disease*
Sore
oriental (leishmaniasis of skin), 133 (1)
veldt, 142 (9)
Sore throat. *See also* Pharyngitis streptococcic, 255 (1)
Sottas-Déjerine neuropathy. *See* Progressive hypertrophic interstitial neuropathy, 431 (9)
Sparganosis, 125 (2)
Spasm. *See also under organ or structure affected*
muscle. *See* Cramp
nodding. *See* Spasmus nutans, 507

Spasm—Continued
occupation: *supplementary term, 505. Diagnose disease*
oculogyric: *supplementary term, 509. Diagnose disease*
supplementary term, 507. Diagnose disease
torsion: *supplementary term, 507. Diagnose disease*
Spasmus nutans, 169 (55)
supplementary term, 507. Diagnose disease
Speech disturbance, 112 (x). *See also* Anarthria; Aphasia; Aphemia; Aphonia; Dysphasia
delayed speech: *supplementary term, 503. Diagnose disease*
disorder due to habit: *supplementary term, 507. Diagnose disease*
interjectional speech: *supplementary term, 505. Diagnose disease*
ungrammatical speech. *See* Paragrammatism: *supplementary term, 505. Diagnose disease*
Spelling disability: *supplementary term, 507. Diagnose disease*
Spermatic cord
abscess, 342 (1)
absence, 342 (0)
constriction
gangrene of epididymis due to, 335 (5)
gangrene of testis due to, 333 (5)
diseases, 342 ff.
fibroma, 342 (8)
hematocele due to unknown cause, 343 (9)
hematoma
due to trauma, 342 (4)
following operation, 342 (4)
hydrocele
congenital, 342 (0)
due to unknown cause, 343 (9)
inflammation. *See* Funiculitis, 342 (1)
injury, 342 (4)
lipoma, 342 (8)
mesothelioma, 342 (8)
myxoma, 342 (8)
neoplasms, 342 (8)
rhabdomyoma, 342 (8)
rhabdomyosarcoma, 342 (8)
sarcoma, 343 (8)

Spermatic cord—Continued
torsion
due to trauma, 342 (4)
not due to trauma, 342 (6)
traumatism due to operation, 342
(4)
tumors, unlisted, 343 (8)
varicocele, 342 (6)
Spermatoblastoma. *Diagnose as* Disgerminoma, 97
Spermatocele, 335 (6)
congenital, 332 (0)
Spermatocytoma. *Diagnose as* Disgerminoma, 97
Spermatorrhea, 344 (55)
Spermatozoa. *See also* Aspermia;
Asthenospermia; Azoospermia;
Necrospermia; Oligospermia;
Spermatorrhea; Spermaturia
count below normal: *supplementary
term,* 499. *Diagnose disease*
Spermaturia: *supplementary term,*
499. *Diagnose disease*
Sphenoid bone
enlargement, congenital, 147 (0)
Sphenoid sinus. *See* Sinuses, accessory; Sinusitis
Sphenopalatine ganglion
neuralgia, 431 (x)
Spherocytosis
hereditary, 230 (9)
Sphincter ani
incontinence
due to paralysis, 285 (55)
due to trauma, 285 (4)
following operation, 285 (4)
laceration, 285 (4)
relaxation, 285 (55)
due to central lesion, 285 (55)
spasm
due to paralysis, 285 (55)
due to reflex action, 285 (55)
Sphincter of Oddi
spasm, 274 (55)
Spider fingers. *See* Arachnodactyly,
114 (0)
Spiegler's tumor. *Diagnose as* Neoplastic cyst, 93
Spiegler-Fendt sarcoid. *Diagnose as*
Hodgkin's disease, 95
Spielmeyer-Stock disease. *See*
Atrophy, retinal, in juvenile
amaurotic familial idiocy, 449 (9)

Spielmeyer-Vogt disease. *See*
Amaurotic familiar idiocy, juvenile, 449 (9)
Spina bifida, 147 (0)
clubfoot, congenital paralytic, in, 157
(0)
contracture of spine due to flaccid
paralysis from, 161 (55)
Spinal accessory nerve
atrophy: *supplementary term,* 509.
Diagnose disease
disturbances: *supplementary term,*
508. *Diagnose disease*
paralysis: *supplementary term,* 509.
Diagnose disease
Spinal cord. *See also* Myelitis; Myelopathy; etc.
absence. *See* Amyelia, 421 (0)
abscess, 421 (1)
aplasia of ventral horn cells, 421
(0)
arteritis, 426 (1)
birth injury, 421 (0)
caudal displacement, 402 (0)
compression
acute, 423 (4)
chronic, 423 (4)
concussion, or commotion, 424 (4)
contusion, 424 (4)
degeneration, 425 (7)
diseases, 421 ff.
electrical shock, 424 (4)
ependymoma, 425 (8)
glioma, 425 (8)
gliosis due to trauma, 424 (4)
hemi-involvement (Brown-Séquard
syndrome): *supplementary term,*
502. *Diagnose disease*
hemisection, 424 (4)
injury, paralysis of bladder due to,
319 (55)
laceration, 424 (4)
birth injury, 421 (0)
muscular atrophy, infantile familial,
425 (9)
necrosis, 425 (9)
neoplasms, 425 (8)
neurofibroma, 425 (8)
rachischisis, 421 (0)
sclerosis
diabetic dorsal, 424 (7)

Spinal cord—Continued
  sclerosis—continued
    dorsal, due to unknown cause, 425
      (9)
  tumors, unlisted, 425 ff.
  varix, 427 (6)
  vessels
    air embolism, 426 (4)
    aneurysm
      arteriosclerotic, 427 (9)
      congenital, 426 (0)
      due to infection, 426 (1)
      due to trauma, 426 (4)
    angiospasm, 426 (55)
    arteriosclerosis, 427 (9)
    arteriovenous aneurysm, 426 (4)
    arteritis and phlebitis, 426 (1)
    atypical distribution, 426 (0)
    developmental defect, 426 (0)
    diseases, 426 ff.
    embolism
      by infected thrombi, 426 (4)
      due to unspecified cause, 426
        (6)
      following operation, 426 (4)
    fat embolism, 426 (4)
    hemangioma, 427 (8) ·
    hemangiosarcoma, 427 (8)
    hemorrhage
      due to arteriosclerosis, 427 (9)
      due to rupture of infectious an-
        eurysm, 426 (1)
      from arteriovenous aneurysm,
        426 (4)
    hypoplasia, 426 (0)
    injury, 426 (4)
    neoplasms, 427 (8)
    thromboangiitis obliterans, 427
      (9)
    thrombosis
      due to infection, 426 (1)
      due to unspecified cause, 426 (6)
      progressive, 427 (9)
    tumors, unlisted, 427 (8)
  wound, 424 (4)
Spinal nerves. *See also* Spinal acces-
    sory nerve
  diseases, 428 ff.
Spine. *See also* Vertebra
  arthritis
    due to tuberculosis, 157 (1)
    rheumatoid, 163 (9)

Spine—Continued
  cervical portion, multiple congenital
    deformities, 146 (0)
  contracture due to flaccid paralysis,
    161 (55)
  craniorachischisis, 146 (0)
  curvature. *See* Kyphosis; Lordosis;
    Scoliosis
  deformity, congenital, 146 (0). *See
    also* Spina bifida, 147 (0)
  intervertebral disk. *See* Herniation
    of nucleus pulposus, 159 (4),
    164 (0)
  lumbosacral, pseudarthrosis follow-
    ing fusion (or arthrodesis), 159
    (4)
**Spinocerebellar atrophy, heredi-
  tary,** 416 (9)
Spiradenoma. *Diagnose as* Sweat
    gland tumor, 94
Splanchnomegaly, 128 (7)
Splanchnoptosis, 128 (6)
Spleen. *See also* Splenitis; Spleno-
    megaly
  abnormality: *supplementary term,
    493. Diagnose disease*
  abscess, 232 (1)
  absence, 232 (0)
  accessory, 232 (0)
  amyloidosis, due to unknown cause,
    233 (9)
  atrophy
    functional, or secondary to sick-
      lemia, 232 (7)
    senile, 232 (7)
  diseases, 211 ff.
    agranulocytosis due to, 228 (5)
  displacement, congenital, 232 (0)
  fibroma, 233 (8)
  floating, 232 (6)
  hemangioma, 233 (8)
  hernia (through diaphragm), con-
    genital, 232 (0)
  Hodgkin's disease, 233 (8)
  infarction
    due to arterial thrombosis, 232
      (5)
    due to embolism, 232 (5)
  injury, 232 (4)
  lobulation, 232 (0)
  lymphosarcoma, 233 (8)
  myeloid metaplasia, 233 (9)
    due to myelofibrosis, 233 (9)

Spleen—Continued
myeloid metaplasia—continued
due to osteopetrosis, 233 (9)
neoplasms, 233 (8)
passive congestion (splenomegaly)
due to portal obstruction, 232 (5)
ptosis. *See* Splenoptosis, 232 (6)
rupture, 232 (4)
sarcoidosis, 232 (1)
sarcoma, reticulum cell, 233 (8)
torsion, 232 (6)
tumors, unlisted, 233 (8)
Splenitis, 232 (1)
Splenomegaly
congestive, 228 (5)
anemia, normocytic, due to, 228
(5)
due to infection, 232 (1)
due to malaria, 232 (1)
due to metabolic disturbance, 232
(7)
supplementary term, 495. *Diagnose
disease*
of undetermined origin, 233 (y)
Splenoptosis, 232 (6)
Spondylolisthesis, 147 (0)
pelvis, 385 (4)
Spondylolysis, 147 (0)
Spongioblastoma. *Diagnose as* Glioblastoma multiforme, 96
ependymal. *Diagnose as* Glioblastoma multiforme, 96
multiforme. *Diagnose as* Glioblastoma multiforme, 96
Spongiocytoma. *Diagnose as* Glioblastoma multiforme, 96
Spongioneuroblastoma. *Diagnose
as* Glioblastoma multiforme, 96
Spoon nails, 141 (9)
Sporotrichosis, 125 (2). *See also
under organ, region or structure
affected*
of skin, 135 (2)
Sprain. *See also* Joints, sprain of
ligament, 159 (4)
of ankle, 159 (4)
Sprengel's deformity. *See* Scapula,
congenital elevation of, 147 (0)
Spring catarrh (vernal conjunctivitis), 469 (3)
Sprue
anemia, normocytic, due to, 229 (7)
nontropical, 269 (7)

Sputum: *supplementary terms,* 490.
Diagnose disease
acid-fast bacilli in, 490
animal parasites in, 490
bronchial casts in, 490
Charcot-Leyden crystals in, 490
Dittrich plugs in, 490
elastic fibers in, 490. *Diagnose disease*
lung stones in, 490
molds and yeasts in, 490
tubercle bacillus in, 490
tumor cells in, 497
Squint. *See* Strabismus
convergent. *See* Esotropia
divergent. *See* Exotropia
upward and downward. *See* Hypertropia
Stab wounds. *See also under organ,
region or structure affected*
multiple, 119 (4)
Stahl's pigment line. *See* Linea corneae senilis, 436 (7)
Stammering. *See* Stuttering: *supplementary term,* 507
Stapedial artery. *See* Arteria stapedia, 477 (0)
Stapes
ankylosis of incustapedial joint due
to infection, 477 (1)
fixation, otosclerosis, with conduction deafness, 480 (7)
Staphyloma
of cornea, 435 (1)
due to poison, 435 (3)
due to trauma, 436 (4)
of sclera due to infection, 438 (1)
Starvation, 119 (7)
encephalopathy due to, 414 (7)
myelopathy due to, 424 (7)
Status following operation, 127 (4)
Status lymphaticus. *See* Lymphatism, 121 (x)
Stealing: *supplementary term,* 486.
Diagnose disease
Stealing personality, 112 (x)
Steatocystoma multiplex. *Diagnose
as* Neoplastic cyst, 93
Steatoma multiplex. *Diagnose as*
Neoplastic cyst, 93
Steatorrhea, 269 (7). *See also* Fat
indigestion, 269 (7)

Steatorrhea—Continued
pancreatic dysfunction, 296 (7)
Steeple head. *See* Acrocephalia, 122
(0)
Stein-Leventhal syndrome, 369 (7)
Stenosis. *See under organ affected*
Stensen's duct
opening, in neck, 252 (0)
Stercoraceous ulcer
of colon, 278 (6)
of rectum, 282 (6)
Sterility
female
due to absence or destruction of
ovary, 349 (7)
due to distortion or displacement
of pelvic organs of unknown
cause, 349 (6)
due to hypopituitarism, 349 (7)
due to obstruction following infection, 349 (1)
due to trauma or operation, 349
(4)
due to unknown cause, 350 (x)
functional
due to decrease in estrogenic
substance, 349 (7)
due to decrease in progesterone,
349 (7)
male, due to infection, 333 (1)
supplementary term, 499. *Diagnose
disease*
Sternberg's disease. *Diagnose as*
Hodgkin's disease, 95
Steven-Johnson syndrome. *See*
Erythema multiforme exudative,
141 (9)
Stewart-Morel syndrome, 155 (9)
Stieda-Pellegrini disease. *See* Calcification of medial collateral
ligament of knee due to trauma,
158 (4)
Still's disease. *See* Arthritis, rheumatoid, multiple, 163 (9)
Stitch abscess, 136 (4)
Stock-Spielmeyer disease. *See*
Atrophy, retinal, in juvenile
amaurotic familial idiocy, 449
(9)
Stokes-Adams syndrome: *supple-
mentary term,* 491. *Diagnose disease*

Stoma, gastroenteric
malfunction, 267 (4)
stenosis, 267 (4)
after enterostomy, 268 (4)
ulcer due to trauma, 273 (4)
Stomach. *See also* Gastritis
abnormally large. *See* Megalogastria, 263 (0)
abnormally small. *See* Microgastria, 263 (0)
abscess of wall, 263 (1)
achlorhydria
due to chronic atrophic gastritis,
265 (9)
due to poison, 264 (3)
supplementary term, 496. *Diagnose
disease*
acid-fast bacilli in gastric contents:
supplementary term, 496. *Diagnose disease*
adenocarcinoma, 265 (8)
adenomyoma, 265 (8)
atony, 264 (55)
blood in gastric contents: *supplementary term,* 496. *Diagnose
disease*
carcinoma, 265 (8)
polypoid, 265 (8)
scirrhous, 265 (8)
congestion, passive, 264 (5)
deformity
due to poison, 264 (3)
due to trauma, 264 (3)
due to ulcer, 265 (9)
dilatation, acute
following operation, 264 (4)
reflex, 264 (55)
diseases, 263 ff.
displacement into thorax, congenital,
263 (0)
diverticulum, 265 (6)
congenital, 263 (0)
due to traction or pulsion, 264
(4)
fibroma, 265 (8)
filling defect: *supplementary term,*
496. *Diagnose disease*
fistula
cholecystogastric
due to calculus, 293 (6)
following operation, 293 (4)
due to trauma, 264 (4)

Stomach—Continued
fistula—continued
following gunshot wound, 264 (4)
gastrocolic
due to tuberculosis, 267 (1)
due to ulcer, 267 (9)
gastrojejunocolic, 267 (9)
foreign body in, nontraumatic, 265 (6)
gastrostomy opening, 264 (4)
gunshot wound, 264 (4)
hair ball in, 265 (6)
hemorrhage
due to ulcer, 265 (9)
following operation, 264 (4)
hernia
congenital, 263 (0)
strangulation due to, 264 (5)
traumatic, transdiaphragmatic, 264 (4)
hourglass
congenital, 263 (0)
due to ulcer, 265 (9)
hypermotility: *supplementary term,* 496. *Diagnose disease*
hypersecretion: *supplementary term,* 496. *Diagnose disease*
hypomotility: *supplementary term,* 496. *Diagnose disease*
inclusion of islands of pancreatic tissue in stomach wall, 263 (0)
injury, 264 (4)
lactic acid in gastric contents: *supplementary term,* 496. *Diagnose disease*
leiomyoma, 265 (8)
lipoma, 265 (8)
lymphosarcoma, 265 (8)
mucosa
herniation, 265 (6)
prolapse, 265 (6)
redundancy, congenital, 263 (0)
neoplasms, 265 (8)
neurofibroma, 265 (8)
odor of gastric contents in newborn: *supplementary term,* 497. *Diagnose disease*
perforation
due to infection, 263 (1)
due to poison, 264 (3)
due to ulcer, 265 (9)
perigastric abscess, 263 (1)

Stomach—Continued
perigastric adhesions due to ulcer, 265 (9)
phytobezoar, 265 (6)
polyp, neoplastic, 265 (8)
prolapse of esophageal mucosa into cardia of, 263 (0)
ptosis. *See* Gastroptosis, 265 (6)
stasis: *supplementary term,* 496. *Diagnose disease*
stenosis of cardia, 265 (9)
transposition, congenital, 263 (0)
tubercle bacilli in gastric contents: *supplementary term,* 497. *Diagnose disease*
tumor cells in gastric secretions: *supplementary term,* 497. *Diagnose disease*
tumors, unlisted, 265 (8)
ulcer, 265 (9)
due to uremia, 264 (3)
gastrojejunal, 267 (9)
varix, 265 (6)
volvulus, 265 (6)
Stomach and intestine combined, diseases, 267
Stomatitis, 241 (1). *See also* Mouth
aphthous, 241 (1)
due to poison, 241 (3)
gangrenous (noma), 241 (1)
Strabismus
congenital, 455 (0)
due to paralysis of ocular muscles, 456 (55)
due to parasite, 455 (2)
due to trauma, 456 (4)
postoperative, 456 (4)
Strain, 127 (4). *See also under organ, region or structure affected*
Strangulation, 119 (4)
Streptococcic infection, 57. *See also under name of specific disease or organ, region or structure affected*
sore throat, 255 (1)
Stress reaction, gross, 112 (x)
Striae atrophic, 140 (9)
Stricture. *See under organ affected*
Stridor: *supplementary term,* 490. *Diagnose disease*
Striocerebellar syndrome: *supplementary term,* 507. *Diagnose disease*
Strongyloidiasis, 268 (2), 272 (2)

Sun fever. *See* Dengue, 115 (1)
Sunburn. *See* Ultraviolet rays
Sunstroke, 119 (4)
Superfecundation: *supplementary term,* 499. *Diagnose disease*
Superfetation: *supplementary term,* 499. *Diagnose disease*
Supernumerary parts, 123 (0). *See also under organ, region or structure affected*
Supranuclear bulbar syndrome: *supplementary term,* 507. *Diagnose disease*
Suprarenal gland. *See* Adrenal gland
Sutton and Gull's disease. *See* Arteriosclerosis, general, 218 (9)
Sutures
coronal, closure, 122 (0)
lamboid, closure, 122 (0)
sagittal, closure, 122 (0)
Sutures, cranial
premature closure, 163 (7)
neuropathy of cranial nerve following, 429 (4)
Swallowing
of air. *See* Aerophagia: *supplementary term,* 496
difficulty in. *See* Dysphagia: *supplementary term,* 496
Sweat
abnormal deficiency. *See* Anhidrosis, 138 (55)
colored. *See* Chromhidrosis, 138 (7)
excessive. *See* Hyperhidrosis, 138 (55)
fetid. *See* Bromhidrosis, 138 (7)
Sweat gland(s)
adenoma (hydradenoma) of skin, 140 (8)
carcinoma of breast, 145 (8)
inflammation. *See* Hidradenitis, 133 (1)
tumor, 94
Swindling: *supplementary term,* 486. *Diagnose disease*
Sycosis pyogenic, 133 (1)
Sydenham's chorea. *See* Chorea, 411 (1)

Symblepharon
congenital, 461 (0)
due to poison, 469 (3)
due to trauma, 470 (4)
due to unknown cause, 471 (x)
following operation, 470 (4)
Symbol(s)
inability to understand. *See* Asymbolia: *supplementary term,* 502
reversal (developmental alexia), 501
Sympathetic nervous system. *See also* Nervous system, vegetative, 432
paralysis, hyperemia of conjunctiva due to, 470 (5)
Sympatheticotonia, 417 (x)
Sympathicoblastoma, 95
of adrenal medulla, 397 (8)
of brain, 415 (8)
retroperitoneal, 301 (8)
of vegetative nervous system, 432 (8)
Sympathicogonioma, 95
of brain, 415 (8)
Sympathicotropic tumor (ovary). *Diagnose as* Virilizing tumor, 93
Sympathoma. *Diagnose as* Sympathicoblastoma, 95
Symphysis pubis
separation, 385 (4)
Syncope
carotid sinus, 206 (55)
supplementary term, 486. *Diagnose disease*
Syncytioma malignum. *Diagnose as* Chorioadenoma, 97
Syndactyly, 132 (0). *See also* Webbed fingers; Webbed toes, 122 (0)
Synechia
anterior
due to infection, 439 (1)
due to trauma, 440 (4)
posterior, 439 (1)
Synesthesia: *supplementary term,* 507. *Diagnose disease*
Synorchism, 332 (0)
Synostosis (incomplete segmentation), 147 (0)
congenital
of humerus and radius, 147 (0)
of lumbosacral vertebra, transitional, 147 (0)
of radius and ulna, 147 (0)

Synovial sarcoma, 97
Synovialoma, 97
Synovioma, 97
  malignant. *Diagnose as* Synovial
    sarcoma, 97
Synovitis. *See also under* Arthritis,
    158 (1)
  pigmented villo-nodular, 163 (7)
Syphilis, 123 (1). *See also under or-
    gan, region or structure affected*
  alopecia due to, 132 (1)
  aneurysm due to
    of aorta, 220 (1)
    of coronary artery, 207 (1)
  atrophy, macular, due to, 132 (1)
  atrophy of optic nerve due to, 450
    (1)
  cerebral, 412 (1)
  cerebrospinal, 402 (1)
    congenital, 402 (0)
  congenital, 123 (1)
  generalized, 116 (1)
  habitual abortion due to, 380 (1)
  leukoplakia of tongue following, 245
    (1)
  meningovascular, 403 (1)
  narrowing of coronary ostium due
    to, 208 (1)
  nephrosis due to, 308 (1)
  perforating ulcer due to, 123 (1)
  poliomyelitis, anterior, chronic, due
    to, 422 (1)
  rupture of artery due to, 216 (1)
  of skin
    congenital, 131 (0)
    primary or secondary, 133 (1)
    tertiary, gumma, 133 (1)
  stricture due to, 123 (1)
  tertiary multiple, 116 (1)
Syphilitic. *For names of diseases pre-
    ceded by this qualifying term, see
    under the principal term, as* Ar-
    thritis, syphilitic; Myocarditis,
    syphilitic
Syphiloma. *See also* Gumma, 123 (1)
  of vulva, 352 (1)
Syphilophobia: *supplementary term,*
    486. *Diagnose disease*
Syringoadenoma. *Diagnose as* Sweat
    gland tumor, 94
Syringobulbia, 416 (9)
Syringocarcinoma. *Diagnose as*
    Sweat gland tumor, 94

Syringocystadenoma; syringocyst-
    adenoma nodularis. *Diagnose
    as* Sweat gland tumor, 94
Syringocystoma. *Diagnose as* Sweat
    gland tumor, 94
Syringoma. *Diagnose as* Sweat gland
    tumor, 94
Syringomyelia, 425 (9)
  atrophy, neurogenic, of bone due to,
    152 (55)
  clawhand due to, 162 (55)
Systolic pressure: *supplementary
    terms. Diagnose disease*
  elevation, 491
  depression, 491

T

Tabes dorsalis, 403 (1)
  atrophy, neurogenic, of bone due to,
    152 (55)
  paresis of bladder in, 320 (55)
Tachycardia
  atrial paroxysmal
    due to unknown cause, 214 (y)
    *supplementary term, 492. Diag-
      nose disease*
  junctional paroxysmal: *supplemen-
    tary term, 492. Diagnose disease*
  paroxysmal
    atrioventricular nodal, due to un-
      known cause, 214 (x)
    unspecified: *supplementary term,
      492. Diagnose disease*
  sinus
    due to unknown cause, 214 (x)
    *supplementary term, 492. Diag-
      nose disease*
  ventricular paroxysmal
    due to unknown cause, 214 (x)
    *supplementary term, 492. Diag-
      nose disease*
Tactile discrimination
  loss or diminution of: *supplemen-
    tary term, 505. Diagnose disease*
Tactile localization
  loss or diminution of: *supplemen-
    tary term, 505. Diagnose dis-
    ease*
Taenia, 65
  saginata, 65

Teeth—Continued
mottled enamel due to fluorine, 248
(3)
necrotic pulp, 247 (1)
neoplasms, 249 (8)
odontogenic cyst. *Diagnose as* Odontogenic tumor, benign, 98
odontogenic tumor, 249 (8)
osteoma (cementoma), 249 (8)
precocious dentition, 247 (0), 249
(9)
pulp capped, 248 (4)
pulpless, 248 (4)
root
idiopathic resorption, 249 (9)
perforated, 248 (4)
resected, 248 (4)
retained, 248 (4)
supernumerary, 247 (0)
tumors, unlisted, 249 (8)
Telangiectasia
familial. *Diagnose as* Hemangiomatosis, 96
hemorrhagica, 219 (9)
hereditary multiple. *Diagnose as*
Hemangiomatosis, 96
Telangioendothelioma. *Diagnose as*
Hemangiosarcoma, 96
Telangioma. *Diagnose as* Hemangioma (angioma), 96
Temperature. *See* Cold; Heat
high. *See* Pyrexia: *supplementary
term,* 486
Temporal bone
elongation of styloid process, 147
(0)
fracture of petrous pyramid and
mastoid, 478 (4)
Temporomandibular joint
malocclusion, otalgia due to, 472 (6)
Tendon(s). *See also* Tenosynovitis
Achilles, short, 167 (4)
due to trauma, 168 (4)
chondroma, 174 (8)
diseases, 173 ff.
dislocation, 174 (4)
division, 174 (4)
fibroma, 174 (8)
hemangioma, 174 (8)
injury, 174 (4)
lipoma, 174 (8)
neoplasms, 174 (8)
rupture, 174 (4)

Tendon(s)—Continued
sheath
abscess, 173 (1)
calcification, 174 (9)
cystic tumor. *Diagnose as* "Ganglion" of tendon sheath, 97
of finger, stenosis, congenital, 173
(0)
"ganglion," 97
giant cell tumor, 174 (8)
sarcoma. *Diagnose as* Synovioma,
97
sloughing, 173 (1)
tumors, unlisted, 174 (8)
xanthoma, 174 (7)
Tendonitis
acute, 173 (1)
chronic, 173 (1)
Tendosynovitis. *See* Tenosynovitis
Tennis elbow, 165 (4)
Tenonitis, 458 (1)
Tenosynovioma. *Diagnose as* Synovioma, 97
Tenosynovitis
acute, due to infection, 173 (1)
adhesive, 173 (1)
crepitans, 174 (9)
due to trauma, 174 (4)
villous, 174 (9)
Tension. *See also* Hypertension; Hypotension
intraocular. *See* Intraocular pressure
premenstrual, 364 (7)
valvular changes due to, 209 (4)
Teratoblastoma. *Diagnose as* Teratoma, 97
Teratocarcinoma
except of testis. *Diagnose as* Teratoma, 97
of testis. *Diagnose as* Embryonal
carcinoma of testis, 98
Teratoid tumor
mixed
except of testis. *Diagnose as* Teratoma, 98
of testis. *Diagnose as* Embryonal
carcinoma of testis, 98
not otherwise specified. *Diagnose as*
Teratoma, 97
Teratoma, 97, 129 (8)
adult. *Diagnose as* Teratoma, 97
cystic. *Diagnose as* Teratoma, 97

Teratoma—Continued
immature. *Diagnose as* Teratoma, 97
mediastinal, 129 (8)
retroperitoneal, 301 (8)
sacrococcygeal, 129 (8)
thyroid, of ovary. *Diagnose as* Teratoma, 97
Term birth; Term delivery, 378
Testis(es)
abscess, 332 (1)
absence (anorchism), 332 (0)
adenocarcinoma, 333 (8)
adenoma, 333 (8)
adenomatoid tumor. *Diagnose as* Embryonal carcinoma of testis, 98
adrenal cortical rest tumor, 94
atrophy
circulatory, 333 (5)
due to unknown cause, 334 (9)
carcinoma
embryonal, 333 (8)
teratoid. *Diagnose as* Embryonal carcinoma of testis, 98
choriocarcinoma, 333 (8)
degeneration due to infection, 332 (1)
diseases, 332 ff.
disgerminoma, 333 (8)
ectopia, 332 (0)
embryoma. *Diagnose as* Embryonal carcinoma of testis, 98
fibroma, 333 (8)
fibrosis following syphilis, 332 (1)
fusion, 332 (0)
gangrene
due to constriction of spermatic cord, 333 (5)
due to infection, 332 (1)
germinal aplasia, 332 (0)
gumma, congenital, 332 (0)
hemangioma, 333 (8)
hematoma due to trauma, 333 (4)
hypergonadism, 333 (7)
hypertrophy, congenital, 332 (0)
hypogonadism, 333 (7)
hypoplasia, congenital, 332 (0)
infarction due to thrombosis, 333 (5)
injury, 333 (4)
interstitial cell tumor, 333 (8)
inversion or retroversion, 332 (0)
leprosy, 332 (1)

Testis(es)—Continued
lipoma, 333 (8)
luxation, 333 (4)
lymphosarcoma, 333 (8)
mixed tumor, not otherwise specified. *Diagnose as* Embryonal carcinoma of testis, 98
myoma, 334 (8)
myxoma, 334 (8)
necrosis due to trauma, 333 (4)
neoplasms, 334 (8)
rest, infantile, 332 (0)
rhabdomyoma, 334 (8)
rudimentary, 332 (0)
rupture due to trauma, 333 (4)
sarcoma, 334 (8)
Sertoli cell tumor, 334 (8)
sinus due to infection, 333 (1)
teratocarcinoma. *Diagnose as* Embryonal carcinoma of testis, 98
teratoid tumor, mixed. *Diagnose as* Embryonal carcinoma of testis, 98
teratoma, 334 (8)
three (polyorchism), 332 (0)
torsion due to unknown cause, 333 (6)
torsion of appendix testis due to unknown cause, 333 (6)
tubular sclerosis, 332 (0)
tubular sclerosis and germinal aplasia combined, 332 (0)
tumors, unlisted, 334 (8)
undescended. *See also* Cryptorchism, 332 (0)
unilateral, 332 (0)
Tests only, 481
Tetanus, 116 (1)
Tetany
associated with rickets, 121 (7)
cataract, 443 (7)
due to alkalosis, 120 (7)
due to deficient absorption of calcium, 120 (7)
due to hyperventilation: *supplementary term,* 486. *Diagnose disease*
of nephritis, 120 (7)
of newborn, 120 (7)
supplementary term, 486. *Diagnose disease*
Tetralogy of Fallot, 203 (0)
Tetraplegia: *supplementary term,* 507. *Diagnose disease*

Thumb
sucking: *supplementary term,* 486.
Diagnose disease
supernumerary, 123 (0)
Thymoma, 98
benign, 392 (8)
malignant, 392 (8)
with myasthenia gravis. *Diagnose as*
Thymoma, malignant, 392 (8)
Thymus
abscess, 392 (1)
atrophy, fatty, 392 (9)
cyst, congenital, 392 (0)
diseases, 392 ff.
failure of involution, 392 (7)
hemorrhage into, 392 (4)
hyperplasia, 392 (9)
hypertrophy, congenital, 392 (0)
inflammation, 392 (1)
neoplasms, 392 (8)
thymoma, 392 (8)
tumors, unlisted, 392 (8)
Thyroglossal cyst, 388 (0)
Thyroglossal duct, persistent, 388
(0)
Thyroid cartilage
abnormal union
with cricoid cartilage, 182 (0)
with hyoid bone, 182 (0)
fracture, 184 (4)
total ventral cleft, congenital, 182
(0)
Thyroid crisis: *supplementary term,*
500. *Diagnose disease*
Thyroid gland. *See also* Goiter
aberrant, lateral, cyst, 388 (6)
abscess, 388 (1)
absence, 388 (0)
accessory, 388 (0)
adenocarcinoma, 389 (8)
adenoma, 389 (8)
functionally hyperactive, 389 (8)
Hürthle cell, 389 (8)
athyrea following operation, 388 (4)
atrophy
congenital (cretinism), 388 (0)
with myxedema, 389 (9)
carcinoma
follicular, 74
giant cell, 389 (8)
Hürthle cell, 389 (8)
cyst, 388 (6)

Thyroid gland—Continued
enzymatic defect of hormone synthe-
sis, 388 (0)
fibrosarcoma, 389 (8)
hyperthyroidism. *See* Hyperthyroidism
hypothyroidism. *See* Hypothyroidism
inflammation. *See* Thyroiditis
injury, 388 (4)
lymphosarcoma, 389 (8)
neoplasms, 389 (8)
roentgen ray injury, 388 (4)
syphilis, congenital, 388 (0)
tissue
aberrant in larynx, 182 (0)
aberrant in trachea, 187 (0)
tumor
functionally hyperactive, 93
of ovary. *Diagnose as* Teratoma,
97
unlisted, 389 (8)
Thyroid gland extract
encephalopathy due to, 412 (3)
Thyroiditis, 388 (1)
chronic, 389 (9)
granulomatous, 389 (9)
lymphomatous, 389 (9)
suppurative, 388 (1)
Thyroxin shock, 117 (3)
Tibia
abscess, 148 (1)
adamantinoma. *Diagnose as* Carcinoma, not otherwise specified,
94
anterior bowing of, 146 (0)
congenital torsion, 146 (0)
osteomyelitis due to typhoid, 148 (1)
torsion due to unknown cause, 152
(6)
tuberosity, osteochondrosis, 155 (9)
vara, due to unknown cause, 155
(9)
Tic
occupation: *supplementary term,* 505.
Diagnose disease
supplementary term, 507. *Diagnose
disease*
Tinea
asbestos-like, 142 (9)
of beard, 135 (2)
capitis, 135 (2)

Tinea—Continued
  corporis, 135 (2)
  favosa. *See* Favus
  of groin, 135 (2)
  imbricata, 135 (2)
  unguium. *See* Onychomycosis, 135
    (2)
  versicolor, 135 (2)
Tinnitus
  supplementary term, 509. *Diagnose
    disease*
Tiphlitis, 277 (1)
Tobacco
  poisoning of heart by, 209 (3)
Toe(s). *See also* Hallux
  bunion, 158 (4)
  failure of segmentation, 122 (0)
  fifth, varus
    congenital, 157 (0)
    due to trauma, 160 (4)
  hammer
    congenital, 156 (0)
    due to trauma, 160 (4)
    due to unknown cause, 164 (9)
    following poliomyelitis, 161 (55)
  hypertrophy, congenital, 122 (0)
  overlapping
    congenital, 123 (0)
    due to footwear, 127 (4)
  supernumerary, 123 (0)
  webbed, 132 (0)
Toenails. *See* Nails
Toluene, 70
Tongue. *See also* Frenulum linguae;
    Hypoglossal nerve; Tonsils, lin-
    gual
  abscess, 245 (1)
  absence, congenital, 245 (0)
  acanthosis, 246 (9)
  adenocarcinoma, 246 (8)
  adhesion to gum or roof of mouth,
    congenital, 245 (0)
  atrophy
    due to avitaminosis, 246 (7)
    of mucous membrane, 246 (9)
    neurogenic, 246 (55)
    senile, 246 (7)
  bifurcation, congenital, 245 (0)
  black, hairy, 246 (9)
  carcinoma, epidermoid, 246 (8)
  chemical burn, 245 (3)
  chondroma, 246 (8)
  cyst, 246 (6)

Tongue—Continued
  cyst, congenital, 245 (0)
  deformity due to unknown cause, 246
    (6)
  diseases, 245 ff.
  displacement downward, congenital,
    245 (0)
  double, congenital, 245 (0)
  erythroplasia of Queyrat, 141 (9)
  fissure, 246 (9)
  fissured, congenital, 245 (0)
  geographic, 246 (9)
  hemangioma, 246 (8)
  hypertrophy, congenital, 245 (0)
  hypoplasia, 245 (0)
  inflammation. *See* Glossitis
  injury, 245 (4)
  leukoplakia
    due to poison, 245 (3)
    due to trauma, 245 (4)
    due to unknown cause, 246 (9)
    following syphilis, 245 (1)
  lipoma, 246 (8)
  lymphangioma, 246 (8)
  myoblastoma, granular cell, 246 (8)
  neoplasms, 246 (8)
  swallowing: *supplementary term,*
    486. *Diagnose disease*
  tongue-tie, 245 (0)
  tumors, unlisted, 246 (8)
  ulcer, 246 (9)
    due to unknown cause, 246 (9)
  Vincent's infection, 245 (1)
de **Toni-Fanconi syndrome:** *sup-
    plementary term,* 485. *Diagnose
    disease*
Tonsil(s)
  abscess, 258 (1)
  calculus in, 259 (6)
  carcinoma
    epidermoid, 259 (8)
    transitional cell. *Diagnose as* Epi-
      dermoid carcinoma, 94
  diseases, 258 ff.
  foreign body in, 258 (4)
  hemorrhage after operation, 258 (4)
  hypertrophy
    due to infection, 258 (1)
    due to unknown cause, 259 (9)
  lingual
    abscess, 258 (1)
    foreign body in, 258 (4)

Tonsil(s)—Continued
lingual—continued
hypertrophy
due to infection, 258 (1)
due to unknown cause, 259 (9)
Vincent's infection, 258 (1)
lymphosarcoma, 259 (8)
necrosis in granulocytopenia, 259
(5)
neoplasms, 259 (8)
papilloma, squamous cell, 259 (8)
peritonsillar tissue
abscess, 258 (1)
cellulitis, 258 (1)
foreign body in, 259 (4)
hemorrhage due to infection, 258
(1)
resected, infection of, 258 (1)
sarcoma, reticulum cell, 259 (8)
tumors, unlisted, 259 (8)
ulcer, 258 (1)
Vincent's infection, 258 (1)
Tonsillitis
acute, 258 (1)
chronic, 258 (1)
lingual, 258 (1)
Tooth. *See* Teeth
Topagnosis (localization agnosia):
supplementary term, 501. *Diagnose disease*
Topographic classification, 3 ff.
Torsion. *See under name of organ affected*
Torsion spasm: *supplementary term,*
507. *Diagnose disease*
Torticollis
acute, due to cold, 168 (4)
chronic, due to trauma, 168 (4)
congenital, 167 (0)
due to ocular imbalance, 169 (55)
intermittent spastic, 416 (9)
spasm: *supplementary term,* 507.
Diagnose disease
Torus. *Diagnose as* Osteoma, 97
Torus mandibulare, 249 (9)
Torus palatinus, 249 (9)
Touch, disturbances of sensation.
See Agnosia, tactile; Agnosia,
texture: *supplementary terms,*
501; Tactile discrimination, loss
or diminution of; Tactile localization, loss or diminution of: *supplementary terms,* 505

Tower skull. *See also* Acrocephalia,
122 (0)
papilledema due to, 451 (4)
Toxemia of pregnancy, 118 (3)
Toxocara canis test reaction: *supplementary term,* 487. *Diagnose disease*
Toxoplasma infection, 116 (1)
Toxoplasma test reaction: *supplementary term,* 487. *Diagnose disease*
Toxoplasmosis infection, congenital, 381 (1)
Trachea
abnormal union with larynx, 182 (0)
absence, congenital, 187 (0)
adenoma, 188 (8)
calcification due to unknown cause,
188 (9)
carcinoma, epidermoid, 188 (8)
chondroma, 188 (8)
diseases, 187 ff.
diverticulum, congenital, 187 (0)
fistula
congenital, 187 (0)
tracheoesophageal, 187 (0)
due to trauma, 187 (4)
foreign body in, 187 (4)
fracture, 187 (4)
fusion of bifurcation of, and esophagus, 187 (0)
injury, 187 (4)
lipoma, 188 (8)
neoplasms, 188 (8)
rings
arrested development, 187 (0)
incomplete separation, 187 (0)
malformation, 187 (0)
stenosis
congenital, 187 (0)
due to infection, 187 (1)
due to poison, 187 (3)
due to pressure, 187 (4)
due to syphilis, 187 (1)
due to trauma, 187 (4)
of tracheotomy wound, 188 (4)
syphilis, 166 (1)
thyroid aberrant tissue in, 187 (0)
thyroid tissue included in, 187 (0)
tuberculosis, 187 (1)
tumors, unlisted, 188 (8)

Tuberculosis—Continued
  verrucosa of skin, 133 (1)
Tuberculous. *For names of diseases
  preceded by this qualifying term,
  see under the principal term, as*
  Pericarditis, tuberculous
Tubes. *See specific name of tube, as*
  Eustachian; Fallopian
Tularemia, 116 (1)
  bronchopneumonia, 193 (1)
Tumor(s). *See* Etiological classification, 93 ff. *See also name of specific tumor in category 8 under
  organ, region or structure affected. If not found, see* "Unlisted
  tumor of . . ." *and complete code
  by specifying appropriate site and
  neoplasm.*
  Abrikossoff's. *Diagnose as* Granu-
    lar cell myoblastoma, 96
  acoustic nerve. *Diagnose as* Schwan-
    noma, 95
  adenomatoid
    of bronchus. *Diagnose as* Ade-
      noma, 94
    except of bronchus and testis. *Di-
      agnose as* Mesothelioma, 97
    of testis. *Diagnose as* Embryonal
      carcinoma of testis, 98
  adrenal clear cell (ovary). *Diagnose
    as* Virilizing tumor, 93
  adrenal cortical rest (testis), 94
  aneurysmal. *Diagnose as* Hemangi-
    oma (angioma), 96
  apocrine. *Diagnose as* Sweat gland
    tumor, 94
  appendage cell (skin). *Diagnose as*
    Adenoma, 94
  argentaffin. *Diagnose as* Argentaf-
    finoma, 95
  basal cell
    of bronchus. *Diagnose as* Specific
      tumors of epithelium, 93
    except of bronchus. *Diagnose as*
      Basal cell carcinoma, 94
  basophilic, 94
  botryoid. *Diagnose as* Mesenchymal
    mixed tumor, 98
  Brenner, 98
  calcified. *Diagnose as* Neoplastic
    cyst, not otherwise specified, 93

Tumor(s)—Continued
  calcifying giant cell. *Diagnose as*
    Chondroblastoma, 97
  carotid body, 98
  cells: *supplementary terms. Diag-
    nose disease*
    in ascitic or peritoneal fluid, 497
    in bronchial secretions (malig-
      nant), 490
    in cerebrospinal fluid, 507
    in cervical or vaginal secretions,
      499
    in gastric secretions, 497
    in kidney secretions, 499
    in pleural fluid (malignant), 490
    in sputum, 497
    in urinary secretions, 499
  central giant cell. *Diagnose as* Giant
    cell tumor of bone, 97
  cerebellopontine angle. *Diagnose as*
    Schwannoma, 95
  chromaffin. *Diagnose as* Pheochro-
    mocytoma, 95
  chromophobe, 94
  clear cell. *Diagnose as* Virilizing
    tumor, 73
  Codman's. *Diagnose as* Chondro-
    blastoma, 97
  compound ovarian. *Diagnose as* Ter-
    atoma, 97
  cystic. *See also* Cyst
    of tendon sheath. *Diagnose as*
      Ganglion of tendon sheath, 97
    serous papillary, 93
  dysontogenetic, 98
  ectopic ovarian. *Diagnose as* Tera-
    toma, 97
  embryonal. *See also* Embryoma
    mixed. *Diagnose as* Mesenchymal
      mixed tumor, 98
  eosinophilic, 94
    of sweat gland. *Diagnose as*
      Sweat gland tumor, 94
  epidermoid
    benign. *Diagnose as* Squamous
      cell papilloma, 94
    malignant. *Diagnose as* Epider-
      moid carcinoma, 94
  epiphyseal giant cell. *Diagnose as*
    Chondroblastoma, 97
  epithelial. *Diagnose as* Epithelioma,
    not otherwise specified, 94

Tumor(s)—Continued

of epithelium, specific, 93

erectile. *Diagnose as* Hemangioma (angioma), 96

Ewing's. *Diagnose as* Ewing's sarcoma, 97

exocrine. *Diagnose as* Sweat gland tumor, 94

fat cell, primitive. *Diagnose as* Fetal fat cell lipoma, 97

fatty. *See also* Tumors of lipoid tissue, 97

benign. *Diagnose as* Lipoma, 97

feminizing, 93

giant cell

of bone, 97

except bone, 97

peripheral (gum). *Diagnose as* Giant cell tumor except bone, 97

glomus. *Diagnose as* Glomangioma, 96

granulosa cell, 93

Grawitz

except of ovary. *Diagnose as* Adenocarcinoma, 94

of ovary. *Diagnose as* Virilizing tumor, 93

hilus cell (ovary). *Diagnose as* Virilizing tumor, 93

Hürthle cell, 94

salivary gland. *Diagnose as* Adenolymphoma, 98

hypernephroid

except of ovary. *Diagnose as* Adenocarcinoma, 94

of ovary. *Diagnose as* Virilizing tumor, 93

interstitial cell, 93

islet cell

functioning, 93

non-functioning, 93

not otherwise specified. *Diagnose as* Non-functioning islet cell tumor, 94

Krukenberg, 93

Langhans'. *Diagnose as* Hürthle cell tumor, 94

large cell, small alveolar (thyroid). *Diagnose as* Hürthle cell tumor, 94

Leydig cell. *Diagnose as* Interstitial cell tumor, 93

Tumor(s)—Continued

lipid or lipoid cell (ovary). *Diagnose as* Virilizing tumor, 93

list, 93 ff.

macrofolliculoid granulosa cell. *Diagnose as* Granulosa cell tumor, 93

malignancy code (behavior), 99

masculinizing. *Diagnose as* Virilizing tumor, 93

medullary, functioning (adrenal). *Diagnose as* Pheochromocytoma, 95

of melanoblast, not otherwise specified, 94

melanotic, malignant. *Diagnose as* Melanoma, 94

mesenchymal. *Diagnose as* Mesenchymal mixed tumor, 98

benign. *Diagnose as* Mesenchymoma, 98

mixed, 98

mesodermal mixed. *Diagnose as* Mesenchymal mixed tumor, 98

microfolliculoid granulosa cell. *Diagnose as* Granulosa cell tumor, 93

of breast. *Diagnose as* Cystosarcoma phyllodes, 97

of bronchus. *Diagnose as* Adenoma, 94

of pharynx. *Diagnose as* Epidermoid carcinoma, 94

salivary gland type, 98

of bronchus. *Diagnose as* Adenoma, 94

of skin. *Diagnose as* Baso-squamous carcinoma, 94

of testis. *Diagnose as* Embryonal carcinoma of testis, 98

monocellular (testis). *Diagnose as* Disgerminoma, 97

mucoepidermoid. *Diagnose as* Myoepithelial tumor, 98

myeloid. *Diagnose as* Plasma cell myeloma, 95

myeloplaxic. *Diagnose as* Giant cell tumor of bone, 97

myoepidermoid. *Diagnose as* Myoepithelial tumor, 98

myoepithelial, 98

Tumor(s)—Continued
Nelaton's. *Diagnose as* Teratoma, 97
nerve sheath, specific. *Diagnose as* Schwannoma, 95
odontogenic
benign, 98
malignant. *Diagnose as* Adamantinocarcinoma, 98
of osseous tissue, 97
osteogenic. *Diagnose as* Osteoma, 97
malignant. *Diagnose as* Osteosarcoma (osteogenic sarcoma), 97
papillary, not otherwise specified, 93
parathyroid, functionally hyperactive, 93
parenchymatous granulosa cell. *Diagnose as* Granulosa cell tumor, 93
pineal. *Diagnose as* Pinealoma, 98
polypoid or papillary, not otherwise specified, 93
pseudoadenomatous granulosa cell. *Diagnose as* Granulosa cell tumor, 93
pseudomucinous cystic, 93
Rathke's pouch. *Diagnose as* Craniopharyngioma, 98
rete cell, 94
rhabdomyoblastic mixed. *Diagnose as* Mesenchymal mixed tumor, 98
Sampson's. *Diagnose as* Adenomyosis, 98
Schneeberg. *Diagnose as* Carcinoma, not otherwise specified, 94
sebaceous, 94
serous papillary cystic, 93
Sertoli cell, 94
solid, of sweat gland. *Diagnose as* Sweat gland tumor, 95
Spiegler's. *Diagnose as* Neoplastic cyst, 93
structural and functional changes due to, 98
sweat gland, 94
sympathicotropic (ovary). *Diagnose as* Virilizing tumor, 93
teratoid. *Diagnose as* Teratoma, 97
mixed, of testis. *Diagnose as* Embryonal carcinoma of testis, 98
theca cell, 93

Tumor(s)—Continued
thyroid. *See* Thyroid gland, tumors
trophoblastic
benign. *Diagnose as* Hydatiform mole, 97
malignant. *Diagnose as* Choriocarcinoma, 97
turban. *Diagnose as* Neoplastic cyst, 93
of vascular tissue origin, 96
virilizing, 93
Warthin's. *Diagnose as* Adenolymphoma, 98
Wilms'. *Diagnose as* Nephroblastoma, 98
Tunica vaginalis
calcification, 338 (9)
calculus, 337 (6)
chylocele
filarial, 337 (2)
non-filarial, 337 (5)
diseases, 337 ff.
fibroma, 338 (8)
hemangioma, 338 (8)
hematocele
congenital, 337 (0)
due to trauma, 337 (4)
due to unknown cause, 338 (9)
induced during delivery, 337 (0)
hydrocele
acute, due to infection, 337 (1)
acute inflammatory, cause unknown, 338 (9)
acute suppurative, 337 (1)
chronic, due to infection, 337 (1)
congenital, 337 (0)
due to trauma, 337 (4)
due to unknown cause, 338 (9)
senile, 337 (7)
infection, acute, 337 (1)
injury, 337 (4)
lipoma, 338 (8)
mesenchymal mixed tumor, 338 (8)
mesothelioma, 338 (8)
myxoma, 338 (8)
neoplasms, 338 (8)
neurofibroma, 338 (8)
rhabdomyoma, 338 (8)
sarcoma, 338 (8)
teratoma, 338 (8)
tumors, unlisted, 338 (8)

Umbilical cord—Continued
lateral insertion, 385 (6)
phlebitis of umbilical vein, 385
prolapse, 385 (6)
rupture due to trauma, 385 (4)
strangulation, 385 (4)
velamentous insertion, 385 (6)
Umbilicus
granuloma, 123 (1)
hernia, 310 (6)
congenital, 298 (0)
recurrent, 300 (4)
inflammation. *See* Omphalitis, 299
(1)
strangulation, 300 (5)
Uncinariasis. *See* Ancylostomiasis,
124 (2)
Undescended testes. *See also* Crypt-
orchidism, 332 (0)
unilateral, 332 (0)
Undulant fever. *See* Brucellosis,
114 (1)
Unguis incarnatus, 137 (4)
Untruthfulness. *See* Mendacity,
pathologic: *supplementary term,*
485
Urachus
abscess, 317 (1)
cyst, 320 (6)
patent, 317 (0)
Urbach-Oppenheim disease. *See*
Necrobiosis lipoidica diabeticorum, 139 (7)
Urea excretion, abnormal: *supplementary term,* 498. *Diagnose disease*
Uremia
amaurosis in, 447 (3)
amblyopia in, 447 (3)
pericarditis in, 209 (3)
supplementary term, 493. *Diagnose
disease*
ulcer of stomach due to, 264 (3)
Ureter(s)
abscess, periureteral, 314 (1)
absence, congenital, 313 (0)
adenocarcinoma, 315 (8)
angulation, 315 (6)
bifurcation, congenital, 313 (0)
calcification due to unknown cause,
316 (9)
calculus, 315 (6)
due to sulfonamide, 314 (3)

Ureter(s)—Continued
carcinoma
epidermoid, 315 (8)
transitional cell, 315 (8)
contracture of ureterovesical orifice
due to infection, 314 (1)
cyst at ureterovesical orifice, congenital, 313 (0)
dilatation, congenital, 313 (0)
diseases, 313 ff.
diverticulum
acquired, due to unknown cause,
315 (6)
congenital, 313 (0)
due to stress, 314 (4)
at ureterovesical orifice, congenital, 313 (0)
double, 313 (0)
with double pelvis, 313 (0)
fibroma, 315 (8)
fistula
due to trauma, 314 (4)
of ureter and common iliac artery due to infection, 314
(1)
ureteroduodenal, 314 (1), 315 (6)
ureterorectal, 314 (4)
ureterosigmoid, 315 (6)
ureterovaginal, 314 (4)
vesicoureteral, 318 (1)
foreign body in, 314 (4)
hemangiosarcoma, 315 (8)
hydroureter, 313 (0), 315 (6)
implantation, anomalous, 313 (0)
injury, 314 (4)
operative, 314 (4)
intussusception, 315 (6)
leiomyosarcoma, 315 (8)
leukoplakia
due to infection, 314 (1)
of pelvis and, due to unknown
cause, 316 (9)
liposarcoma, 315 (8)
lymphangioma, 315 (8)
lymphangiosarcoma, 315 (8)
malacoplakia, 314 (1)
neoplasms, 316 (8)
neurofibroma, 315 (8)
obstruction by pressure, 314 (4)
occlusion
congenital, 313 (0)
by pressure, 314 (4)

Ureter(s)—Continued

opening, displacement, congenital, 313 (0)

papilloma, squamous cell, 315 (8)

polyp, 315 (8)

prolapse, 315 (6)

pyoureter, 314 (1)

redundancy, congenital, 313 (0)

retrocaval, 313 (0)

rupture due to trauma, 314 (4)

sarcoma, 315 (8)

spastic constriction, 314 (55)

stricture

  congenital, 313 (0)

  due to infection, 314 (1)

  due to trauma, 314 (4)

  following operation, 314 (4)

teratoma, 315 (8)

triplication, 313 (0)

tumors, unlisted, 316 (8)

valve formation, 315 (6)

  congenital, 313 (0)

Ureteritis. *See also* Periureteritis, 314 (1)

acute, 314 (1)

chronic, 314 (1)

cystica, 316 (9)

due to calculus, 315 (6)

due to catheter, 314 (4)

due to diathermy, 314 (4)

due to poison, 314 (3)

due to radium, 314 (4)

Ureterocele

acquired, 315 (6)

congenital, 313 (0)

Urethra

abscess, 322 (1)

absence, congenital, 322 (0)

adenocarcinoma, 325 (8)

adhesions of prostatic portion following operation, 324 (4)

atresia, congenital, 322 (0)

calculus, 325 (6)

carcinoma

  epidermoid, 325 (8)

  papillary, 325 (8)

caruncle, 325 (9)

cellulitis, periurethral, 323 (1)

chancroid (Ducrey's bacillus), 323 (1)

chill and fever, urethral, due to trauma, 324 (4)

deformity, acquired, due to unknown cause, 325 (6)

Urethra—Continued

dilatation, acquired, due to unknown cause, 325 (6)

diseases, 322 ff.

diverticulum

  congenital, 322 (0)

  due to trauma, 324 (4)

  following operation, 324 (4)

double (bifurcation), 322 (0)

double meatus urinarius, 322 (0)

electric burn, 324 (4)

fibroma, 325 (8)

fistula

  congenital, 322 (0)

  due to trauma, 324 (4)

  penile, due to infection, 323 (1)

  urethroperineal, 323 (1)

    following operations, 324 (4)

  urethrorectal

    congenital, 322 (0)

    due to infection, 323 (1)

    due to trauma, 324 (4)

    following operations, 324 (4)

  urethroscrotal, 323 (1)

  urethrovaginal

    following operations, 324 (4)

    following parturition, 324 (4)

foreign body in (exogenous), 324 (4)

hemangioma, 325 (8)

hemorrhage

  due to unknown cause, 325 (9)

infection due to trauma, 324 (4)

inflammation. *See* Urethritis

injury, 324 (4)

laceration following parturition, 324 (4)

leukoplakia

  due to infection, 323 (1)

  due to unknown cause, 326 (9)

malacoplakia, 323 (1)

meatitis, 323 (1)

melanoma, 325 (8)

neoplasms, 325 (8)

  squamous cell, 325 (8)

paramedial vesicourethral orifice, 317 (0)

paraurethral ducts, infection, 323 (1)

polyp, 325 (8)

prolapse

  of bladder mucosa into, 317 (0)

  congenital, 322 (0)

  following parturition, 324 (4)

Urethra—Continued
prolapse—continued
of meatus urinarius, 325 (6)
radium burn, 324 (4)
rupture
due to infection, 323 (1)
due to trauma, 324 (4)
sarcoma, 325 (8)
shortening, congenital, 322 (0)
stricture
congenital, 322 (0)
due to infection, 323 (1)
due to medication, 324 (3)
due to trauma, 325 (4)
following operation, 324 (4)
of meatus urinarius, 322 (0)
spasmodic, due to trauma, 325 (4)
syphilis (including chancre), 323
(1)
teratoma, 325 (8)
tumors, unlisted, 325 (8)
ulcer of meatus urinarius, 326 (9)
valve formation, congenital, 322 (0)
varix, 325 (6)
wound caused by instrument, 324
(4)
Urethral glands
abscess, 322 (1)
cyst, 323 (1)
Urethritis
acute, 323 (1)
allergic, 324 (3)
anterior, chronic, 323 (1)
chronic, 323 (1)
polypoid, 324 (1)
with conjunctivitis and arthritis
(Reiter's disease), 116 (1)
due to Gonococcus, 323 (1)
due to medication, 324 (3)
due to remote infection, 323 (1)
following gonococcic infection, 323
(1)
granular, 323 (1)
posterior, chronic, 323 (1)
Urethrocele, 325 (4)
Urhidrosis, 139 (7)
Uricacidemia: *supplementary term,*
495. *Diagnose disease*
Urinary system
diseases, 307 ff.
pain referable to: *supplementary
term,* 499. *Diagnose disease*

Urinary system—Continued
tumor cells in secretions: *supplementary term,* 499. *Diagnose
disease*
Urination
frequency of micturition: *supplementary term,* 498. *Diagnose
disease*
painful. *See* Dysuria: *supplementary term,* 498
suppressed. *See* Anuria: *supplementary term,* 498
Urine
abnormal chemical substances in:
supplementary term, 499. *Diagnose disease*
acetone bodies in. *See* Acetonuria:
supplementary term, 498
acid-fast bacilli, nonpathogenic, in:
supplementary term, 498. *Diagnose disease*
acidity, abnormal: *supplementary
term,* 498. *Diagnose disease*
albumin in. *See* Albuminuria, 498
alkalinity, abnormal: *supplementary
term,* 498. *Diagnose disease*
ammoniacal: *supplementary term,*
498. *Diagnose disease*
bacteria in. *See* Bacteriuria: *supplementary term,* 498
Bence-Jones protein in: *supplementary term,* 498. *Diagnose disease*
bile pigments in: *supplementary
term,* 498. *Diagnose disease*
blood in. *See* Hematuria, 498
casts in: *supplementary term,* 498.
Diagnose disease
cystine in. *See* Cystinosis, 120 (7)
electrolyte content, abnormal: *supplementary term,* 498. *Diagnose
disease*
epithelial cells in: *supplementary
term,* 498. *Diagnose disease*
extravasation, 320 (6)
incontinence
stress, 319 (4)
supplementary term, 498. *Diagnose
disease*
pentose in. *See* Pentosuria, 120 (7)
pus in. *See* Pyuria: *supplementary
term,* 499

Urine—Continued
retention: *supplementary term,* 499.
Diagnose disease
sugar in. *See* Glycosuria
tubercle bacillus in: *supplementary
term,* 499. *Diagnose disease*
yeast cells in: *supplementary term,*
499. *Diagnose disease*
Urogenital system
congenital defects, 306 (0)
diseases, 306 ff.
psychophysiologic genito-urinary reaction, 111 (55)
Urticaria, 136 (3)
of conjunctiva, 469 (3)
giant. *See* Angioneurotic edema, 138
(55)
of larynx, 184 (3)
papular, 136 (3)
pigmentosa, 132 (0)
Usher-Senear disease. *See* Pemphigus erythematosus, 141 (9)
Uterine vessels. *See* Uterus, blood
vessels
Uterus. *See also* Cervix uteri; Endometritis; Endometrium; Metritis;
Myometrium, hyperplasia
abnormal communication
with anterior abdominal wall, 306
(0)
with bladder, 306 (0)
between rectum and, 327 (0)
abscess, parauterine, 360 (1)
absence, 360 (0)
with absence of vagina, 355 (0)
actinomycosis, 364 (8)
adenocarcinoma, 364 (8)
adhesions, parauterine, 360 (1)
due to trauma, 361 (4)
following parturition, 362 (4)
anteflexion
due to infection, 360 (1)
due to unknown or uncertain
cause, 362 (6)
following parturition, 361 (4)
atony due to unknown cause, 376
(x)
atresia
congenital, 360 (0)
due to infection, 361 (1)
atrophy
puerperal lactation, 375 (7)
senile, 364 (7)

Uterus—Continued
bicornis, 360 (0)
double vagina with, 355 (0)
blood in. *See* Hematometra, 362 (6)
blood vessels, arteriosclerosis, 364
(9)
carcinosarcoma, 364 (8)
contraction, abnormal, due to obstructed labor, 375 (6)
contraction or constriction ring, 375
(55)
cyst, embryonal, 360 (0)
didelphys, 360 (0)
diseases, 360 ff.
displacement
due to infection, 360 (1)
following operation, 361 (4)
following parturition, 361 (4)
metrorrhagia due to, 362 (6)
embryoma. *Diagnose as* Mesenchymal mixed tumor, 98
fetalis, 360 (0)
fibroma; fibromyoma. *Diagnose as*
Leiomyoma, 96
fistula
due to infection, 361 (1)
uterorectal, due to infection, 361
(1)
vesicouterine, due to infection, 318
(1)
hemorrhage
due to lacerations, 375 (4)
due to partial separation of placenta, 375 (6)
due to retained secundines, 375 (6)
due to trauma, 375 (4)
due to undetermined cause, 376
(y)
postpartum, due to uterine inertia,
375 (55)
hyperinvolution, 375 (7)
hypoplasia due to ovarian hypofunction, 364 (7)
inertia
intrapartum, 375 (55)
postpartum hemorrhage due to,
375 (5)
infantile, 364 (7)
injury, 361 (4)
innervation, disturbance of sympathetic and parasympathetic, 362
(55)

Uterus—Continued
instrumentation wound, 361 (4)
inversion
  due to traction, 361 (4)
  following parturition, 361 (4)
lateral flexion
  due to infection, 360 (1)
  due to unknown or uncertain
    cause, 362 (6)
  following parturition, 361 (4)
lateral version
  due to unknown or uncertain cause,
    362 (6)
  following parturition, 361 (4)
laterocession due to unknown or uncertain cause, 362 (6)
leiomyosarcoma, 364 (8)
myofibroma. *Diagnose as* Leiomyoma, 96
myoma (fibroid), 364 (8)
neoplasms, 364 (8)
polyp
  neoplastic, 364 (8)
  simple, 365 (9)
pregnant
  atony due to anesthetic, 374 (3)
  contraction, abnormal, 375 (55)
    due to ergot, 374 (3)
    due to pituitary extract, 374
      (3)
  hernia, 375 (6)
  injury, 374 (4)
  inversion due to unknown cause,
    375 (6)
  penetration by instrument, 374 (4)
  prolapse, 375 (6)
  retrodisplacement, 375 (6)
  retroflexion, 375 (6)
  retroversion, 375 (6)
  rupture, 375 (4)
    due to obstructed labor, 375 (6)
    due to uterine scar, 374 (4)
  sacculation, 375 (6)
  torsion, 375 (6)
  tumor, 376 (8)
prolapse
  congenital, 360 (0)
  due to unknown or uncertain
    cause, 362 (6)
  following parturition, 361 (4)

Uterus—Continued
puerperal
  inversion
    due to traction, 374 (4)
    due to trauma, 374 (4)
pus in. *See* Pyometra, 361 (1)
retrodisplacement due to unknown
  or uncertain cause, 362 (6)
retroflexion
  congenital, 360 (0)
  due to infection, 360 (1)
  due to unknown or uncertain
    cause, 362 (6)
  following parturition, 361 (4)
retroversion
  congenital, 360 (0)
  due to infection, 360 (1)
  due to unknown or uncertain
    cause, 362 (6)
  following parturition, 361 (4)
rudimentary, 360 (0)
  in male, 327 (0)
rupture. *See* Uterus, pregnant, rupture
scar following operation, 362 (4)
squamous epithelium in uterine mucosa, 360 (0)
stricture
  due to infection, 361 (1)
  following operation, 362 (4)
subinvolution, 375 (7)
tumors, unlisted, 364 (8)
two distinct uteri, 360 (0)
unicornis, 360 (0)
unilateral vagina with, 355 (0)
Utricle, prostatic. *See* Utriculus
  masculinus
Utriculus masculinus
cyst due to infection, 324 (1)
infection, 324 (1)
Uvea. *See* Uveal tract; Uveitis
Uveal tract
infection, detachment of retina due
  to, 447 (1)
melanoma, malignant, 440 (8)
Uveitis
cataract due to, 442 (1)
due to phaco-anaphylactic, 440 (3)
melanosis of cornea following, 435
  (1)

Uveitis—Continued
  sympathetic, 439 (1)
Uvula
  abscess, 250 (1)
  absence, congenital, 250 (0)
  carcinoma
    basal cell, 251 (8)
    epidermoid, 251 (8)
    transitional cell, 251 (8)
  deformity due to infection, 250 (1)
  diseases, 250 ff.
  duplication (bifid uvula), 250 (0)
  elongation
    acquired, 251 (6)
    congenital, 250 (0)
  lymphosarcoma, 251 (8)
  neoplasms, 251 (8)
  paralysis
    due to lead, 250 (3)
    due to pressure on nerves, 250 (55)
    following diphtheria, 250 (1)
    supplementary term, 497. *Diagnose disease*
  sarcoma, 251 (8)
  shortening, congenital, 250 (0)
  tumors, unlisted, 251 (8)
Uvulitis, 250 (1)

V

Vaccination
  reaction, general, 118 (3)
  smallpox, reactions to: *supplementary terms,* 487
  successful: *supplementary term,* 488. *Diagnose disease*
Vaccine
  meningismus, or aseptic meningitis, due to, 406 (3)
Vaccinia, 116 (1)
  of conjunctiva, 469 (1)
  lesions of lid in, 462 (1)
  localized, 124 (1)
  supplementary term, 488. *Diagnose disease*
Vagabondage: *supplementary term,* 486. *Diagnose disease*
Vagal nerve. *See* Vagus nerve
Vagina
  aberrant sebaceous glands at junction of vulva and, 351 (0)

Vagina—Continued
  abscess
    paravaginal, 355 (1)
    of wall, 355 (1)
  absence, congenital, with absence of uterus, 355 (0)
  atresia, 355 (0)
    senile, 357 (7)
    vaginitis due to, 357 (6)
  atrophy, senile, 357 (7)
  bleeding: *supplementary term,* 499. *Diagnose disease*
  blood in. *See* Hematocolpos, 357 (6)
  carcinoma, epidermoid, 357 (8)
  chemical burn, 356 (3)
  cyst, 356 (6)
    embryonal, 355 (0)
  diphtheria, 355 (1)
  diseases, 355 ff.
  double, 355 (0)
  embryoma. *Diagnose as* Mesenchymal mixed tumor, 98
  fibroma, 357 (8)
  fibromyxoma. *Diagnose as* Mesenchymal mixed tumor, 98
  fibromyxosarcoma. *Diagnose as* Mesenchymal mixed tumor, 98
  fistula
    anovaginal, following parturition, 356 (4)
    rectovaginal
      congenital, 355 (0)
      due to infection, 355 (1)
      due to radium, 356 (4)
      due to trauma, 356 (4)
      following operation, 356 (4)
      obstetric, 375 (4)
    ureterovaginal
      due to trauma, 314 (4)
      following operation, 314 (4)
    urethrovaginal
      due to infection, 323 (1)
      following operation, 324 (4)
      following parturition, 324 (4)
    vaginocutaneous, following parturition, 356 (4)
    vesicovaginal
      congenital, 355 (0)
      due to infection, 318 (1)
      due to trauma, 356 (4)

Vagina—Continued
fistula, vesicovaginal—continued
  obstetric, 375 (4)
  postoperative, 356 (4)
foreign body in, 357 (6)
inclusion cyst following operation,
  356 (4)
inflammation. *See* Colpitis; Vaginitis
injury (not obstetric), 356 (4)
kraurosis, 357 (9)
laceration, obstetric, 374 (4)
melanoma, malignant, 357 (8)
mesenchymal mixed tumor, malignant, 357 (8)
moniliasis (candidiasis), 356 (2)
myosarcoma of infant's. *Diagnose as*
  Mesenchymal mixed tumor, 98
myxofibroma. *Diagnose as* Mesenchymal mixed tumor, 98
myxofibrosarcoma. *Diagnose as*
  Mesenchymal mixed tumor, 98
myxoma. *Diagnose as* Mesenchymal
  mixed tumor, 98
myxosarcoma. *Diagnose as* Mesenchymal mixed tumor, 98
necrosis in granulocytopenia, 356
  (5)
neoplasms, 357 (8)
parasitic infection, 356 (2)
prolapse, 357 (6)
pus in. *See* Pyocolpos, 355 (1)
rectovaginal septum, tear, 356 (4)
rudimentary, 355 (0)
septum, congenital, 355 (0)
stenosis, congenital, 355 (0)
stricture
  due to infection, 355 (1)
  due to trauma, 356 (4)
tear, 356 (4)
Trichomonas infection, 355 (1)
tumor cells in secretions: *supplementary term,* 499. *Diagnose
  disease*
tumors, unlisted, 357 (8)
ulceration due to prolapse, 356 (6)
unilateral (with uterus unicornis),
  355 (0)
urogenital sinus communication
  with, 327 (0)

Vaginismus, 356 (55)
supplementary term, 499. *Diagnose
  disease*
Vaginitis, 355 (1). *See also* Colpitis;
  Vulvovaginitis
due to foreign body, 356 (4)
due to obstruction (atresia), 357
  (6)
due to pressure, 356 (4)
emphysematous, 355 (1)
exfoliative, due to trauma, 356 (4)
paravaginitis, 355 (1)
senile, 357 (7)
Vagotonia, 417 (x)
Vagrancy: *supplementary term,* 486.
  Diagnose disease
Vagus nerve
disturbances: *supplementary term,*
  508. *Diagnose disease*
Valley fever. *See* Coccidioidosis, generalized, 114 (1)
Valves, cardiac. *See* Heart, valves;
  and under specific name of valve
Valvulitis. *See* Heart, valvulitis
Vapors
suffocation by nonpoisonous, 119 (4)
Vaquez-Osler disease. *See* Polycythemia vera, 230 (8)
Varicella. *See* Chickenpox, 114 (1)
Varicocele, 342 (6)
thrombosed, 342 (6)
Varicose veins. *See also* Varicosities; Varix
of breast, 144 (6)
due to unknown cause, 225 (9)
with infection, 225 (6)
of leg, 225 (6)
of nasal septum, 178 (6)
Varicosities. *See also* Varicose
  veins; Varix
of urethra, 325 (6)
of vessels of mouth, 241 (6)
of vulva due to pregnancy, 375 (4)
Variola. *See* Smallpox, 116 (1)
Varix. *See also* Varicose veins; Varicosities, 128 (6)
aneurysmal, of vein, 225 (0)
of bladder, 320 (6)
of colon, 278 (6)
compression of spinal cord by, 423
  (4)
due to passive congestion, 225 (5)

Varix—Continued
due to trauma, constant or intermittent, 225 (4)
of esophagus, 261 (6)
congenital, 260 (0)
gastric, 265 (6)
of orbit, 459 (6)
congenital, 458 (0)
of renal papilla, 310 (6)
rupture, 225 (4)
of trachea, 188 (6)
of vocal cord, 185 (6)
of vulva, 353 (6)
Vas deferens
absence, congenital, 341 (0)
atresia, congenital, 341 (0)
diseases, 341 ff.
infection, 341 (1)
inflammation due to poison, 341 (3)
injury, 341 (4)
rupture, 341 (4)
stricture
due to infection, 341 (1)
due to trauma, 341 (4)
Vasa previa, 383 (6)
Vascular disease. *See also* Blood
vessels; Cardiovascular system
hypertensive, 217 (5)
Vasitis
due to infection, 341 (1)
due to poison, 341 (3)
Vasomotor disturbances
hydrorrhea due to, 178 (5)
supplementary term, 507. *Diagnose disease*
Vasovagal attacks, paroxysmal, 417 (x)
Vater, ampulla of
variations of common bile duct and
pancreatic duct openings into,
292 (0)
Vegetative nervous system. *See*
Nervous system, vegetative
Vein(s). *See also name of specific vein*
anomaly, 224 (0)
collateral distention, 225 (5)
diseases, 224 ff.
inflammation. *See* Phlebitis
injury, 224 (4)
obstruction, 225 (6)
edema due to, 128 (5)

Vein(s)—Continued
phlebolith, 225 (6)
poisoning, 224 (3)
recanalization: *supplementary term,*
492. *Diagnose disease*
sclerosis. *See* Phlebosclerosis, 225
(9)
thrombosis
due to polycythemia, 225 (5)
due to thrombocytosis, 225 (5)
due to trauma, 225 (4)
due to unspecified cause, 225 (6)
elephantiasis due to, 128 (5)
following operation, 225 (4)
tuberculosis, 224 (1)
varix, 225 (0)
Veldt sore, 142 (9)
Vena cava
persistent left superior, 205 (0)
superior, absence, 205 (0)
Venereal disease. *See under name of
specific disease and organ or region affected*
Venom poisoning, 118 (3)
Venous hemangioma. *Diagnose as*
Hemangioma (angioma), 96
Ventral hernia, 298 (0), 300 (4)
Ventral horn cells. *See* Spinal cord,
cells
Ventricles of brain. *See* Brain, ventricles
fifth. *See* Cavum septi pellucidi
Ventricular abnormalities, 203 (0)
Ventricular arrhythmia
unspecified: *supplementary term,*
492. *Diagnose disease*
Ventricular escape
due to unknown cause, 214 (x)
supplementary term, 492. *Diagnose
disease*
Ventricular fibrillation
due to unknown cause, 214 (x)
supplementary term, 492. *Diagnose
disease*
Ventricular paroxysmal tachycardia
due to unknown cause, 214 (x)
supplementary term, 492. *Diagnose
disease*

Ventricular premature contractions
due to unknown cause, 214 (x)
supplementary term, 492. Diagnose disease
Ventricular septal defects, 203 (0)
Ventricular standstill
due to unknown cause, 214 (x)
supplementary term, 492. Diagnose disease
Verruca
acuminata, 134 (1). *See also* Condyloma acuminatum
peruana or peruviana. *See* Verruga peruana, 134 (1)
plana, 134 (1)
wart, 134 (1)
Verruga peruana, 134 (1)
Vertebra(e). *See also* Spine
absence, congenital, 146 (0)
arch, fusion defect, 147 (0)
atrophy
due to infection, 147 (1)
neurogenic, due to tabes dorsalis, 152 (55)
senile, 153 (7)
compression of spinal cord by, 423 (4)
dislocation, compression of spinal cord by, 423 (4)
fracture, compression of spinal cord by, 423 (4)
hemivertebra, 146 (0)
lumbosacral, transitional, 156 (0)
multiple dysplasia, 147 (0)
osteochondrosis with thoracic kyphosis, 155 (9)
sacralization of fifth lumbar, with sciatica and scoliosis (Bertolotti's syndrome), 156 (0)
supernumerary, 146 (0)
tuberculosis, 149 (1)
Vertex presentation, 382 (6)
Vertigo: *supplementary term, 510. Diagnose disease*
aural. *See* Ménière's syndrome, 480 (9) ; *supplementary term,* 509
Verumontanum. *See also* Colliculitis, 323 (1)
cyst, 325 (6)
hypertrophy, 326 (9)
Vesical; vesico-. *See* Bladder

Vesicles, seminal. *See* Seminal vesicles
Vesiculitis. *See* Seminal vesiculitis, 344 (1)
Vessels. *See* Blood vessels
Vestiges, branchial. *See* Branchial vestiges, 255 (0)
Vibratory sensibility
absence : *supplementary term, 501. Diagnose disease*
diminution : *supplementary term, 503. Diagnose disease*
Vicarious menstruation
nasal, 178 (7)
Villaret syndrome: *supplementary terms, 506. Diagnose disease*
Vincent's gingivitis, 247 (1)
Vincent's infection
of larynx (laryngitis due to Borrelia vincenti), 183 (1)
of mouth, 241 (1)
of tongue, 245 (1)
of tonsils, 258 (1)
Vinson-Plummer syndrome. *See* Anemia, hypochromic microcytic, due to deficient intake, absorption or metabolism of iron, 229 (7)
Violent personality, 112 (x)
Virilism
adrenal cortical hyperfunction with, 397 (7)
with female pseudohermaphroditism, 396 (0)
with male macrogenitosomio precox, 396 (0)
Virilizing tumor, 93
clear cell. *Diagnose as* Virilizing tumor, 93
Virus
bronchopneumonia, 193 (1)
infection of undetermined origin, 116 (1)
myocarditis due to, 208 (1)
Viscera
abdominal
ectopia due to defect in abdominal wall, 240 (0)
transposition, 263 (0). *See also* Situs transversus, 114 (0)
enlargement. *See* Splanchnomegaly, 128 (7)
Visceral larva migrans, 125 (2)

Vomiting—Continued
pernicious, in pregnancy, 118 (3)
supplementary term, 497. *Diagnose disease*
von Gierke's disease, 120 (7)
glycogen infiltration of myocardium in, 211 (7)
hepatic glycogenosis in, 289 (7)
Vossius' ring, 442 (4)
Voyeur-exhibitionist personality, 112 (x)
Vulva
aberrant sebaceous glands at junction of vagina and, 351 (0)
abscess, 352 (1)
absence, 351 (0)
adenocarcinoma, 354 (8)
adenoma, 354 (8)
atresia, superficial, congenital, 351 (0)
atrophy, senile, 353 (7)
carcinoma
basal cell, 354 (8)
epidermoid, 354 (8)
cellulitis, 352 (1)
chancroid (due to Ducrey's bacillus), 352 (1)
condyloma acuminatum due to infection, 352 (1)
cyst
due to lacerations, 353 (4)
embryonal, 351 (0)
diphtheria, 352 (1)
diseases, 351 ff.
edema, obstetric, acute, 374 (4)
elephantiasis, nonfilarial, 353 (5)
epidermophytosis, 352 (2)
erythroplasia of Queyrat, 141 (9)
fibroma, 354 (8)
fistula, vulvorectal
congenital, 351 (0)
due to infection, 352 (1)
due to trauma, 353 (4)
following operation, 353 (4)
gangrene
due to infection, 352 (1)
due to trauma, 353 (4)
hemangioma, 354 (8)
hematoma
during pregnancy, 374 (4)
nonpuerperal, 353 (4)
hemorrhage not due to trauma, 353 (5)

Vulva—Continued
herpes, 352 (1)
hypertrophy due to unknown cause, 354 (9)
infantile, 351 (0)
inflammation. *See* Vulvitis; Vulvovaginitis
injury, 353 (4)
kraurosis, 354 (9)
laceration, obstetric, 374 (4)
leiomyoma, 354 (8)
leukoplakia, 354 (9)
lipoma, 354 (8)
melanoma, 354 (8)
malignant, 354 (8)
mesenchymal mixed tumor, malignant, 354 (8)
neoplasms, 354 (8)
neurofibroma, 354 (8)
pediculosis, 352 (2)
pigmented nevus, 354 (8)
polyp, 354 (8)
pruritus, neurogenic, 353 (55)
sarcoma, 354 (8)
scabies, 352 (2)
sebaceous cyst, 354 (8)
sweat gland tumor, 354 (8)
syphiloma, 352 (1)
thrush, 352 (2)
tumors, unlisted, 354 (8)
ulcer
due to infection, 352 (1)
due to unknown cause, 354 (9)
varix, 353 (6)
due to pregnancy, 375 (4)
vitiligo, 353 (7)
Vulvitis
acute, 352 (1)
due primarily to uncleanliness, 353 (4)
adhesive, congenital, 351 (0)
chronic, 352 (1)
diabetic, 353 (7)
intertriginous, 353 (4)
Vulvovaginitis, 352 (1)

W

Wandering kidney, 308 (0)
Wandering pacemaker
due to unknown cause, 214 (x)
supplementary term, 492. *Diagnose disease*

War gases, poisoning, 118 (3)
Wart. *See also* Verruca, 134 (1)
  venereal. *See* Condyloma acumina-
    tum
Warthin's tumor. *Diagnose as* Ade-
    nolymphoma, 98
Water
  deprivation of, 119 (7)
  intoxication, 120 (7)
  metabolism, disorders, 120 (7)
Wax in ear. *See* Cerumen, impacted,
    476 (6)
Webbed fingers and toes, 132 (0).
    See also Segmentation, failure of,
    122 (0)
Weber, circles of: *supplementary
    term,* 505. *Diagnose disease*
Weber paralysis: *supplementary
    term,* 505. *Diagnose disease*
Weber-Christian disease. *See* Nod-
    ular nonsuppurative panniculitis,
    133 (1)
Weber-Osler-Rendu syndrome,
    219 (9)
Weight
  gain in: *supplementary term,* 485.
    Diagnose disease
  loss in: *supplementary term,* 485.
    Diagnose disease
  sense, loss of. *See* Agnosia, weight:
    supplementary term, 501
Weil's disease. *See* Jaundice, spiro-
    chetal, 115 (1)
Weil-Felix reaction, positive: *sup-
    plementary term,* 486. *Diagnose
    disease*
Wen. *Diagnose as* Neoplastic cyst, not
    otherwise specified, 93
Werlhof's disease. *See* Thrombocy-
    topenic purpura, 229 (7)
**Westphal-Strümpell pseudosclero-
    sis.** *See* Pseudosclerosis, 416 (9)
Wharton's duct
  dilatation due to closure of opening
    in mouth, congenital, 252 (0)
  displacement of opening in mouth,
    252 (0)
  fusion with sublingual duct at open-
    ing in mouth, congenital, 252 (0)
Whipple's disease. *See* Intestinal
    lipodystrophy, 269 (7)
Whitlow, melanotic. *Diagnose as*
    Melanoma, 94

Whitmore's disease. *See* Melioido-
    sis, 114 (7)
Whooping cough (pertussis), 115
    (1)
Wilms' tumor. *Diagnose as* Nephro-
    blastoma, 98
**Wilson's hepatolenticular degener-
    ation.** *See* Hepatolenticular de-
    generation, 414 (7)
Wilson-Kimmelstiel syndrome. *See*
    Intercapillary glomerulosclerosis,
    310 (7)
Witzelsucht (moria): *supplementary
    term,* 485. *Diagnose disease*
Wolff-Parkinson-White syndrome,
    202 (0)
Wolffian adenoma. *Diagnose as* Vir-
    ilizing tumor, 93
Wolffian duct, vestigial cyst, 306
    (0)
Wood alcohol. *See* Methyl alcohol
Word(s)
  blindness: *supplementary term,* 510.
    Diagnose disease
  deafness: *supplementary term,* 510.
    Diagnose disease
  developmental, 510
  misuse. *See* Paraphasia: *supplemen-
    tary term,* 506
  repetition. *See* Palilalia: *supplemen-
    tary term,* 505
  urge to say: *supplementary term,*
    486. *Diagnose disease*
Wound(s), 127 (4). *See also* In-
    juries; *and under organ, region
    or structure affected*
  bullet, multiple, 118 (4)
  infection, 123 (1), 127 (4)
    Bacillus welchi or gas bacillus,
      123 (1)
    diphtheritic, 123 (1)
  operative
    abscess of, 125 (4)
    disruption of, 127 (4)
  penetrating, 127 (4)
  postoperative, 127 (4)
    infected, 127 (4)
  of skin, 137 (4)
  stab, multiple, 119 (4)
Wrist
  arthritis due to pneumococcic infec-
    tion, 157 (1)

Wrist—Continued
 contracture due to spastic paralysis,
 162 (55)
Writer's cramp, 168 (4)
Writing disability. *See* Agraphia,
 501
Wryneck. *See* Torticollis

X

Xanthelasma
 of eyelid, 464 (7)
Xanthofibroma. *Diagnose as* Fibroma, 96
Xanthoma
 diabeticorum, 139 (7)
 disseminatum, 139 (7)
 eruptive, 139 (7)
 fibrous. *Diagnose as* Fibroma, 96
 giant cell. *Diagnose as* Giant cell
 tumor except bone, 97
 of joint, 163 (7)
 of tendon, 174 (7)
 tuberosum multiplex, 139 (7)
Xanthomatosis, 128 (7)
 of bone, 153 (7)
 symptomatic: *supplementary term,*
 486. *Diagnose disease*
Xanthosarcoma, giant cell. *Diagnose as* Giant cell tumor except
 bone, 97
Xeroderma
 follicular. *See* Keratosis pilaris, 141
 (9)
 pigmented, 132 (0)
Xerophthalmia
 night blindness due to, 448 (7)

Xerosis
 of conjunctiva, 470 (7)
 of skin, 132 (0)
Xerostomia, *supplementary term,* 497.
 Diagnose disease
X-rays. *See* Roentgen rays

Y

Yaws. *See* Treponematosis, 116 (1)
Yeast
 cells in urine: *supplementary term,*
 499. *Diagnose disease*
 and molds in feces: *supplementary
 term,* 497. *Diagnose disease*
 and molds in sputum: *supplementary
 term,* 490. *Diagnose disease*
Yellow fever, 116 (1)

Z

Zeiss's gland. *See* Gland of Zeiss
Zinc
 incrustation of cornea, 435 (3)
Zondek-Aschheim test
 reactions to: *supplementary terms,*
 499. *Diagnose disease*
Zoster, 134(1)
 of bladder, 318 (1)
 of conjunctiva, 469 (1)
 herpes, 134 (1)
 of iris, 439 (1)
 ophthalmicus, 450 (1)
 supplementary term, 488. *Diagnosis
 disease*

INDEX
TO
NOMENCLATURE OF OPERATIONS

OPERATIONS INDEX

The number in parentheses refers to the type of operative procedure.

A

Abdomen
drainage, 569 (0)
operations on, 569. *See also specific name of operation*
paracentesis, 570 (0)
wall
  debridement, 571 (6)
  excision of lesion, 570 (1)
  incision and drainage, 570 (0)
  incision and removal of foreign body, 570 (0)
  suture, 571 (7)
Abortion, therapeutic. *See* Pregnancy, termination, 585 (1)
Accessory sinuses. *See* Sinuses, accessory
Acoustic nerve
neurotomy, 594 (0)
Adenoid(s)
operations on, 557. *See also specific name of operation*
tag, excision, 557 (1)
Adenoidectomy, 557 (1)
Adrenal gland(s)
operations on, 589
Adrenalectomy, 589 (1)
Advanced flap
plastic closure of wound by, 526 (5)
Air
filling of extrapleural space with, 546 (3)
injection, 518 (3)
  intraperitoneal, 570 (3)
  intrapleural, 546 (3)
  into lateral ventricles, 593 (3)
  retroperitoneal, 570 (3)
  into subarachnoid space, 591 (3)
Air cells, petrous pyramid. *See under* Operations on middle ear, 604
Albee's operation. *See* Spinal fusion, 533 (5)
Alcohol, injection, 518 (3)
Alimentary tract. *See* Operations on digestive system, 553
Alveolectomy, 555 (1)
Alveolus
incision and drainage, 554 (0)

Alveolus—Continued
plastic repair, 554 (5)
Ampulla of Vater
excision, 567 (1)
Amputation. *See also under organ or structure involved*
of extremities, list, 537 (2), 538 (2)
Anal. *See* Anus
Analgesics, local, 607
Anastomosis, 520 (5). *See also specific name of operation or organ or structure involved*
arterial, 549 (5)
venous, 549 (5)
Anesthesia, 607 ff.
agents, 607
methods, 608
Aneurysm
arterial, excision, 549 (1)
arteriovenous, excision, 549 (1)
operations for, 549, 550. *See also specific name of operation*
suture, 550 (7)
Aneurysmectomy, 549 (1)
Aneurysmorrhaphy, 550 (7)
Angiectomy. *See* Arteriectomy, 549 (1); Phlebectomy, 549 (1)
Angiocardiography, 547 (4)
Angiography, 549 (3)
Angioplasty. *See* Arterioplasty, 549 (5); Lymphangioplasty, 551 (5)
Angiorrhaphy. *See* Arteriorrhaphy, 550 (7); Phleborrhaphy, 550 (7)
Angiotomy. *See* Arteriotomy, 548 (0); Phlebotomy, 548 (0)
Angulation
correction of, 531 (5)
Ankle, amputation at, 538 (2)
Ankylosis
fusion to produce. *See* Arthrodesis, 533 (5); Spinal fusion, 533 (5)
Anoplasty, 566 (5)
Anoscopy
various types, 566 (4)
Anterior tibial tendons
reattachment, 536 (5)
Antibiotic, injection, 518 (3)

Auricle. *See under* Operations on external ear, 604
Auricular ligation, 547 (1)

B

Bacitracin, injection, 518 (3)
Bag
collapsible, insertion, 519 (3)
dilation of esophagus by, 559 (8)
intracervical insertion, 585 (3)
vaginal, insertion, 582 (3)
Balanoplasty, 577 (5)
Barbiturates, 607
Bartholin's gland
excision, 581 (1)
incision and drainage, 581 (0)
Basal hypnotic agents, 607
Basal narcotic agents, 607
Basiotripsy, 587 (6)
Bassini's operation. *See* Hernioplasty, 570 (5)
Bile duct(s)
anastomosis, 568 (5)
excision of cystic remnant, 568 (1)
excision of lesion, 567 (1)
exploration, 567 (0)
incision, 567 (0)
operations on. *See under* Operations on biliary tract, 567 ff.; *and specific name of operation*
plastic repair or reconstruction, 568 (5)
suture, 568 (7)
Biliary tract
biopsy, 568 (1)
fistula, closure, 568 (7)
fistulous, implantation into stomach or intestine, 568 (5)
operations on, 567 ff. *See also specific name of operation*
Billroth's operation. *See* Gastrectomy, 559 (1)
Biopsy. *See also under organ, region or structure involved*
endoscopic, 519 (4)
various types, 525 (1)
Bladder
anastomosis of ureter to, 573 (5)
biopsy, 574 (1)
calculus, crushing, 574 (6)
excision of lesion, 574 (1)

Bladder—Continued
fistula, closure, 575 (7)
rectovesical, 565 (7)
vesicovaginal, 575 (7)
operations on, 574. *See also specific name of operation*
plastic or reconstruction operation on, 575 (5)
reimplantation of ureter into, 573 (5)
suture, 574 (7)
Blalock's anastomosis, 549 (5)
Blepharectomy, 601 (1)
Blepharoplasty, 601 (5)
Blepharorrhaphy, 602 (7)
Blepharotomy, 601 (0)
Blood circulation
collateral, in portal obstruction, omentofixation for, 571 (5)
Blood transfusion
various types, 518 (3), 549 (3)
Blood vessel(s)
graft, 520 (5)
operations on, 548. *See also specific name of operation*
Body regions
operations on, 525 ff.
Bone(s). *See also* Fracture
biopsy, 530 (1)
block, stabilization of joint by, 533 (5)
cutting, division or transection, 530 (0)
debridement, 531 (6)
drainage, 530 (0)
drilling or "windowing" of cortex, 530 (0)
excision for graft, 531 (1)
excision of lesion, 530 (1)
exploration, 530 (0)
freeing of adhesions, etc., 531 (6)
fusion, 531 (5)
graft, 526 (5), 531 (5)
arthroplasty with, 533 (5)
autogenous, 525 (5)
heterologous, 525 (5)
homologous, 525 (5)
plastic operation on skull with, 590 (5)
growth arrest, longitudinal, 531 (5)
insertion or application of traction device, 531 (3)
lengthening, 531 (5)

Canthorrhaphy, 602 (7)
Canthotomy, 601 (0)
Canthus
  division, 601 (0)
  palpebral fissure, suture of, 602 (7)
  plastic repair, 602 (5)
Canula
  insertion into accessory sinus (for
    aspiration or irrigation), 541
    (3)
Capsule of joint
  cutting or division, 532 (0)
  operations on, 532. *See also specific
    name of operation*
  suture or repair, 533 (7)
Capsulectomy
  lens, 599 (1)
  renal, 572 (1)
Capsulorrhaphy (joint), 533 (7)
Capsulotomy
  joint, 532 (0)
  lens, 599 (0)
Cardiac. *See* Heart
Cardiac sphincter, dilation, 559 (8)
Cardiocentesis, 547 (0)
Cardiography, 547 (3)
Cardiolysis, 548 (6)
Cardiopericardiopexy, 547 (3)
Cardioplasty, 558 (5)
Cardiorrhaphy, 548 (7)
Cardiotomy, 547 (0)
Cardiovascular system
  operations on, 547 ff. *See also spe-
    cific name of operation*
Carotid gland, operations on, 589
Carpectomy, 530 (1)
Cartilage(s)
  division of, 532 (0)
  excision, 532 (1)
  graft, 526 (5)
    autogenous, 526 (5)
    heterologous, 526 (5)
    homologous, 526 (5)
  operations on, 532. *See also specific
    name of operation*
Cast, application
  for fracture, 532 (8)
  and manipulation of joint, 533 (8)
  and manipulation of muscle, 535 (8)
Castration
  female, 584 (1)
  male, 577 (1)

Catheter, insertion, 519 (3)
  in bronchus, bronchoscopy with, 543
    (4)
  endoscopic, 519 (4)
  urethroscopy with, 576 (4)
Catheterization, 519 (3)
  of eustachian tube, 605 (3)
  of heart, 547 (3)
Cauterization, 526 (6) ; *footnote,* 517
  of lesion of anus, 566 (6)
Cavernostomy, 544 (0)
Cecectomy, 561 (1)
Cecocolostomy, 562 (5)
Cecopexy, 562 (5)
Cecosigmoidostomy, 562 (5)
Cecostomy, 562 (5)
  closure, 563 (7)
Cecotomy, 561 (0)
Cecum
  fistula, fecal, closure, 563 (7)
  fixation to abdominal wall, 562 (5)
  operations on. *See under* Operations
    on intestine, 560 ff.; *and specific
    name of operation*
Celiotomy, exploratory, 569 (0)
Cephalic version, *footnote,* 587
Cerebral arteriography (angiography), 549 (3)
Cerebral nerves
  excision of mixed ganglia associated
    with, 596 (1)
  neurectomy, 594 (1)
  neurotomy, 594 (0)
  operations on, 594. *See also specific
    name of operation*
Cervicectomy, 584 (1)
Cervix uteri. *See also* Uterus
  amputation, 584 (1)
  biopsy, 585 (1)
  conization, 585 (1)
  dilation, 585 (8)
  excision
    local, of lesion, 584 (1)
    partial, 585 (1)
  insertion, intracervical
    of bag, 585 (3)
    of pack, 585 (3)
    of radioactive substance, 585 (3)
  operations on, 584 ff. *See also spe-
    cific name of operation*
  plastic repair, 585 (5)
  suture, 585 (7)

Dye
 injection
  nonopaque, 518 (3)
  into nose, 539 (3)

E

Ear
 amputation, 604 (1)
 application of ultrasonics to canals
  of, 606 (6)
 biopsy, 604 (1)
 division of adhesions, 606 (6)
 division of otosclerotic processes,
  606 (6)
 excision, 604 (1)
 external, operations on, 604. *See also
  specific name of operation*
 incision and drainage, 604 (0)
 insertion
  of pack or tampon, 605 (3)
  of plastic tube, 605 (3)
  of wire loop, 605 (3)
 internal, operations on, 606. *See also
  specific name of operation*
 middle, operations on, 604. *See also
  specific name of operation*
 plastic repair, 605 (5)
 reconstruction with graft, 604 (5)
 removal of packing, 606 (8)
 suture, 604 (7)
Eggars procedure, 536 (5)
Elbow
 disarticulation, 537 (2)
Electrocoagulation, *footnote,* 517
 of prostate, 580 (4)
 of semicircular canals, 606 (6)
Elliot's operation, 598 (1)
Elongation. *See* Lengthening
Emasculation. *See* Castration, 577
 (1) ; Radical excision of penis, 577
 (1)
Embolectomy
 with aortotomy, 548 (0)
 with arteriotomy, 548 (0)
Embryo, removal, 586 (1)
Embryotomy, 586 (6)
Encephalography, 591 (3)
Endarterectomy, 549 (1)
Endocrine products
 introduction or implantation, 519 (3)
Endocrine system
 biopsy of endocrine gland, 589 (1)

Endocrine system—Continued
 exploration of endocrine gland, 589
  (0)
 local excision of lesion of endocrine
  gland, 589 (1)
 operations on, 588. *See also specific
  name of gland and of operation*
Endoscopy. *See under organ or re-
  gion involved*
 types, 519 (4)
Endothermy, *footnote,* 519
Enterectomy, 561 (1)
Enteroanastomosis, 562 (5)
Enteroenterostomy, 562 (5)
Enterolysis, 562 (6)
Enteropexy. *See* Cecopexy, 562 (5) ;
  Sigmoidopexy, 562 (5)
Enterorrhaphy, 563 (7)
Enterostomy, 562 (5)
 closure, 563 (7)
 dilation, 563 (7)
 reduction of prolapse, 563 (8)
Enterotomy, 560 (0)
Enucleation of eyeball, 597 (1)
Epididymectomy, 578 (1)
Epididymis
 anastomosis to vas deferens, 578 (5)
 biopsy, 578 (1)
 excision of lesion, 578 (1)
 operations on, 578. *See also specific
  name of operation*
Epididymotomy, 578 (0)
Epididymovasostomy, 578 (5)
Epidural space
 cerebral, drainage, 591 (0)
 spinal, drainage, 591 (0)
Epigastric hernioplasty, 570 (5)
Epiglottidectomy, 541 (1)
Epiglottis. *See under* Operations on
  larynx, 541 ff.
Epilation of eyelid, 601 (1)
Epiphysial arrest, 531 (5)
Epiphysial-diaphysial fusion, 531
  (5)
Epiploectomy, 570 (1)
Epiplopexy, 571 (5)
Epiplorrhaphy, 571 (7)
Episioperineoplasty, 581 (5)
Episioperineorrhaphy, 581 (7)
Episioplasty, 581 (5)
Episiorrhaphy, 581 (7)
Episiotomy, 581 (0)

Fundectomy
of stomach, 559 (1)
uterine, 584 (1)
Fusion, 521 (5)
of bone, 531 (5)
epiphysial-diaphysial, 531 (5)
of joint to produce ankylosis, 533 (5)
lumbosacral, 531 (5)
spinal, 531 (5)

G

Gallbladder. *See also under* Operations on biliary tract, 567
calculus, removal, 567 (0)
fistula, closure, 568 (7)
Gallstone(s), removal, 567 (0). *See also* Choledocholithotomy; Hepaticolithotomy
outside of gallbladder or bile ducts, 567 (0)
Ganglion(a)
cerebral, operations on, 594
mixed, associated with cerebral nerves, excision, 596 (1)
operations on, 594, 595, 596. *See also specific name of operation*
Ganglionectomy, 594 (1), 595 (1)
gasserian, 594 (1)
sphenopalatine (Meckel's), 596 (1)
Gas, injection, 518 (3)
Gastrectomy
various types, 559 (1)
Gastric varices
injection, 559 (0)
Gastrocnemius, tenotomy, 535 (0)
Gastroduodectomy, 559 (1)
Gastroduodenostomy, 560 (5)
closure or taking down of, 560 (7)
Gastrogastrostomy, 560 (5)
Gastroileal anastomosis
closure, 560 (7)
Gastrointestinal tract. *See* Intestine; Stomach
Gastrojejunostomy, 560 (5)
closure or taking down of, 560 (7)
Gastromyotomy. *See* Pyloromyotomy, 559 (0)
Gastroplasty, 560 (5)
Gastrorrhaphy, 560 (7)
Gastroscopy, 560 (4)

Gastrostomy, 560 (5)
closure, 560 (7)
Gastrotomy, 559 (0)
Genital system
operations on, 577 ff. *See also specific name of operation*
Genitourinary system
operations on, 572 ff. *See also specific name of operation*
Genyplasty. *See* Plastic operation on cheek, 525 (5)
Gifford's operation, 597 (0)
Gillies' graft. *See* Tube graft, 520 (5), 525 (5)
Gingiva
biopsy, 555 (1)
enucleation of cyst, 555 (1)
excision, 555 (1)
operation on, 554. *See also specific name of operation*
removal of cyst (partial), 555 (1)
restoration of, 520 (5), 555 (5)
suture, 555 (7)
Gingivectomy, 555 (1)
Gland(s)
endocrine. *See* Endocrine system; *and specific name of gland*
of skin, operations on, 528
Glans penis. *See under* Operations on penis, 577
Glass, insertion, 519 (3)
Globe. *See* Eyeball
Glossectomy, 554 (1)
Glossopharyngeal neurotomy, 594 (0)
Glossoplasty, 554 (5)
Glossorrhaphy, 554 (7)
Glossotomy, 554 (0)
Gluteus medius
myotomy of, 534 (0)
Gluteus minimus
myotomy of, 534 (0)
Goniotomy, 597 (0)
Graft. *See also specific name of graft; and organ, region or structure involved*
arthroplasty with, 533 (5)
cartilage, 533 (5)
donor site, regional, 526 (5)
excision of bone for, 530 (1)
excision of tissue for, 518 (1)
fascial, 520 (5), 525 (5), 536 (5)
muscle, 535 (5)

L

Labia. *See under* Operations on vulva, 581
Labyrinthectomy, 606 (1)
Labyrinthotomy, 606 (0)
Lacrimal tract
catheterization of lacrimonasal duct, 603 (3)
dilation of punctum, 603 (8)
drainage
of lacrimal gland, 603 (0)
of lacrimal sac, 603 (0)
excision
of lacrimal gland, 603 (1)
of lacrimal sac, 603 (1)
fistulization of lacrimal sac into nasal cavity, 603 (5)
operations on, 603. *See also specific name of operation*
plastic operation on canaliculi, 603 (5)
probing of lacrimonasal duct, 603 (8)
splitting of lacrimal papilla, 603 (0)
Lacrimonasal duct. *See under* Lacrimal tract
Lagrange's operation, 598 (1)
Laminectomy, 590 (1)
Laminotomy, 530 (0)
Lane plate
open reduction of fracture with, 531 (5)
Laparorrhaphy, 571 (7)
Laparotomy
exploratory, 569 (0)
reopening of, 570 (0)
Laparotrachelotomy. *See* Low cervical cesarean section, 586 (0)
Large intestine. *See under* Operations on intestine, 560 ff.; *and under* Operations on rectum, 564
Laryngectomy, 541 (1)
Laryngocentesis, 541 (0)
Laryngofissure, 541 (0)
Laryngopharyngectomy, 541 (1)
Laryngoplasty, 542 (5)
Laryngorrhaphy, 542 (7)
Laryngoscopy, 542 (4)
Laryngostomy, 542 (5)
Laryngotomy, 541 (0)
Laryngotracheotomy, 542 (0)

Larynx
biopsy, 541 (1)
excision of lesion (by laryngotomy), 541 (1)
fistula, closure, 542 (7)
fistulization, 542 (5)
incision and drainage, 541 (0)
insertion of tube into, 541 (3)
operations on, 541 ff. *See also specific name of operation*
puncture, 541 (0)
suture, 542 (7)
Lateral sinus
drainage, 591 (0)
Le Fort's operation. *See* Colpectomy, partial, 582 (1)
Leg, amputation, 538 (2)
Lengthening
of bone, 531 (5)
of tendon, 536 (5)
Lens, crystalline
extraction, 599 (1)
needling, 599 (0)
operations on, 599. *See also specific name of operation*
Leucotomy, 592 (0)
Levator palpebrae muscle, tenotomy, 601 (0)
Lid. *See* Eyelid
Ligament(s)
cutting or division of, 532 (0)
excision or resection, 532 (1)
operations on, 532. *See also specific name of operation*
suture, 533 (7)
Ligamentopexy. *See* Hysteropexy with shortening of round ligaments or with shortening of sacrouterine ligaments, 585 (5)
Ligation, 521 (7). *See also under organ or structure involved*
Limitation of motion of joint. *See* Stabilization of joint by bone block, 533 (5)
Lingual tonsil, excision, 557 (1)
Lip(s)
biopsy, 553 (1)
excision of lesion, 553 (1)
incision and drainage, 553 (1)
operations on, 553. *See also specific name of operation*
suture, 554 (7)

Obstetric forceps
application of, or delivery by, 587 (8)
Obturator hernioplasty, 571 (5)
Occlusion, 521 (7). *See also under organ, region or structure involved*
Ocular muscle(s)
advancement, 600 (5)
operations on, 600. *See also specific name of operation*
recession, 600 (5)
shortening, 600 (5)
transplantation, 600 (5)
Ocular tendon(s). *See under* Operations on ocular muscles, 600
Oddi, sphincter of
incision, 567 (0)
Odontogenic tumor
removal, 555 (1)
Odontomy, 554 (0)
Oil, injection, 518 (3)
intrapleural, 546 (3)
radiopaque
bronchoscopy with, 543 (4)
laryngoscopy with, 542 (4)
into larynx, 542 (4)
tracheoscopy with, 543 (4)
Oleothorax, 546 (3)
Omental drainage, 569 (0)
Omentectomy, 570 (1)
Omentofixation, 571 (5)
Omentopexy, 571 (5)
Omentorrhaphy, 571 (7)
Omentum
operations on, 569. *See also specific name of operation*
reduction of torsion, 571 (5)
suture, 571 (7)
Omphalectomy, 570 (1)
Onychectomy. *See* Excision of nail, nail bed or nail fold, 528 (1)
Onychotomy. *See* Incision of nail bed or fold, 528 (0)
Oophorectomy, 584 (1)
Oophorocystectomy, 584 (1)
Open reduction
of dislocation or fracture-dislocation of joint, 533 (5)
of fracture, 531 (5)
of skull, 590 (1)
Operative procedures, classification, 517 ff.

Orbit
biopsy, 601 (5)
decompression
antral approach, 601 (0)
intracranial approach, 590 (0)
excision of lesion, 601 (1)
exenteration or evisceration of contents, 601 (1)
implant, 597 (3)
operations on, 601
plastic repair, 601 (5)
Orbitotomy, 601 (0)
Orchidectomy. See Orchiectomy, 577 (1)
Orchidorrhaphy. *See* Orchiopexy, 577 (5)
Orchidotomy. *See* Incision and drainage of testis, 577 (0)
Orchiectomy, 577 (1)
Orchiopexy, 577 (5)
Orchioplasty, 577 (5)
Organs of special sense
operations on, 597
Orthodontic appliance, 519 (3), 555 (3)
Ossiculectomy, 605 (1)
Ostectomy, 530 (1)
of skull. See Craniectomy, 590 (1)
Osteochondritis dissecans, 533 (1)
Osteoclasis, 531 (6)
Osteoperiosteal graft, 531 (5)
Osteoplasty, 531 (5)
Osteorrhaphy, 531 (5)
Osteosynthesis, 531 (5)
Osteotomy, 530 (0)
of nasal bones, 539 (0)
Otoplasty, 604 (5)
Otosclerotic processes
divisions of, 606 (6)
Otoscopy, 604 (4)
Ovary(ies)
excision of lesion, 584 (1)
operations on, 583. *See also specific name of operation*
wedge resection, 584 (1)
Oviduct. *See* Fallopian tube

P

Pack, insertion, 519 (3)
intracervical, 585 (3)
intrauterine, 585 (3)
vaginal, 582 (3)

Space maintainer, 519 (3), 555 (3)
Special sense, organs of
operations on, 597
Spermatic cord
excision of hydrocele, 579 (1)
excision of varicocele, 579 (1)
incision and drainage, 579 (0)
operations on, 579
transection, 579 (0)
Sphenoid sinus
operations on, 540
Sphenoid sinusotomy, 540 (0)
Sphenoidotomy, 540 (0)
Sphincter
anal. *See under* Anus, 566
of Oddi, incision, 567 (0)
Sphincteroplasty, anal, 566 (5)
Sphincterotomy
anal, 565 (0)
of iris, 598 (0)
Oddi, 567 (0)
Spinal accessory-facial neuroanastomosis, 595 (5)
Spinal accessory-hypoglossal neuroanastomosis, 595 (5)
Spinal canal, exploration, 590 (0)
Spinal cord
biopsy, 594 (1)
decompression, 593 (0)
drainage, 593 (0)
excision of lesion, 594 (1)
exploration, 593 (0)
operations on, 593. *See also specific
name of operation*
structures overlying, operations on,
590
Spinal fusion, 533 (5)
Spinal nerves
neurectomy, 594 (1)
neurotomy, 594 (0)
Spinal puncture, 591 (0)
Spine
repair of defect of vertebral arch
and, 590 (5)
Spineography. *See* Myelography,
592 (3)
Splanchnicectomy, 595 (1)
Splanchnicotomy, 595 (0)
Spleen
biopsy, 551 (1)
fixation, 551 (5)
operations on, 551. *See also specific
name of operation*

Spleen—Continued
suture, 551 (7)
Splenectomy, 551 (1)
Splenic puncture, 551 (0)
Splenopexy, 551 (5)
Splenorenal anastomosis, 550 (5)
Splenorenal shunt. *See* Splenorenal
anastomosis, 550 (5)
Splenorrhaphy, 551 (7)
Splenotomy, 551 (0)
Splint, application
for fracture, 532 (8)
and manipulation of joint, 535 (8)
Spondylosyndesis, 531 (5)
Stabilization, 521 (5)
of joint by bone block, 533 (5)
Stabilizing appliance, 519 (3), 555
(3)
Stapedectomy
with insertion of prosthesis, 605 (5)
with tissue graft, 605 (5)
Stapes
fracture of, 606 (6)
mobilization, 605 (5)
Steindler procedure, 536 (5)
Steinmann pin
insertion (without incision), 531 (3)
Sternal puncture
by aspiration, 531 (1)
by curettage, 531 (1)
Sternotomy, 530 (0)
Stomach
anastomosis of bile duct to, 568 (5)
biopsy, 559 (1)
fistula, closure
cholecystogastric, 568 (7)
gastrocolic, 560 (7)
gastrojejunocolic, 560 (7)
implantation of biliary fistulous
tract, 568 (5)
operations on, 559. *See also specific
name of operation*
Stomatoplasty, 553 (5)
Streptomycin, injection, 518 (3)
Stretching
of iris, 599 (8)
of muscle, 535 (8)
of nerve, 595 (8)
Stripping, 521 (6). *See also under
organ or structure involved*
Subarachnoid space
drainage, 591 (0)

APPENDIX

ABRIDGED STATISTICAL
CLASSIFICATION
FOR
CLINICAL INDEXING

APPENDIX TO THE STANDARD NOMENCLATURE AND THE ABRIDGED STATISTICAL CLASSIFICATION FOR CLINICAL INDEXING BASED ON STANDARD NOMENCLATURE OF DISEASES AND OPERATIONS

The Clinical Statistical Classification consists of four-digit rubrics ranging from 0000 to 9999. This permits grouping to 10,000 specific groups. Even under the most detailed grouping it is estimated that not more than 1,500 rubrics will ever be used. Generally the first two digits are identical with the first two digits of the topographic code and the last two digits identical with the first two digits of the etiologic categories of the Standard Nomenclature of Diseases and Operations. Some arbitrary assignments are necessary.

The classification as presented herein lists only a limited number of rubrics. The listing may be used in its entirety or it may be used selectively. The simplest pattern of use is to record diseases under the major general rubrics only. General rubrics are recognized by ending in 00. For example, all diseases of the cardiovascular system may be recorded under the general rubric 4000, Diseases of the Cardiovascular System. If greater detail of classification is desired, entities may be recorded under rubrics ending in 0 or 01. If still greater specificity is desired, entities may be recorded under the rubrics listed for specific conditions. Thus all vascular disorders of the myocardium may be recorded under the rubric 4350, Vascular disorders of myocardium, and greater specificity may be obtained by recording the particular vascular disorder under the specific rubric, thus 4351, Myocardial infarction.

Any combination of the rubrics listed may be selected to meet the special needs of the Institution. Specialized facilities, such as Mental Institutions may desire to classify diseases of the Psychobiologic Unit with greater specificity, whereas the facility may consider it advisable to group diseases of other systems under general or broader groups. The user because of this flexibility may group broadly or specifically in detail according to the user's specific need for statistical grouping.

Since only a limited number of four-digit rubrics are used, presentation of need or demand for additional specific groupings can be readily met by adding additional rubrics to the final section.

This classification can be kept current without difficulty by the Standard Nomenclature Department, and as the need for additional grouping is evidenced, such rubrics can be scientifically established compatible with the Standard Nomenclature of Diseases and Operations.

851

ABRIDGED STATISTICAL CLASSIFICATION

0001 Acute brain disorders

0000–100	000–332122	000–7▲▲
000–100	000–4▲▲	000–8▲▲
000–3▲▲	000–5▲▲	000–900
000–33212	000–550	000–xx0
000–332121		

0002 Mental deficiency

000–x90	000–x93	000–x97
000–x91	000–x95	000–x98
000–x92	000–x96	

0006 Psychophysiologic autonomic visceral disorders

000–580	004–580	008–580
001–580	005–580	009–580
002–580	006–580	00x–580
003–580	007–580	

0007 Psychoneurotic disorders

000–x00	000–x03	000–x06
000–x01	000–x04	000–x09
000–x02	000–x05	002–7861

0008 Personality disorders

000–x40	000–x60	000–x72
000–x41	000–x61	000–x73
000–x42	000–x615	000–x74
000–x43	000–x616	000–x79
000–x44	000–x617	000–x80
000–x45	000–x619	000–x81
000–x46	000–x62	000–x82
000–x465	000–x63	000–x83
000–x466	000–x635	000–x84
000–x467	000–x636	000–x85
000–x47	000–x639	000–x86
000–x48	000–x70	
000–x59	000–x71	

0009 Chronic brain disorders

009–0▲▲	0095–147	009–4▲▲
009–016	009–1▲▲	009–415
009–071	009–300	009–462
009–052	009–3▲▲	009–470
009–147	009–33212	009–516
0091–147	009–050	009–5▲▲
0092–147	009–400	009–550

0009   Chronic brain disorders (Continued)

009–79x	009–746.x4	009–900
009–700	009–8▲▲	009–xx0

0030   Addiction

000–x64

0031   Alcohol addiction

000–x641

0032   Drug addiction

000–x642

0033   Combined alcohol and drug addiction

000–x643

0050   Psychotic disorders

000–x39
000–x3x

0051   Affective reactions

000–x10	000–x13
000–x11	000–x14
000–x12	000–x15

0052   Schizophrenic reaction

000–x20	000–x24	000–x28
000–x21	000–x25	000–x29
000–x22	000–x26	000–x2x
000–x23	000–x27	

0053   Paranoid reactions

000–x30

0100   DISEASES OF THE BODY AS A WHOLE

0101   Congenital conditions of the body as a whole

013–010	010–025	010–071
010–032	010–012	011–076
010–076	015–077	014–02x
010–013	010–070	014–02x1

0110   Infections of the body as a whole

010–100.2	010–136	010–186
010–151	010–120	012–187
014–100.9	018–1▲▲	010–162
014–123.9	010–1763	016–195
012–118	010–129	010–134
012–100	012–158	010–190

0110   Infections of the body as a whole (Continued)

010–160	010–172	010–1x0
010–1605	010–114▲	010–1761
010–192	010–109	010–119
010–113	010–108	010–1577
010–126	010–106	010–1833
010–193	010–1686	010–146
013–166	010–197	010–153
010–142	010–1603	010–1531
010–152	010–173	010–1532
010–166.0	010–1832	010–183
010–124	010–174	012–123
010–1302	010–1341	010–107
010–157▲	013–100.0	010–115
010–127	010–1411	018–115
012–104	010–1412	010–184
010–16x	010–1814	010–1762
013–160	010–1811	010–19y
010–170	010–165	010–178

0111   Inoculation state

019–100	019–169	0193–100
019–125	019–108	0194–100
019–171	0191–100	
019–119	0192–100	

0112   Scarlet fever

010–102

0113   Mononucleosis

010–1301

0114   Syphilis

012–147	110–147	130–147.6
014–147	110–147.6	

0116   Measles

010–169

0117   Brucellosis

010–117▲

0118   Influenza

010–168

0119   Septicemia

013–190

0120   Fungus and parasitic infections of the body as a whole

012–219
012–2▲▲
012–201

0121   Histoplasmosis

010–220

0130   Toxic disorders of the body as a whole

014–393▲	010–3990	010–3932
010–390	010–399	010–391
010–395	010–3▲▲.0	014–390
011–300	010–3931	

0131   Poisoning, general, of the body as a whole

010–3141	011–3196	010–3483
010–3▲▲.x	010–33152	010–33221
010–382	010–34129	010–34648
010–38271	010–315▲	010–34651
010–38211	010–33231	010–3253
010–3▲▲	010–33212	010–36731
010–33▲	011–33212	010–3432
010–33613	010–33156	010–3257
010–34814	010–33111	010–3485x
010–321	010–3238	010–369
011–321	010–3243	010–38x
010–3196	010–33211	010–3843

0135   Carbon monoxide poisoning

010–3151

0137   Barbiturate poisoning

010–34851

0139   Venom poisoning

010–381▲

0140   Injuries; multiple injuries

010–414	010–481	010–4xx
010–480	010–443	010–411
010–402	010–400	

0141   Crushing, general

010–482
010–404

0142   Drowning

010–423
010–49x
010–499

0144   Freezing, general

010–447
010–448

0145   Heat prostration, sunstroke

010–445
010–453

0146   Electric shock

010–460	010–464
010–462	010–463

0147   Radioactivity, general

010–47▲1
010–47▲
010–471

0149   Suffocation

014–421	010–433	010–493
010–422	010–492	

0155   Innervation disorders, general

010–576

0160   Disorders due to mechanical abnormalities, general

010–640

0170   Metabolic disorders, of the body as a whole

010–711	010–740	010–752
010–717.x	010–746	010–70x2
010–721	010–749	014–797
010–722	010–754	010–797
010–722.x	010–75x	010–707
012–731	013–755	010–705
010–731	010–7551	010–7011
010–73▲	013–752	010–708
010–736	010–751	017–735
010–743	010–755	010–712
010–741	010–757	010–718
010–742	010–759	

0171   Malnutrition

011–709	013–711	010–701
012–709	014–711	010–701.8

0175   Obesity

010–70x
010–70y
010–753

0176   Avitaminosis

010–7621	010–7623	010–763
010–761	010–7622	010–76▲
010–766	010–764	
010–760	010–764.x	

0180   Neoplasms, general

012–8▲▲▲
012–8▲▲▲

0190   Diseases due to unknown cause of the body as a whole

011–940	013–930	010–x30
013–997	010–971	

0192   Amyloidosis, general

014–922

0193   Rheumatic fever

010–932

0195   Lupus erythematosus, systemic

013–955

0201   Congenital anomalies of head and face

021–01x	0213–01x	027–076
0211–01x	027–019	027–022
0212–01x		

0212   Subgaleal abscess

0261–100.2

0240   Decapitation

020–405

0301   Congenital anomalies of neck, thorax, and mediastinum

039–064

0310   Infection of mediastinum

039–190
039–100
039–123

0340   Collapse of thorax following operation

034–415.4   039–427
039–435.4   034–415.3

0341   Wound of chest wall

034–410
033–4111

0380   Mediastinal neoplasms

039–882

0401   Congenital anomaly of abdomen

069–02x
06▲–025.4

0402   Congenital hernia

044–027
042–027

0410   Infection of abdomen, generalized

044–100.6   044–100.0   041–100
044–100   042–100.3

0412   Abscess of abdomen

042–100.2
041–100.2

0440   Injuries of abdomen

042–415.3
042–400.3
042–496

0441   Wound of abdominal wall

042–410
040–4111

0442   Injury of pelvic floor

047–43x   047–4123
047–4x9   047–4122

0445   Hernia of abdomen, traumatic

042–4x9   042–4x9.5
042–415.9   0421–4x9

0450   Vascular disorders of abdomen

044–514

0463   Hernia epigastric

| 043–639 | 044–639 | 048–641 |
| 043–639.5 | 044–639.5 | |

0480   Generalized abdominal carcinomatosis

040–8▲▲▲I

0490   Diseases of the abdomen due to unknown cause

040–941
040–9x1

0501   Pilonidal sinus (or cyst)

0582–029

0563   Hernia, ischiatic

| 057–639 | 056–639 |
| 057–639.5 | 056–639.5 |

0580   Sacrococcygeal neoplasms

058–882

0601   Congenital anomaly of abdomen and peritoneum

067–025
06▲–025

0602   Congenital hernia

0602–027
0601–027

0610   Infection of intestine

| 06▲–1x4 | 060–1x7 |
| 060–158 | 065–100 |

0611   Peritonitis

060–100	060–112	060–100.0
060–101	063–100	060–123
060–102	066–100	060–123.8
060–105	0661–100	066–100.4

0612   Abscess of pelvic peritoneum

067–100.2	064–100.2	066–100.2
06▲–100.2	065–100.2	
063–100.2	0651–100.2	

0620   Parasitic and fungus infections of peritoneum

060–240.6
060–260.6

0630   Toxic disorders of peritoneum

060–382
060–3▲▲
060–380

0640   Injuries of peritoneum

06▲–415.4	060–415.7	060–420
06▲–4x4	060–4x7	069–4x9
060–438.6	060–4▲▲	066–415.4

0645   Hernia, peritoneal, traumatic

0601–4x9
066–4x9

0650   Vascular disorders of peritoneum

060–522.8	060–501
060–502	067–514

0660   Splanchnoptosis

069–631

0663   Hernia of peritoneum

0602–639	0601–6392	066–639.5
066–639	0601–639.5	067–639
0602–639.5	0601–639.6	067–637
0601–639	650–639	
0601–6393	650–639.5	

0670   Metabolic disorders of peritoneum

060–794
069–776

0680   Neoplasms of peritoneum

060–850A	065–840A	065–8431
060–850F	065–866A	065–841F
067–830	065–872A	065–882
060–830	065–872F	06▲–879
060–8772A	065–830	06▲–8▲▲▲

0690   Diseases of the peritoneum due to unknown cause

067–9x7
068–9x8

0701   Congenital anomaly of perineum

074–017

0710   Infection of perineum

074–100.2
074–100.3

0740   Injury of perineum

074–415.3

0741   Wound of perineum

074–410

0801   Congenital anomaly of upper extremities

| 083–013 | 080–076 | 0861–031 |
| 086–03x | 086–031 | 097–031 |

0830   Sulfuric acid burn of hand

085–3116

0855   Causalgia of arm

08x–572

0870   Clubbed fingers

086–704

0901   Congenital anomalies of lower extremities

097–03x	097–075	0975–022
099–03x	090–016	096–034
096–075	097–022	085–034

0920   Fungus and parasitic infections of lower extremities

093–205
096–205

0930   Lime burn of foot

096–3126

0940   Injuries of lower extremities

097–433

0950   Vascular disturbances of lower extremities

099–518
090–522.8

0955   Causalgia of leg

09x–572

0963   Hernia, obturator

091–639

0990   Ainhum

097–9x1

0▲01   Congenital anomaly of . . . . *Specify site*

▲▲▲–011
▲▲▲–025
▲▲▲–0▲▲
▲▲▲–0y0
▲▲▲–050
▲▲▲–050.0
▲▲▲–050.7
▲▲▲–039
▲▲▲–013
0▲▲–03x
0▲▲–075
▲▲▲–014
0▲▲–076
0▲▲–031

0▲10   Infection of . . . . *Specify site*

▲▲▲–100.3
▲▲▲–103
▲▲▲–100.6
▲▲▲–147.6
0▲▲–100
0▲▲–125
0▲▲–11x
0▲▲–122
▲▲▲–1x0
▲▲▲–100.4
▲▲▲–147.4
▲▲▲–147
▲▲▲–1471
▲▲▲–147.3
▲▲▲–154
▲▲▲–1236
▲▲▲–123
▲▲▲–1237
0▲▲–100.9
0▲▲–1762

0▲11   Gangrene of . . . . *Specify site*

▲▲▲–100.1

0▲12   Abscess of . . . . *Specify site*

▲▲▲–100.2

0▲20   Parasitic and fungus infections. *Specify site*

▲▲▲–202
▲▲▲–243
▲▲▲–241
▲▲▲–226
▲▲▲–2171
▲▲▲–2172
▲▲▲–219
▲▲▲–218
▲▲▲–258
▲▲▲–257
▲▲▲–214
▲▲▲–2161
▲▲▲–220
▲▲▲–20▲
▲▲▲–209
▲▲▲–232
▲▲▲–2▲▲
▲▲▲–24▲
▲▲▲–201
▲▲▲–231
▲▲▲–278
▲▲▲–216
▲▲▲–26▲
▲▲▲–266
▲▲▲–267
▲▲▲–265
▲▲▲–270
▲▲▲–2542
▲▲▲–240

0▲30   Toxic disorders of . . . . *Specify site*

0▲▲–393
0▲▲–382
▲▲▲–32▲
▲▲▲–300.4
▲▲▲–3▲▲.1
▲▲▲–312▲1
▲▲▲–3322▲1
▲▲▲–34637
▲▲▲–3▲▲
▲▲▲–300.3

0▲40   Injury of . . . . *Specify site*

▲▲▲–415.2
▲▲▲–400.2
▲▲▲–415.x
▲▲▲–400.x
0▲▲–405
0▲▲0–4xx
0860–4xx
0▲▲–413▲
0▲▲–4413
0▲▲–446
▲▲▲–400.4
▲▲▲–415.4
▲▲▲–441.4
0▲▲–400.8
0▲▲–427
▲▲▲–47▲.3
▲▲▲–415.3
▲▲▲–400.3

0▲40   Injury of . . . . *Specify site* (Continued)

▲▲▲–496	▲▲▲–47▲2	▲▲▲–47▲.0
▲▲▲–438.6	▲▲▲–4712	▲▲▲–47▲1
0▲▲–448	▲▲▲–4722	▲▲▲–4711
▲▲▲–400.1	▲▲▲–47▲.1	▲▲▲–4721
0▲▲–448.1	▲▲▲–400.6	▲▲▲–444
0▲▲–441.1	▲▲▲–47▲	▲▲▲–400.4
0▲▲–44x	▲▲▲–471	▲▲▲–415.4
▲▲▲–4▲▲	▲▲▲–472	0▲▲–43x

0▲41   Wound of . . . . *Specify site*

0▲▲–410	0▲▲–415.5	0▲▲–415
0▲▲–410.0	0▲▲–4111	0▲▲–415.0

0▲43   Hematoma of . . . . *Specify site*

▲▲▲–402.7
▲▲▲–4x7
▲▲▲–400.7
▲▲▲–415.7

0▲44   Burn of . . . electric. *Specify site*

▲▲▲–461
0▲▲–461.1

0▲45   Hernia of . . . traumatic. *Specify site*

0▲▲–415.9

0▲50   Vascular disorders of . . . . *Specify site*

▲▲▲–520.2	▲▲▲–515.1	▲▲▲–511.1
▲▲▲–522	▲▲▲–516.1	▲▲▲–549.7
▲▲▲–501	▲▲▲–512.1	▲▲▲–520.6
▲▲▲–522.6	▲▲▲–513.1	▲▲▲–510
▲▲▲–502	▲▲▲–514.1	0▲▲–516.9
▲▲▲–500.1	▲▲▲–51x.1	

0▲55   Innervation disorders of . . . . *Specify site*

0▲▲–565.9

0▲60   Disorders of . . . due to mechanical abnormality. *Specify site*

▲▲▲–641

0▲63   Hernia of . . . . *Specify site*

▲▲▲–639

0▲70   Metabolic disorders of . . . . *Specify site*

0▲▲–785.1	▲▲▲–754	0▲▲–753
0▲▲–785.9	▲▲▲–748	▲▲▲–755

0▲80   Neoplasm, regional . . . . *Specify site*

▲▲▲–8532	▲▲▲–8531	▲▲▲–8▲▲▲I
▲▲▲–850B	▲▲▲–832	▲▲▲–882
▲▲▲–850A	▲▲▲–854A	▲▲▲–8▲▲▲
▲▲▲–851	▲▲▲–852	

0▲90   Diseases of . . . due to unknown cause. *Specify site*

▲▲▲–922	▲▲▲–959	▲▲▲–929
▲▲▲–923	▲▲▲–943	▲▲▲–944
▲▲▲–921	▲▲▲–941	▲▲▲–913
▲▲▲–910	▲▲▲–92x	

1100   DISEASES OF THE SKIN AND SKIN APPENDAGES

1101   Congenital disorders of skin

112–079	111–014	111–070
114–077	112–014	110–1471
114–092	110–097	110–045
116–076	112–074	110–044
110–077	114–074	

1110   Infections of skin proper

110–118	110–105.1	110–1231
116–147.9	110–149	110–1232
111–1005	111–130	110–1233
110–105	114–130	110–1234
110–130	117–1x0	110–1235
111–190	114–123	110–1236
110–1x9	102–123	110–1238
110–1x91	110–123	110–1239
111–185	11x–190	114–1x0
110–190	110–1230	

1111   Impetigo

111–105	13▲–105	1▲▲–100.1
111–105.8	110–1021	

1120   Fungus and parasitic diseases of skin proper

110–283	110–29▲	110–2912
110–218	110–244	110–292
112–211	110–292.0	110–2831
112–2011	114–211	110–216
110–240	110–2911	112–208

1130   Toxic disorders of skin

113–3253	111–390	113–3x1
110–321.6	116–300.8	113–3x0
111–394	11x–3x7	110–396

1131   Contact dermatitis

110–300

1132   Dermatitis medicamentosa

113–3▲▲
110–3▲▲

1133   Urticaria

11x–390
11x–3901

1140   Injuries of skin

112–430	11x–445	110–446
110–470	112–451	110–452
110–451	111–437	
110–400	11x–440	

1150   Vascular disorders of skin proper

110–521.6	110–515	114–501
110–5x0	110–518	

1155   Innervation disorders of skin

11x–580	110–572
110–565	110–573

1160   Disorders of skin proper due to mechanical abnormalities

112–6x8
132–6x8

1170   Metabolic disorders of skin proper

110–776	112–799	112–747
110–798	111–799	114–785
110–718	112–745	114–7571
112–770	110–742	114–7572
110–749	110–770	114–757

1190   Diseases of skin due to unknown cause

110–960	111–985	110–965
110–910	110–943	111–9662
110–922	110–96x	111–966
116–973	110–974	111–9661
114–929	11x–943	111–963
115–943	11x–971	111–989
116–9x6	111–964	111–983
110–966	1▲▲–9x6	111–981
110–969	111–984	111–982
110–985	113–978	111–980

1190   Diseases of skin due to unknown cause (Continued)

111–987	112–995	114–970
11x–931	110–963	110–9x1
110–986	110–964	104–x90
111–962	116–911	11x–x95
110–968	100–971	
112–970	114–971	

1196   Psoriasis

111–961	111–9612	111–9614
111–9611	111–9613	111–9615

1200   Diseases of mucous membranes

12▲▲–023	122–943	124–941
123–943	122–951	124–944
12▲–943	1231–023	129–747
12▲–941	124–960	129–943
12▲–965	124–910	122–190
122–1x1	124–957	

1301   Congenital disorders of regions of skin

13▲–012	141–03x	132–079
131–014	148–03x	13▲–023.8
149–097	132–013	
149–093	132–014	

1310   Infections of regions of skin

141–100	13▲–179	132–130
13▲–151	13▲–1791	132–1236
13▲–10x	13▲–1792	132–1762
13▲–125	144–166	132–1761
13▲–100.1	144–100.9	132–1764
146–137	142–100	13▲–100.4
13▲–152	132–100.4	1▲▲–1764
13▲–1x9	132–166	13▲–100.6
13▲–124	132–100	
130–147.6	132–185	

1313   Erysipelas

13▲–102
13▲–130

1316   Herpes simplex

1▲▲–166

1320   Fungus and parasitic diseases of regions of skin

13▲–210	131–211	13▲–211
13▲–266	141–209	145–2831
13▲–299	13▲–209	144–292
13▲–2833	13▲–2172	144–2831
13▲–2▲▲	130–211	132–213
13▲–213	146–215	

1330   Toxic disorders of regions of skin

13▲–300.4	149–300	132–321▲
13▲–320	132–390	132–3▲▲
143–3001	132–3253	

1340   Injuries of skin

13▲–4x8	13▲–448	13▲–410
13▲–441.4	13▲–400.1	145–4x6
13▲–433	13▲–441.1	132–400.4
13▲–450	13▲–448.1	132–454
13▲–49▲▲	13▲–400.4	132–415.4
13▲–4962	13▲–4x9	

1341   Ulcer of skin due to trauma

13▲–430

1342   Abrasion of skin

13▲–401

1343   Burn, first degree

13▲–4411

1344   Burn, second degree

13▲–4442

1350   Vascular disorders of skin

147–5xx	147–5x2	13▲–544.9
13▲–501	133–521.6	132–521
147–501	131–521.0	

1352   Ulcus hypostatic

147–522.9
13▲–522.9

1355   Innervation disorders of regions of skin, regionally

132–580	149–573	148–5651.9
132–581	13▲–565.9	148–567.9
132–582	148–565.9	148–566.9

1370 Metabolic disorders of skin regionally

132–711	132–7xx	13▲–772
132–789	132–770	13▲–785
132–771	132–747	13▲–754
132–748	132–757	
132–742	133–7x0	

1380 Neoplasms of skin

13▲–8192	13▲–8701A	13▲–8171
13▲–834	13▲–866A	13▲–814A
13▲–8532	114–829	13▲–831
13▲–868A	13▲–854A	13▲–879
13▲–8882	13▲–830	13▲–8075
13▲–850B	13▲–8895	13▲–8061
13▲–850A	13▲–8032A	1▲▲–8▲▲▲
13▲–850G	13▲–852	
13▲–832	13▲–8851A	

1381 Epidermoid carcinoma of skin

13▲–814
13▲–814E

1382 Basal cell carcinoma of skin

13▲–8175
13▲–812F
132–812F

1383 Melanoma of skin

13▲–8173

1384 Neurofibroma of skin

110–8453
13▲–8451
132–8451

1385 Pigmented nevus of skin

13▲–8170
132–8170

1390 Diseases of skin regionally due to unknown cause

131–943	149–988	13▲–975
131–976	13▲–965.9	132–911
13▲–954	130–943	132–929

1500   Diseases of glands of skin

150–042	152–565	152–740
152–100	152–580	155–900
153–445	151–7x0	152–977
153–4451	152–7xx1	
153–4452	152–7xx	

1600   Diseases of the hair

160–011	160–747	16x–792
160–075	161–7x8	164–022
160–077	160–792	164–014
161–034	160–744	164–012
162–388	160–794	163–074
162–409	161–940	164–079
160–580	162–992	164–400.4
162–580	161–943	164–794
160–5801	161–952	163–747
160–5802	162–940	164–747

1610   Infections of hair

161–1x3	161–1x6	166–133
162–190	161–190	164–105
162–115.9	161–100.2	164–100.1
162–147.9	162–130	164–1x4
162–168.9	161–105	

1611   Furuncles

16▲–100.0
161–100.0

1620   Fungus and parasitic infections of hair regionally

162–213.9	164–292	162–211
16▲–2832	160–204	
162–213	165–211	

1700   Diseases of nails

170–011	176–100	170–961
170–021	170–518	170–962
170–022	173–549	170–943
170–014	170–565	170–961
170–031	170–796	170–960
173–100	170–700	170–092

1720   Fungus and parasitic infection of nails

170–2▲▲

1740   Injury of nails

170–4▲▲
173–4x7

1743   Unguis incarnatus

176–433

1800   Diseases of subcutaneous tissue

18▲–3▲▲	18▲–4x7	18▲–639
18▲–3▲▲.9	18▲–4x8	180–770
185–3827.9	181–427	184–415.6
18▲–400.2	182–427	18▲–427
180–4x9	184–427	

1810   Infections of subcutaneous tissue

18▲–190

1811   Cellulitis

18▲–100
129–100

1812   Carbuncles

18▲–100.3

1813   Abscess of subcutaneous tissue

18▲–100.2

1880   Neoplasms of subcutaneous tissue

18▲–872A

1900   Diseases of breast

194–209
190–32▲
190–510

1901   Congenital disorders of breast

190–021	194–023	194–031
190–012	199–075	
190–016	190–031	

1910   Infections of breast

193–100.8	193–100.4	194–100
190–100.3	19x–100.7	

1911   Mastitis

190–190	190–190.0	190–100
190–170	192–190	

1912   Abscess of breast

190–100.2
196–100.2
197–100.2

1940   Injuries of breast

193–400.8   190–4x7   194–4x0
190–4x9   190–4▲▲

1960   Disorders of breast due to mechanical abnormalities

19x–641

1968   Cystic breast

190–6x8

1970   Metabolic disorders of breast

199–788   193–796   190–793
199–793   190–7x0   190–789
191–789   190–786

1980   Neoplasms of breast

190–8832   190–830   190–8▲▲▲
190–850G   190–879

1981   Carcinoma of breast

190–8091   190–8062G
193–8031F   190–8061

1982   Adenofibroma of breast

190–8831A

1990   Diseases of breast due to unknown cause

190–940   190–993   198–x40
193–957   193–958   198–x10
192–956   198–x30   198–x20

1995   Fissure of nipple

194–9x5

2000   DISEASES OF MUSCULOSKELETAL SYSTEM

2100   DISEASES OF BONES

2101   Congenital conditions of bones

2▲▲–011   220–012   2394–031
235–011   220–012.4   2331–031
2▲▲–012   2▲▲–031   229–031

2101   Congenital conditions of bones (Continued)

220–031	200–002	23x1–016
200–001	220–077	2▲▲–021
2101–038	2▲▲–007	226–021
2▲▲–077	200–008	200–004
221–077	2133–013	200–005
2351–077	200–003	200–007
2351–0776	2▲▲–097	200–0071
2351–0777	200–006	2▲▲–076
231–077	2▲▲–037	236–076
237–022	236–037	2▲▲–03x
237–0221	23x1.0–037	2x51–03x
229–077	2x51–024	223–03x
229–0771	2▲▲.4–014	2x1–03x
2▲▲–026	215–013	210–012
236–026	2▲▲–016	210–016

2102   Spondylolisthesis

2205–037
2203–037
2203–0371

2103   Spina bifida

220▲–037

2110   Infections of bones, excluding tuberculosis and osteo-
        myelitis

2▲▲–100.2	2▲▲–100.6	2▲▲.4–100
2▲▲–130.2	2391–103.6	230.4–102
2▲▲–100.7	2▲▲–100.3	2▲▲.4–100.0
220–100.7	2▲▲–100.5	2▲▲–100.1
2135–100.9	230–147.5	2361–100.6
2▲▲–100.4	2▲▲–100.x	20x–100
2351–100.4	235–102.x	2▲▲.2–147
2▲▲.2–100.4	2▲▲–124	x51–100
235▲2–100.4	2▲▲–190.6	210.4–100

2120   Fungus and parasitic infections of bones

2▲▲–2▲▲

2130   Toxic disorders of bones

2▲▲–38253	200–3238	200–3185.6
2▲▲–3▲▲	219–3185	
200–3195	2▲▲–3185.1	

2140   Injuries of bones, except fracture

2▲▲–437	2▲▲.2–409	2▲▲–480
210–437	235▲2–409	2▲▲.4–402.9

2140   Injuries of bones, except fracture (Continued)

2▲▲–416.0	2▲▲–408	2▲▲–47▲.1
236–4x9	2▲▲–400.6	229–4x0
2▲▲–400.4	2▲▲–496	2▲▲–400.0
2351–400.4	2▲▲–41▲.x	2▲▲–400.9
2351–4001.4	2▲▲.4–4x7	2▲▲.4–400.0
210–431	21▲.4–4x7	236–40x
210–408	2▲▲–4▲▲	2361–4x6
2▲▲–406	2▲▲–400.1	
2▲▲–407	2▲▲–438.1	

2150   Vascular disorders of bone

2▲▲–510	2▲▲–515.9	2▲▲▲2–510.1
2▲▲–516.9	2▲▲–511	
2▲▲–512	2▲▲–510.1	

2155   Innervation disorders of bone

210–565	2▲▲–566	2▲▲–564.9
2▲▲–565	220–566	

2160   Disorders of bone due to mechanical abnormalities

229–630
226–630
237–637

2170   Metabolic disorders of bones

2▲▲–713	2▲▲–764.4	2▲▲–770
2▲▲–755.6	2x2–764.4	2▲▲–787
2▲▲–711	2▲▲–7642.5	22▲–798
200–704	2▲▲–764.5	220–798
200–720	200–7642	220–798.4
200–734	200–7644	210–794
2▲▲–755	200–7643	219–791
2▲▲–781	2▲▲–776	216–793
2▲▲–7641	2351–773.4	21▲–792
2▲▲.4–763	2▲▲–773.5	

2180   Neoplasms of bone

2▲▲–873A	2▲▲–874	2▲▲–833
2▲▲–873B	2▲▲–874F	2▲▲–831
2▲▲–873F	2▲▲–850A	2▲▲–8▲▲▲
2▲▲.4–870A	2▲▲–850G	
2▲▲–870F	2▲▲–8451	

2182   Ewing's sarcoma
2▲▲–875G

2187   Osteoma
2▲▲–876A

2190　　Diseases of bone due to unknown cause

22x5–9x9	216–952	2▲▲–992
2▲▲–922	2▲▲–943	2▲▲–992.5
2▲▲–9▲▲.8	211–943	2▲▲–992.4
2▲▲–9x8.5	211–9431	220–9x4
2▲▲–947	2▲▲–940	237–9x4
2▲▲▲2–942	2▲▲–915	2▲▲–914.8
2▲▲▲2–912	200–9x9	210–943
23512–912	2▲▲–9401	
231–950	2103–912	

2191　　Osteochondrosis

2▲▲–911	2333–911	220–911
2391–911	23x–911	220–911.4
23512–911	2394–911	2▲▲–911.5
22x1–911	23717–911	

2194　　Osteoporosis

200–947

2212　　Tuberculosis of bones

220–123

2311　　Osteomyelitis of bones

237–105.2	237–115	2▲▲–100.0
23514–105	2▲▲–100	2▲▲–100.9

2341　　Fracture of upper extremity

2x12–41▲▲
2x1–41▲▲

2346　　Fracture of lower extremity

2x22–41▲▲
2x225–41▲▲
23512–400.4

2347　　Fracture of bones, excluding upper and lower extremities

2▲▲–4167	2▲▲–403.5	2▲▲–41▲.5
2▲▲–416▲	2▲▲–41▲.9	2▲▲–415.5
2▲▲–417	2▲▲–41▲.4	2▲▲–4x5.5
2▲▲–417.5	2▲▲–414.5	2▲▲▲2–400.4
2▲▲–419	2x▲–41▲.4	
2▲▲–418▲	2▲▲–41▲.7	
2▲▲–4185	2▲▲–41▲.6	

2400   DISEASES OF JOINTS

2401   Congenital conditions of joints, general

240–022
253–013

2402   Congenital deformity of joints

24▲–022	248–022	24▲–042
245–022	248–0223	24▲–026
2414–022	248–0224	247–026
2414–0221	24x1–0221	2493–026
2414–0224	24x1–022	
2414–025	24x5–022	

2404   Talipes, congenital

2493–022	2493–0225	2493–0229
2493–0227	2493–0220	24x–042
2493–0226	2493–0224	2494–022
2493–0221	2493–0222	
2493–0228	2494–0223	

2410   Infections of joints

24▲–100.4	24▲–100.5
24x1–100.4	24▲–100.3

2411   Arthritis

24▲–100
248–103
244–101

2412   Arthritis, tuberculous

241–123
241–123.4

2430   Toxic disorders of joints

24▲–390

2440   Injuries of joints, excluding dislocations

24▲–4x4	241–435	24▲–415.9
24▲–400.4	24▲–496	2414–415.7
24▲–415.4	24▲–4x4.5	24▲–415.7
24▲–400.0	24x1–400.9	24▲–400.x
248–402.0	24x1–433	24▲–415.x
243–40x.0	24x1–4001.9	24x–43x
243–416.0	24x1–400.6	24x–415.9
24x1–4x0.0	24▲–4x7	24▲.4–412
24▲–400.9	24▲–4▲▲	242.4–412
241–400.9	269–412	24x5–433
241–4001.9	24▲–4x9	

2441 Dislocation of joint, excluding shoulder, elbow and hip

248–40x
2493–408

2442 Dislocation of shoulder

242–408

2443 Dislocation of elbow

243–407

2444 Dislocation of hip

247–406

2455 Innervation disorders of joints

24▲–564	241–564	245–561
24x–564	241–5642	2468–561
24x–5641	2413–564	242–561
24x–5647	241–5641	241–561
24x–5646	24x1–564	244–561
24x–5648	26x–5641	24▲–564.5
24x–5644	241–569	24▲–560.5
24x–5645	24▲–560	24▲–561.5
24x–5640	24x–560	24▲–569.5
24x–5642	247–560	24▲–564.x
24x–5643	248–560	24▲–565
247–564	2468–560	245–565
247–5643	2468–5601	248–566
247–5644	2468–5602	24▲–564.9
247–5642	2468–5603	248–564.9
247–5646	241–560	24▲–560.9
247–5641	24x1–560	248–560.9
247–5645	24▲–561	
248–564	24x–561	

2460 Disorders of joint due to mechanical abnormalities

24▲.7–600.8	248–639	248–611
248.7–600.8	24▲–611	297–630

2470 Metabolic disorders of joint

24▲–741	24▲–7642	24▲–755
24▲–764.4	24▲▲–794	
248–764.4	24▲.7–755	

2480 Neoplasms of joint

24▲–871B
24▲–8771
2▲▲–8▲▲▲

2490   Diseases of joint due to unknown cause

240–932	24▲–911	24▲–x40
248–9x6	24▲–930	24▲–x90.4
24x1–940	240–991	24▲–x90.7
24x1–9x4	241–9x4	
24▲–9x8	24x–9x4	

2491   Osteoarthritis

240–912

2492   Arthritis, rheumatoid

24▲–952
240–952
241–952

2500   Diseases of cartilages and bursas

253–600.8
2501–630

2510   Infections of cartilages and bursas

25▲–100.2	25▲–190	25▲–100
25▲–100.1	251–190	25▲–190.0
251–100.9	25▲–190	

2512   Tuberculosis of cartilages and bursas

251–123

2540   Injuries of cartilages and bursas

25▲–430	25▲–4x0	258–430
25▲–402.9	25▲–43x	25▲–4▲▲
25▲–4x9	24x1–4x0.0	257–430
25▲–4▲▲	24x▲–4x0.0	259–430
2531–409	25▲–4x0.0	2511–400.9
2532–412	25▲–4x0.9	

2570   Metabolic disorders of cartilages and bursas

25▲–797
25▲–741
25▲–731

2580   Neoplasms of cartilages and bursas

25▲–873B	25▲–870A	25▲–8▲▲▲
251–873B	25▲–871B	
25▲–873F	25▲–879	

2590   Diseases of cartilages and bursas due to unknown cause

25▲–911	26x–9x6	25▲–923
25▲–943	2511–9x9	
253–943	25▲–930	

2600   Diseases of ligaments

26▲–017	2681–400.9	26x–9x4
26x–017	26▲–400.4	261–9x6
261–017	267–400.4	26x–x10
26▲–013	267–4001.4	26x–x30
268–013	267–4002.4	26x–042
26▲–100.4	26x–900.4	

2640   Injuries of ligaments

26▲–412	2682–412	2684–412
2681–412	2683–412	26x–434

2700   DISEASES OF MUSCLES

2701   Congenital conditions of muscles

27▲–011	270–0441	2751–027
27▲–031	27▲–050	275–016
270–090	270–043	27▲–012
27▲–017	272–017	2719–012
278–017	2x72–042	27▲–04▲
27▲–037	275–012	27▲▲–050
27325–037	275–027	2716–042
28819–013	275–021	
270–044	275–037	

2710   Infections of muscles

27▲–100.2	3052–100.3	2750–100
27▲–100.4	3072–100.3	2716–1xx
275–100.3	3061–100.3	

2711   Myositis

27▲–100
27▲–100.0
275–100

2740   Injuries of muscles

27▲–402	27▲–44x	27▲–400.4
27▲–400.4	27▲–432	272–44x
279–431.4	27x–432	272–4x4
279–400.4	27▲–4x6	27▲–410
270–499	276–4x6	27▲–410.0
270–445	27817–4x6	275–409
27▲–4▲▲.5	27819–4x6	275–414
27325–43x.5	27▲–43x	275–424
27325–415.5	27▲–430	275–43x
27▲–438	27▲–416	275–436
27▲–4x7	27▲–412	275–415
27▲–4x9	27▲–415.4	275–416

2740   Injuries of muscles (Continued)

275–411	27110–415.9	2716–410
27▲–43x	27▲▲–400.9	
27▲▲–415.9	2719–400.9	

2750   Vascular disorders of muscles

27▲–514

2755   Innervation disorders of muscles

2747–551	27▲–569	275–569
27▲–590.x	27▲–561	275–595
270–562	272–550	2716–561
27▲–564	272–590	2716–560
27▲–568	275–560	
27▲–567	275–564	

2760   Disorders of muscles due to mechanical abnormalities

2751–639
275–639

2770   Metabolic disorders of muscles

27▲–713	270–712
270–731	270–748

2780   Neoplasms of muscles

27▲–870A	27▲–872F	27▲–876F
27▲–870F	27▲–868A	27▲–8▲▲▲
27▲–850A	27▲–8451	
27▲–872A	27▲–867A	

2790   Diseases of muscles due to unknown cause

2x4–920	270–9x94	270–x30
27▲–930	270–x95	27112–x201
270–9x9	270–x20	27112–x202

2800   DISEASES OF TENDONS

2801   Congenital conditions of tendons

287–017

2810   Infections of tendons

28▲–100.2	28▲–100	28▲.9–100
28▲–100.1	28▲–100.0	28▲.9–100.4

2840   Injuries of tendons

28▲–4▲▲	28▲–405	293–424
28▲–406	28▲–416	28▲.9–43x

2860 Disorders of tendons due to mechanical abnormalities

287–646

2870 Metabolic disorders of tendons

28▲–755

2880 Neoplasms of tendons

28▲–873B	28▲–8741A	28▲–872A
28▲–870A	28▲–850A	28▲–8▲▲▲

2890 Diseases of tendons due to unknown cause

28▲.9–923
28▲.9–940
28▲.9–952

2900 DISEASES OF FASCIA

2910 Infections of fascia

2964–100.2	2966–100	29▲–100.2
29▲–100	29▲–100.1	

2940 Injuries of fascia

29▲–400.4	296–430	293–424
29▲–430	299–430	

2990 Diseases of fascia due to unknown cause

29▲–9x4
296–9x6

3000 DISEASES OF THE RESPIRATORY SYSTEM

3010 Infections of upper respiratory system

3001–19y

3011 Common cold

300–100

3012 Acute diffuse upper respiratory infection

3001–100

3040 Injuries of respiratory system, general

3054–438.3
3054–400.3

3044 Inhalation burn

3▲▲–494

3100   DISEASES OF NOSE

3101   Congenital conditions of nose

310–011	310–037	310–010
31▲–012	313–022	312–017
312–018	310–022	

3110   Infections of nose

318–100.2	125–100.0	310–100
3181–100.2	317–190	310–1x6
313–100.2	310–126	310–16▲
312–100.4	310–124	133–130
x00–100.x	313–100.3	310–147.4
3181–100.8	313–147.3	310–123
310–100.4	313–123.3	310–100.9
313–100.4	316–1x6	

3111   Nasopharyngitis

318–125
318–100

3120   Fungus and parasitic infections of nose

3011–200.3
310–231

3130   Toxic disorders of nose

310–3▲▲
310–319
310–300.6

3139   Allergic rhinitis (hay fever)

310–391▲

3140   Injuries of nose

312–400.4	310–402.7	310–438.0
312–415.4	31▲–4▲▲	313–4x6
216–400.4	313–430.3	318–415.4
216–408	313–415.3	310–400.9
310–448	310–438	

3141   Epistaxis due to trauma

310–400.7

3142   Deflection of septum due to trauma

313–400.4

3143   Foreign body in nose

310–496

3150   Vascular disorders of nose

31x–533.5
310–518
313–522.9

3160   Disorders of nose due to mechanical abnormalities

313–600.8   312–611   31x–641
316–6x8   310–615

3164   Deflection of septum due to unknown cause

313–640

3170   Metabolic disorders of nose

216–794
310–786

3180   Neoplasms of nose

310–8091   310–850A   310–814A
310–8091A   310–830   310–811
310–814   310–8451   310–8▲▲▲
310–870F   310–833

3190   Disease of nose due to unknown cause

310–957   310–951   310–x30
313–900.6   x00–x10
31▲–940   31x–x30

3194   Polyp of nose, simple

31▲–944

3200   DISEASES OF ACCESSORY SINUSES

3201   Congenital conditions of accessory sinuses

32▲–039   32▲–014   32▲–019
32▲–032   32▲–012

3210   Infections of accessory sinuses

302–100.3   32▲–100.6
3021–100.3   32▲–100.8

3211   Sinusitis

32▲–100   320–190   32▲–123
32▲–100.0   32▲–130
320–100   320–100.0

3220   Fungus and parasitic infection of accessory sinuses

32▲–2952

3230   Toxic disorders of accessory sinuses

320–3▲▲

3240   Injuries of accessory sinuses

3021–415.3
32▲–400.6
32▲–4▲▲

3248   Basosinusitis

321–481.0

3260   Disorders of accessory sinuses due to mechanical
          abnormalities

32▲–615
32▲–600

3290   Diseases of accessory sinuses due to unknown cause

32▲–9x8

3294   Polyp formation, simple, sinus

32▲–944

3300   DISEASES OF LARYNX

3301   Congenital conditions of larynx

33▲–011	331–034	333–037
330–018	331–016	330–023
330–017	3031–025	337–027
334–025	331–013	337–026
33▲–064	333–025	330–077

3310   Infections of larynx

330–100.2	303▲–100.3	335–147
3381–100.4	33▲–100.6	330–1x0
3381–100	330–166	330–100.4
332–100.8	330–124	330–123
331–100	335–100	

3311   Laryngitis

330–125	330–100.0	330–1x0.6
330–100	330–1x0.9	330–1413

3312   Laryngotracheitis

3031–100
3031–100.0

3320   Fungus and parasitic infections of larynx

330–29▲
33▲–2▲▲

3330   Toxic disorders of larynx

330–3▲▲	336–3x0	339–300.4
330–300.0	339–3238.x	330–300.4
332–300.8	330–3931	330–390

3340   Injuries of larynx

330–441	303▲–400.3	330–43x
330–472.0	303▲–415.3	335–4x0
330–471.0	330–414	335–47▲
336–43x	33▲–4x7	330–411
338–406	21x–416	330–415.4
3381–406	336–430	330–4▲▲.4
3382–406	336–430.9	330–4702.4
332–408	33▲–4▲▲	336–416
331–401	336–43x.6	
331–441	337–4x9	

3343   Foreign body in larynx

330–496
339–438.4

3350   Vascular disorders of larynx

332–505.8
330–554.1

3355   Innervation disorders of larynx

330–593	339–569	339–567
339–5631	3391–569	339–590
3391–5631	3392–569	330–567.4
3392–5631	3393–569	330–560.4
3393–5631	3394–569	
3394–5631	336–569	

3360   Disorders of larynx due to mechanical abnormalities

330–600.8	330–611	33x–641
330–631	337–631	

3370   Metabolic disorders of larynx

330–776
330–776.4

3380   Neoplasms of larynx

337–8091	33▲–814	330–8▲▲▲
330–8091A	330–870A	
330–873B	330–872A	

3390   Diseases of larynx due to unknown cause

330–913	330–940	330–954
330–957	330–900.8	336–941
330–923	336–900.6	3301–940

3394   Polyp of larynx, simple

330–944
336–944

3400   DISEASES OF TRACHEA

3401   Congenital conditions of trachea

340–011	3041–024	340–023
341–076	341–024	3041–029
340–036	341–010	
304▲–029	340–017	

3410   Infections of trachea

340–100.4
340–147.4
340–123

3411   Tracheitis

340–100

3430   Toxic disorders of trachea

340–3▲▲
340–300.4

3440   Injuries of trachea

340–496	340–4▲▲.4	340–441.9
340–4▲▲	340–415.4	340–435.9
340–416	340–438	340–438.9
3041–400.3	340–438.0	
340–435	340–400.9	

3460   Disorders of trachea due to mechanical abnormalities

34x–641

3480   Neoplasms of trachea

340–8091A	340–814	340–8▲▲▲
340–873B	340–872A	

3490   Diseases of trachea due to unknown cause

340–923

3500   DISEASES OF BRONCHI

3501   Congenital conditions of the bronchi

350–011	350–015	350–077
350–018	350–036	

3510   Infection of bronchi and bronchioles

350–100.8	3051–100.3	350–147
3053–100.3	350–100.4	

3511   Bronchitis

353–100	350–100
353–100.4	350–100.0

3512   Tuberculosis of bronchi and bronchioles

350–123.9	3051–123.3
3053–123.3	350–123

3513   Pertussis, epidemic

350–108

3514   Bronchiectasis

350–100.6
350–123.6
353–100.6

3520   Fungus and parasitic infections of bronchi and bronchioles

350–220.9
35▲–2▲▲

3530   Toxic disorders of bronchi and bronchioles

350–3▲▲	350–300.8	350–300.4
353–319	353–300.4	

3539   Asthma

350–390

3540   Injuries of bronchi and bronchioles

350–430	305▲–415.3	350–435
350–400.8	350–4▲▲	350–400.9

3543   Foreign body in bronchus

350–438.6
350–496
350–438.9

3560   Disorders of bronchi and bronchioles due to mechanical
          abnormalities

350–615
350–600.8

3580   Neoplasms of bronchi and bronchioles

350–8091   350–814   350–8191G
350–8091A   350–870A   350–8▲▲▲

3590   Diseases of bronchi and bronchioles due to unknown
          cause

350–923
350–956
350–900.9

3600   DISEASES OF LUNG

3601   Congenital conditions of lung

360–034   360–019   36▲–015
360–077   3071–029   360–064
36▲–031   361–064   360–027
361–031   360–034.8   360–016
360–031   300–032   300–075
360–011   360–023

3610   Infections of lung

362–100.4   36x–1x0.4   360–100.6
360–100.9   368–100.6   360–1x0
360–123.9   368–123.0   360–147
360–100.8   360–100.1

3611   Pneumonia, bacterial

360–118   360–100   360–100.0
368–100   360–101
368–100.0   360–102

3612   Tuberculosis of lung

361–123.6   360–1235   361–1236
3601–123   360–1236   3063–123
360–123   360–1237   3063–1231
360–1231   360–1238   3063–1232
360–1232   360–1239   3063–1233
360–1233   360–123x   362–123.4
360–1234   361–1233   361–123.0

3613   Abscess

360–100.2
360–101.2
360–151

3614   Bronchopneumonia

361–190   361–173   361–100.0
361–168   361–102   361–107
361–101   361–100

3616   Viral pneumonia

361–160
360–160

3620   Fungus and parasitic infections of lung

360–2▲▲.2   360–241   360–2▲▲.8
360–2▲▲.6   360–219   360–267
360–2▲▲   360–201   361–2▲▲.8

3621   Actinomycosis of lung

360–202

3622   Blastomycosis of lung

360–217

3623   Histoplasmosis

360–220

3630   Toxic disorders of lung

360–3224   368–3224   360–3▲▲
360–390   360–3▲▲.8

3631   Pneumonia due to toxins

368–319

3640   Injuries of lung

360–400.2   360–440   360–496
360–438.2   360–400.8   360–400.1
360–496.2   360–415.8   360–4x9
362–435   36x–429   360–406
362–415.4   36x–427   360–424
360–400.4   36x–426   360–4▲▲
360–415.4   36x–425   360–436
361–496.0   362–434   360–415.3
361–4961.0   368–427   360–471.0
361–415.0   360–438.6
360–428   360–4712.6

3643   Pneumoconiosis

368–438▲   368–4384   362–438
368–4382   368–4389   368–498.0
368–4381   368–4386

3650   Vascular disorders of lung

360–500.1
360–535.7

3651   Infarction of lung

360–510
360–511

3652   Passive congestion

360–520
360–522

3653   Embolism of lung

360–512.1
36x–500.4
360–512

3660   Disorders of lung due to mechanical abnormalities

360–611.4
362–600.8
36x–618

3661   Emphysema

360–641
362–600.6
362–610

3670   Metabolic disorders of lung

362–797

3680   Neoplasms of lung

360–8091	360–814	360–8▲▲▲
360–8072	360–8882	
360–8191	360–8191G	

3690   Diseases of lung due to unknown cause

360–923	360–932	362–941
362–9x6	362–923	

3691   Fibrosis of lung

368–9x6
368–9xx1

3692   Hyaline membrane of lung

360–9x0

3700   DISEASES OF PLEURA

3701   **Congenital conditions of pleura**

370–0▲▲

3710   **Infections of pleura**

370–1x4	30754–1x4.5	370–17x4
370–100.9	370–100.7	
370–123.9	30752–100	

3711   **Pleurisy**

370–190
370–190.8
370–190.0

3712   **Pleurisy, tuberculous**

370–123.8
370–123.0
370–1237

3713   **Pneumothorax due to infection**

30751–100.5	30753–100
30751–100.4	30753–100.5

3714   **Pneumothorax due to tuberculosis**

30751–123.4	30751–123.5
30753–123	30752–123

3715   **Empyema**

370–100	373–100
3074–100.3	375–100

3716   **Empyema, tuberculous**

370–1231
370–1232

3720   **Fungus and parasitic infections of pleura**

370–2▲▲.8	30571–2▲▲
370–2▲▲	30753–2▲▲

3740   **Injuries of pleura**

370–400.4	30751–415.8	370–490
370–438.2	370–400.7	370–420
370–415.2	370–4▲▲	370–4x0
370–4x6	370–436	

3741   **Pneumothorax, traumatic**

30754–4x4.5	30752–4001	3075–415.4
30752–400	30752–415	30751–43x.5

3741   Pneumothorax, traumatic (Continued)

30751–400	30751–4151	30753–4001
30751–4001	30751–400.4	30753–415
30751–415	30753–400	30753–4151

3750   Vascular disorders of pleura

370–502
370–532
370–522

3760   Disorders of pleura due to unknown cause

30754–641.5
376–641

3780   Neoplasms of pleura

370–8▲▲.8	370–7451
370–8772A	370–879

3790   Diseases of pleura due to unknown cause

30754–900
30751–900
30752–9x5

4000   DISEASES OF THE CARDIOVASCULAR SYSTEM

4050   Vascular disorders of cardiovascular system

400–533

4070   Metabolic disorders of cardiovascular system

400–78x

4100   DISEASES OF HEART

4101   Congenital anomalies of heart, excluding septal defects

410–011	412–039	455–018
41▲–0▲▲	412–0391	455–0242
4151–0▲▲	430–01x	453–0242
4195–0▲▲	413–015	454–032
410–037	457–030	452–032
410–021	437–030	452–021
410–0211	413–039	455–038
410–022	413–0391	453–038
410–026	440–042	455–024
410–0261	435–019	453–024
410–0262	4443–042	454–017
410–0263	413–0▲▲	454–015
410–091	4442–042	455–031
456–013	436–019	453–031
410–0y0	454–031	452–015
410–013	452–031	452–017

4101   Congenital anomalies of heart, excluding septal defects
             (Continued)

451–0▲▲	41x2–011	41x–026
40x–0x5	41x1–011	41x–010
40x–0x0.6	41x–031	41x2–010
40x–0x8	41x1–015	41x1–010
40x–0x0	41x–021	

4102   Septal defects of heart

412–0xx	412–0▲▲	413–0x0
412–030	413–0x8	413–0▲▲
412–0x9	413–030	411–0x8
412–0x2	413–0x3	411–0x5
412–0x1	413–0x4	411–0xx
411–0x6	413–0x5	40x–0x3

4110   Infections of heart

41x–147.6	410–100	41x–147.4
410–100.6	410–100.0	41▲–147
41x–100	41x–1x0.6	410–100.5

4130   Toxic disorders of heart

410–3▲▲	410–33152.9	410–34382
410–34819	410–3471	410–3844
410–321	410–3185	
410–33152	410–34649	

4140   Injuries of heart

410–427	410–4x4	410–43x.6
410–402.x	410–43x	410–416
410–435.x	410–414	410–411

4150   Vascular disorders of heart

410–540	410–535.6	410–522
41▲–516.6	410–540.9	410–5x7.5
416–535.6	41▲–511.6	

4151   Arteriosclerotic heart disease

410–516

4155   Innervation disorders of heart

41x–584

4160   Disorders of heart due to mechanical abnormalities

410–600.x
41▲–619

4161   Coronary artery embolism

41x–618

4170   Metabolic disorders of heart

410–701   410–754   410–772
410–7621   410–771   410–798

4180   Neoplasms of heart

410–870A   410–8871   410–882
410–850A   410–879   410–8▲▲▲

4190   Diseases of heart due to unknown cause

410–922   410–9x6   410–9x9
410–911   41x–956   410–925
410–923   410–917   41x–932

4193   Rheumatic heart disease

410–932
410–932.0

4194   Arteriosclerosis of coronary artery

41x–942   41x–942.4
41x–942.6   41x–942.7

4200   DISEASES OF PERICARDIUM

4201   Congenital conditions of pericardium

420–011
420–012
420–036

4210   Infections of pericardium

420–100.3   410–100.5   420–123.9
420–1001.3   404–123
420–1002.3   420–123.4

4211   Pericardial effusion

420–102.8   420–100.2   420–123.8
420–115.8   420–100.8
420–100   420–100.0

4230   Toxic disorders of pericardium

420–389

4240   Injuries of pericardium

420–496   420–4001.7   420–400.4
420–400.7   420–4002.8   420–400.3

4250   Vascular disorders of pericardium

420–532   420–522.8
420–531.5   420–511.0

4280   Neoplasms of pericardium

420–879

4290   Diseases of pericardium due to unknown cause

420–900.4	420–932	404–900.4
420–923	420–932.8	404–932
420–900.8	420–932.4	
420–930	420–932.0	

4300   DISEASES OF MYOCARDIUM

4310   Infections of myocardium, excluding myocarditis

437–100.5
430–1x0
430–100.2

4311   Myocarditis

430–100	430–115	430–123
430–168	430–160	
430–102	430–100.0	

4350   Vascular disorders of myocardium

430–5x9.6
430–5x7.6

4351   Myocardial infarction

430–516.7
430–515.7
430–512.7

4355   Innervation disorders of myocardium

430–563.0

4370   Metabolic disorders of myocardium

430–751
430–748

4380   Neoplasms of myocardium

430–871B
430–867A
430–867F

4390   Diseases of myocardium due to unknown cause

430–932.6	431–x26	434–x43
430–955	431–x25	434–x45
430–9x7	431–x24	434–x42
430–930	431–x23	434–x41
430–932	431–x22	434–x44
430–932.0	431–x21	

4395   Myocarditis of unknown cause (Fiedler)
430–950

4400   DISEASES OF CONDUCTION SYSTEM

4410   Infections of conduction system
440–147

4450   Vascular disorders of conduction system
444▲–516.x

4455   Innervation disorders of conduction system

443–584.x	440–590	440–584
440–580	440–585	

4490   Diseases of conduction system due to unknown cause

444▲–932.x	4443–x37	441–x12
444▲–x31	4442–x37	441–x13
444–x36	443–x32	441–x14
444–x35	443–x31	4441–x37
444–x34	441–x16	441–x15
443–x33	441–x11	

4500   DISEASES OF ENDOCARDIUM, VALVES,
AND CHORDAE TENDINEAE

4510   Infections of endocardium, valves, and chordae tendineae

45▲–1x0.6	45▲–1x0.3	45▲–147.4
45▲–100.6	45▲–147.3	457–100.5
45▲–100.3	457–100.5	

4511   Endocarditis
450–100
450–100.0

4540   Injuries of endocardium, valves, and chordae tendineae
451–43x

4590   Diseases of endocardium, valves, and chordae tendineae
due to unknown cause

455–923	450–925	45▲–932.4
456–955	456–925	450–932.0
45▲.▲–941	450–940.7	45▲–932.6
45▲–941.4	450–932	
45▲–9x9	456–932	

4600 DISEASES OF ARTERIES

4601 Congenital conditions of arteries

4612–015	4611–016	46▲–010
4612–015.5	461–019	463–010
461–0181	4613–019	4623–010
461–0183	4613–0192	402–029
461–0181.6	4051–01x	4621–021
461–0181.5	4611–02x	4622–021
461–018	4051–02x	4623–021
4611–0x3	4051–02x1	
461–016	46▲–015	

4610 Infections of arteries

46▲–100.2	46▲–147.5	4032–100.5
46▲–1x0.6	46▲–100.7	4051–100.5
46▲–147.6	461–100.6	4033–100.5
46▲–100.6	461–147.6	4051–147.5
402▲–100.6	461–100.9	466–100.6
46▲–1x0.4	461–100.5	468–100.1
46▲–100.5	4034–100.5	

4611 Arteritis

46▲–100	46▲–123	46▲–147
46▲–100.0	461–100	
4602–147	461–190	

4630 Toxic disorders of arteries

460–3▲▲
460–3238

4640 Injuries of arteries

46▲–427	46▲–4▲▲	466–400.6
46▲–400.6	46▲–416	466–400.4
402▲–400.6	46▲–415.5	466–425
402–400.3	46▲–400.7	469–400.4
46▲–420.4	46▲–415.7	469–425
46▲–425	461–4▲▲	469–4▲▲
46▲–426	461–416	468–400.7

4650 Vascular disorders of arteries

47x–513	46▲–547	461–533.9
460–534	46▲–5x7.4	

4653 Hypertensive vascular disease

460–533

4655   Innervation disorders of arteries

402–564
47x–581
47x–582

4661   Embolism of artery

46▲–618
466–618
469–618

4662   Thrombosis of artery

46▲–619
469–619

4663   Aneurysm of artery

46▲–615.6
46▲–618.6

4665   Embolism of aorta

4616–618

4670   Metabolic disorders of arteries

460–781   460–782
460–776   461–754

4690   Diseases of arteries due to unknown cause

46▲–9x6   401–992   461–941.6
46▲–942.6   402–930   461–915.6
46▲–942.5   46▲–942.7   461.2–955
460–923   460–x10   461.2–955.5
402–931   461–932   4051–942.5
46▲–931.6   461.2–915.6   466–900.7
46▲–931.5   461–942.6   466–931
46▲–931.7   4616–942.6   469–931
46▲–932   4615–942.6   469–931.7

4694   Arteriosclerosis

460–942   4616–942   469–942
4602–955   461–942.5   469–942.7
46x.2–955   461–942.4   469–942.4
460–952   461–942.7   468–942
46▲–941   471–942   468–942.7
47x–943   4711–942.6
461–942   466–942

4699   Essential vascular hypertension

47x–x30

4700   DISEASES OF LESSER CIRCULATION

4701   Congenital conditions of lesser circulation

4711–031	471–015	4711–02x
4711–021	4711–015	486–021
4711–018	471–016	486–022

4710   Infections of lesser circulation

471–100.6
471–123

4740   Injuries of lesser circulation

4711–4▲▲
471–425

4750   Vascular disorders of lesser circulation

400–535	471–533	471–522.7
471–522.4	471–533.3	486–522.7

4760   Disorders of lesser circulation due to mechanical abnormalities

4711–610.9
4711–641
486–619

4761   Embolism of pulmonary artery

471–618

4762   Thrombosis of pulmonary artery

4711–619

4800   DISEASES OF VEINS

4801   Congenital conditions of veins

4811–011	48▲–010	480–015
4811–01x	482–010	

4810   Infections of veins, excluding phlebitis

487–100.7	482–1x7.3
482–100.7	48▲–123

4811   Phlebitis

487–100	48▲–124	482–100
48▲–190	48▲–184	485–190
48▲–115	482–190	484–190

4812   Thrombophlebitis, thrombosis

48▲–100.7
482–100.7
485–100.7

4830   Toxic disorders of veins

48▲–3▲▲

4840   Injuries of veins

48▲–4▲▲	48▲–400.7	48▲–432.6
48▲–415.0	482–4▲▲	48▲–431.6
48▲–400.0	482–435	48▲–434.6
48▲–4x6.5	48▲–430.6	48▲–435.6
48▲–415.7	48▲–433.6	

4850   Vascular disorders of veins

480–520	48▲–541.7	482–547.7
48▲–547	48▲–522	

4860   Disorders of veins due to mechanical abnormalities

481–610	48▲–619.0	485–619
48▲–615	48▲–619	

4864   Varicose veins

48▲–641
48x–641
48x–641.0

4890   Diseases of veins due to unknown cause

480–930	48▲–9x6	482–900.7
480–952	482–952	485–900.7
48▲–931.7	482–952.7	485–952

4900   DISEASES OF CAPILLARIES

4910   Infections of capillaries

490–100.5

4930   Toxic disorders of capillaries

490–300.5

4940   Injuries of capillaries

490–400.5

4950   Vascular disorders of capillaries

490–5x5.5
490–512.5

4970   Metabolic disorders of capillaries

490–700.5

4990   Diseases of capillaries due to unknown cause

490–991	490–995
490–992.5	490–993.5

5000   DISEASES OF THE HEMIC AND LYMPHATIC
SYSTEMS

5001   Congenital conditions of blood and blood-forming organs

500–016
501–016
507–076

5010   Infections of blood and blood-forming organs

500–100.9	501–100	507–1▲▲
501–100.9	501–157	

5020   Fungus and parasitic infections of blood and blood-
forming organs

501–200

5030   Toxic disorders of blood and blood-forming organs

501–3▲▲	501–3991	500–33131
501–397	501–3992	507–3▲▲
501–3432	502–300	
501–399	500–3▲▲.9	

5040   Injuries of blood and blood-forming organs

500–470.9
500–47▲.9
500–471.9

5041   Anemia due to acute blood loss

501–400.7

5050   Vascular disorders of blood and blood-forming organs

502–536	500–5361	501–5x6
500–536	501–5x7.5	501–5x9

5070   Metabolic disorders of blood and blood-forming organs

502–790	501–7034	501–709
501–794	501–790.9	501–772
501–703	500–790.9	501–704.6
501–7031	500–7901.9	505–755
501–7032	501–700	505–756
501–7033	501–715	505–758

5071   Anemia, pernicious

501–7035

5073   Anemia, microcytic

501–736
501–736.7
501–736.x

5079   Thrombocytic disease

507–792.6   507–791   507–790.9
507–7921.6   507–7911

5080   Neoplasms of blood and blood-forming organs

503–834   500–839   504–8282
502▲–822▲   503–830   501–8271
505–832   507–8281   505–831
500–829   506–821   500–8283
503–820   504–833   5▲▲–8▲▲▲

5090   Diseases of blood and blood-forming organs due to un-
          known cause

501–991.5   501–9912.5   505–9x9
500–995   501–9912.4   501–9913.5
501–991   501–991.4   501–9913.4
501–9915   501–9911.5   507–920
501–9916   501–9911.4   507–9x7
501–9913   501–9x6   507–x90.5
501–9914   502–9x6

5091   Anemia normocytic

501–9x0
501–920.1

5101   Congenital conditions of plasma constituents

5122–011

5130   Toxic disorders of plasma constituents

514▲–3▲▲
5132–3▲▲
515–3▲▲

5140   Injuries of plasma constituents

5145–404
5141–44x
515–450

5150   Vascular disorders of plasma constituents

513▲–549

5170   Metabolic disorders of plasma constituents

5142–7671
5141–712
515–749

5190   Diseases of plasma constituents due to unknown cause

5122–x80	5131–x90	5122–x81
519–x80	5134–x90	5141–x80
5135–x80	5132–x95	515–x80
5131–x95	519–x81	

5200   DISEASES OF SPLEEN

5201   Congenital conditions of spleen

520–011	520–021	520–010
520–031	520–027	

5210   Infections of spleen

520–100.2	520–100	520–157.6
520–1x0	520–100.6	

5240   Injuries of spleen (fixed cells)

520–4▲▲
520–416

5250   Vascular disorders of spleen (fixed cells)

520–511
520–512
520–536

5260   Disorders of spleen (fixed cells) due to mechanical
abnormalities

520–630
520–631
520–637

5270   Metabolic disorders of spleen (fixed cells)

520–796
520–798
520–700.6

5280   Neoplasms of spleen (fixed cells)

520–870A	520–832	520–831
520–850A	520–830	520–8▲▲

5290   Disorders of spleen (fixed cells) due to unknown cause

520–922	520–958.4
520–958	520–958.9

5300   DISEASES OF MARROW

5310   Infections of marrow

530–123

5380   Neoplasms of marrow

530–875G   530–831
530–832   530–8▲▲▲

5390   Diseases of marrow due to unknown cause

530–941
530–922
530–942

5400   DISEASES OF LYMPHATIC CHANNELS

5401   Congenital condition of lymphatic channels

542–019.8

5410   Infections of lymphatic channels and lymph

541–100.3   54▲–100.4
54▲–100.6   54▲–100.5

5411   Lymphangitis

54▲–100   54▲–123   545–103
54▲–100.0   545–100   545–100.0

5420   Fungus and parasitic infections of lymphatic channels
           and lymph

54▲–257

5440   Injuries of lymphatic channels and lymph

541–400.3   54▲–400.4
54▲–4▲▲   54▲–415.4

5480   Neoplasms of lymphatic channels and lymph

54▲–845A
54▲–854G
54▲–854B

5490   Diseases of lymphatic channels and lymph due to un-
           known cause

546–900.8

5500   DISEASES OF LYMPH NODES (FIXED CELLS)

5510   Infections of lymph nodes (fixed cells)

55▲–100.9   55▲–198
55▲–123.9   559–198

5511   Lymphadenitis

55▲–100
55▲–100.0
55▲–100.1

5512   Abscess of lymph nodes

558–190.8	558–103.8	55▲–100.2
558–10x.8	558–147.8	

5513   Nonbacterial regional lymphadenitis (cat scratch fever)

55▲–130

5530   Toxic disorders of lymph nodes (fixed cells)

55▲–3▲▲

5540   Injuries of lymph nodes (fixed cells)

55▲–496
55▲–438
55▲–400.0

5580   Neoplasms of lymph nodes (fixed cells)

55▲–838A	55▲–839	55▲–831
55▲–834	55▲–830	55▲–8▲▲▲
55▲–832	55▲–833	

5590   Diseases of lymph nodes (fixed cells) due to unknown cause

55▲–959

5594   Hyperplasia of lymph node

55▲–943

5600   OBSTETRICAL CONDITIONS

5602   Pregnancy, not delivered

7x2–789

5610   Infections of pregnancy

7x9–100.2	7x52–100	7x2–100
7x94–100	7x51–100	78x–100.7
7x9–100	7x5–100	
7x3–100.4	7x21–100	

5630   Toxic disorders of pregnancy

7x2–33▲▲	010–388	014–388
7x2–34637	015–388	x23–388
7x2–3824	013–388	x3x–388

5640   Injuries of pregnancy

7x3–409	7x4–435	7x3–412
7x3–415.4	7x4–4x7	7x41–412
7x3–412.4	7x2–400	7xx–400.5
7x3–400.4	7x2–43x	7xx–412
7x3–430	7x2–400.9	7x1–412

5640   Injuries of pregnancy (Continued)

7x4–412	7x2–416	7x2–412.7
7x2–415	7x2–416.4	77x–435.6
70x2–412.3	7x2–400.7	7031–412.3

5655   Innervation disorders of pregnancy

7x3–561	7x2–561	7x2–560
7x2–560.7	7x21–561	

5660   Disorders of pregnancy due to mechanical abnormalities

7x2–600.7	7x2–636	7x2–610.5
7x2–614.7	7x2–643	7x2–6x6
7x2–639	7x2–63x	7x2–6x4
7x2–938	7x3–646	7x2–637
7x2–631	7xx–646	

5670   Metabolic disorders of pregnancy

7x2–796
7x2–7x9
7x2–795

5680   Neoplasms of pregnancy
7x2–8▲▲▲

5690   Diseases of pregnancy due to unknown cause

7x2–x90
7x2–911
7x2–9x9

5700   False labor

7x2–7891
7x2–7892

5702   Pregnancy, abnormal site

060–789	7892–789	7x7–789.6
060–789.5	7x8–789	7x7–789.5
7x3–789	7x22–789	
7x21–789	7x7–789	

5710   Pregnancy, delivered

7x2–000
7x2–001
7x2–002

5712   Pregnancy, delivered, term multiple

7x2–050	7x2–051	7x2–052
7x2–0501	7x2–0511	7x2–0521
7x2–0502	7x2–0512	7x2–0522

5712   Pregnancy, delivered, term multiple (Continued)

7x2–053	7x2–055	7x2–058
7x2–0531	7x2–056	7x2–059
7x2–0532	7x2–057	7x2–05x

5713   Pregnancy, delivered prematurely

7x2–004	7x2–005
7x2–0041	7x2–006

5714   Pregnancy, delivered prematurely, multiple

7x2–054	7x2–0545	7x2–0561
7x2–0541	7x2–0546	7x2–0571
7x2–0542	7x2–0547	7x2–0581
7x2–0543	7x2–0548	7x2–0591
7x2–0544	7x2–0551	7x2–05x1

5715   Pregnancy, delivered immaturely

7x2–008	7x2–0083	7x2–0086
7x2–0085	7x2–0081	7x2–007
7x2–0082	7x2–0084	

5716   Pregnancy, delivered postmaturely

7x2–00x
7x2–00x1
7x2–00x2

5720   Abortions

7x2–009	7x2–0093	7x2–0096
7x2–0095	7x2–0091	7x2–y00.9
7x2–0092	7x2–0094	7x2–147.9

5730   Births

790–000

5732   Premature, immature birth, living child

790–007
790–004

5733   Postmature birth

790–00x

5734   Multiple birth

790–050	790–0541	790–058
790–0501	790–0542	790–0581
790–0502	790–055	
790–054	790–0551	

5741   Disorders of bony pelvis

22x–021	22x–6511	22x–6405
22x–123.4	22x–646	22x–6406
22x–435	22x–640	22x–650
22x–436	22x–6408	22x–657
22x–43x	22x–6401	22x–652
246–408	22x–6402	22x–771
22x–434	22x–6403	22x–787
22x–564	22x–6409	22x–764
22x–651	22x–6404	22x–940
22x–6510	22x–6407	

5750   Complications of puerperium

0662–100	198–100.3	198–100.2
198–400.8	198–100	195–100
198–100.8	48▲–1901	

5751   Septicemia, puerperal

014–190

5752   Disorders of umbilical cord

799–638	799–100	799–146
799–792	799–6301	799–794
799–790	799–190	799–422
799–400.7	799–631	799–643
799–639	799–6311	799–630

5760   Diseases of infants

790–514	790–421	790–165
790–430	7991–019	790–1577

5770   Presentation

790–650	790–673	790–680
790–660	790–672	790–681
790–661	790–674	790–682
790–662	790–677	790–683
790–663	790–678	790–684
790–664	790–679	790–695
790–665	790–690	790–696
790–666	790–691	790–697
790–670	790–692	790–698
790–676	790–693	790–699
790–675	790–694	790–6y0
790–671	790–69x	

5800   DISEASES OF THE EAR

5801   Congenital conditions of auricle

x72–011	x72–016	x83–017
x72–010	x76–018	x80–017
x72–021	x76–093	x8x–019
x75–011	x72–031	x81–031
x75–018	x72–019	x88–011
x75–017	x72–064	x85–011
x72–029	x72–022	x85–018
x78–011	x72–01x	x88–022
x78–032	x83–021	x88–0421
x78–013	x80–011	x88–0422
x78–034	x81–011	x88–0423
x78–016	x81–077	x85–092
x78–031	x83–036	x94–092
x72–013	x81–024	x94–015

5810   Infections of ear

x72–100.2	x75–100	x83–100.0
x72–105.2	x77–100	x83–100.4
x75–100.2	x77–100.8	x85–100
x72–118	x77–100.0	x85–104
x72–100.4	x74–100	x85–1x0.0
x72–125	x81–100.4	x85–1x8
x75–100.0	x80–100.6	x93–100.3
x72–100.1	x8x–100	x89–100
x72–100	x83–100	

5811   Otitis

x71–100	x80–100	x80–100.0
x71–123	x80–101	x80–123
x80–190	x80–105	x81–100.1
x80–190.0	x80–102	

5812   Mastoiditis

x84–100	x84–1x6	x84–100.0
x84–101	x84–1x7	x84–1x0
x84–102	x84–1x1	x84–123

5820   Fungus and parasitic infection of ear

x75–297
x75–2▲▲

5830   Toxic disorders of ear

x72–32▲	x75–3122.4	x85–3▲▲
x77–32▲	x80–390	x88–3▲▲.x
x75–300.0	x85–390	

5840   Injuries of ear

x70–400	x72–4▲▲	x84–416
x77–482	x75–4▲▲	x80–415.0
x77–482.5	x77–4x0	x80–481
x72–441	x77–416	x85–482
x72–400.4	x75–400.4	x93–415.3
x75–44x.6	x75–415.4	x86–416
x75–496	x81–482	x85–4x0
x76–416	x81–400.5	x88–400.x
x72–448	x84–415.3	
x72–4x7	x84–496	

5850   Vascular disorders of ear

x72–501	x85–532
x85–520	x85–510

5855   Innervation disorders of ear

x71–593
x72–573

5860   Disorders of ear due to mechanical abnormalities

x71–646
x75–616

5870   Metabolic disorders of ear

x86–7x9.4	x86–7x1	x88–7x9.8
x86–7x9	966–79x	
x86–7x9.6	x88–79x	

5880   Neoplasms of ear

x71–8091	x71–870A	x72–854A
x71–8091A	x71–870F	x72–8451
x71–812	x71–8532	x71–8170
x71–873B	x72–850A	x71–879
x71–814	x71–872A	x71–8▲▲▲

5890   Diseases of ear due to unknown cause

x74–923	x80–956	x85–9x8
x74–940	x80–956.5	x85–910
x76–944	966–9x9	
x77–941	x93–9x3	

5900   DISEASES OF THE EYE

5901   Congenital conditions of the eye

x11–011	x11–076	x12–012
x11–024	x11–012	x12–0223
x11–050	x12–092	x12–0224

5901   Congenital conditions of the eye (Continued)

x12–019	x22–019	x11–010
x12–027	x23–041	x11–016
x12–050	x23–042	x11–0131
x12–1471	x2x–024	x30–045
x12–013	x25–016	x32–043
x12–074	x2x–029	x11–022
x12–016	x3x–019	x46–015
x13–074	x1x–019	x52–022
x15–079	x23–019	x52–011
x15–012	x24–019	x52–012
x16–01x	x23–0x4	x52–024
x15–016	x23–0x0	x52–027
x15–01x	x23–0x1	x52–017
x15–026	x23–0x2	x52–01x
x15–064	x23–0x3	x52–018
x15–027	x23–064	x54–013
x15–074	x25–092	x52–013
x15–0161	x23–074	x54–016
x15–019	x23–045	x52–019
x15–034	x1x–013	x64–011
x17–01x	x2x–010	x63–018
x24–016	x2x–019	x67–018
x20–011	x2x–032	x67–031.8
x20–077	x29–016	x64–021
x20–01x	x29–015	x62–031
x20–026	x29–039	x67–031
x20–016	x29–074	x29–02x
x4x–019	x29–013	x56–025
x22–01x	x11–017	x56–050

5910   Infections of the eye

x11–100.1	x12–100.8	x15–1x4
x11–100	x12–100.9	x151–1x4
x12–100.2	x12▲–1x91	x152–100.4
x124–100.9	x121–1x93	x14–130
x12–100.6	x12–101.9	x15–1764
x12–100.3	x12–1764	x17–100
x12–190	x13–190	x17–100.5
x12–1x6	x13–100.6	x22–100.2
x12–1x0.9	x13–100	x22–1x6
x12–100.4	x13–100.8	x22–100.5
x12–1x41	x15–100.9	x22–1x0
x12–1x42	x14–100	x221–1x9
x12–1x43	x15–100.7	x222–1x9
x12–194.6	x15–100	x22–100.4
x12–1x9.3	x15–100.6	x23–100.9

5910 Infections of the eye (Continued)

x23–1x9.5	x68–100.2	x66–100.0
x24–100	x52–119	x64–100.6
x23–100.5	x52–105	x62–100.3
x1x–100	x52–105.9	x66–100.3
x3x–100.5	x52–100.4	x65–100.6
x1x–190	x55–100.4	x66–100.6
x12–1xx	x52–146	x63–100
x3▲–100	x61–105	x62–100.5
x51–100.2	x52–152	x66–130
x50–190	x52–124	x65–100.4
x51–100.6	x55–100	x67–100.4
x51–100.4	x62–100.6	x56–100.2
x50–100.3	x62–123.6	x59–100.2
x50–100.6	x62–100	x56–190
x111–100	x62–100.0	
x52–100.2	x66–100	

5911 Conjunctivitis

x56–100.0	x56–105	x56–194.0
x56–100.8	x56–102	x56–194.4
x56–100	x56–125	x56–123
x56–111	x56x–190	x56–100.9
x56–107	x56–166	x56–1762
x56–103	x56–124	x56–1761
x56–1101	x56–147	x56–1764
x56–101	x56–194	

5912 Retinitis

x23–100	x24–1471	x23–123
x24–1x0	x23–1472	

5913 Keratitis

x12–166	x122–1762	x12–124
x12–147	x122–130	x12–123
x123–147	x121–1235	
x123–130	x127–18x2	

5920 Fungus and parasitic infections of eye

x12–2▲▲	x22–240	x56–2542.8
x20–2▲▲	x23–266.5	x56–299
x22–2▲▲	x40–200.x	x56–2952

5930 Toxic disorders of eye

x11–3▲▲	x12–3231	x12–3▲▲.4
x11–3237	x12–3▲▲	x12–33613
x121–390.6	x12–3238	x12–3237
x12–3253	x12–300	x12–300.8

5930 Toxic disorders of eye (Continued)

x12–3263	x22–3237	x56–3902
x13–390	x23–340	x56–3▲▲
x15–390	x3x–3151	x56–31▲
x38–3483	x23–351.6	x56–3162
x38–34649	932–389	x56–34651
x38–34648	932–3891	x56–380
x38–38▲	x52–3▲▲	x56–3123
x38–34652	x52–32131	x56–319▲
x38–34611	x52–34651	x56–3126
x14–390	x52–3243	x56–3253
x14–393	x56–390	x57–300.4
x15–3237	x56–3901	x57–3126.4
x20–3231	x56–3903	
x20–3237	x56–395	

5940 Injuries of eye

x11–415.x	x12–4101	x22–400.7
x11–400.9	x13–496	x22–400.9
x11–409	x13–4▲▲	x22–4▲▲
x19–496	x13–410	x22–4111
x11–4▲▲	x13–416	x22–406
x11–4111	x13–430.5	x22–4061
x11–415	x15–400.4	x23–428
x12–401	x15–415.1	x24–4x0
x12–441	x15–496	x23–400.9
x12–472.0	x15–400.8	x23–4▲▲
x12–471.0	x15–4▲▲	x23–414
x126–400.4	x15–4101	x23–4x3
x12–402	x15–405	x29–43x.9
x126–400.8	x15–4xx	x29–4x8
x124–416	x15–4x9	x29–435
x12–4x9	x15–4x91	x29–435.9
x12–400.3	x15–4x93	x29–434
x12–496	x15–4x94	x10–400
x12–4▲▲	x15–416	x32–4▲▲.x
x12–430	x17–400.5	x33–4▲▲.x
x12–430.5	x17–415.5	x45–400.6
x12–444	x17–4▲▲	x51–415.4
x12–400.4	x17–416	x11–436
x12–400.8	x20–400.x	x50–4x8
x12–451	x20–415.x	x51–427
x12–400.9	x20–496	x11–4x1
x12–41▲	x20–4▲▲	x11–415.1
x12–412	x21–402	x50–496
x12–415	x22–400.2	210–416
x12–4111	x22–496	x50–4x7

5940   Injuries of eye (Continued)

x50–4▲▲	x66–496	x56–415.0
x52–415.x	x62–406	x56–420.7
x52–415.4	x65–400.4	x56–43x
x52–427	x67–400.4	x56–4▲▲
x55–415.4	x63–415.4	x56–401
x55–400.4	x65–410	x56–412
x52–4x7	x62–410	x57–438.1
x52–4▲▲	x66–410	x56–467
x521–4▲▲	x56–441	x56–451
x522–4▲▲	x56–4x0	x56–439
x62–400.3	x56–494	x58–415.6
x66–400.3	x56–430	x56–472.1
x67–400.3	x56–400.8	x56–471.0
x62–435	x56–415.9	x57–400.4
x62–4x6	x56–427	x57–415.4
x65–496	x56–496	x29–43x

5945   Detachment of retina

x23–415.5
x23–400.5

5950   Vascular disorders of eye

x19–5x7	x2x–549.5	x29–532
x12–532	x2x–533	x29–501
x24–5x9	x23–5x7	x50–5x8
x17–532	x23–511	x11–522
x22–500.7	x23–512	x46–5x7
x22–5x7.9	x23–516.7	x50–522
x23–516	x28–532	x52–501
x23–500.9	x23–532.5	x56–521
x23–511.9	x27–532	x56–5x2
x23–512.9	x23–510	x56–500.7
x23–532	x29–500.9	x56–501
x2x–540.5	x29–540	

5955   Innervation disorders of eye

x12–565	x32–5973	27▲▲–56▲
x38–580	x33–597	x39–561
x38–587	x33–5973	x30–560
x38–586	x36–597	x31–567
x3x–582	x30–577.x	x32–5671
x3x–590	x40–567	x32–5672
x32–595	x40–5672	x33–5672
x32–596	x40–5691	x34–567
x37–597	x40–5692	x34–5671
x32–597	x40–5693	x35–567

5955   Innervation disorders of eye (Continued)

x35–5671	x52–561	x56–565
x69–590	x69–561	x56x–581
x52–560	x69–560	

5960   Disorders of eye due to mechanical abnormalities

x20–630	x11–654	x20–6xx
x20–6301	x11–656	x11–6521
x20–6302	x11–6561	x10–650
x25–652	x20–637	x51–600.8
x3x–618	x11–65x	x11–630
x2x–619	x11–651	x44–641
x2x–619.5	x20–636.x	x60–600.8
x12–657	x11–652	x61–615
x11–655	x11–653	x62–615
x11–6551	x20–635.x	x62–600.8

5961   Glaucoma

x18–600.8	x18–6xx	x18–610
x18–616	x18–610.x	x18–6x0

5970   Metabolic disorders of eye

x11–771	x23–755	x11–708
x127–7x1	x25–798	x11–798
x12–761	x28–794	x51–798
x12–798	x23–761	x52–711
x12–745	x25–797	x52–798
x15–798.5	x23–785	x52–7x1
x22–797	x20–785.x	x52–797
x23–757	x20–79x	x64–797
x2x–763	x30–712	x56–798
x2x–785.5	x11–711	x56–761

5971   Chalazion

x61–7x8

5972   Cataract

x20–100.9	x20–47▲	x20–774
x20–390	x20–400.0	x20–9x6
x20–3▲▲	x20–772	x20–992
x20–415.6	x20–785	
x20–4▲▲.x	x20–797	

5980   Neoplasms of eye

x12–814	x12–8451	x13–8▲▲▲
x12–8701A	x12–8▲▲▲	x15–850A

5980   Neoplasms of eye (Continued)

x15–866A	x51–830	x52–8▲▲▲
x14–8173	x51–8173	x62–8091
x16–8170	x51–8451	x62–814
x15–8170	210–876A	x62–830
x15–8▲▲▲	x51–8170	x62–8852
x17–850A	x51–867A	x62–8032A
x17–8173	x51–8▲▲▲	x62–8▲▲▲
x17–8451	x60–8091A	x56–812
x17–8170	x52–8091A	x56–814
x17–8▲▲▲	x61–8091A	x56–870A
x23–850A	x68▲–812	x56–850A
x23–851	x52–873B	x56–872A
x23–842F	x68▲–814	x56–854A
x23–8▲▲▲	x52–870A	x56–839
x51–870A	x52–850A	x56–830
x51–870F	x52–872A	x56–8173
x51–850A	x52–854A	x56–8451
x51–866A	x52–830	x56–8170
x51–866F	x52–8173	x56–879
x51–872A	x52–8024A	x56–8▲▲▲
x51–872F	x52–867A	
x51–839	x52–879	

5990   Diseases of eye due to unknown cause

x11–9x9	x22–920	x33–x21
x126–950	x3x–942	x32–x15
x12–995	x3x–942.5	x33–x15
x12–9951	x23–992	x36–x15
x12–9952	x23–992.5	x45–942.6
x12–9953	x27–996	x46–9x6
x12–910	x28–996	x61–x20
x12–9101	x23–9x5	x62–954
x12–9102	x23–9x5.5	x62–x20
x12–9103	x1x–942	x56–922
x12–9x8	x1x–942.5	x56–923
x12–912	x25–911	x56–928
x121–923	x25–9x8	x56–980
x12–921	x24–992	x58–929
x12–952	x25–9111	x56–944
x12–924	x25–996	x58–9x4
x13–996	x26–996	x58–956
x17–942	x25–956	x57–9x4
x17–911	x29–928	x21–x21
x17–929	x37–x30	
x17–928	x32–x21	

6000   DISEASES OF DIGESTIVE SYSTEM

6001   Congenital conditions of the digestive system

600–011
600–012
600–026

6010   Infections of digestive system

6014–123.3	604–155	604–1x0
60▲–100.4	6048–100.3	604–156

6011   Enterocolitis

604–100	604–105	604–1232
604–100.0	604–1231	

6012   Gastroenteritis

601–190	601–1142
601–105	6012–190

6020   Fungus and parasitic infections of digestive tract

604–242
604–246

6030   Toxic disorders of digestive system

601–300	601–390	604–3▲▲.0
601–384	604–3▲▲	6012–300

6040   Injuries of digestive system

604–4x9	60▲▲–400.3	601▲–415
6049–400.9	604–4▲▲	601▲–415.x
60▲▲–415.3	6049–415.4	601▲–415.4

6041   Intestinal adhesions, postoperative

60▲–415.4

6050   Vascular disorders of digestive tract

604–510
604–510.4
604–522

6060   Disorders of digestive system due to mechanical abnor-
          malities

604–631	604–611.4
604–611	604–611.6

6061   Diverticulosis, general, intestinal

604–642

6070   Metabolic disorders of digestive system

600–716	6024–753.6	604–715
604–714	604–716	

6080   Neoplasms of digestive tract

604–830

6090   Diseases of digestive system due to unknown cause

601–930
604–930

6091   Constipation

604–x11

6092   Gastrointestinal ulcer

6013–951
6014–951.3
6015–951.3

6100   DISEASES OF ORAL CAVITY

6101   Congenital conditions of oral cavity

6111–0▲▲	612–032	613–051
611–022	6121–013	6135–012
611–029	612–010	613–075
611–013	612–013	613–031
611–034	612–016	617–011
611–017	6145–010	616–064
612–025	6135–011	617–037
612–011	61431–037	617–013
6121–017	6142–064	617–016
612–035	6134–077	616–016
612–064	613–077	
612–021	613–024	

6102   Harelip, cleft lip

6112–037	6112–0373	616–0371
6112–0371	6112–0374	616–0372
6112–0372	616–037	

6110   Infections of oral cavity

610–100.2	611–100.2	612–1413
6102–100	611–190	6142–100.2
610–190.1	611–166	6142–100
610–166	612–100.2	6142–102
610–100.3	612–100	6143–100.6
610–190	612–100.0	6143–100.8
610–1413	124–147.6	6132–100.0

6110   Infections of oral cavity (Continued)

614–100.3	6132–100.9	617–125.x
6142–166	6145–100.9	616–147
6132–100.1	616–100.2	616–147.3
6142–1413	617–100.2	617–190
6132–100	617–100.4	

6111   Apical infection

6143–100

6112   Periodontitis, periodontal abscess

614–100.2

6114   Caries of teeth

613–100.1

6120   Fungus and parasitic infections of oral cavity

610–209

6130   Toxic disorders of oral cavity

610–3▲▲	6142–3116	6142–3111
611–3▲▲	613–3▲▲▲.1	6133–3215
612–3▲▲	6142–33731	616–3▲▲
124–300.6	6142–3112	617–3238.x

6140   Injuries of oral cavity

6101–415.3	61353–415.1	6142–4▲▲
6101–400.3	61354–415.1	6136–415.3
610–4▲▲	61351–415.1	614–495
610–414	61352–415.1	614–434
610–411	6143–415.0	6132–496
610–400.3	613–438.1	613–415.1
611–415.4	613–437.1	6145–430
611–451	6132–415	6136–416.0
611–400.4	613▲–418	613–405.1
611–4▲▲	6143–400.7	616–415.4
612–4▲▲	6143–415.7	616–4▲▲
124–400.6	6142–415.0	

6141   Avulsion of tooth

6143–415

6155   Innervation disorders of oral cavity

612–565
617–569

6160   Disorders of oral cavity due to mechanical abnormalities

610–600.8	612–600.8	6135–63▲
61x–641	612–640	6142–610.0
156–600.8	613–615	616–640
611–640	613–63▲	617–649

6170   Metabolic disorders of oral cavity

611–7622	6131–793	6135–7931
612–760	6142–793	6135–793
612–798	6132–793	6132–700.6
613–7x4	6133–793	6135–791
6142–770	6133–791	6135–7911
6142–700.9	614–798	6142–763

6179   Impacted tooth

613–794

6180   Neoplasms of oral cavity

618–814	611▲–8852	6▲▲▲–8▲▲
122–8032A	611▲–8451	61▲–812
610–870A	611▲–8▲▲▲	616–873B
610–870F	612–8091	616–8887
610–854A	612–873B	61▲–814
610–8852	612–814	616–870A
610–8▲▲▲	612–868A	616–850A
611▲–8091	612–850A	61▲–830
611▲–812	612–872A	616–8852
611▲–873B	612–854A	218–876A
611▲–814	612–8▲▲▲	616–8170
611▲–870A	6133–886E	616–833
611▲–868A	6131–886A	61▲–879
611▲–850A	6142–814	61▲–811
611▲–872A	614–8741	6▲▲–8▲▲▲
611▲–854A	613–886A	

6190   Diseases of oral cavity due to unknown cause

611–9x5	612–951	219▲–900.6
611–951	6131–900.4	218▲–900.6
612–9x5	613–9x1	616–951
612–9x6	6143–900.8	
612–940	6136–900.1	

6200   DISEASES OF SALIVARY GLANDS

6201   Congenital conditions of salivary glands

620–011	621–031	623–064
621–011	622–018	622–064
623–011	623–018	6231–021

6201   Congenital conditions of salivary glands (Continued)

621–021	621–016	62▲–100.2
622–029	623–026	62▲–190
623–029	621–026	62▲–100.3
620–024	6211–021	62▲–100.4
6201–024	622–061	622–021
622–013	62▲–100	6231–063

6210   Infections of salivary glands

62▲–100	62▲–190	62▲–100.4
62▲–100.2	62▲–100.3	

6230   Toxic disorders of salivary glands

62▲–3197
62▲–3▲▲

6240   Injuries of salivary glands

62▲–400.3
62▲–4▲▲
621–415.0

6260   Disorders of salivary glands due to mechanical abnormalities

62▲–615
62▲–600.8
622–600.8

6280   Neoplasms of salivary glands

62▲–8091	621–8842	62▲–8851A
62▲–8091A	62▲–8852	62▲–8▲▲▲

6290   Diseases of salivary glands due to unknown cause

62▲–943

6300   DISEASES OF PHARYNX AND ESOPHAGUS

6301   Congenital conditions of pharynx and esophagus

6311–064	637–064	3054–029
6311–01x	637–012	637–013
6311–019	637–015	637–016
6311–01x.3	638–023	637–017
637–011	637–036	63x–015
637–018	637–032	

6310   Infections of pharynx and esophagus

631–100.2	639–123.2	636–100.2
631–100.4	635–100.2	636–100
639–100.2	634–100.2	636–100.7

6310   Infections of pharynx and esophagus (Continued)

| 634–100.9 | 637–100 | 637–100.4 |
| 637–100.2 | 637–100.3 | 637–100.9 |

6311   Pharyngitis

631–100
631–100.0

6312   Tonsillitis

| 634–100 | 635–100 | 635–1413 |
| 634–100.0 | 6340–100 | 634–1413 |

6313   Streptococcic sore throat

631–102

6314   Adenoiditis

633–100
633–100.0
633–100.6

6315   Hypertrophied tonsils and adenoids due to infection

635–100.6
634–100.6
632–100.6

6320   Fungus and parasitic infections of pharynx and esophagus

631–209

6330   Toxic disorders of pharynx and esophagus

631–3▲▲	637–3▲▲	637–300.4
631–3▲▲	637–382x	637–300.9
631–300.0	637–300.3	631–319▲
631–300.4	637–300.5	

6340   Injuries of pharynx and esophagus

631–4▲▲	634–496	637–400.4
631–438	634–415.7	637–438.9
631–444	633–415.7	637–430
630–430	637–496	637–4x0
631–400.4	637–4▲▲	6004–400.3
635–496	637–438.5	637–400.3
636–496	637–43x.5	637–438.3

6350   Vascular disorders of pharynx and esophagus

631–544.1
634–544.1
637–500.9

6355   Innervation disorders of pharynx and esophagus

631–590	6376–599	637–586
6373–580	6373–590	6375–580.6

6360   Disorders of pharynx and esophagus due to mechanical abnormalities

631–611	637–641	637–630.5
634–615	637–642	63x–641

6380   Neoplasms of pharynx and esophagus

631–812	631–8852	634–831
631–873B	631–8170	634–814A
631–8887	631–833	634–8▲▲
631–814	631–879	637–8091
631–870A	631–811	637–814
631–850A	631–8▲▲	637–814A
631–872A	634–814	637–8▲▲▲
631–830	634–830	

6390   Diseases of pharynx and esophagus due to unknown cause

631–931	637–941	637–944
631–940	637–971	637–951
632–943	637–971.9	

6391   Hypertrophied tonsils and adenoids due to unknown cause

632–940	635–940
633–940	634–940

6400   DISEASES OF STOMACH

6401   Congenital conditions of stomach

641–043	640–023	645–043
640–026	640–013	647–075
640–036	640–016	640–02x
640–017	647–023	

6402   Pylorus, hypertrophic stenosis, congenital

645–093

6410   Infections of stomach

640–100.2	649–100
640–100.3	649–100.2

6411   Gastritis

640–190
640–190.9
640–190.0

6430   Toxic disorders of stomach

642–300.x	640–3▲▲	640–389.9
640–300.4	640–300.3	

6440   Injuries of stomach

640–400.4	6011–414.3	640–424
640–415.6	640–415.0	640–4▲▲
640–430	6011–415	640–414
6011–400.3	640–415.7	645–415.4

6450   Vascular disorders of stomach

640–522
640–514

6455   Innervation disorders of stomach

640–599
640–586

6459   Pylorospasm

645–590

6460   Disorders of stomach due to mechanical abnormalities

640–642	640–631	640–617
640–611	640–612	647–631
64x–641	647–639	640–637

6480   Neoplasms of stomach

640–8091	640–866A	640–8023A
640–8881A	640–872A	640–8023F
640–8191	640–830	640–8076G
640–870A	640–8451	640–8▲▲▲

6490   Diseases of stomach due to unknown cause

640–940	640–940.9	641–954
640–940.6	642–940.9	645–954

6495   Ulcer of stomach

640–951	640–951.3	649–951.4
640–951.7	647–951	640–951.4

6500   DISEASES OF SMALL INTESTINE AND MESENTERY

6501   Congenital conditions of small intestine and mesentery

650–018	650–047.4	65▲–075
650–036	650–023	65▲–066
651–036	651–023	650–065

6502   Meckel's diverticulum

658–019	658–013	658–091
658–063	658–067	658–417.5
658–023	658–036	
658–027	658–065	

6510   Infections of small intestine and mesentery

650–100.2	650–100.x	650–130.6
657–100.4	650–101.x	65▲–100.4
650–100.9	659–100.4	
650–118	65▲–100.3	

6511   Enteritis

651–190
650–100
650–100.0

6512   Diverticulitis

658–190
658–190.3

6520   Fungus and parasitic infections of small intestine and mesentery

650–243	650–270	650–246
650–241	650–240.4	650–2▲▲

6530   Toxic disorders of small intestine and mesentery

650–3▲▲	659–382
650–300.0	650–300.0

6540   Injuries of small intestine and mesentery

651–449.9	65▲–4▲▲	659–415.4
650–415.3	657–415.4	65▲–416
650–400.3	657–400.4	654–415.x
659–4x7	650–400.7	65▲–415.4
650–415.x	650–415.4	
659–4▲▲	6013–415.9	

6550   Vascular disorders of small intestine and mesentery

651–500.x	650–544	65▲–512
659–502	65▲–510	650–514
650–510.1	65▲–511	

6555   Innervation disorders of small intestine and mesentery

651–560
650–560
6511–590

6560   Disorders of small intestine and mesentery due to
          mechanical abnormalities

659–600.8   651–6x3   659–637
650–615   6021–646
650–639.4   650–600.8

6561   Diverticulosis of small intestine

65▲–642
65▲–642.0

6563   Intussusception

604–630
6036–630

6564   Volvulus

6▲▲–637
604–637.3

6580   Neoplasms of small intestine and mesentery

650–8091   659–850A   650–8023
650–844   659–866A   650–831
650–814   650–872A   650–879
650–870A   659–872A   659–879
659–870A   659–854A   650–8▲▲▲
650–850A   650–830

6590   Diseases of small intestine and mesentery due to un-
          known cause

651–930   659–9x8   654–952
650–930   650–945   651–944

6595   Ulcer of small intestine

651–951   651–951.7   650–951.4
651–951.3   653–951
651–951.4   653–951.3

6600   DISEASES OF COLON

6601   Congenital conditions of colon

662–026   662–028   661–011
660–063   660–028   661–021
660–036   660–075   661–013
662–032   662–050   661–016
660–032   660–02x   661–02x
660–027   660–033   668–018
660–016   660–062   668–028

6602   Megacolon, congenital

660–015

6610   Infections of large intestine

660–100.2	6691–100.2	669–123.3
66▲–1x4	6692–100.2	66x–100
66▲–100.3	6693–100.2	668–103.4
66▲–100.5	668–10x	668–100.5
66▲–100.4	668–100.3	668–100.4
669–100.2	668–123.3	668–1732.4
669–105.2	669–100.3	668–100.9

6611   Appendicitis

661–100	661–100.3	6613–100
661–100.2	661–100.0	
661–100.1	661–190.3	

6613   Proctitis

668–151	668–100.0
668–100	668–103

6615   Colitis

660–100	660–116▲	662–100
660–151	660–100.0	
660–159	666–190	

6620   Fungus and parasitic infections of large intestine

660–2▲▲	660–242	661–240.4
660–209	660–254	

6630   Toxic disorders of large intestine

660–3▲▲	668–3▲▲	668–300.9
660–3▲▲.0	668–3▲▲.4	

6640   Injuries of large intestine

660–415.3	668–4▲▲	668–47▲▲.0
660–4▲▲	668–435	668–416
660–415.4	668–415	668–415.4
661–4▲▲	668–438.3	668–400.4
668–441	668–4111	668–400.9

6641   Colostomy

6038–415
6038–415.x

6642   Rectocele

668–4x9

6650   Vascular disorders of large intestine

667–510.1	667–511	668–522.9
660–510.1	660–514	
660–544	661–514	

6655   Innervation disorders of large intestine

660–586
660–585

6658   Irritability of colon

660–580

6660   Disorders of large intestine due to mechanical abnormalities

661–642	6682–631	660–630
661–616	668–611	66▲–631
661–611	668–616.9	660–616.9
661–630	660–600.8	66x–641
661–643	660–641	66▲–637
661–610.8	660–615	
668–631	6055–615.3	

6661   Impacted feces

660–611

6664   Diverticulosis of large intestine

660–642.0	66▲–642.3
660–642	66▲–642.4

6670   Metabolic disorders of large intestine

661–796

6680   Neoplasms of large intestine

660–8091	668–8091	668–830
660–8023	668–8091A	668–8173
660–8▲▲▲	668–844	668–8023
661–8091	668–814	668–8▲▲▲
661–844	668–872A	
661–8▲▲▲	668–838A	

6690   Diseases of large intestine due to unknown cause

660–951.4	6611–943	668–951
660–945	668–945	668–x00

6694   Polyp simple of colon

668–944

6695   Ulcerative colitis

66▲–952	660–951.3	663–951
6045–951	66▲–951	6035–951
6046–951	660–951	

6700   DISEASES OF ANUS

6701   Congenital conditions of anus

670–011	709–018	670–0181
670–012	7085–018	670–029
70x5–018	670–018	1271–023
70x2–018	670–0182	

6710   Infections of anus

6731–100	675–100	670–147.6
670–10x	676–100	67x–100.7
670–100.4	670–100.2	
670–100.6	670–1x4.4	

6711   Fistula in anus

670–100.3

6712   Abscess, perianal tissue

677–100.2	6773–100.2
6771–100.2	6772–100.2

6720   Fungus and parasitic infections of anus

6731–209

6730   Toxic disorders of anus

670–3▲▲
670–300.4
670–300.9

6740   Injuries of anus

670–415.2	672–400.x	672–412
143–430	672–415.x	670–415.4
670–496	670–4▲▲	
675–496	670–412	

6745   Fissure in anus

670–400.1

6755   Innervation disorders of anus

672–560	672–586	672–590
2747–551	672–588	
143–573	672–561	

6760   Disorders of anus due to mechanical abnormalities

67x–641.6
673–631

6764   Hemorrhoids

67x–641
67x–631
67x–619

6780   Neoplasms of anus

670–8091   670–870A   670–8▲▲▲
670–814   670–8170

6790   Diseases of anus due to unknown cause

675–9401   143–943
676–940   670–951

6800   DISEASES OF LIVER

6801   Congenital conditions of liver

680–011   682–011   686–013
680–031   687–011   687–029
682–091   684–031   687–027
680–091   687–035   687–017
680–064   687–061   687–091
680–027   685–015   686–065
680–016   687–021   682–018
680–023   685–032   685–016
680–010   686–032   686–016
686–023   687–032   687–065
684–023   685–013   688–021

6810   Infections of liver and biliary tract

680–100.2   3062–100.3   687–100.3
680–1x2.3   680–1x0   68▲–100.4
680–151.2   680–147.0   680–100.9
680–100.6   6871–100.2   68x–190
6095–100.3   687–100.6   68x–100
3056–100.3   6052–100.3   68x–147
3073–100.3   68▲–100.3   68x–100.7

6811   Hepatitis

680–100   680–158   681–100
680–151   680–160
680–100.0   680–1891

6812   Cholecystitis

683–100   687–114   687–100.5
682–100   687–115   687–100.1
687–100   687–100.0   687–100.2

6820   Fungus and parasitic infections of liver and biliary tract

680–266	680–267	682–270
680–270	680–285	68▲–2▲▲.4

6830   Toxic disorders of liver and biliary tract

680–3▲▲	680–3151	680–3154
680–33212	680–33154	680–3313
680–3322	680–34850	680–33152
680–321	680–3231	680–3185

6840   Injuries of liver and biliary tract

680–400.2	687–4x0	687–4▲▲
680–4▲▲	6051–415.3	68▲–415.4
68▲–415.6	68▲–415.3	68▲–435
687–415.6	687–415.3	68▲–400.4
687–400.6	68▲–4▲▲	685–430

6850   Vascular disorders of liver and biliary tract

680–522.6	680–511	680–522
680–512	680–515	68x–533

6855   Innervation disorders of liver and biliary tract

680–563
687–580

6860   Disorders of liver and biliary tract due to mechanical abnormalities

680–6x8.0	680–631	687–600.8
680–615.8	682–6xx	68x–600.7
680–615	68▲–611	
680–6x6	687–637	

6861   Cholelithiasis

68▲–615	6052–615.3	685–615.9
687–615	68▲–615.3	687–615.9
687–615.x	68▲–615.0	
6051–615.3	68▲–615.4	

6870   Metabolic disorders of liver and biliary tract

680–701	680–748
680–753	680–751

6880   Neoplasms of liver and biliary tract

680–8091	680–8063	68▲–8073
680–8091A	680–8833	68▲–814
680–8073	680–8▲▲▲	68▲–8▲▲▲
680–870A	68▲–8091	
680–850A	68▲–8091A	

6890   **Diseases of liver and biliary tract due to unknown cause**

680–911	680–x72	687–943.8
680–915	680–x70	68x–930
680–922	687–923	68x–900.7
680–x71	687–921	

6891   Cirrhosis

680–953	680–9x6
680–952	680–956

6900   DISEASES OF PANCREAS

6901   Congenital conditions of pancreas

690–021	690–035	692–017
690–031	690–010.6	
690–010	690–045	

6910   Infections of pancreas

690–100.2	690–100	690–1x0.6
690–190	690–190.0	
690–190.7	690–100.1	

6920   Fungus and parasitic infections of pancreas

690–2▲▲▲.4

6930   Toxic disorders of pancreas

690–3▲▲
690–3▲▲.0

6940   Injuries of pancreas

690–400.3	690–400.1	690–416
690–4▲▲	690–4x1.6	

6950   Vascular disorders of pancreas

690–512.7	690–510.1
690–540.7	690–516

6960   Disorders of pancreas due to mechanical abnormalities

690–600.9	690–6x0	69x–618
692–615	690–600.8	

6970   Metabolic disorders of pancreas

690–763	690–716
690–713	690–798

6980   Neoplasms of pancreas

690–8091	690–8044	690–8▲▲▲
690–8091A	690–8074	

6990   Diseases of pancreas due to unknown cause

690–930	69x–942	690–956
69x–942.6	690–923	690–926

7000   DISEASES OF THE UROGENITAL SYSTEM

7001   Congenital conditions of urogenital system

70x7–029	70x3–029	770–019
7032–029	705–011	705–019
7061–019	705–010	760–01x
704–019	705–01x	7052–019
700–01x	750–019	

7010   Infections of urogenital system

705–1xx

7040   Injuries of urogenital system

705–4xx

7055   Innervation disorders of urogenital system

705–588

7060   Disorders of urogenital system due to mechanical abnormalities

705–6xx

7070   Metabolic disorders of urogenital system

705–791	705–787	705–7872
705–7862	705–777	705–7xx
705–7872	705–7871	

7090   Diseases of urogenital system due to unknown cause

705–x11	705–x13	705–x10
705–x12	705–x32	

7100   DISEASES OF KIDNEY

7101   Congenital conditions of kidney

710–011	710–0281	710–019
710–012	719–063	710–050
71x–031	710–014	710–031
71x–026	710–013	710–1471
71x–021	710–016	710–033
719–061	710–022	710–021
710–028	710–027	710–072

7102   Fused kidney; double kidney

719–032
710–024
710–025

7103   Cyst of kidney, congenital

710–010
710–064

7110   Infections of kidney

710–100.2	710–100.9	716–100.0
710–105.2	710–100.4	71x–190
716–100.2	710–100.3	
716–1x4	716–100	

7111   Nephritis

710–100	712–1x4	713–147.0
714–100.0	712–190	719–100
712–100	714–100	719–112
712–103	713–100.0	719–100.1
712–100.0	713–123.0	719–1x0.1

7130   Toxic disorders of kidney

713–300.9
713–38x.9
719–3▲▲

7140   Injuries of kidney

710–435	710–4x7	710–4▲▲
710–400.8	710–415.7	710–406
710–415.3	710–415.9	713–449
710–400.3	719–435.8	710–4▲▲.5
710–496	710–420.5	
716–4x7	710–4x0	

7150   Vascular disorders of kidney

710–517	710–512	710–516
710–5171	710–5x7	
710–511	710–522	

7155   Innervation disorders of kidney

710–563

7160   Disorders of kidney due to mechanical abnormalities

710–6xx	71x–618	71x–619
710–600.8	719–639	718–637
710–6x8	710–631	71x–641
710–630	710–610	

7161   Calculus in kidney

722–615
721–615.8

7169   Hydronephrosis

719–6▲▲.8
719–6x8.0
719–6x8.4

7170   Metabolic disorders of kidney

710–741.7	713–700.9	713–720.9
712–7x9	713–785.9	710–798

7180   Neoplasms of kidney

710–8091	710–850G	718–871B
710–8091A	710–850A	718–871G
710–812	710–866A	710–8834
710–8191	710–866F	710–8021
710–8831F	718–872A	710–879
710–8034	710–872A	710–882
710–870A	716–872A	7▲▲–8▲▲▲
710–870F	716–872F	

7190   Diseases of kidney due to unknown cause

710–922	710–900.5	710–x10
710–923	715–955	71x–x30
710–959	713–x40.9	
71x–931	713–x40	

7200   DISEASES OF RENAL PELVIS AND URETER

7201   Congenital conditions of renal pelvis and ureter

722–034	723–036	723–075
721–036	720–032	723–0211
723–011	723–032	724–017
723–012	723–063	727–017
723–035	723–021	723–033
723–064	723–018	726–027
723–015	723–017	724–062
727–036	727–021	727–062

7210   Infections of renal pelvis and ureter

722–100.2	723–1x6	7071–100.3
725–100.2	723–1x9	722–1x6
727–100.4	723–100.4	722–1x9
7023–100.3	724–100.4	

7211   Pyelitis

722–100
722–103

7212   Ureteritis

725–100	723–100	723–100.0
723–100.2	723–103	

7230   Toxic disorders of renal pelvis and ureter

722–3▲▲
723–3432
723–3▲▲

7240   Injuries of renal pelvis and ureter

722–496	723–4▲▲	723–415.4
723–43x.6	723–416	723–401.0
723–400.3	723–415	723–449
7075–400.3	723–435	723–472
7022–400.3	723–435.4	
723–496	723–400.4	

7255   Innervation disorders of renal pelvis and ureter

723–584

7260   Disorders of renal pelvis and ureter due to mechanical abnormalities

721–641	723–641	723–615.0
723–643	723–600.8	726–645
723–642	723–630	723–644
7071–6x3	723–650	
7074–6x3	723–631	

7261   Calculus in ureter

723–615

7280   Neoplasms of renal pelvis and ureter

722–814	723–870A	723–8023A
722–872F	723–850G	723–879
722–8690A	723–866F	723–814A
722–8023	723–872F	723–882
721–811	723–854A	723–881
723–8091	723–854G	723–8▲▲▲
723–814	723–8023	

7290   Diseases of renal pelvis and ureter due to unknown cause

722–9x8	723–959	723–9x8
723–923	720–941	

7300   DISEASES OF BLADDER

7301   Congenital conditions of bladder

730–011   730–026   733–021
730–015   730–012   7301–046
730–036   730–027   736–021
730–032   7311–013   733–017

7310   Infections of bladder

730–100.2   730–100.3   736–1x6
7301–100.2   7033–100.3   737–1x9
739–100.2   708▲–100.3   7084–100.3
730–151   7011–100.3   7083–100.3
733–100.4   7032–100.3

7311   Cystitis

730–100   730–100.0   739–100
730–103   736–100.0   731–100
730–100.8   736–100.8   730–1764
730–100.7   730–100.1

7320   Fungus and parasitic infections of bladder

730–2▲▲
730–2952

7330   Toxic disorders of bladder

730–3▲▲.9
730–3▲▲
730–390

7340   Injuries of bladder

732–415.4   7302–415.3   736–415.9
733–400.4   7303–415.3   7085–415.3
730–4x0   730–496   7085–400.3
7086–415   730–400.7   730–43x.6
730–43x   730–415.7   730–472.9
7083–400.3   730–4▲▲   730–400.x
7083–415.3   730–416
730–400.3   730–415

7341   Cystocele

730–4x9

7350   Vascular disorders of bladder

730–512
730–512.0
730–514

7355   Innervation disorders of bladder

730–589	749–591	733–561
730–560	749–560	730–566
730–591	749–561	749–580
730–569	733–560	
730–561	733–591	

7360   Disorders of bladder due to mechanical abnormalities

730–600.8	730–642	730–638
7301–600.8	730–642.0	730–631
730–600.0	739–613	733–615.4
730–640	730–611	73x–641
730–641	730–639	
730–630	739–639	

7361   Calculus in bladder

730–615
730–615.0

7370   Metabolic disorders of bladder

730–7xx

7380   Neoplasms of bladder

730–8091	730–854A	730–8023
730–8091A	730–854G	730–8023A
730–873F	730–8871	730–867A
730–814	730–8872A	730–867F
730–870A	730–8012	730–879
730–850A	730–871B	730–882
730–866A	730–871G	730–811
730–866F	730–8451	730–8▲▲▲
730–872A	730–876A	

7390   Diseases of bladder due to unknown cause

730–922	730–957	730–944
730–9x8	730–957.9	730–900.5
736–9x8	730–941	730–951
730–959	736–965	

7400   DISEASES OF URETHRA

7401   Congenital conditions of urethra

740–011	740–0122	740–027
740–018	740–01221	740–016
740–036	740–01222	746–017
746–032	740–01223	740–017
740–032	740–01224	709–037
740–0121	740–01225	740–062
740–029	740–01226	

7410   Infections of urethra

747–100.2	748–100	746–100.4
747–103.2	740–10x	740–100.5
748–100.2	745–100	740–100.4
7471–100.2	7471–100.8	740–103.4
7471–103.2	744–100.3	740–147
747–100	7044–100.3	747–123
747–103	7042–100.3	7402–100
747–100.0	709–100.3	7402–100.8
747–103.0	740–1x6	748–103.2
7461–100	7401–1x9	

7411   Urethritis

7403–100	744–100.0	740–100.6
746–100	740–100.0	741–100.0
740–100	740–1x0	740–1x0.8
740–103	740–103.0	

7430   Toxic disorders of urethra

745–3▲▲	740–390
740–3▲▲.4	740–3▲▲

7440   Injuries of urethra

741–415.4	709–415.3	740–415
740–420	7042–412.3	740–412.9
740–400.6	740–496	740–415.4
740–415.6	740–4x0	740–400.4
740–461	740–4▲▲	749–400.4
740–400.3	740–412	740–4x9
7044–415.3	740–472.0	7042–415.3
709–400.3	740–416	

7460   Disorders of urethra due to mechanical abnormalities

740–615	740–640	74x–641
747–6x8	740–641	
745–6x8	128–631	

7480   Neoplasms of urethra

747–8091	740–850A	740–879
740–8091	740–8173	740–814A
740–814	740–8023	740–882
740–870A	740–8023A	740–8▲▲▲

7490   Disorders of urethra due to unknown cause

740–930	745–9x6	746–951
74x–900.7	740–941	

7500   DISEASES OF EXTERNAL MALE ORGANS

7501   Congenital conditions of external male organs

751–011	755–026	755–012
751–025	755–1471	755–064
751–034	755–013	755–024
751–021	755–016	757–095
753–064	755–0161	757–050
752–032	755–0162	758–074
751–032	755–0163	758–012
1281–023	755–022	758–019
751–022	755–031	761–011
755–011	755–023	761–018

7502   Phimosis, congenital

753–017

7503   Cryptorchism

755–028
755–0281

7510   Infections of external male organs

754–100.2	755–100.1	758–100
751–100.2	755–124	758–10x
753–100.4	755–190	758–102
753–100	755–170	758–100.3
753–103	755–100.0	758–100.1
751–10x	755–100	758–166
754–100.4	755–1x3	758–190
754–103.4	755–1xx	758–190.0
751–1792	756–100.8	761–100
754–100	756–100.6	761–100.4
751–1732	756–100.3	761–100.0
753–100.6	757–100	145–100
751–147	757–100.8	145–166
755–100.2	757–100.2	145–1x6
755–100.9	757–1x8.0	
755–147.6	758–100.2	

7511   Epididymitis

756–100.2	756–170	756–123.3
756–100	756–100.0	
756–103	756–100.1	

7520   Fungus and parasitic infections of external male organs

757–257
758–215

7530　　Toxic disorders of external male organs

756–3▲▲
758–390
761–3▲▲

7540　　Injuries of external male organs

753–495	751-422	757–4x7
751–448	755–4x7	757–400.8
751–400.1	755–4▲▲	757–4▲▲
751–402.7	755–406	758–448
751–400.7	755–416	758–400.7
751–4▲▲	755–400.1	758–4▲▲
751–406	755–4x0	761–4▲▲
751–400.9	756–4x7	761–416
753–415.6	756–4▲▲	761–400.4
751–416	756–4x0	

7550　　Vascular disorders of external male organs

750–501	755–511	757–502
755–510	756–510	758–501
755–514.1	756–514.1	

7555　　Innervation disorders of external male organs

751–584
758–573

7560　　Disorders of external male organs due to mechanical abnormalities

753–615	75x–619	756–615
751–640	751–637	756–600.8
75x–618	755–637	7561–637
753–600.4	7551–637	757–615

7570　　Metabolic disorders of external male organs

753–794	755–787	758–792
755–786	757–797.8	

7579　　Redundant prepuce

753–792

7580　　Neoplasms of external male organs

751–812	751–872A	755–8091A
752–814	751–8173	755–880F
751–814	751–876A	755–881
753–814	751–8170	755–8835
751–870A	751–879	755–870A
751–850A	751–8▲▲▲	755–850A
751–866A	755–8091	755–8043

7580   Neoplasms of external male organs (Continued)

755–872A	756–8451	757–8▲▲▲
755–830	756–8077	758–812
755–8690A	756–879	758–814
755–871B	756–882	758–870A
755–867A	756–8▲▲▲	758–850A
755–879	757–870A	758–866A
755–8068	757–850A	758–872A
755–882	757–872A	758–854A
755–8▲▲▲	757–8871	758–8173
756–8091A	757–8772A	758–8170
756–8091	757–871B	758–879
756–870A	757–8451	758–814A
756–850A	757–867A	758–882
756–872A	757–879	758–8▲▲▲
756–8871	757–882	756–8772A

7590   Diseases of external male organs due to unknown cause

754–923	755–911	757–9x7
754–942	756–900.8	
752–943	757–923	

7591   Hydrocele

757–930.8
757–900.8

7600   DISEASES OF INTERNAL MALE ORGANS

7601   Congenital conditions of internal male organs

762–011	764–011	764–075
762–095	765–018	
765–011	764–076	

7610   Infections of spermatic cord

762–100.2	763–151	765–100.6
762–100	763–100.6	764–100.6
762–100.0	7631–100	764–100.3
762–130	7631–100.4	764–1x0.6
763–100.2	763–100	765–100.4
763–103.2	763–100.0	
763–100.4	766–100.4	

7611   Prostatitis

766–100.2	764–151	764–103
764–100.2	764–100	764–100.0
764–103.2	764–117	764–154

7620   Fungus and parasitic infections of internal male organs

764–219

7630   Toxic disorders of internal male organs

763–300.0

7640   Injuries of internal male organs

762–4x7	762–415	764–410
762–415.7	764–400.3	764–416
762–4▲▲	764–415.7	764–4x0
762–4x4	764–4▲▲	

7650   Vascular disorders of internal male organs

764–521	764–512
764–511	764–522

7655   Innervation disorders of internal male organs

763–580
764–580

7660   Disorders of internal male organs due to mechanical
          abnormalities

76x–619	763–600.8	764–600.8
762–637	763–610.6	767–641
76x–6x6	764–616	
763–615	764–615	

7679   Hypertrophy of prostate

764–799

7680   Neoplasms of internal male organs

762–870A	763–870A	764–870A
762–872A	763–866A	764–866A
762–8772A	763–8772A	764–866F
762–871B	763–8690A	764–830
762–867A	763–879	764–8871
762–867F	763–882	764–8012
762–879	763–8▲▲▲	764–867F
762–8▲▲▲	764–8091	764–879
763–8091	764–8831A	764–8▲▲▲
763–8091A	764–8091A	
763–814	764–873F	

7690   Diseases of internal male organs due to unknown cause

762–9x7	764–911
762–900.8	764–942

7700 DISEASES OF EXTERNAL FEMALE ORGANS

7701 Congenital conditions of external female organs

774–011	776–021	772–013
774–018	776–034	772–024
779–019	776–077	773–011
775–011	776–013	773–025
775–034	776–010	7812–023
775–013	776–030	774–064
776–011	740–012	774–019
776–024	772–011	774–091
776–064	772–025	70x1–037

7710 Infection of external female organs

772–100.2	70x4–100.3	774–100.9
774–100.2	70x1–100.3	774–100
776–100.4	774–100.1	774–103
774–10x	777–100.8	774–100.0
774–1792	774–147.6	

7711 Vulvovaginitis

7052–100

7712 Abscess of Bartholin's gland

777–100.2
777–100
777–103

7720 Fungus and parasitic infections of external female organs

774–215
774–209

7740 Injuries of external female organs

774–495.6	774–400.1	774–495
776–412.8	774–4x7	774–437
774–412.8	776–4▲▲	70x1–400.3
773–43x	774–4▲▲	70x1–415.3

7750 Vascular disorders of external female organs

774–501
774–500.7

7755 Innervation disorders of external female organs

774–570

7760 Disorders of external female organs due to mechanical abnormalities

775–615	775–600.8	772–600.8
779–600.8	776–600.8	77x–641

7763   Cyst of Bartholin's gland

777–600.8

7770   Metabolic disorders of external female organs

774–785
774–798

7780   Neoplasms of external female organs

774–8091	774–850A	774–8170
774–8091A	774–866A	774–8023
774–812	774–872A	774–879
775–814	774–8173F	774–8075
774–814E	774–8173	774–8061
774–814	774–8871	774–8▲▲▲
774–870A	774–8451	

7790   Diseases of external female organs due to unknown cause

779–900.8	774–9x6	774–951
775–9x6	776–940	

7800 DISEASES OF INTERNAL FEMALE ORGANS

7801   Congenital conditions of internal female organs

781–012	783–016	787–021
781–011	783–015	787–032
781–018	783–019	787–013
781–091	783–021	787–018
781–064	783–023	787–023
781–032	780–011	787–031
781–030	782–018	787–033
70x2–037	782–064	788–011
781–016	782–0212	788–032
781–034	782–022	788–025
781–017	782–016	788–064
7031–029	782–023	788–021
783–011	782–032	788–091
783–012	782–037	788–027
7051–025	782–019	788–013
783–018	782–012	788–016
785–021	787–0111	788–01x
783–036	787–011	788–031
783–034	787–012	788–065
783–064	787–019	
783–013	787–064	

7810   Infections of internal female organs

780–100	781–100.2	781–100.x
780–100.0	7811–100.2	70x2–100.3

7810　Infections of internal female organs (Continued)

781–1732	782–1x43	788–103.2
781–100.8	782–1x44	788–100.7
781–100.4	782–100.3	788–1x6
781–103.4	70x3–100.3	7892–100.2
783–100.2	785–1xx	789–100.2
783–100.6	782–100.7	7892–100
783–1x6	785–100.9	789–100
783–100.4	785–1x6	783–100
784–100.2	782–100.2	783–103
784–100.4	785–100.4	783–100.0
782–100.4	787–100.4	783–100.9
782–1x41	7803–100.2	783–154
782–1x42	788–100.2	

7811　Vaginitis

781–125	781–154	781–190
7811–190	781–100	

7813　Endometritis; metritis

785–190	785–100	784–100
785–103	782–190	
785–190.0	782–190.0	

7814　Salpingitis

787–100	787–100.7	787–103.2
787–103	7871–100	787–1x2.5
787–100.0	787–100.2	

7815　Oophoritis

788–100	788–100.0
788–170	7886–100

7820　Fungus and parasitic infections of internal female organs

781–209
781–2▲▲

7830　Toxic disorders of internal female organs

781–3▲▲
783–3▲▲.9
785–3▲▲.9

7840　Injuries of internal female organs

70x2–412.3	781–415.8	781–400.4
781–415.x	781–4▲▲	70x21–412
781–400.x	70x2–415.3	7022–400.3
781–400.1	70x2–400.3	7042–400.3
781–441.1	70x2–472.3	781–412

7840   Injuries of internal female organs (Continued)

781–438	783–415.7	784–412.4
781–439	783–4x6	785–415.4
7053–412.3	783–400.6	786–415.4
7031–400.3	783–4▲▲	7804–415.3
7031–415.3	783–412	787–400.7
7051–412.4	783–415.9	787–4▲▲
783–400.0	7832–400.4	787–415.4
783–438	7832–415.4	788–400.7
783–400.4	7832–412.4	788–4▲▲
783–412.4	782–415.x	788–471
783–415.4	785–470	788–472
783–400.8	782–4▲▲	788–415
783–409	782–415	788–415.x
783–400.9	782–43x	7892–435.7
783–412.6	784–4x4	70x6–4x9

7841   Uterine displacement, traumatic

782–415.4	782–4x47	782–4x46
782–4x4	782–4x44	782–4x41
782–4x43	782–4x45	782–4x42

7850   Vascular disorders of internal female organs

781–544.1	788–522	788–514
788–532	788–510.1	789–532

7855   Innervation disorders of internal female organs

781–594
782–580

7860   Disorders of internal female organs due to mechanical abnormalities

781–600.8	781–6x0	787–637
781–610.x	780–6x7	788–630
781–611	782–61x	788–639
781–61x	787–630	788–637
781–631	787–6x8	78x–641
781–631.9	787–61x	

7864   Uterine displacement

782–6431	785–630.7	782–63x
782–6432	782–630.7	782–636
782–6371	782–631	
782–633	782–643	

7865   Cyst, Nabothian

783–600.8

7870   Metabolic disorders of internal female organs

781–797.4	785–70x	787–798
781–798	785–7862	788–777
781–797	785–787	788–796.7
783–787	782–787	788–786
783–798	782–791	788–787
783–797	782–798	788–798
785–712	787–796	

7875   Endometrial dysfunction

785–771	785–7761	785–7763
785–772	785–777	785–786.6
785–781	785–7861	786–786.6
785–782	785–7871	

7877   Cyst of ovary

788–795	7881–795	7881–7701
7888–795	7882–795	7881–770

7880   Neoplasms of internal female organs

781–814	782–8▲▲▲	788–8021B
781–870A	787–8091	788–882
781–8173	787–8772A	788–882.8
781–8871	7887–8042	788–8052
781–8▲▲	788–8836	788–8▲▲▲
782–8091	788–8033	7892–870A
782–8881A	788–8033F	7892–866A
782–8831F	788–881	784–866A
783–814E	788–870A	7891–866A
783–814	788–8053	7893–866A
782–866F	788–8013	789▲–8772A
782–866A	788–8884	789–8▲▲▲
782–8023	788–8011	787–8▲▲▲
783–879	788–8012	
785–879	788–8021F	

7890   Diseases of internal female organs due to unknown cause

781–943	78x–942	788–959
781–x30	785–995	7883–9x8
783–954	785–911	7884–9x8
783–923	787–941	788–x10
783–941	788–923	7892–959
783–958	788–952	7891–900.8
78x▲2–955	788–911	

7900 DISEASES OF THE FETUS AND FETAL STRUCTURES

7910 Infections of fetal structures

795–100
794–100

7940 Injuries of fetal structures

794–4x5

7955 Innervation disorders of fetal structures

794–5x7
794–511

7891 Polyp of endometrium simple

785–944
787–944

7893 Endometriosis

782–959
787–959

7894 Polyp of cervix, simple

783–944
785–943
786–956

7895 Erosion of cervix

783–951

7896 Functional uterine disorder

785–x10   782–x30
785–x20   780–x32

7960 Disorders of fetal structures due to mechanical abnor-
          malities

794–6x4   795–600.5   7951–614
794–631   7x52–614   79x–631
794–6311   794–614   795–614
794–6312   7941–614
794–6313   7942–614

7970 Metabolic disorders of fetal structures

795–794   794–7942   794–7945
794–794   794–7943   794–791
794–7941   794–7944   794–7911

7980 Neoplasms of fetal structures

796–880E   797–880B
796–880F   79▲–8▲▲▲

7990   Disorders of fetal structures due to unknown cause

795–900.8	794–9x4	795–x10
794–900.8	794–900.5	795–x20
794–940	795–x30	

8000   DISEASES OF THE ENDOCRINE SYSTEM

8090   Diseases of endocrine system due to unknown cause

800–953

8100   DISEASES OF THYROID GLAND

8101   Congenital conditions of thyroid gland

810–031	810–093	815–064.0
810–1471	815–019	
810–070	815–064	

8102   Cretinism

810–016

8110   Infections of thyroid gland

810–100.2
810–100
810–190

8130   Toxic disorders of thyroid gland

810–300
810–38214

8140   Injuries of thyroid gland

810–4▲▲	810–415.6	810–471.6
810–415	810–471	

8160   Disorders of thyroid gland due to mechanical abnormalities

814–600.8
810–600.8

8170   Metabolic disorders of thyroid gland

810–739

8177   Hyperthyroidism

810–771
810–776

8178   Hypothyroidism

810–7721
810–7722
810–777

8180   Neoplasms of thyroid gland

810–8091	810–8047F	810–830
810–8091A	810–8066	810–8▲▲▲
810–870F	810–8065A	
810–8047A	810–8065F	

8190   Diseases of thyroid gland due to unknown cause

| 810–911 | 810–941 |
| 810–942 | 810–942.1 |

8194   Goitre

| 810–943 | 810–943.6 |
| 810–952 | 810–952.6 |

8200   DISEASES OF PARATHYROID GLANDS

8240   Injuries of parathyroid glands

| 820–4▲▲ | 820–415.x | 820–773 |
| 820–415 | 820–47▲.x | |

8250   Vascular disorders of parathyroid glands

820–5x7

8280   Neoplasms of parathyroid glands

| 820–8091 | 820–8046A | 820–8▲▲▲ |
| 820–8091A | 820–8046F | |

8290   Diseases of parathyroid glands due to unknown cause

| 820–943 | 820–940 |
| 820–934.6 | 820–x10 |

8300   DISEASES OF THYMUS GLAND

8301   Congenital conditions of thymus gland

830–064
830–013

8310   Infections of thymus gland

830–100.2
830–100

8340   Injuries of thymus gland

830–4x7

8370   Metabolic disorders of thymus gland

830–795

8380   Neoplasms of thymus gland

830–8841A
830–8841F
830–8▲▲▲

8390   Diseases of thymus gland due to unknown cause

830–921
830–943

8400   DISEASES OF PITUITARY GLAND

8401   Congenital conditions of pituitary gland

844–064

8410   Infections of pituitary gland

840–100.2
840–100.9

8440   Injuries of pituitary gland

840–400.9
840–436
840–4▲▲

8450   Vascular disorders of pituitary gland

840–512.9
841–530
840–512

8460   Disorders of pituitary gland due to mechanical abnor-
            malities

840–600.8
840–615

8470   Metabolic disorders of pituitary gland

841–776	841–7765	841–7774
841–7761	841–777	841–7775
841–7762	841–7771	841–7776
841–7763	841–7772	842–779
841–7764	841–7773	

8480   Neoplasms of pituitary gland

841–8091	841–8067A	841–8045A
841–8091A	841–8067	841–8▲▲▲
841–8055A	841–8887	

8490   Diseases of pituitary gland due to unknown cause

840–900.9
840–x10

8500   DISEASES OF PINEAL GLAND

8540   Injuries of pineal gland

850–4▲▲

8570   Metabolic disorders of pineal gland

850–780

8580   Neoplasms of pineal gland

850–8475	850–882
850–8982	850–8▲▲▲

8590   Disorders of pineal gland due to unknown cause

850–923

8600   DISEASES OF ADRENAL GLAND

8601   Congenital conditions of adrenal glands

860–012	860–021	860–0161
860–031	860–014	860–0162
860–050	860–013	
860–064	860–016	

8610   Infections of adrenal glands

860–100	860–100.7	860–123
860–100.0	860–147.x	
860–100.9	860–123.x	

8640   Injuries of adrenal glands

860–4x7
860–4▲▲

8650   Vascular disorders of adrenal glands

860–505.7
860–540.7
860–500.1

8678   Adrenal cortical hyperfunction

861–781	861–7813	861–7811
861–7814	861–7822	861–7812

8679   Adrenal cortical hypofunction

861–782
861–788
861–7821

8680   Neoplasms of adrenal glands

860–8091	860–8091A	860–8051F
860–8091.x	860–8091A.x	860–8051A

8680   Neoplasms of adrenal glands (Continued)

862–840A	862–841F	860–8041A
862–8431	860–8041F	860–8▲▲▲

8690   Diseases of adrenal glands due to unknown cause

861–911

8770   Metabolic disorders of pancreas

870–784

8778   Diabetes

870–771	870–781	870–953.6
870–772	870–782	870–x10
870–776	870–770	
870–777	870–785	

8780   Neoplasms of pancreas

870–8091	870–8044A	870–8▲▲▲
870–8091A	870–8074F	
870–8044F	870–8074A	

8790   Diseases of pancreas due to unknown cause

870–953

8800   Diseases of gonads

880–011
880–016
880–0161

8980   Neoplasms of carotid gland

890–8881A
890–8981
890–8▲▲▲

9000   DISEASES OF THE NERVOUS SYSTEM

9001   Congenital conditions of the nervous system

903–092	906–1471
906–021	901–027.8

9010   Infections of the nervous system

906–175	901–100	91x–147
906–100	9011–1577	906–147
906–100.0	9011–100.0	
90x–147	900–147	

9020   Fungus and parasitic infections of nervous system

901–218
9▲▲–2▲▲

9030   Toxic disorders of nervous system

906–3▲▲	900–3▲▲
946–399	901–3▲▲

9040   Injuries of nervous system

9▲▲–4▲▲
900–485
901–400.4

9070   Metabolic disorders of nervous system

902–755	902–7551	906–7623
902–7554	902–7553	
902–7552	906–785	

9080   Neoplasms of the nervous system

90x–851
9▲▲–8▲▲▲
9▲▲–8453A

9090   Diseases of the nervous system

9062–953	90x–930	9▲▲–x30
90x–952	90x–931	

9091   Multiple sclerosis

906–953

9092   Amyotrophic lateral sclerosis

904–953	904–9532	904–9534
904–9531	904–9533	9041–953

9100   DISEASES OF MENINGES

9101   Congenital conditions of meninges

9▲▲–039	91▲▲–029	91x▲–050
910x–025	914▲–064	91x▲–015
91x▲–0▲▲	91▲▲–027	91x▲–077
91▲▲–050	91x–016.5	

9110   Infections of meninges

915▲–100.2	91x▲–100.4	91x7–100.7
9153–102.2	91x▲–190	91x▲–1x0.7
913▲–100.2	91x5–190	91x4–101.7
913▲–1x8	91x▲–1x6.5	
91x▲–100	91x▲–100.7	

9111   Meningitis

91▲–100	912–100	91▲–100.0
914–100	911–100	914–100.0

9111   Meningitis (Continued)

912–100.0	911–190	912–100.8
911–100.0	91▲–1x0.4	91▲–1x0.8
910–189	914–1x0.4	912–1x0.8
91▲–190	912–1x0.4	91▲–100.6
914–190	911–1x0.4	91▲–160
912–190	91▲–100.8	91▲–170

9120   Fungus and parasitic infections of meninges

9▲▲–2▲▲
910–209

9130   Toxic disorders of meninges

912–3931
912–3932

9140   Injuries of meninges

913▲–4x7	910▲–400.4	91x1–400.6
915▲–4x7	91061–404.4	91x▲–4x6
915▲–427	918–415.8	91x▲–4x6.5
910▲–496	913–4x7.0	91x▲–4▲▲
910▲–4▲▲	913–4x7.9	91x2–416
91041–412	913▲–4x8	91x1–412
912–438	91x▲–400.6	

9150   Vascular disorders of meninges

91x▲–534.7
91x5–534.7
91x–533.7

9160   Disorders of meninges due to mechanical abnormalities

91x▲–619

9180   Neoplasms of meninges

91▲▲▲–872A	91▲▲–846	91x▲–8▲▲▲
9▲▲▲–8173	91▲▲–8▲▲▲	
91▲▲–846A	91x▲–850A	

9190   Diseases of meninges due to unknown cause

91▲▲–923	910–x20	91x▲–900.7
913▲–9x7	91x▲–9x6	

9200   DISEASES OF VENTRICLES

9201   Congenital conditions of ventricles

92▲▲▲–018	926–064
924–031	926–015

9202   Hydrocephalus, congenital

920–063
920–064

9210   Infections of ventricles and central canal

927▲–100
9272–105
927–100.0

9212   Hydrocephalus due to infection

927–100.8
928▲–1x4.8

9230   Toxic disorders of ventricles and central canal

927–3▲▲
927–3931

9240   Injuries of ventricles and central canal

927–4742

9261   Hydrocephalus due to trauma

914–415.8

9290   Diseases of ventricles and central canal due to unknown
             cause

92x–923

9300   DISEASES OF BRAIN

9301   Congenital conditions of brain

93y–050	93▲▲–027	946–011
932–045	930–021	930–090
930–051	932–013	946–092
930–053	901–019	9▲▲▲–050
930–048	901–019.8	958–011
930–050.x	932–076	930–076.6
930–012	930–010	9334–076

9310   Infections of brain

930–196	930–147.9	930–115.6
9301–147.9	930–100.6	930–147.6

9311   Encephalitis

930–100	930–1▲▲.x	955–1755
930–115	930–169.x	930–1753
930–100.0	930–1761.x	955–1751
930–166	930–1▲▲.x	930–1756
930–175	930–115.x	930–175.0
955–175	955–1752	

9312   Brain abscess

9▲▲–100.2   933–100.2
958–100.2   935–100.2

9320   Fungus and parasitic infections of brain

9▲▲–2▲▲

9330   Toxic disorders of brain

908–388   930–39322   930–3821
930–3932   930–3▲▲   930–300.7
930–39321   930–321

9340   Injuries of brain

9▲▲–435   9▲▲–4x9   9▲▲–4x6
9▲▲–438   930–481   93▲–400.9
9▲▲–436   930–436   93▲▲–4x7
9▲▲–4362.x   930–438   9▲▲–4362
930–428   930–445   9▲▲–412
9▲▲–402   930–480   930–427
935–402   930–420.x   9▲▲–4x8.3
9▲▲–4▲▲.8   930–453   9▲▲–414
958–414.8   9▲▲–4x4   9▲▲–410
930–460   9▲▲–496   9▲▲–411

9350   Vascular disorders of brain

930–519   930–516   932–500
930–533   9▲▲–549.7

9351   Encephalomalacia

9▲▲–5x0   945–532   9▲▲▲▲–516
946–512   955–511

9360   Disorders of brain due to mechanical abnormalities

93▲▲–639.7

9370   Metabolic disorders of brain

935–791   930–701   953–762▲
930–705   930–760
930–784   9463–740

9380   Neoplasms of brain

9▲▲–8091   9▲▲–814   95x–850A
9▲▲–8473   9▲▲–870A   9▲▲–872A
9▲▲–812   9▲▲–870F   9▲▲–830
9▲▲–873B   9▲▲–8471   9▲▲–842G
9▲▲–8886   9▲▲–8474   9▲▲–8173
9▲▲–8887   9▲▲–8475   9▲▲–846
9▲▲–848   9▲▲–850B   9▲▲–842F

9380   Neoplasms of brain (Continued)

9▲▲–8451	9▲▲–841F	9▲▲–8▲▲▲
9▲▲–8472	9▲▲–841G	
9▲▲–879	9▲▲–882	

9390   Diseases of brain due to unknown cause

958–953	908–992	959–992
930–910	950–9535	957–9x8
939▲▲–910	942–992	930–997
9461–953	9591–953	990–x53
908–953	9586–911	930–x50
930–995	931–9x1	930–x51
958–9531	954–953	954–x30
950–9532	9462–9531	930–x30
9273–956	9385–953	990–x41
906–992	950–9533	990–x20

9391   Epilepsy

93▲▲▲–x02	935–x02	930–x05
9334–x02	930–x08	930–x12
930–x0x	930–x01	930–x52
9341–x02	930–x07	
933–x021	930–x06	

9393   Migraine

930–x40	930–x48	930–x49
930–x46	930–x42	930–x41
930–x45	930–x43	

9395   Paralysis agitans

9464–953

9500   DISEASES OF CEREBRAL VESSELS

9501   Congenital conditions of cerebral vessels

477▲–015	92x▲–01x	477▲–050
477▲–015.5	95x–029	
95x▲–010	95x▲–019	

9510   Infections of cerebral vessels

95x▲–100.6	477–100.6	477▲–1x6.5
477▲–190	477▲–100.6	95x▲–157
477▲–190.5	477▲–100.4	

9520   Fungus and parasitic infections of cerebral vessels

94x▲–2x6

9540   Injuries of cerebral vessels
477▲–400.6
95x▲–400.6

9541   Hemorrhage from cerebral vessels, traumatic
95x▲–4x6.5
95x▲–416

9542   Embolism of cerebral vessels, traumatic
477▲–427
477▲–425
477▲–426

9551   Cerebral hemorrhage, nontraumatic
477▲–533.5

9553   Cerebral thrombosis, nontraumatic
477▲–541.7
477▲–547.7

9555   Innervation disorders of cerebral vessels
97x▲▲–582

9556   Angiospasm of cerebral vessels
477▲–582

9562   Embolism of cerebral arteries due to unspecified cause
477▲–618
477▲–611

9563   Thrombosis of cerebral arteries due to unspecified cause
477▲–619

9580   Neoplasms of cerebral vessels
477▲–850A
477▲–850F
94x▲–8▲▲▲

9590   Diseases of cerebral vessels due to unknown cause
477▲–9x6   477–930   477▲–900.7
95x▲–9x6   477▲▲–930

9594   Cerebral arteriosclerosis
90x–942   477▲–942.6   477▲–942.7
477▲–942   477▲–942.5   477▲–997

9600   DISEASES OF CRANIAL NERVES

9601   Congenital conditions of cranial nerves

962–01x

9610   Infections of cranial nerves

96▲▲–100.9	962–147.9	962–100
96▲▲–1764	9641–1764	9623–100
962–100.9	962–104	

9630   Toxic disorders of cranial nerves

9623–3▲▲.9	9623–3845	9623–34382
9623–3238.9	9623–3▲▲.x	9623–3257
9623–3238	9623–33211.x	9623–33212.x
9623–3313▲	9623–36171.x	9623–33131.x

9640   Injuries of cranial nerves

96▲▲–4353	962–409	9623–435
96▲▲–415.x	962–404	962–414
962–430	962–496	96▲▲–4351
962–400.9	962–4▲▲	965–430

9655   Innervation disorders of cranial nerves

9636–5631

9670   Metabolic disorders of cranial nerves

962–713

9680   Neoplasms of cranial nerves

962–8475
962–8451
962–8▲▲▲

9690   Diseases of cranial nerves due to unknown cause

9624–911	964–x30	9624–995
965–x40	9641–x30	962–940
965–x20	9642–x30	9623–953
9651–x30	9643–x30	99x2–x30
967–x30	9644–x30	
967–x301	962–900.9	

9700   DISEASES OF SPINAL CORD

9701   Congenital conditions of the spinal cord

970–011	972▲–011	970–034
972–090	970–012	970–021
97▲–011	909▲▲–050	97▲▲▲–093

9701   Congenital conditions of the spinal cord (Continued)

970–076	978▲▲▲–0681	97x▲▲–010
97▲▲–077	978▲▲▲–068	97x▲▲–076
909–027	97x▲▲–015	929–015
970–037	97x▲▲–019	

9710   Infections of spinal cord

970▲▲–100.2	970–100	979–160
97031–105.2	97034–102	97x▲▲–100.6
970–102	970▲▲–100	97x▲▲–1x6.5
9783▲▲–1764.x	971–100	97x–100
9783▲▲–1764	970–100.0	97x▲▲–100.4
909–100	972▲▲–147.0	97x▲▲–100.7
909–101	974▲▲–100	97x▲▲–1x0.7
909–100.0	907–160	
909–147	978▲▲–100	

9711   Anterior poliomyelitis

972–171	972▲▲–171.0
972▲▲–171	906–171

9720   Fungus and parasitic infections of spinal cord

909▲▲–2▲▲
909▲▲–2▲▲

9730   Toxic disorders of spinal cord

970–3▲▲	970–3238	978▲▲–3▲▲
970–321	97▲▲–3▲▲	
970–33212	907▲▲–3▲▲	

9740   Injuries of spinal cord

97844–4x4	970▲▲–4352	970▲▲–4051
978▲▲–409	970▲▲–4362	970▲▲–4▲▲
970▲▲–403	970▲▲–4351	970▲▲–412
970▲▲–43▲	970▲▲–434	970–480
970▲▲–437	970▲▲–436	970–481
970▲▲–435	978▲▲–4354	970▲▲–410
970▲▲–4361	970–428	97x▲▲–427
970▲▲–43x	970▲▲–428	97x▲▲–400.6
970▲▲–439	970▲▲–402	97x–4x6
970▲▲–4341	970–460	97x▲▲–425
970–438	970▲▲–4x6	97x▲▲–426
970▲▲–4353	970▲▲–4x7	97x▲▲–4▲▲

9750   Vascular disorders of spinal cord

970▲▲–516	970▲▲–515	970▲▲–532
970–51▲	970▲▲–512	970▲▲–511

9755   Innervation disorders of spinal cord

97x▲▲–582

9760   Disorders of spinal cord due to mechanical abnormalities

97x▲▲–618
97x▲▲–619
97x4▲▲–641

9770   Metabolic disorders of spinal cord

975–785	970–760	907▲▲–785
970–704	970–7621	977–7625
970–711	970–7623	
970–701	970–7625	

9780   Neoplasms of spinal cord

970▲▲–848	97x▲▲–850A	970▲▲–8▲▲▲
970▲▲–8475	97x▲▲–850G	
970▲▲–8451	97x▲▲–8▲▲▲	

9790   Diseases of spinal cord due to unknown cause

975–953	970–915	97x▲▲–942
972–992	907▲▲–953	97x▲▲–942.5
971–953	970▲▲–9x8	97x–930
971–9531	97x▲▲–942.6	97x▲▲–930
971–9530	97x–942	97x▲–900.7

9800   DISEASES OF PERIPHERAL NERVES AND PLEXUSES

9801   Congenital conditions of peripheral nerves and plexuses

98▲▲–011	98▲▲–050	983–0212
98▲▲–019	983–021	983–0211

9810   Infections of peripheral nerves and plexuses

980–100
98▲▲–100
98▲▲–100.0

9830   Toxic disorders of peripheral nerves and plexuses

98▲▲–300.x	98▲▲–321	98▲▲–3238
98▲▲–3▲▲	98▲▲–33212	

9840   Injuries of peripheral nerves and plexuses

98▲▲–409	98▲▲–4341	98▲▲–4362
98▲▲–403	9833–4341	98▲▲–402
98▲▲–435	98▲▲–438	98▲▲–460
98▲▲–4x7	98▲▲–436	98▲▲–400.9
98▲▲–434	98▲▲–43x	98▲▲–4▲▲

9840   Injuries of peripheral nerves and plexuses (Continued)

98▲▲–4363   98▲▲–400.x   98▲▲–436
98▲▲–412   98▲▲–4x6
98▲▲–430   98▲▲–4091

9850   Vascular disorders of peripheral nerves and plexuses

98▲▲–514
98▲▲–532

9855   Innervation disorders of peripheral nerves and plexuses

98▲▲–563.x
98▲▲–563

9870   Metabolic disorders of peripheral nerves and plexuses

98▲▲–785   98▲▲–784   98▲▲–702
98▲▲–711   98▲▲–76▲▲
98▲▲–781   98▲▲–749

9880   Neoplasms of peripheral nerves and plexuses

98▲–8451   98▲–8453B   98▲–8▲▲
98▲–8453A   98▲–8452

9890   Diseases of peripheral nerves and plexuses due to unknown cause

980–x10
98▲▲–922
980–997

9900   DISEASES OF VEGETATIVE NERVOUS SYSTEM

9940   Injuries of vegetative nervous system

994–4▲▲.x   994–415.x
994–430.x   99▲–4▲▲

9980   Neoplasms of vegetative nervous system

990–840A   990–8432   990–841F
990–842F   990–8431   990–8▲▲▲

9990   Diseases of vegetative nervous system due to unknown cause

994–x30
994–x20
994–x40

9▲01   Dysplasia, aplasia, hypoplasia, atrophy, and hyperplasia. *Specify site*

9▲▲–077
9▲▲▲–093

0060   Undiagnosed disease of body as a whole
    01x–y00
    y00–y10
    y00–y00

0061   Undiagnosed disease of integumentary system
    162–y00   13▲–yx1
    110–y10   13▲–yx9
    161–yx2   198–yx8

0062   Undiagnosed disease of musculoskeletal system
    25▲–yx9

0063   Undiagnosed disease of respiratory system
    360–yx2   360–yx4
    362–yx4   360–y00.8
    361–y10   360–y00.6

0064   Undiagnosed disease of cardiovascular system
    410–y00
    451–y00

0065   Undiagnosed disease of hemic and lymphatic systems
    501–y00.1
    520–yx6
    550–y10

0066   Undiagnosed disease of digestive system
    640–yx7   604–yx4   680–yx6
    604–yx9   060–yx7   680–yx7
    604–yx7   680–yx0

0067   Undiagnosed disease of genitourinary system
    776–yx4
    7x2–yx7

0068   Undiagnosed disease of endocrine system

0069   Undiagnosed disease of nervous system
    477▲–yx7

0070   Undiagnosed disease of psychobiologic unit

0071   Undiagnosed disease of eye

0072   Undiagnosed disease of ear